Aquaculture for Vete

Fish Husbandry and M.

D1586987

Pergamon Veterinary Handbook Series

Series Editor: A.T.B. Edney BA BVetMed MRCVS

This series of practical and authoritative handbooks covers topics of interest to the practising veterinary surgeon, to veterinary students and to veterinary nurses. The text is authoritative, yet written in a clear and accessible form, and there are numerous photographs and specially commissioned line drawings to enhance understanding. The volumes in this Series will be valuable additions to any practice bookshelf.

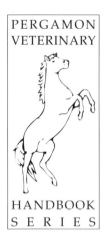

ANDERSON & EDNEY
Practical Animal Handling

EMILY & PENMAN
Handbook of Small Animal Dentistry

GORREL, PENMAN and EMILY
Handbook of Small Animal Oral Emergencies

SHERIDAN & McCAFFERTY
The Business of Veterinary Practice

WHITE & WILLIAMSON
The Foal

WILLS & WOLF
Handbook of Feline Medicine

Other Pergamon publications of related interest

Books

BURGER
The Waltham Book of Companion Animal Nutrition

GOLDSCHMIDT & SHOFER
Skin Tumors of the Dog and Cat

IHRKE, MASON & WHITE
Advances in Veterinary Dermatology, Volume 2

LANE
Jones's Animal Nursing, 5th Edition

ROBINSON
Genetics for Cat Breeders, 3rd Edition
Genetics for Dog Breeders, 2nd Edition

THORNE
The Waltham Book of Dog and Cat Behaviour

Journals

Annual Review of Fish Diseases
Veterinary Dermatology
The official journal of the European Society of Veterinary Dermatology
and the American College of Veterinary Dermatology

Aquaculture for Veterinarians

Fish Husbandry and Medicine

Edited by

LYDIA BROWN
Abbott Laboratories, North Chicago, USA

PERGAMON PRESS

OXFORD · NEW YORK · SEOUL · TOKYO

U.K.	Pergamon Press Ltd, Headington Hill Hall, Oxford OX3 0BW, England
U.S.A.	Pergamon Press, Inc., 660 White Plains Road, Tarrytown, New York 10591-5153, U.S.A.
KOREA	Pergamon Press Korea, KPO Box 315, Seoul 110-603, Korea
JAPAN	Pergamon Press Japan, Tsunashima Building Annex, 3-2-12 Yushima, Bunkyo-ku, Tokyo 113, Japan

First edition 1993

Library of Congress Cataloging-in-Publication Data

Aquaculture for veterinarians: fish husbandry and medicine/edited by Lydia Brown. -- 1st ed. p. cm. -- (Pergamon veterinary handbook series)
Includes index.
1. Fishes--Diseases. I. Brown, Lydia. II. Series.
SH171.A68 1993 639.3--dc20   92-41237

British Library Cataloguing in Publication Data

A catalogue record for this book is available from the British Library

ISBN 0 08 040835 4 Hardcover
ISBN 0 08 040836 2 Flexicover

DISCLAIMER

Whilst every effort is made by the Publishers to see that no misleading data, opinion or statement appears in this book, they wish to make it clear that the data and opinions appearing in the articles herein are the sole responsibility of the contributor concerned. Accordingly, the Publishers and their employees, officers and agents accept no responsibility or liability whatsoever for the consequences of any such inaccurate or misleading data, opinion or statement.

Drug and Dosage Section: The Authors have made every effort to ensure the accuracy of the information herein, particularly with regard to drug selection and dose. However, appropriate information sources should be consulted, especially for new or unfamiliar drugs or procedures. It is the responsibility of every veterinarian to evaluate the appropriateness of a particular opinion in the context of actual clinical situations, and with due consideration to new developments.

Printed in Great Britain by BPCC Wheatons Ltd, Exeter

Contents

Foreword   ix
R. J. ROBERTS

Preface   xi

List of Contributors   xiii

1 Basic Anatomy and Physiology   1
       EDWARD BRANSON

2 Basic Husbandry on Fish Farms   31
       ANDREW GRANT

3 Aquaculture Systems   43
       JONATHAN SHEPHERD

4 Environmental Aspects of Aquaculture   57
       EDWARD BRANSON

5 Principles of Disease Diagnosis   69
       RICHARD COLLINS

6 Disease in Aquaculture   91
       PETE SOUTHGATE

7 Therapy in Aquaculture   131
       PETER SCOTT

8 Nutrition in Aquaculture   153
       AUD SKRUDLAND

9 Anaesthesia   161
       MICHAEL STOSKOPF

10   Welfare Aspects of Aquatic Veterinary Medicine   169
       GRAHAM CAWLEY

11   Legislation Affecting Farmed Fish   173
       KEITH TREVES BROWN and ALASTAIR GRAY

12   The Veterinary Approach to Salmon Farming in Norway   179
       ROLF NORDMO

13   The Veterinary Approach to Salmon Farming in Scotland   193
       TONY WALL

14   The Veterinary Approach to Trout   223
       ANDY HOLLIMAN

15   The Veterinary Approach to Channel Catfish   249
       MIKE JOHNSON

16   The Veterinary Approach to Marine Prawns   271
       IAN ANDERSON

17   The Veterinary Approach to Carp   297
       RUDOLF HOFFMANN

18   The Veterinary Approach to Eels   311
       EVERT LIEWES and OLGA HAENEN

19   The Veterinary Approach to Turbot   327
       RONNIE SOUTAR

20   The Veterinary Approach to Halibut   339
       MARY BRANCKER

21   The Veterinary Approach to Cod   345
       OLE TORRISEN, INGEGJERD OPSTAD, and ODD MAGNE RØDSETH

22   The Veterinary Approach to Ornamental Fish   357
       RAY BUTCHER

23   The Veterinary Approach to Sea-bass and Sea-bream   379
       PANOS CHRISTOFILOGIANNIS

24   The Veterinary Approach to Game Fish   395
       RUTH FRANCIS-FLOYD

       Appendices   409
       Index   411

Foreword

When I first began to work on the pathology of farmed and wild fishes in the early 1960s, not only was our understanding of disease in fishes very much in its infancy but really, despite its antiquity, so was the subject of aquaculture itself. Veterinarians had virtually no clinical involvement in the area and, apart from the very distinguished contributions of Marianne Plehn in Germany and, later, Nikola Fijan in Yugoslavia, they had made virtually no contribution to its science, such as it was.

There had, however, been recognition of the role that the clinically trained scientist can make to the subject, with the involvement of Professor Mackie at the medical school of the University of Edinburgh, Scotland, in the major advances in our knowledge of fish bacterial diseases during the 1930s. The work of Professor Mackie and his medical colleagues for the Furunculosis Committee set up by the British Government in1930, marked the first real recognition of the economic importance of fish diseases and provided what Stanislaus Snieszko, the doyen of American fish pathologists (who himself received part of his training at the Jagelonian University Veterinary School, Poland), referred to as 'a "must" for anyone who intends to study communicable diseases of fish'.

Since the 1960s, however, driven by the economic imperative of the commercial expansion of fish culture, our knowledge of fish diseases has expanded beyond all bounds. This expansion has been a scientific endeavour which has involved research workers of many disciplines. It is however noteworthy that the contribution of the veterinary scientists has been significant both in its volume and in its quality. Two major advantages that the veterinarians have been able to bring to the discipline are the comparative dimension, the ability to relate disease patterns seen in fish populations to the whole spectrum of such conditions in the vertebrate phylum, and thus to gain insights which would otherwise be very difficult to acquire; and the breadth of integrated knowledge derived from a training in both aetiologies and host responses. It is possibly this latter area, the understanding of the disease processes and host responses of the individual fish, which has been the most significant single contribution that the veterinary scientist has made.

It is the role of the clinician to relate all of this hard-won scientific knowledge to the circumstances of a particular disease problem in the field. In most countries of the world this is a role which the veterinary clinician, once presented with the necessary corpus of scientific information by his veterinary and other scientific colleagues, has increasingly been able to service. In contrast to the situation in the 1960s, when the embryonic fish farmer had virtually no one to turn to (except in the USA where extension services were often very good). Nowadays, practising veterinary surgeons are servicing aquaculture just as any other sector of livestock production and being seen to be an essential adjunct to intensive fish production.

One of the features of farmed fish clinical medicine is the generally low value of the individual fish. Thus it is usually possible to sacrifice a few clinical examples to gain diagnostic information which is often of a much higher order of sophistication than in species where the individual is the subject rather than the flock or school. Thus the fish veterinarian has to link clinical observation to clinical pathology and microbiology in the context of environmental and husbandry conditions if he is properly to contribute his skills.

This book, written by veterinarians for veterinarians, should I believe greatly contribute to the advance of the veterinarian's role in fish clinical medicine. It provides a sequential introduction into all of the different areas of knowledge essential to allow the trained veterinarian to acquire the specific details which he requires to orient his expertise towards the aquatic sector.

Of particular importance in this respect, of course, is an understanding of the aquatic environment, and of the husbandry systems in which the fish are being maintained. Of no less importance, however, is the understanding of the differences in pathophysiology and immune response, which a poikilothermic existence imposes on fishes.

All of these areas are well covered in the book and it even moves further from mainstream veterinary science, in its embracement of the cultured crustaceans and their problems, particularly in South East Asia, where veterinarians have given, and indeed continue to give, considerable support to a very large and important export industry.

In the past it was, on occasion, a concern within the veterinary profession as to whether fish were a proper concern for them. The contribution which veterinarians have subsequently made, which is very clearly demonstrated in this book, must surely demonstrate that as with any other livestock production system, the veterinarian, by training, by legislative rights and responsibilities, and by experience is the appropriate professional to practise the diagnostic skills derived from the integration of the collaborative scientific efforts of the aetiologists, pathologists and fish biologists of whatever discipline is necessary, who have created the corpus of primary knowledge.

I commend this book to the veterinary profession throughout the world. I am proud that so many of its authors have trained in my own institute and wish them well in their contribution to man's effort to manage the waters as well as the land.

RONALD J. ROBERTS
Institute of Aquaculture
University of Stirling
Stirling, Scotland

Preface

Aquaculture, the farming of aquatic organisms, either for food or for hobbyists, is a relatively new industry. Man has held fish in ponds and harvested the fruits of the sea for centuries but the knowledge of intensive production methods only developed from the early part of this century.

As the rapid increase in production of farmed fish has occurred, so too have the problems. Intensive systems lead to higher stocking densities and increasing stress. When animals are stressed, disease outbreaks often occur.

For agricultural animals, a farmer goes to his veterinarian for advice on husbandry, disease and therapy. Sadly this has not generally been the case in aquaculture although many highly gifted non-veterinary fish pathologists have ably advised in this area.

Veterinarians are now realising that their responsibilities do not cease with warm-blooded animals. They are uniquely qualified to assess disease and production practices in the context of both welfare for the animal and profitability for the client.

Very little postgraduate education is available to veterinarians wishing to work in aquaculture. Professor Roberts, who has written the foreword to this book, is the Founder and Director of the Institute of Aquaculture at Stirling University where such training is available. There is a great need for veterinary students as well as practising veterinarians to master the basic principles of their work as it specifically relates to aquatic animals.

The aim of this text is to ensure that such basics are available in one easily readable book. There are two sections to the book, the first of which deals with basic principles and approaches to aquaculture (Chapters 1–11). It is recommended that the reader studies this section in detail. The second section (Chapters 12–24) contains specific information which will be useful to veterinarians working in particular regions of the world. The authors have drawn on their own, considerable, practical experience. The reader should be aware, however, that local conditions, especially water quality, can affect fish medicine markedly. The veterinarian should thus ensure that suggested dosages are correct for the particular situation.

The major portion of this book is devoted to fin fish. A section on shrimp farming has been included since this represents 75% of the world's aquaculture. Ornamental (non-food) fish have also been given a chapter to recognise that some special procedures apply for these fish compared with their food fish counterparts. It is important to remember that the practising veterinarian will often get his first experience with aquatic animals through his aquarist clients rather than from those clients producing fish farmed for food.

This book is a first step for the land-based veterinarian who wishes to test the waters of aquatic animal practice.

I would like to express grateful appreciation to my colleagues in the Animal Health Business Unit at Abbott Laboratories for their patience and forbearance during the production of this book.

Finally, on behalf of all the contributors, I wish to thank Pergamon Press for their friendly and efficient help in the production of this book. Particular thanks must go to Mrs Marion Jowett and her colleagues.

LYDIA BROWN

List of Contributors

Ian Anderson Oonoonba Veterinary Laboratory, Abbott Street, Townsville, PO Box 1085, Townsville, Queensland 4810, Australia

Mary Brancker 38 Streetly Lane, Sutton Coldfield, West Midlands, B74 4TU, UK

Lydia Brown Aquaculture and Animal Health, Abbott Laboratories, 1401 Sheridan Road, North Chicago, Illinois 60064, USA

Edward Branson Garden Cottage, Eastnor, Ledbury, Herefordshire, HR8 1RL, UK

Ray Butcher 196 Hall Lane, Upminster, Essex, RM14 1TD, UK

Graham Cawley Grampian Pharmaceuticals Research, Talkin, Brampton, Cumbria CAB 1LE, UK

Panos Christofilogiannis Institute of Aquaculture, The University of Stirling, Stirling FK9 4LA, UK

Richard Collins Veterinary Investigation Centre, Drummondhill, Stratherrick Road, Inverness IV2 4JZ, UK

Ruth Francis-Floyd Institute of Food and Agricultural Sciences, School of Forest Resources and Conservation, University of Florida, 7922 N. W. Street, Gainesville, Florida 32606–0300, USA

Andrew Grant Marine Harvest, Lochailort, Inverness-shire, PH38 4LZ, UK

Alastair Gray The Veterinary Medicines Directorate, Central Veterinary Laboratory, New Haw, Weybridge, Surrey, KT15 3NB, UK

Olga Haenen C. D. I. Postbus 65, 8200 AB Lelystad, The Netherlands

Rudolph Hoffmann Institut fur Zoologie und Hydrobiologie, University of Munich, Kaulbachstrasse 37, D-8000, Munchen 22, Germany

Andy Holliman MAFF VI Centre, Merrythought, Calthwaite, Penrith, Cumbria, CA11 9RR, UK

Mike Johnson College of Veterinary Medicine, PO Drawer V, Mississippi State, MS 39762, USA

Evert Liewes HVA Fish Farm Development b.v., PO Box 503, 1110 Am Diemen, The Netherlands

Rolf Nordmo VESO Vikan AkvaVet, Alhusstrand, Namsos, N–7810, Norway

Ingegjerd Opstad Austevoll Aquaculture Research Station, N–5392 Storebø, Norway

Odd Magne Rødseth Institute of Marine Research, Division of Aquaculture, N–5024 Bergen, Norway

Peter Scott Zoo and Aquatic Veterinary Group, PO Box 60, Winchester, Hants, SO23 9XN, UK

Jonathan Shepherd ECOline Ltd, Bridge House, 69 London Road, Twickenham, Middlesex, TW1 1EE, UK

Aud Skrudland T Skretting a/s, Bruhagen, N-6530, Norway

Ronnie Soutar Golden Sea Produce, South Shian, Connel, Argyll, PA37 1SB, UK

Pete Southgate 11 Princes Avenue, Maylandsea, Chelmsford, Essex, CM3 6BA, UK

Michael Stoskopf Department of Companion Animal Medicine and Special Species Medicine, School of Veterinary Medicine, North Carolina State University, 4700 Hillsborough Street at William Moore Drive, Raleigh, North Carolina 27606, USA

Ole Torrisen Institute of Marine Research, N-5198, Matredal, Norway.

Keith Treves Brown The Veterinary Medicines Directorate, Central Veterinary Laboratory, New Haw, Weybridge, Surrey KT15 3NB, UK

Tony Wall Veterinary Surgery, Rogart, Highland, IV28 3UA, UK

1

Basic Anatomy and Physiology

EDWARD BRANSON

Fish are often considered to be the forebears of modern terrestrial vertebrates and very primitive in evolutionary terms. To a certain extent this is true, but after the first fish 'crawled out on to dry land', the remainder did not cease development. In fact many fish have developed very advanced systems and have adapted to fill a large range of very different niches. Most modern fish should be looked upon as sharing a common ancestor with terrestrial vertebrates rather than being that ancestor.

Fish have evolved in a variety of ways, but the group containing more than 90% of the fish species living today is the class Osteichthyes or bony fish. The teleosts — the higher bony fish in evolutionary terms — constitute the largest group within the class. This group contains all those species of fin fish farmed today, and most of the ornamental fish species found in ponds and aquaria.

Crustaceans belong to another phylum entirely, and have evolved along quite different lines. They will be considered in rather less detail at the end of this chapter.

Teleosts can be divided roughly into two main groups, the soft-rayed and spiny-rayed fish, of interest mainly because they signify relative evolutionary advancement. The soft-rayed fish tend to be the more primitive, and typically have fins supported only by soft rays, possess cycloid scales and have a swim-bladder opening into the oesophagus (physostome). They also tend to have a fusiform body shape, with pectoral fins caudal in position. Typical of this group are the salmonids, carp and eels.

The spiny-rayed fish are more advanced and typically have bony spines in some fins, possess ctenoid scales and have a swim-bladder which lacks a connection with the oesophagus (physoclist). Bodies tend to be deeper, with pectoral fins high up on the body wall and pelvic fins set cranially,

often below, or even in front of, the pectorals. Typical of this group are the perches and flatfish.

Life in an aquatic environment presents its own set of problems distinct from those experienced by terrestrial animals, not least of which are the much greater ionic and osmoregulatory challenges that occur in water. In additon, microbial multiplication and challenge are more likely to occur in water than in air. Despite this, most of the organ systems of teleosts are similar to those found in mammals although they have developed along different lines in order to deal with their particular problems. For the purposes of this book, the main organ systems will be described in general terms for teleosts, with differences between the main relevant species highlighted where appropriate.

It should be remembered that almost all fish are poikilotherms, that is their body temperature varies passively with that of the surrounding water. The exceptions are some of the fast ocean swimming species. Due to the consequent relatively low and often variable body temperature, definite statements concerning growth, heart rate, digestion and other processes cannot be made, since all are affected by temperature. Usually, however, body systems will show a 50% increase in activity for every 5°C rise in temperature.

Teleosts are quite adaptable to temperature as a group and can be found in temperatures ranging from 0 to 45°C. Generally each species will have its preferred range, and will not react well to movement outside this range or to rapid changes within it.

External Features

The shape of a fish is generally determined by the need to minimise drag while swimming. It is commonly fusiform with an ovoid cross section

1

FIG. 1.1 (a) Body layout of lower teleost, e.g. salmonid. (b) Body layout of higher teleost, e.g. perch.

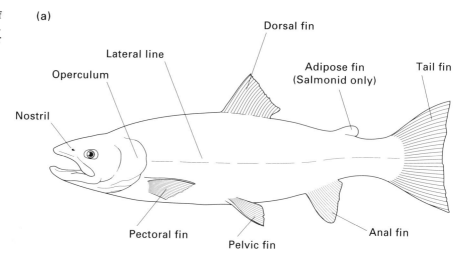

(a)

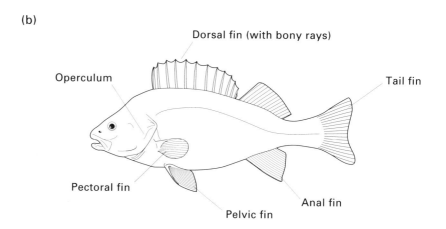

(b)

(Fig 1.1) and this plan is adapted in many cases to suit a particular environmental niche.

Most fish are covered in scales, but some may be scaleless. Lips are usually membranous, but may be fleshy or contain cartilaginous plates; they are generally scaleless. Teleosts have gill covers (opercula) which serve to protect the gills and assist with respiratory effort. The vent is usually found in the ventral mid-line in the caudal half of the body, just cranial to the anal fin.

The lateral line, a sensory organ consisting of a series of small pores in the skin, runs bilaterally, approximately midway down each side. It is usually seen as a single line from caudal fin to head, but it may branch and extend over the head. Around the mouth there may be barbels, which

have a sensory capability and are used in feeding. Paired external nares usually occur on the dorso-lateral aspect of the snout. Eyes are lidless and usually bilateral.

Musculoskeletal System

Skeleton

The axial skeleton consists of a rigid cranium, which supports the bones related to the gill apparatus and jaws, and a vertebral column.

The number of vertebrae is not constant within a given species and is affected by environmental conditions during larval development. Vertebrae are all very similar in shape, except for the atlas and axis which are modified to connect the skull to the spine.

The body of each vertebra is a simple cylinder with concave ends which carry intervertebral pads. All vertebrae have a neural arch and spine. The caudal vertebrae also have a ventral spine and a ventral arch which partly encases the main axial blood vessels. In the thoracic region the vertebrae have lateral processes carrying ribs. In many species, for example the salmonids and carp, small splint bones of various arrangements radiate out from the vertebral column in the intermuscular septa.

The vertebral column is simpler than in mammals with adjacent vertebrae connected by ligaments. There are also longitudinal elastic ligaments which run dorsal and ventral to the vertebrae. The complex articulations seen in mammals are not present, and it is probably the support given by the water which makes this simpler system possible.

Fins

In teleosts, fins are median or paired. Median fins usually consist of dorsal, caudal and anal; pectoral and pelvic fins are paired. Pectoral fins are supported on a bony pectoral girdle which is suspended immediately behind the opercular region of the skull. The pelvic fins are also supported by a bony girdle which, in the lower teleosts such as salmonids, is embedded in the ventral body musculature in the caudal part of the body. In the evolutionary process this girdle has migrated cranially, and in the higher bony fish they may even be in contact with the pectoral fin girdle, which tends to move dorsally.

Unpaired fins are not supported by girdles. Dorsal and anal fins tend to be supported on small bones within the intermuscular septa, which continue the line of the dorsal and ventral vertebral processes. The caudal fin is supported by the final few vertebrae fused together.

Fin rays are of two types, spiny or soft. The spiny rays of the more advanced species are simple single bones, as seen in the first dorsal fin of the perch. The fins of the more primitive species are all soft-rayed, as are the caudal fins of all teleosts. The soft rays are segmented, often branched, and are formed of two lateral components joined at the mid-line.

Some soft-rayed species, such as the catfish and carp, may have modifications to this arrangement with resulting spinous processes. These are distinct from spiny processes, and are made up by a fusion of the soft elements rather than of bone as seen in the spiny-rayed group.

Bone

Bone has a similar microscopic structure to that of the other vertebrates. Generally there are two types of bone: cellular and acellular. Cellular bone contains osteocytes and is found in the less advanced species. Acellular bone is found only in the more advanced teleosts, and is unique to this group of vertebrates. It is usually a solid feature-less matrix containing no osteocytes. Because of this absence of cells, calcium, resorption cannot occur and consequently this bone cannot be used as a functional calcium reserve. No haemopoietic tissue is present within the spaces which occur in some bones of both types.

Muscle

As with other vertebrates, three types of muscle are found: smooth, cardiac and striated skeletal, with the latter occurring in two forms.

The main skeleton musculature forms muscle blocks arranged in quadrants delineated by a vertical median septum and a transverse horizontal septum. The two dorsal blocks are termed the epaxial musculature, the two ventral the hypaxial musculature. This arrangement is obvious in cross section.

The muscle blocks are made up of myomeres which arise segmentally in embryos, and in the adult fish appear typically sigma-shaped super-ficially. Beneath this they are complexly folded and nested together in such a way that a line passing at right angles through the skin, moving towards the vertebral column, would pass through several different myomeres. This relationship can be seen clearly in cross-sections of a fish body, especially near the tail.

This complex inter-relationship of the myomeres means that during contraction individual myomeres influence others in close contact. This results in smooth sequential contractions passing along the body of a swimming fish, producing a wave of increasing amplitude passing caudally along the body. Co-ordination of these waves of contraction results in lateral oscillation of the body, most clearly evident in eels, and this gives rise to the name of this type of motion: anguilliform movement. In shorter bodied fish these movements are less obvious, and the only oscillation really apparent is that of the tail, described as carangiform locomotion. Some fish swim by a sculling or waving motion of certain fins, in which case the appropriate muscles are highly developed and the main myomeres may be considerably reduced: this is particularly evident in the seahorse.

Myomeres contain a range of fibre types which, in many species, are arranged into distinct zones. The two main types of fibre are red and white, and there are several minor types. Red muscle is used during slow cruising: the fibres are well vascularised, aerobic and slow contracting, similar to the skeletal muscle of mammals. They have *en grappe* nerve endings within the fibre. In many species these fibres are located as a wedge beneath the lateral line.

White muscle is used during strenuous bursts of swimming: the fibres are poorly vascularised, anaerobic and fast contracting, but a consequence of this is that they are also fast fatiguing. White fibres, which have *en platte* nerve endings, have a wide range of diameters especially in growing fish, but the diameter of both red and white fibres may vary with exercise, starvation and stage of development. In the higher teleosts white fibres have polyneuronal innervation, a feature unique to this group. The neurotransmitter is acetylcholine.

'Pink' fibres also occur, and these appear to be intermediate in form. Usually they are found separating the red and white fibres but are more widespread in some species.

Skin

Skin is the primary protection against the environment, and it acts as an osmotic barrier and the first line of defence against disease. Any minor lesion may rapidly progress to a major one, due to waterlogging of the underlying tissues; the skin is quite delicate and thus more susceptible to damage than that of mammals. It contains sensory receptors tuned to the surroundings, and to some degree has excretory, respiratory and osmoregula-

tory functions. Great inter-species differences occur in the skin structure, and there are often large variations within a species, and even within different locations on the same fish. Age, sex and time of year can also cause variations within an individual animal.

The skin is made up of several layers (Fig. 1.2). The two main layers are the epidermis overlaid by a cuticle, and the dermis, with an underlying hypodermis.

Cuticle

The cuticle is the outermost layer of the epidermis. It is approximately 1 µm thick and mainly mucopolysaccharide, being a combination of cellular material, sloughed cells and mucus that has been secreted onto the surface. The physical consistency varies greatly with species. It also contains specific immunoglobulins, lysozyme and free fatty acids, all of which are thought to have some anti-pathogenic activity.

Mucus is an important feature of the skin. It assists in osmoregulation by making the skin less permeable, helps to reduce frictional drag, protects against abrasion, and carries away microorganisms and irritants as it is sloughed off. Chemicals contained in mucus have fungicidal and bactericidal roles, and other chemicals may be present for communication. An example of this is the alarm substance secreted from the Schreckstoff cells in the skin of the carp.

Epidermis

This is a non-keratinising, stratified squamous epithelium with the basic malpighian cell common to all vertebrates. Thickness varies from 3 or 4 cells up to approximately 20, and tends to vary with age, species, site and, in some, the stage of the reproductive cycle. Thickness tends to be greater in those fish with less scale cover, for example eels, and also over the fins, which are well supplied with nerve endings and mucus cells.

Malpighian cells are rounded and very similar at all levels except the outer, where they tend to be flattened. Cell multiplication occurs in the deepest layer, the stratum germinativum, which rests on a basement membrane, but all layers are living and capable of mitotic division.

(a)

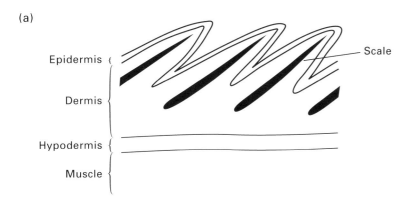

Epidermis

Dermis

Hypodermis

Muscle

Scale

Fig. 1.2 (a) Diagrammatic representation of a section through fish skin. (b) Diagrammatic representation of fish skin structure.

(b)

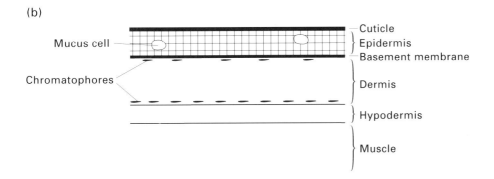

Mucus cell

Chromatophores

Cuticle
Epidermis
Basement membrane

Dermis

Hypodermis

Muscle

Wound repair might be expected to be temperature dependent and thus very slow at low temperatures. In fact, due to an unusual feature of fish skin, malpighian cells migrate across the wound surface in a temperature independent manner when the epidermis is breached. The result is that the wound is quite quickly covered with an epidermal layer at least one cell thick. The surrounding epidermis, from which the cells have migrated, is of course made thinner by this migration. More fundamental repair is then carried out at a rate that is temperature dependent.

As well as malpighian cells, a variety of other types occur. Mucus or goblet cells secrete mucus on to the skin surface, their numbers varying with species and site. They usually originate in the middle layers of the epidermis and increase in size as they approach the surface. Club cells are large, eosinophilic and usually rounded. They are found in the lower and middle layers of the epidermis of some species, typically carp where they secrete alarm substances (Schreckstoff cells). Many other species have similar cells but they do not appear

to be related to fright reactions and their function is not clear. Eosinophilic granular cells occur in some species (function unknown), and other cells found include lymphocytes, macrophages and large clear cyst-like structures which are especially prominent in the cod. Specialised structures such as taste buds are also found.

Dermis

The dermis consists of two layers: the upper stratum spongiosum, and the deeper stratum compactum. The stratum spongiosum, a loose network of collagen and reticulin fibres connected to the epidermal basement membrane, contains pigment cells (chromatophores), mast cells and scale pockets. The stratum compactum is a dense collagenous matrix giving the skin structural strength.

Colour is used principally for camouflage (e.g. protection from predators) and communication (e.g. sexual activity). Background colour is given by underlying tissues and body fluids, with other colour being produced by the interplay of chromatophores in the dermis. Large numbers of different types of chromatophore are present at different levels in the dermis. These include melanophores, lipophores and iridocytes, the effect of which is due to their absorptive and reflective properties.

Scales are a major feature of most teleosts, although some have few or none. They originate in scale pockets in the dermis and are covered by a layer of epidermis. Loss of scales therefore means loss of epidermis, and this can have important consequences with respect to osmotic control.

Scales are calcified flexible plates which have an outer ridged bony part, and an inner fibrous connective tissue part that is uncalcified in some species and partly calcified in others. This inner part consists of parallel collagen fibres in an organic matrix. Scales are a ready source of calcium in times of deprivation.

The two main types of importance here are ctenoid scales, found on the spiny-rayed fish, and cycloid scales, found on most soft-rayed fish. The caudal edge of the ctenoid scale carries variable numbers of tooth-like processes, which are lacking in cycloid scales. Both types grow along with the rest of the body and consequently have growth rings on the surface, allowing estimates of age in many species.

Hypodermis

The hypodermis is a loose, well vascularised, adipose layer connecting the skin to underlying structures. Due to its loose structure, any pathogen penetrating the skin, and any associated inflammation, is able to spread easily along this layer.

Respiration

Water contains only about 5% of the amount of oxygen that is available in air. This level falls even further as temperature and ionic concentration increase. A consequence of this is that the respiratory apparatus of fish must be very efficient to take advantage of the available oxygen. This has been achieved by the development of gills over which there is a constant flow of water from which oxygen is extracted.

Some gaseous exchange may take place in the skin of some scaleless fish. The skin is usually very important for this purpose in most fish embryos before gills develop. Some species have developed the ability to breathe air, but the primary organ for gaseous exchange in most fish is the gill.

The gill surface consists of a thin epithelium carried on lamellae, providing an intimate interface for the uptake of oxygen and excretion of carbon dioxide. This epithelium can have a surface area of up to ten times that of the rest of the body, the actual size determined by the lifestyle of the fish and its respiratory demands. Sluggish bottom dwellers tend to have relatively small respiratory surfaces compared with fast-swimming predators such as the salmonids.

In addition to gaseous exchange, the gill is involved in acid–base balance, osmoregulation and the excretion of nitrogenous waste products (mainly in the form of ammonia in teleosts).

Because of the thinness of the respiratory surface, the gill is extremely vulnerable to damage and invasion by pathogens. Any structural damage will lead to disruption of all the gill's functions.

Gill Structure

A typical teleost gill consists of two sets of four gills arches or holobranchs, each set forming one side of the pharynx. Each arch is supported on a bony skeleton and carries two diverging hemibranchs (rows of filaments) on its caudal edge. The free tips of the hemibranchs on each arch are so arranged that they touch those of the adjacent holobranch (Fig. 1.3).

The hemibranch filaments, known as primary lamellae, are long and thin, and radiate out from the gill arch like the teeth of a comb. These primary lamellae are supported by bony gill rays arising from the gill arch.

On dorsal and ventral surfaces of the primary lamellae, mounted at right angles to the long axis, are semi-circular folds of epithelium, the secondary lamellae. These are the site of gaseous exchange. The dorsal and ventral secondary lamellae on adjacent primary lamellae are so positioned that they interdigitate with one another, so that each side of the pharynx is effectively a mesh through which water must pass.

Gill rakers are present on each of the gill arches. These structures are on the opposite side of the

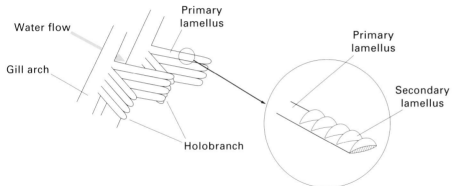

FIG. 1.3 Arrangement of lamellae on the gill arch (based on Lagler *et al.*, 1977).

arch to the primary lamellae and are directed cranially. They serve to prevent entry of food particles into the gill cavity from the mouth, and are particularly well developed in plankton or filter feeders.

The gill arch is covered by typical teleost epithelium, which is usually much thicker at the origin of primary lamellae, and is usually well endowed with mucus cells. Primary lamellae are covered by a mucoid epidermis which may contain chloride cells (salt-secreting cells), especially at the base of the secondary lamellae. These cells are usually more numerous in marine species. Beneath the epidermis can be seen lymphocytes, eosinophilic granular cells, phagocytic cells (which vary in number with species) and rodlet cells. Rodlet cells are found in many species and in many tissues but their function is unknown.

The secondary lamellae are essentially epithelial envelopes with the basement membrane of the epithelium on the inside of the envelope. The epithelium is usually one or two cells thick. The two sides of the envelope are separated and supported by pillar cells arranged in rows. These pillar cells attach to the basement membrane of the envelope epithelium, and at the point of attachment spread along the basement membrane until they come into contact with adjacent pillar cells. This arrangement forms the lining of the lamellar blood channels, and erythrocytes move through the spaces created. There is evidence to suggest the presence of a distinct marginal blood channel around the edge of the secondary lamellae, and this is probably the preferred route of blood flow.

The epithelial cell surfaces have micro-ridges which increase the surface area further and may also aid the flow and attachment of mucus. Epithelial cell replacement in the secondary lamellae is from the base: cells migrate along the lamellae to the tip, where they are shed. Pillar cells replicate *in situ*.

Oxygen Uptake

The gill arches contain branchial blood vessels. The afferent arteries arise from the ventral aorta and the efferent arteries supply the dorsal aorta. The afferent filament arteries run along the edge of the primary lamellae downstream of the water-flow. Blood enters the blood spaces of the secondary lamellae from these vessels via short afferent lamellar arteries. This deoxygenated blood then flows through the secondary lamellar blood spaces, primarily in the marginal channels, in the opposite direction to the water-flow which is passing out from the buccal cavity. This arrangement creates a counter-current flow system (Fig. 1.4) which can lead to up to 80% of the oxygen in the water being transferred to the blood. This figure varies with species and water and gill conditions. Oxygenated blood then leaves the secondary lamellae by efferent lamellar arteries to feed the dorsal aorta by way of the efferent filament and efferent branchial arteries.

The oxygen requirement of a fish changes with variations in activity, and the area of gill in use at any one time can be altered to meet that change in demand. It has been shown that the functional area can increase by a factor of 6 between standard to maximum aerobic metabolic rates. At rest many secondary lamellae are not perfused with blood,

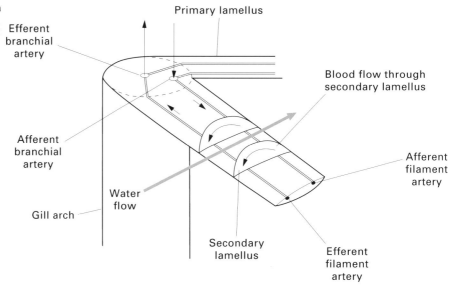

FIG. 1.4 Blood flow through the gill, water flow over gill surface, and consequent countercurrent effect.

Primary lamellus

Efferent branchial artery

Blood flow through secondary lamellus

Afferent branchial artery

Afferent filament artery

Water flow

Gill arch

Secondary lamellus

Efferent filament artery

and the increase in function is achieved mainly by an increase in the number of secondary lamellae in use.

Changes in the angle of gill arches to the body axis are possible by the use of adductor muscles, and this has the effect of altering water-flow through the hemibranchs. Under situations of increased oxygen demand the arches can be moved in such a way as to allow recruitment of more primary lamellae for oxygen uptake, probably the more dorsal ones. Secondary lamellae may be differentially perfused with blood. Under resting conditions only the secondary lamellae on the proximal parts of the primary lamellae are perfused, usually the ventral rather than dorsal. Thus more secondary lamellae can be recruited under conditions of high demand.

Regulation of branchial blood flow is poorly understood but autonomic control through neurotransmitters and endocrines has been shown to have an effect on branchial resistance to blood flow.

Carbon dioxide is readily soluble in water, and freely moves from the blood into the water passing across the gills. Excretion of nitrogenous waste products and the gill's role in osmoregulation will be dealt with under Excretion and Osmoregulatory Control.

Water-flow

Water-flow over the gills is continuous and unidirectional, and is achieved by means of a double pump system. This operates by the co-ordinated opening and closing of the mouth and opercula, and expansion and contraction of the buccal and opercular cavities. The result of this process is that water is drawn in through the mouth and expelled through the operculae, passing over the gills en route. This system gives a continuous flow of water over the gill, unlike the tidal system which occurs in mammals (Fig. 1.5).

The energy required for oxygen extraction is very high when compared with mammals. Up to 10% of the oxygen uptake of a fish at rest may be required for the muscular activity involved in ventilation. In conditions of warm or polluted water where oxygen levels are low, oxygen needs for extraction can be greater than the oxygen uptake — the so-called Respiratory Distress Syndrome, which can be lethal.

Different species may modify the pumping system according to their way of life. In some fast swimmers, such as mackerel, the pumps have been dispensed with entirely and the fish relies on forward motion to supply enough water to the gills. This is known as ram ventilation.

Blood flow is pulsatile and enters the blood spaces of the secondary lamellae under pressure as it comes directly from the ventral aorta. Because of this there is always a danger that the delicate secondary lamellae may be damaged. Pillar cells contain contractile proteins which help to resist damage to a degree, but there is also

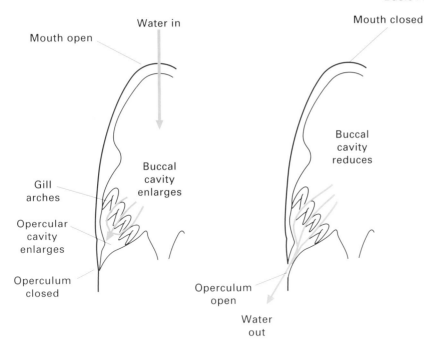

Fig. 1.5 Simplified buccal pump mechanism.

Water in

Mouth open

Mouth closed

Buccal cavity reduces

Buccal cavity enlarges

Gill arches

Opercular cavity enlarges

Operculum closed

Operculum open

Water out

synchronisation of water-flow through the gills with blood flow. Thus an increase in blood pressure is compensated for by a corresponding increase in water pressure.

Ventilation control is by proprioceptors and mechanoreceptors which respond to changes in water-flow, and can initiate changes in water-flow and heart rate. If branchial water-flow is artificially arrested, a reflex cardiac inhibition occurs. The presence of irritants can stimulate a 'cough reflex' where water-flow is reversed through the gills, resulting in back-flushing. Low pO_2 and high pCO_2 cause an increase of heart rate and ventilation rate.

Pseudobranch

These organs are found on the dorsal part of the inner aspect of each operculum and are modified hemibranchs. In some species, such as carp, they are deeply embedded in the opercular tissue; in others they are superficial and may even protrude above the epithelial surface. They are absent from some fish, such as some eels.

Their function is uncertain but they are perfused with oxygenated blood from the first gill arch and may be associated with monitoring arterial pO_2. This blood then passes to the choroid rete in the eye, which may indicate an involvement with the

supply to the retina of well oxygenated blood. Its considerable afferent innervation from the glossopharyngeal nerve means that it probably plays a sensory role, and it may also have an endocrine function.

Swim-bladder

Most teleosts have a swim-bladder, the primary function of which is the maintenance of buoyancy. In some species it may also be involved with sound reception and production, pressure reception, and occasionally even respiratory function. It may be absent, very reduced, or even lipid filled in some species such as bottom dwellers. Grossly the organ may constitute up to 7% of body volume in fresh water, 5% in the sea. It is found dorsally in the abdomen and may be divided into two or even three chambers.

Embryologically the swim-bladder arises as a diverticulum of the fore-gut. A patent connection with the gut is still present as the pneumatic duct in many adult fish; these fish are known as physostomes, and include most of the soft-rayed teleosts, such as the salmonids. The duct is closed in the spiny-rayed fish, and these are therefore known as physoclists.

The swim-bladder wall is made up of two main

layers, an inner tunica interna, and a tunica externa. The tunica interna has a transitional epithelium which lines the bladder, overlying a muscularis mucosa, which itself overlays a sub-mucosa of loose vascular connective tissue. The tunica externa consists of an outer serosa over a tough fibrous layer in which muscle and elastic connective tissue are found. In multi-chambered swim-bladders the cranial chamber is usually concerned with gas reception and retention and as a consequence has a thick wall. The caudal chamber, involved with gas reabsorption, has a thinner wall.

Nerve endings in the swim-bladder walls respond to stretching and slackening, and both secretory and absorptive functions are under vagal control.

Buoyancy

In order to maintain and control buoyancy, the amount of gas within the swim-bladder is adjusted according to need. Inflation of the bladder in physostomes can be achieved by the oral intake of air which is then forced along the pneumatic duct into the swim-bladder. Gas may also be voided by the same route. This process is not possible in physoclists (or physostomes with no access to air), and inflation of the bladder is achieved by the release of gas from arterial blood passing through the gas gland, a rete mirabile, in the tunica interna of the cranio-ventral area of the swim-bladder. This gland is present in all physoclists and many physostomes as well.

Release of gas into the swim-bladder by the gas gland is due to several factors, but mainly an increase in blood acidity in this area, activating the Bohr and Root effects in the blood. Gas reabsorption occurs by means of the oval, a capillary plexus arising from the dorsal aorta. The oval has an impervious muscular diaphragm which controls the area of exposed plexus, and thus the area available for gas absorption. The presence of purine crystals in the tunica interna helps to reduce the absorptive capacity of the rest of the swim-bladder wall.

The gases present in the swim-bladder are oxygen, nitrogen and carbon dioxide, but they are usually in different proportions to air. For example, the swim-bladders of cyprinids (which are physostomes) contain almost pure nitrogen.

Sound and Pressure

Sound in water consists of pressure waves, so any pressure sensitive organ should be able to detect it. The gas-filled swim-bladder will respond to pressure changes by corresponding changes in volume, and thus it is a useful sensor of pressure change and consequently sound. Pressure changes of less than 0.5% of ambient pressure can be detected by fish with swim-bladders.

Fish can detect sound up to about 400 Hz by

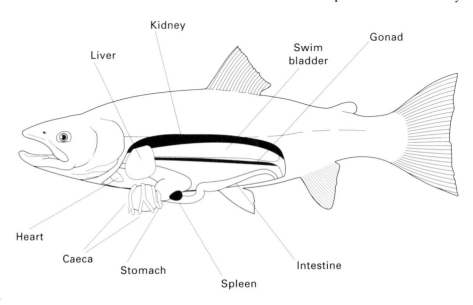

FIG. 1.6 Internal organs.

use of the otolith organ and lateral line, but detection can increase markedly in fish with a swim-bladder. Where the bladder has no connection to the inner ear, such as in the cod, its presence can increase the detection level to 520 Hz. Where there is a direct connection, such as in the ictalurids and cyprinids, detection levels can be raised to as high as 7000 Hz. This connection takes the form of a series of three small bones derived from the vertebrae — the Weberian ossicles — which transmit vibrations to the perilymph around the inner ear.

Some fish produce sound by vibration of the swim-bladder wall, using special muscles.

Excretion and Osmoregulatory Control

Compared with terrestrial animals, fish are exposed to much greater ionic and osmoregulatory challenges, and regulation of internal body fluid composition is a complex process. There is little movement of water or ions across the skin of an adult fish, but they can easily pass across gill surfaces, which means that this organ is very important in osmoregulatory control. Other sites where transfer can occur are the gut wall and kidney.

In addition to being involved with respiration and osmoregulatory control, gills are also primarily responsible for the excretion of nitrogenous waste products. A small amount of these will be present in the urine, but the kidney plays only a minor role in this function.

Excretory Kidney

The teleost kidney is a composite organ made up of haemopoietic, reticuloendothelial, endocrine and excretory tissues. It arises embryologically as a paired organ, but has become completely fused in some species such as the salmonids. The degree and pattern of fusion are variable between species.

Lying against the vertebral column just ventral to the dorsal aorta, the kidney is retroperitoneal and usually extends the length of the body cavity (Fig. 1.6).There is no cortex and medulla, but there is a divison between the anterior or head kidney, and posterior kidney. Urine drains from the collecting ducts to paired ureters which may fuse caudally, and in some fish may enlarge to form a urinary bladder. The urine then leaves the body via the vent.

The head kidney contains predominantly haemopoietic and lymphoid tissue, with some endocrine elements. The posterior kidney contains the excretory tissue along wth varying levels of haemopoietic and lymphoid tissue. Nephron structure tends to vary with habitat, with marine, euryhaline and freshwater forms reflecting the differing physiological requirements.

The endocrine elements present within the kidney are inter-renal tissue (equivalent to the adrenal cortex), chromaffin cells (equivalent to the adrenal medulla) surrounding the major blood vessels, and the Corpuscles of Stannius (associated with calcium balance).

A typical freshwater nephron has a well vascularised glomerulus, a ciliated neck, two distinct proximal segments (one with a prominent brush border, one with numerous mitochondria but a less well developed brush border), a narrow ciliated intermediate segment, a distal segment and collecting duct system. The distal segment is where dilution of the tubular filtrate takes place.

Marine species tend to have fewer glomeruli (which are smaller than in freshwater species) and some species have no glomeruli at all. This difference reflects the reduced need for urine production in the marine fish. A typical marine nephron has a glomerulus (which is usually less well developed than its freshwater counterpart), neck and proximal segments (which constitute the major component), an intermediate segment and the collecting duct system.

The reticuloendothelial element of the kidney occurs in sinusoids in the head kidney and within the peritubular capillaries, all these areas being lined with highly phagocytic cells which can rapidly clear particulate matter from the blood.

The kidney has a dual blood supply from a renal artery and renal portal veins. The renal artery is derived directly from the dorsal aorta and supplies high pressure blood to the glomerular capillary bed via afferent arterioles, this blood producing the glomerular filtrate. The efferent vessels from the glomerulae then supply the capillary network around the kidney tubules which, in many species, also receives blood from the renal portal veins. This portal system carries blood and lymph draining

Fig. 1.7 Osmoregulation in
(a) fresh water and (b) sea
water.

(a)

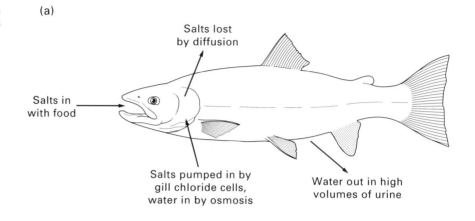

Salts lost
by diffusion

Salts in
with food

Salts pumped in by
gill chloride cells,
water in by osmosis

Water out in high
volumes of urine

(b)

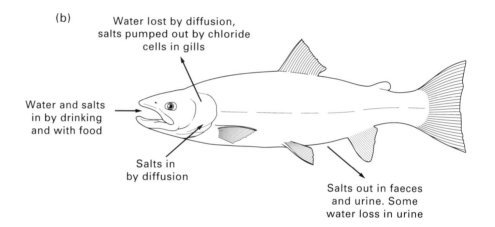

Water lost by diffusion,
salts pumped out by chloride
cells in gills

Water and salts
in by drinking
and with food

Salts in
by diffusion

Salts out in faeces
and urine. Some
water loss in urine

from the tail region of the fish. All blood leaves through the post-cardinal veins.

Osmotic and Ionic Balance

Homeostasis must be maintained in the fish body and an important part of this process is the maintenance of the osmotic balance of the blood. The tissue fluids of teleosts have a concentration intermediate between that of sea and fresh water. In fresh water the blood of fish is hyper-osmotic with respect to the environment, whereas in the marine situation it tends to be hypo-osmotic. Both these situations require some form of compensatory mechanisms, different in each case (Fig. 1.7).

Fish in fresh water suffer a constant inflow of water into the blood through the gills and an outflow of salts, mainly sodium and chloride, by the same route. This is overcome to a certain extent by the production of large volumes of dilute urine which can be up to 20% of body-weight per day. The production of this urine results in the loss of further ions, although there is active resorption of sodium and chloride in the kidney. Loss of ions is compensated for by active uptake from the water by chloride cells in the gills, and by uptake from food in the gut. This uptake relies on Na^+/NH_4^+, Na^+/H^+ and Cl^-/HCO_3^- ion exchange mechanisms. Thus the main work of the kidney in the freshwater fish is excretion of water, and this is reflected by the presence of a large number of well vascularised glomeruli.

In fish in the marine environment there is a constant fight against deyhdration due to the passive loss of water across gills by osmosis. This dehydration is countered by the ingestion of water, (fish drinking up to 15% of their body-weight per day) but this ingestion also increases the salt content of the body. Divalent ions are not usually absorbed by the gut and are excreted with the faeces, so the main problem occurs with mono-valent ions, predominantly sodium and chloride. Ions also move into the blood by diffusion across the gills.

The nephron of the teleost is unable to concentrate urine which is, at best, iso-osmotic with blood. Because of the need to conserve water in marine fish, only small amounts of urine are produced, and thus only small amounts of salt can be eliminated from the body by the kidneys. The excess sodium and chloride ions are eliminated by active excretion by the chloride cells in the gills, the same cells which pump salts inwards in fresh water. Many more chloride cells are found in the gills of marine fish than freshwater fish. Any divalent ions excess to requirements are actively excreted in the urine.

Euryhaline fish (that is, those which can tolerate wide ranges of salinity) can alternate between the mechanisms of freshwater and marine species as required. Examples are the anadromous salmon which move from the sea to fresh water in order to breed, and catadromous eels which do the opposite. The glomerular apparatus of some species degenerates once in the marine environment.

Control of filtration and reabsorption is by hormonal action, and changes in habitat are usually accompanied, or preceded, by changes in endocrine activity. Sexual development is usually the reason for such changes of habitat, and changes in endocrines associated with sexual maturation can affect the ionic and osmoregulatory mechanisms.

Circulatory System

The fish has a single circulatory system (Fig. 1.8), the heart pumping blood through the gills for aeration, and thence to the capillaries in the tissues. Venous blood returns to the heart, although that from the tail and gut first passes through the capillaries of the renal and hepatic portal systems respectively.

Heart

The heart is usually immediately behind the gills in a cranio-ventral position. It is separated from the peritoneal cavity by a thin septum which forms the posterior part of the enveloping pericardial sac. The whole heart is intimately covered by a pericardium within the pericardial sac; serous fluid separates the two membranes.

Venous blood enters the heart via the sinus venosus. This structure has a thin wall, usually made of connective tissue, but in some species it can be muscular and contractile. It serves to collect venous blood (though its volume is only a fraction of that of the atrium) which then passes through the sino-atrial valves to enter the atrium.

The atrium has a thin muscular wall, and muscular trabeculae cross the lumen to form a

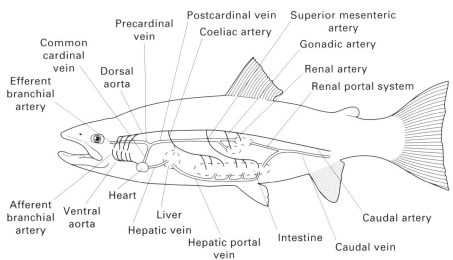

FIG. 1.8 The basic circulatory system.

loose mesh within the chamber. Because of this structure, the endothelial lining of the atrium has a very large surface area and, in many species, this lining has phagocytic activity as part of the reticuloendothelial system. The muscle fibres are so arranged that contraction of the atrium tends to move blood towards the atrio-ventricular valves and thus to the ventricle, which lies ventral to the atrium.

The ventricle has much thicker walls than the atrium, commonly having two layers of muscle: a superficial compact cortical layer and an inner spongy one. The ventricular chamber is lined with an endothelium similar to that seen in the atrium, but with less phagocytic activity.

Where both layers of muscle are present they are usually separated by a thin connective tissue septum. The thickness of the compact layer is determined by normal levels of physical activity. It can be a significant proportion of the heart weight in actively swimming fish and may be almost absent in less active species. Variations in the proportions of these muscle types can occur with different stages of the life cycle. Cardiac muscle fibres are about half the thickness of mammalian fibres (approximately 6 μ) but are otherwise similar in structure.

Two groups of coronary vessels are supplied by the efferent branchial arteries and run over the outside of the ventricle, supplying the compact muscle. Coronary veins carry the blood to the sinus venosus or atrium. Spongy muscle obtains most of its requirements from the 'venous' blood in the lumen. When venous oxygen levels become very low during periods of intense activity, cardiac myoglobin gives some protection against anoxia.

From the ventricle, blood passes through a pair of semilunar valves into the highly distensible and non-contractile bulbus arteriosus. This has a thick wall consisting of a mixture of elastic tissue and smooth muscle. The elasticity of the bulbus enables it to act as a passive elastic reservoir which helps to smooth out pressure pulses from the ventricle, and ensures a continuous flow of blood in the ventral aorta throughout the cardiac cycle.

Arteries

The ventral aorta lies in the midline beneath the gills, running cranially, and its wall can dilate or contract to make adjustments in blood flow. The ventral aorta supplies blood to each gill arch via afferent branchial arteries. These have a structure in common with other vertebrates, consisting of three layers: an adventitia, media and intima with an endothelial lining. The intima consists largely of elastic tissue and an endothelium. This endothelium, with its extremely thin basement membrane, is so thin that it is often only noticeable by the presence of nuclei bulging into the lumen. The media is made up of elastic tissue interleaved with smooth muscle cells. The outer adventitia is thin and made mainly of collagen fibres.

Oxygenated blood leaves the gill capillaries by the efferent branchial arteries, and these converge above the pharynx to form the dorsal aorta. The carotid arteries, which are the main supply to the head region, also arise from here. Some blood from the first efferent branchial artery flows via the pseudobranch to the eye.

A considerable pressure drop occurs across the gills due to the dispersal of the blood through the capillary beds. This reduction in pressure varies with species, but typical values of dorsal aortic pressure as a percentage of ventral aortic pressure range from 15 to 60. Because of this lower pressure, the efferent vessel walls are thinner than those of the afferent vessels, with less elastic tissue and muscle.

The dorsal aorta is the main vessel for distribution to the rest of the body. In fish it is effectively half way between an artery and a vein in structure compared to other vertebrates. In some lower teleosts, such as the salmonids, an elastic ligament stretches along the length of the aortic lumen. This is said to act as an auxiliary 'heart', automatically increasing circulation to the muscles during swimming movements.

The dorsal aorta runs along the entire length of the abdominal cavity just ventral to the vertebral column. It is known as the caudal artery in the tail region. Along its length it gives off branches to the body musculature and organs. The viscera are mainly supplied by the anterior mesenteric artery.

After passing through the tissue capillary beds, the deoxygenated blood is collected by the venous system and returned to the sinus venosus along with lymph.

Veins

As in the case of other vertebrates, the veins are relatively inelastic, with walls constructed mainly of collagen. The major veins are large in diameter and pressures are low. Valves are not common in the teleost system. Blood from the tail region is collected in the caudal vein which then drains into the kidney — the renal portal system. There is also a typical hepatic portal sytem from the viscera.

Capillaries

Capillaries in teleosts are much more permeable than in mammals, and a consequence of this is that plasma can move quite freely across the capillary wall. The interstitial fluid therefore has a high protein concentration, and loss of blood protein can be relatively easily made up from the tissues.

Circulation Control

Heart rates are governed by a sino-atrial pace-maker, but temperature has a significant effect on heart rate. The ECG is similar to that of other vertebrates.

Cardiac output is mainly altered by changes to stroke volume rather than heart rate. The heart has a vagal innervation giving an inhibitory effect, and also a weak excitatory adrenergic innervation in some teleosts. The heart obeys Starling's law where there is an increase in cardiac output in response to an increase in venous return.

General increases in circulation during exercise can be accounted for by the action of circulating catecholamines on alpha-receptors in various parts of the body. Vasomotor nerves have also been demonstrated and, although there are many differences, many of the mechanisms seen in mammals have their counterparts in fish.

Lymph

The lymph drainage system is very extensive, probably due to the high capillary permeability. Lymph volume is about four times that of blood, and the composition is almost identical to blood plasma. Most of the white muscle is poorly vascularised, and the lymphatic system is effectively its only circulation.

Lymph vessels are thin-walled sinuses and are not easily seen on dissection. There are no lymph nodes. Three main lymph ducts are present in the body: the dorsal, lateral and ventral subcutaneous lymph trunks. The lymph finally rejoins the main circulation in one of the veins just before the sinus venosus, the exact site varying with species.

A false lymph heart relying on gill movements helps to propel the lymph in species such as eels, and some species have true lymph hearts with valves and cardiac muscle-like fibres. Double chambered, valved lymph hearts are found in the tail of both eels and salmon.

Digestive Tract

Teleosts occupy a great diversity of ecological habitats. Their digestive tract, which is broadly similar in arrangement to those of all vertebrates, tends to be modified by the wide range of feeding habits and diet associated with those niches.

The overall length of the tract varies with species, and other specialisations occur such as dentition, absence of stomach, etc. Predators usually have well developed grasping teeth, a well defined stomach with strong acid secretions, and an intestine generally shorter in length than in herbivores of comparable size. Herbivores tend to have teeth within the oral cavity; they may have no stomach at all, and tend to have a relatively long intestine.

Mucus membrane lines the entire digestive tract, and the tract wall is liberally supplied with mucus-secreting glands to lubricate the passage of food and protect the gut lining. As with most vertebrates, food is moved through the gut by peristaltic waves of muscular contraction.

Physiological changes occur in the digestive tract of many species during periods of starvation, migration, spawning, etc. This is especially obvious in some euryhaline species such as European eels and Atlantic salmon. In these, there tends to be flattening of epithelial folding, shrinkage and often necrosis of epithelial cells.

Digestive organs are under nervous and endo-crine control. Innervation by the sympathetic system and the parasympathetic via the vagus nerve occurs, and several hormones are involved.

Mouth

The jaws of most fish are for biting, and in predators the lips are usually quite thin and undeveloped. Lips can be much more fleshy and mobile in some fish, and many have well developed sensory barbels bordering the mouth which assist with food location. Modifications of mouth shape for specialised feeding purposes are also seen.

The oral cavity and pharynx are lined with stratified squamous epithelium on a thick basement membrane with a dense dermis binding it to underlying bone and muscle. Many mucus-secreting glands are present, but no salivary glands except in very specialised species. The lining is well supplied with sensory nerve endings. Chewing is not usually a feature of teleosts except in a few highly developed herbivores, but teeth do occur which are variable in type and location.

Teeth are thought to have arisen from scales, and in teleosts three types occur, named according to location: jaw, mouth and pharyngeal. Jaw teeth are found on the jaw margins and can be of a variety of forms. They are present in the channel catfish, many sea-bass and sea-bream, and salmonids. Mouth teeth are found within the oral cavity on the roof, sides and floor, often including the tongue. Pharyngeal teeth occur as pads on various gill arch elements in many species, and typical of this arrangement is the carp where teeth develop from the last gill arch. Tooth-like modifications of the gill rakers also occur in some predatory species.

Gill rakers protect the gill filaments from damage due to ingested material, but are also specialised in relation to the feeding habits of some fish. They range from quite short and simple in omnivores to elongated and complex in filter feeders, where they prevent the loss of food particles.

Oesophagus

The oesophagus is usually short, thick-walled, and very distensible so that anything that can be taken into the mouth can be swallowed. Longitudinal folding along its length make this distension possible. The wall is very muscular with interweaving skeletal muscle fibres which may extend as far as the stomach. The lining is a stratified cuboidal epithelium, well supplied with mucus cells.

Stomach

The stomach shows adaptations according to habits, and varies from elongate in piscivorous fish to sac-like in omnivorous fish. About 15% of teleosts have no stomach at all. Where the stomach exists, most pronounced in carnivores, it is typically a sigmoid shape, with numerous folds in the lining and is a highly muscular organ. The striated muscle of the oesophagus changes to the smooth muscle of the stomach at the cardia. The wall consists of a number of muscle layers, a submucosa containing large numbers of eosinophilic granular cells, blood vessels and nerve fibres, and a gastric mucosa which is folded and very mucoid with numerous glands (including fundic and pyloric) at the base of the folds. The main secretions into the stomach, apart from mucus, are pepsinogen and hydrochloric acid, and a pH as low as 2.4 has been measured.

Pyloric Caeca

Pyloric caeca occur in many species, most notably the salmonids where they may number 70 or more. These structures are blind-ended finger-like projections that extend outwards from the pyloric valve region of the stomach and the anterior intestine. Their structure and function resemble the intestine rather than the stomach, and they have a multi-folded intestinal type epithelium. The enzyme lactase has been found in the caeca of trout, and a high level of saccharase in carp. Pyloric caeca and intestinal mucosae are sources of lipase, which breaks down fats into fatty acids and glycerine. As well as digestion, some absorption may occur in these organs.

Intestine

The intestine is quite short in carnivorous species and longer in herbivores. It is usually a simple tube, with no enlargement into a colon distally, and may be straight or coiled depending on abdominal shape. The lining is a simple columnar mucoid epithelium overlaying a submucosa. Lymphocytes and rodlet cells, of unknown function, are often seen in the mucosa. Only a few species have anything resembling the intestinal villi of mammals, but the simple columnar epithelial cells do possess a brush border of microvilli. The submucosa contains variable quantities of lymphoid tissue and often many eosinophilic granular cells. Beneath this is a dense muscular layer and then a fibroelastic layer.

The intestinal epithelium is not divided into regions histologically, but there may be functional differentiation, different areas specialising in lipid, protein and ionic regulation respectively. Digestive products are readily absorbed, and this process is facilitated by the folding of the wall along the tract. This folding increases the surface area available for absorption and also helps to slow down the passage of food through the gut, giving more time for absorption.

The small intestine contains the openings for the bile and pancreatic ducts. Intestinal enzymes are secreted as inactive forms which are activated within the lumen, and the enzymes entering this part of the gut work best at neutral to alkaline pH.

Rectum

The rectum, which connects with the vent, has a thicker muscular wall than the intestine and is capable of considerable distension.

Liver

The liver is a relatively large organ, usually reddish-brown in carnivores and a lighter brown in herbivores. In farmed fish, where diets may be less than ideal, it may be lighter in colour than in equivalent wild fish. It is usually in the cranial abdomen, but in some species processes extend the length of the abdomen or are closely applied to other viscera. It is not regularly divided into lobules as in mammals. In some species, such as carp, it is a compound organ with the pancreas and is known as the hepatopancreas.

The liver acts as a storage organ for carbohydrates (as glycogen) and fats. It is also involved with blood cell destruction and blood chemistry, as well as other metabolic functions such as the production of urea and other compounds concerned with nitrogen excretion. Fat storage varies

with species, but in flatfish and cod, for example, the liver is the primary site of fat storage.

The histology of the liver varies from the mammalian form in that there is less of a tendency for the hepatocytes to be arranged in cords or lobules. Sinusoids are fewer in number, and do not contain functional Kuppfer cells; they are lined with endothelial cells with very prominent nuclei. The space between sinusoid cells and hepatocytes (the space of Disse) contains microvilli from both sets of cells and a number of fat storage cells (the cells of Ito) which also store vitamin A and produce collagen. They are involved in cirrhotic responses, as in mammals.

Hepatocytes are polygonal with a distinctive central nucleus which has densely staining chromatin margins and a prominent nucleolus. Their appearance can vary greatly between species and also with age, sex, exposure to pollution, nutritional status and other factors. They are often swollen with glycogen or neutral fat when nutrition is less than ideal. During cyclical starvation periods, which may be part of normal physiological cycles, the cells may be shrunken and the entire liver loaded with yellow ceroid pigments.

The liver is supplied with blood by the hepatic portal vein from the gastro-intestinal tract and the hepatic artery, both of which supply blood to the sinusoids. The blood then drains into the central vein and thence to the hepatic vein.

The liver produces bile which, as with mammals, contains fat-emulsifying bile salts along with bile pigments biliverdin and bilirubin, and is greenish-yellow in colour. Bile salts emulsify fats and help to adjust intestinal pH for digestion. Bile is collected via intracellular canaliculi which eventually anastomose to form typical bile ducts. In most species these fuse to form a gall bladder with a lining of transitional epithelium which often contains rodlet cells. Bile enters the intestine via the common bile duct in the pyloric region.

Haemopoietic tissue, complete with melano-macrophage centres, is often found in varying amounts around the larger vessels of the liver.

Pancreas

The pancreas has exocrine and endocrine activity. Its position varies with species but some sites are prevalent. It is usually found in nodules which may be interspersed among the fat cells in the mesentery of the pyloric caeca (in the case of salmonids), or dispersed within the liver to form the hepato-pancreas, usually around the hepatic portal vein (such as in the carp), or even in the subcapsular tissue of the spleen.

The cellular structure of the exocrine pancreas is similar to that of mammals. It consists of acinar cells with a very dark basophilic cytoplasm which, in actively feeding fish, contain bright eosinophilic secretory granules. The pancreatic duct usually joins the common bile duct somewhere along its length.

The endocrine element consists of the Islets of Langerhans, whose distribution varies with species. These organs are composed of a number of poorly staining structures within a thin capusle, formed of small fusiform α, β and δ cells.

Other Organs

The swim-bladder, thyroid, thymus and ultimo-branchial organs are all derived from the digestive tract, but none have any digestive function and are considered elsewhere.

Digestion

The digestive enzymes are essentially the same as in the higher vertebrates. Stomach evacuation rate, digestion and assimilation rate are all temperature dependant, and the processes involved all require energy — the 'specific dynamic action'. This energy requirement, and the associated need for oxygen can lead to hypoxia and death can occur when oxygen levels are too low.

Protein requirements are directly related to growth and gonad development. In those species of fish studied so far, the same essential amino acids are required as in terrestrial animals. Protein can also be used as a primary energy source. Protein absorption takes place in the intestine.

Lipids are used as a source of energy, and to maintain the structure and function of cellular membranes. Because of the low body temperatures found in fish, lipids with low melting points are required so that they remain liquid at normal body temperatures. These materials are used as a primary energy reserve, instead of carbohydrates as in mammals. Lipid has a 'protein sparing' action in that, if it is used as the primary energy source, protein will not be used for this purpose. Therefore a certain minimum level of lipid is required in the diet in order to maximise the efficiency of use of dietary protein; that is, the protein can be used entirely for growth. However, excess dietary lipid can cause 'fatty livers' and consequent hepatic damage, especially true in salmonids. Fats can be absorbed as fatty acids and glycerol or, in some species, as complete fats direct into the lymphatic system. Such absorption occurs in the pyloric caeca of salmonids.

Carbohydrate can be utilised by some fish as well as lipids as an energy source, but it is not an important part of the diet. Fish energy metabolism resembles that of a diabetic mammal, and ingestion of glucose results in persistent hyperglycaemia. Insulin will lower this level but it is not normally used to reduce blood levels. In starved fish, liver glycogen levels remain unchanged for long periods and some other substrate, such as non-essential amino acids and lipids, is used in preference as an energy source. The capacity of fish to metabolise glucose aerobically is consequently very low compared with mammals. Nervous tissue, which apparently does use glucose as a primary fuel, produces it by gluconeogenesis rather than glycogenolysis.

Blood, Blood Forming Organs, the Reticulo-endothelial System

Blood Composition

Blood volumes in fish are in the region of 2–4% of body-weight, compared with values of 5–8% for other vertebrates. Serum composition is very similar to that seen in mammals. Protein levels in plasma are generally lower than those seen in higher vertebrates, but their immunological and other functions are similar.

Assessment of blood parameters is difficult due to the disproportion in volume between blood and lymph. As noted earlier, lymph volume is approximately four times larger than that of blood, and lymph has a composition very similar to that of plasma. Thus relatively small changes in lymph formation can lead to large changes in blood composition, and this will be reflected mainly in haematocrit values. Blood parameters may also be affected by other factors such as age, sex, diet, species, time of year, water temperature and osmotic disruption.

Erythrocytes

Erythrocytes are similar to those found in other vertebrates, except for mammals, and are nucleated with a flattened ellipsoid shape. Non-nucleated cells are seen in some species. The cells are usually in the region of 11×9 μm in size, but this varies considerably with species. Numbers of erythrocytes in the blood can vary with species, stage of life cycle and environmental conditions, and a few fish have none. Erythrocytes usually contain haemoglobin, but amounts and type can vary.

Leucocytes

These cells can form up to 10% of the blood cell population, with lymphocytes by far the most abundant.

Neutrophils or polymorphs are inappropriately named in fish as their nucleus is not often lobulated, and the intra-cellular granules are not necessarily neutral staining. They are found at sites of inflammation, and their function is probably the same as that in mammals, but they may have little phagocytic activity. Their origin is probably the haemopoietic tissue of the kidney and, to a lesser extent, the spleen. They form a much smaller part of the blood leucocyte population in fish than in mammals, but they are present in similar actual numbers. Neutrophilia occurs as a non-specific response to a variety of stress stimuli in fish in the same way as in mammals.

Monocytes are similar to those found in mammals and, in the right circumstances, will develop into mature phagocytic cells of the reticulo-endothelial system, or the **macrophages** of inflammatory lesions. They are also phagocytic in their own right. They arise from the renal haemopoietic tissue.

Thrombocytes are responsible for blood clotting with cytoplasm very similar to that of the mammalian platelet.

Eosinophils are almost certainly different to the eosinophilic granular cells found in other tissues. They are implicated in inflammatory reactions and may be phagocytic.

Basophils and mast cells probably occur in fish, but their role is unclear.

Lymphocytes are the most common white cells found in fish and their numbers are significantly higher than those in mammals. They are similar to mammalian lymphocytes in form, and are responsible for the immune response. They circulate in the blood and tend to concentrate in the organs which filter body fluids, and are activated by the presence of their specific antigens.

Gas Transport

When blood temperatures are quite low, relatively high levels of oxygen can be carried in the plasma in simple solution. However, most teleost erythrocytes contain haemoglobin which accounts for, in the region of, 99% of oxygen transport.

More than one type of haemoglobin occurs in fish, often determined by habitat. For example, fish that can live in water with low oxygen levels, such as the eel, tend to have haemoglobins with a higher oxygen affinity than those which normally live in water with high levels of oxygen, such as the mackerel. Also different types of haemoglobin can be found within the same individual, and some species have different haemoglobins at different stages of their life cycle.

Changes in the dissociation characteristics of the blood haemoglobin occur in certain circumstances. An increase in pCO_2 or reduction in pH results in a reduction in the affinity of haemoglobin for oxygen (the Bohr effect). This produces a shift in the dissociation characteristics of the haemoglobin which facilitates the unloading of oxygen in the tissues where pCO_2 levels are high and pH levels tend to be low. This is of particular use to fish adapted to conditions of high oxygen and low carbon dioxide.

Another system, unique to teleosts, occurs in some species. This mechanism (the Root effect) involves a reduction in the total oxygen carrying capacity of the haemoglobin in conditions of low pH. The consequence is a speeding up of the unloading of oxygen in the tissues where the pH tends to be low.

A result of these effects is that, in the gill, at a pH of approximately 7.4, the rate of oxygenation tends to be about four times faster than the rate of deoxygenation, whereas in actively metabolising tissue with a typically much lower pH, the rate of deoxygenation is 400 times faster than that of oxygenation. These effects are particularly important in tissues such as the gas gland of the swim-bladder and the choroid rete of the eye where high levels of oxygen are required.

There can be a major drawback with these systems. In conditions of high environmental carbon dioxide, oxygen uptake can be impaired even when environmental oxygen levels remain good.

Carbon dioxide is carried by the blood mainly in the form of bicarbonate, with little carried in direct combination with haemoglobin. For this reason erythrocytes contain a high level of carbonic anhydrase, which aids the conversion of carbon dioxide to bicarbonate. Deoxygenated blood has a significantly higher carrying capacity of carbon dioxide than oxygenated blood, but this capacity is reduced considerably with increases in temperature. At low temperatures the slope of the carbon dioxide dissociation curve is also greater.

Haemopoietic Tissue

Fish have no lymph nodes and haemopoietic tissue is not found in the medullary cavity of bones as in the case of mammals. Haemopoiesis in fish occurs mainly in the spleen and kidney, but may also occur to a degree in the peri-portal area of the liver and the intestinal submucosa. The thymus, a completely lymphoid organ, is also involved.

Spleen

The spleen is usually a single organ but may consist of several parts. It is located close to the stomach and is dark red in colour. There are three major constituent parts: ellipsoids, pulp and melanomacrophage centres (MMCs). In teleosts it is the organ most like a lymph node, and acts as an important filter in the circulatory system.

The splenic capsule is thin and fibrous with no muscle fibres. Unlike the mammalian spleen, there are no extensions of this capsule into the body of the spleen. In some species, such as the cod, the pancreas is found as a subcapsular layer.

Within the spleen the splenic arterioles divide until they produce thick-walled capillaries within the ellipsoids. On leaving the ellipsoids the capillaries open into the pulp spaces. Each ellipsoid consists of a central splenic capillary lined by an endothelium, outside which is a sheath of reticular cells supported by reticulin fibres. Finally these are surrounded by sinusoidal blood spaces, lined with endothelium, containing erythrocytes and phagocytic cells. The ellipsoid system is capable of removing large quantities of particulate matter from the blood as it passes through. Once replete, macrophages responsible for this trapping migrate to melanomacrophage centres (MMCs).

The pulp is quite diffuse and consists of a network of phagocytic tissue, in the form of sinusoids, which contains haemopoietic tissue and large numbers of erythrocytes. The haemopoietic tissue tends to be predominantly lymphopoietic. MMCs, which are found here (usually close to the blood vessels), are discrete groups of cells contained within a capsule, and these structures are also found in the kidney, liver and occasionally other sites. In lower teleosts, such as salmonids, the cells simply form loose aggregates within the tissues and are not contained within a capsule. These structures serve as storage sites for the end products of cell breakdown, antigens and other particulate matter, and replete macrophages tend to move towards and be absorbed by them. The colour of the cells can vary from pinkish to black, depending on the predominant pigment present. The degree of melanisation tends to increase with age so that cells tend to be darker in older or sick fish. The melanin or related pigments may well be part of a defensive mechanism due to their ability to produce hydrogen peroxide. Particulate matter trapped anywhere in the body, which may include bacteria, is usually transferred eventually to the splenic MMCs, probably via the macrophages.

Kidney

Haemopoietic tissue is present throughout the kidney; it surrounds the nephrons in the posterior kidney, and is almost exclusive in the head kidney. Blast cells are held in a network of reticulo-endothelial tissue in the form of a system of sinuses, similar to that seen in the spleen. Blood from the renal portal system passes through these sinuses; new erythrocytes are released into them and old ones are removed. MMCs occur here in many species. Endocrine tissue, in the form of inter-renal tissue, chromaffin cells and Corpuscles of Stannius, is also present within the haemopoietic tissue (see later).

Thymus

This is a paired organ found subcutaneously on the dorsal part of the branchial cavity. It occurs in fry in most species, but in others at a later stage: for example, it appears in plaice at metamorphosis. It is primary lymphoid tissue which, in section, appears as a collection of small lymphocytes with a fibrous capsule and fine connective tissue stroma. Its main role seems to be the production of lymphocytes for export to other tissues. Macrophages are very numerous in some fish and in these cases they may be related to the production of immunity. Structures which may correspond to the Hassl's corpuscles of mammals also occur.

Reticulo-endothelial System

The reticulo-endothelial system consists of highly phagocytic cells, dispersed throughout the body. They are responsible for the removal of effete erythrocytes and particulate matter from the circulation. The system is made up predominantly of the cells found in the sinusoids and peri-tubular capillaries of the kidneys, the sheaths of the splenic ellipsoids, the lining of the atrium and, to a lesser extent, the ventricle, and in the peritoneal cavity as free cells. The liver is not involved in this system: functional Kupffer cells, as found in mammals, are absent. Other cells with more limited phagocytic activity are also found throughout the body.

It is important to remember the atrium in this system because of its vulnerability. When bacteria or toxic materials are phagocytosed from the circulation, concentration of such material in the lining of the atrium can result in damage to the atrium with severe consequences.

The fixed macrophages of this system are probably derived from circulating monocytes and their precursors, but this is not certain. Macrophages from the reticulo-endothelial system move towards the MMCs once replete, but may form aggregations within or around chronic inflammatory lesions.

Nervous System

The nervous system of fish has the same basic layout as that of other vertebrates, with central, peripheral and autonomic systems. The autonomic system is involved in the control of peristalsis and other smooth muscle functions, heart rate, chromatophore control etc.

Neurons resemble those of other species except that some, such as the Mauthnerian groups, are very large compared with those of mammals. Supporting neuroglial cells, astrocytes, oligodendrocytes and, possibly, microglia are also present.

The central nervous system is divided into grey and white matter. There is evidence to suggest that mature cells within the brain retain their ability to differentiate, and this may indicate that damaged brain tissue can be repaired. The brain and spinal cord are protected by a single primitive meningeal layer containing cerebrospinal fluid. This fluid is produced by brain plexuses, usually found in different sites to those of the mammal due to developmental differences. Roots of the spinal nerves are usually overlaid by clusters of eosinophilic granular cells.

Brain

The fish brain is similar in its basic layout to that of higher vertebrates, but many differences occur. The cerebral hemispheres tend to be small compared with mammals, and the most obvious portion of the brain to be seen on removal of the cranium is the mesencephalon, the optic lobes. The cerebellum is not very prominent, but varies with species.

Spinal Cord

The spinal cord originates through the foramen magnum and extends the length of the body within the vertebral canal. In higher teleosts it ends in an endocrine organ, the urophysis.

Grey and white matter is well demarcated and becomes more complex with evolutionary development. The grey matter forms an inverted Y in cross section. The resulting single dorsal horn and two ventrolateral horns do not have a demarcation of motor and sensory nerves as in higher vertebrates, all tracts containing a mixture of nerve types. In some species, including salmonids, the number of neurons increases with body growth.

A major feature of the cord is the group of very large Mauthner axons which run from the medulla just beneath the arms of the Y and ventral to the central canal. Excitation of these nerves results in a powerful tail flip, the so-called Mauthner-initiated startle response.

Peripheral Nerves

Ten cranial nerves are present in fish. These supply the motor, voluntary and involuntary, and sensory functions of the head. A parasympathetic innervation to the main visceral organs is also supplied by the vagus nerve.

Sensory Organs

Eye

The fish eye is very similar in basic layout to the eyes of other vertebrates, but there are significant differences. Eyes generally appear to have adapted according to evolutionary niche rather than according to phylogenetic group. The normal eye is a slightly flattened sphere resulting in a relatively flat cornea. This shape is possible in the aqueous environment because the refractive index of the cornea is very similar to that of water. The result of this is that the cornea is irrelevant as an optical surface, and even contour irregularities which would cause incapacity in terrestrial animals have little or no effect on vision.

The globe, which varies in size according to habitat, is maintained in position by three pairs of oculomotor muscles which attach to the sclera and are innervated by the third cranial nerve. However, the eye does not move to follow objects, as with mammals; instead, the whole body is moved.

The sclera is similar to that of other vertebrates with a laminated fibrous layer reinforced with hyaline cartilage. Scleral ossicles may occur in some species.

Eyelids and lacrimal apparatus are not present, there being no need for these organs in the aquatic environment. The cornea is similar to that of mammals with a surface non-keratinised stratified squamous epithelium resting on a basement or Bowman's membrane. Beneath this is a substantia propria and an internal basement membrane and endothelial layer (Descemet's membrane and endothelium).

The lens is usually completely spherical and bulges through the iris to provide a very wide angle of view. The short focal length also means the fish has a large depth of focus. The lens has little elasticity and consequently accommodation cannot be achieved by changes in lens shape but rather by movement of the lens along the visual axis. In fact, due to the relative positions of the retractor lentis muscle and the lens suspensory ligament, any such movement tends to be hinge-like, so that not only is the lens–retina distance altered, but also the edge of the lens is moved into the visual axis. This latter movement can have a significant effect on focusing because the lens is not optically uniform throughout its body. Despite this, histologically it appears very similar to the mammalian lens.

The body of the lens is a matrix of interlocking fibres surrounded by a simple cuboidal epithelium with an external basement membrane. This epithelium enters the cortex at the back of the lens to form the nuclear bow, the source of the lens fibres.

The iris is virtually fixed with poorly developed sphincter muscles, probably because in most fish there is little need for rapid adaptation to changes in light levels. Where this is necessary, modifications occur. Cells containing melanin are present within the iris and, in some species, guanophores which produce a silvery appearance.

The ciliary body is rudimentary, there being no need for development as the lens shape is not altered for accommodation. Aqueous and vitreous humours are very similar to those in higher animals.

Choroid vessels supply blood to the retina and are present as a vascular network between the sclera and the retina as in other vertebrates. Within the choroid is a choroid gland, a network of capillaries which actively secrete oxygen into the eye, thus ensuring a high level of oxygen for the retina. Oxygen is secreted in the same way as in the gas gland of the swim bladder. The choroid gland may also have other functions, such as blood monitoring, but this is not known.

Some form of tapetum is usually present in most fish, but it is best developed in species which live in conditions of low light intensity. It operates by reflecting light back to the retina, thus doubly stimulating the retinal cells.

The retina is similar to that of other vertebrates. Retinal nourishment is aided by the falciform process, a vascular ridge similar to the pectin of birds, which protrudes through the floor of the globe. Optic discs vary in number, shape and location.

The reception of light varies with habitat, but generally most shallow-water fish have colour vision and deep-water fish do not. The latter also tend to have large eyes and well developed tapeta in order to maximise the use of available light. Visual pigments tend to be most sensitive to the wavelengths best transmitted by the water in which the fish live.

Fish with efficient tapeta may suffer damage when exposed to bright light, and in the absence of a mobile iris, other methods have arisen to give protection. The first is occlusible tapeta: melanin granules, contained within the reflective tapetal cells are concentrated in the centre of the cell in normal conditions, but in strong light they can be dispersed within the cell in order to obstruct the reflective granules. The second method is photo-receptor motility: in conditions of bright light, photoreceptor cells (usually rods) are withdrawn into deep recesses within the retina, thus reducing exposure to the light.

Labyrinth or inner ear

This organ is involved with maintenance of equilibrium and 'hearing'. It consists of semi-circular canals (with a similar layout to that in mammals) and otolith organs, both filled with endolymph. The semicircular canals are used to detect angular acceleration, the otolith organs the force of gravity and low frequency sound waves. Frequencies of up to about 400 Hz can be detected by this organ alone, but if operating in conjunction

with the swim-bladder this figure can be increased to as high as 7000 Hz.

The otolith organ consists of three interconnecting chambers known as the membranous labyrinth (utriculus, sacculus and lagena), with the semicircular canals inserting into the utriculus. Otoliths, white calcified 'stones', are present in each chamber, connected to the hairs of patches of sensory cells.

Lateral line

This organ is found only in fish and the aquatic stages of amphibians. Although it has connections to the brain by the same afferent pathways as the labyrinth, it is a separate system. The main components are the paired lateral line canals, but in some species these canals branch and form head canals. Each canal is a groove along the body of the fish from operculum to caudal fin, one on each side. It has a bony support, and is covered by epidermis containing pores along its length.

Mechanoreceptors are present within the canal, alternating with the position of pores. They consist of neuromasts — patches of receptor cells with sensory hair-like extensions attached to a gelatinous cupula. Localised disturbances caused by small currents and vibrations up to 200 Hz cause movement of the water within the lateral line and thus disturb and stimulate the neuromasts. The system is involved in location of moving objects such as predators and prey, and in the sensing of fixed objects that reflect the water movements caused by the swimming fish itself.

Olfactory organ

Olfactory organs are paired and contained within sacs, water being directed to the organs via nasal orifices. These orifices are usually on the snout, and there is considerable variation in arrangement. There may be two apertures for each organ, or just one, and this may have a piece of tissue dividing the entrance into an anterior inlet and posterior exhaust.

Swimming and breathing movements cause the passage of water through the sacs, passing en route over sensory tissue in the form of a rosette of folded olfactory epithelium. This epithelium consists of focal groups of receptor cells surrounded by mucoid and ciliated columnar epithelium. In many species the loose sub-epidermal tissue of the nasal mucosa contains many eosinophilic granular cells.

Organic substances of interest to fish are detected through the olfactory epithelium, although some are detected by taste buds. The sense of smell is quite important when smell gradients are followed, such as in the case of salmon returning to their home rivers to spawn.

Cutaneous senses

Taste buds are found in the epidermis of the mouth, lips, barbels, pharynx and gill arches. Some species have additional taste buds on other parts of the body such as head and fins. In some species they may be spread over the entire body surface. The buds consist of receptor, supporting and basal cells, arranged like the segments of an orange and have short hair-like processes extending into the water. In especially sensitive areas, free nerve endings from supplying nerves may be present in the surrounding skin.

Other free nerve endings also occur in the teleost epidermis and these are probably related to detection of temperature, pressure and, possibly, touch.

Endocrine System

The basic layout of the endocrine system in fish is similar to that of higher vertebrates, but some peculiarities do occur, including the presence of some organs with no parallel in mammals whose functions are little understood. Nervous and endocrine systems are often highly interdependent and often act together.

Pituitary

This complex neuro-epithelial structure is very similar within the major classes of fish. As with other vertebrates, its components are the neurohypophysis, which originates as a down-growth of the brain, and the adenohypophysis, an up-growth of the roof of the mouth. In the adult this composite organ is enclosed by the diencephalon above, and a bony cavity below.

The neurohypophysis is made up of glial cells called pituicytes, and neurosecretory axons which have their cell bodies in the hypothalamus. Pituicytes are probably phagocytic. Various different hormones have been found in this organ in different fish, but little is known of their function.

The adenohypophysis is made up of a pars distalis and a pars intermedia. Stellate cells, found in the pars distalis, probably also have a phagocytic function. The hormones produced either have a stimulating effect on other endocrine organs, for example thyroid (TSH), gonads (gonadotrophins) and adrenal (ACTH), or influence physiological processes, for example melanophore behaviour (melanocyte stimulating hormone, MSH), osmoregulation, metabolism and growth. Pituitary extracts have been used to stimulate spawning behaviour in cultivated species. Prolactin is thought to have a role in freshwater osmoregulation, probably by affecting gill permeability, and may have an effect on metabolic rate. Growth hormone helps to control metabolic rate as well as being involved in growth.

A simple hypothalamo-hypophyseal portal system is found in some fish, but hypothalamic control of the pituitary is more likely to be by direct innervation or deposition of releasing factors in close proximity to the adenohypophysis by axons of the hypothalamic neurones.

Pineal Gland

This light-sensitive gland is found beneath a thinning of the cranial cartilage in the mid-line between the eyes. It is covered by a well vascularised capsule, and secretes melatonin as in mammals. Its function appears to be associated with photoperiod and the control of seasonal cycles such as breeding.

Thyroid

This organ is diffuse in most fish, unlike in mammals. Follicles of the gland are found mainly around the ventral aorta, but may also occur at other sites such as the eye, kidney, spleen, etc. In most teleosts they are encapsulated. The basic structure is similar to that of mammals. The follicles are round to oval in shape, with cuboidal epithelial cells surrounding a colloid-filled lumen.

The epithelial cells have microvilli and occasional cilia projecting into the lumen.

Thyroxine (T4) is the major product of this gland. Conversion to T3 occurs in the liver and kidney. Control of T3 and T4 is via the pituitary hormone TSH. Thyroid hormones have a stimulatory effect on many metabolic processes. They have a role in growth regulation, especially of muscle, bone and cartilage, and are involved with pigment deposition, such as during the smoltification of salmon, and ovarian function. They may also have an effect on osmoregulation during seawater adaptation of euryhaline species.

Interrenals

The interrenal cells are found along the major blood vessels in the head kidney, and are the equivalent of the mammalian adrenal cortex. They are cuboidal in shape and pale staining with an eosinophilic granular cytoplasm. Corticosteroids are produced, the most important in teleosts being cortisol: their role is little understood, but they appear to have similar functions to those in the higher vertebrates. They are involved with intermediate metabolism, and may have an influence on seawater adaptation in euryhaline species. Release of cortisol appears to increase in response to certain types of stress, and also seems to lower resistance to disease. Synthesis and release of the corticosteroids are controlled by pituitary ACTH, but MSH also has an effect.

Chromaffin Cells

These cells are the equivalent of the adrenal medulla of mammals. They are found with the interrenal cells in the head kidney, or associated with sympathetic ganglia, or as clumps of tissue between the kidney and spine. They tend to be paler than the interrenal cells, with a larger nucleus, and they produce epinephrine and norepinephrine. These hormones are released as the primary stress response: they increase cardiac output and produce systemic vasoconstriction and gill lamellar vasodilation.

Renin–angiotensin System

This system is found in almost all vertebrates. The enzyme renin is produced in juxtaglomerular cells and released into the blood, where it is converted into angiotensin. In some species renin is released in response to a fall in renal perfusion pressure, and so it is likely that angiotensin is involved with blood pressure control, as in mammals.

Corpuscles of Stannius

These organs are usually paired discrete encapsulated structures found within the kidney parenchyma. Their usual position is midway along the length of the kidney. In some species they are deeply embedded in the kidney tissue; in others, such as the salmonids, they are superficial and appear as white nodules. They are formed of lobules separated by thin connective tissue septa which carry blood vessels and nerves. The large, clear endocrine cells appear to secrete into the centre of the organ. They are supplied by the renal portal system, the blood then passing into the kidney.

Their function is not clear, but hormones involved with calcium homeostasis are produced. These hormones block branchial uptake of calcium. Substances similar to renin are also produced in some species.

Ultimobranchial Gland

Originating from the fifth gill arch of the embryo, this gland is found just ventral to the oesophagus in the septum separating the heart from the abdominal cavity. It is similar in action to the parathyroid of mammals and may be single or, in most species, paired. In structure it consists of small follicles of columnar cells, supplied with blood by a capillary network which drains directly into the sinus venosus.

Calcitonin, which has the effect of reducing blood calcium levels, is produced. Along with prolactin and the product of the Corpuscles of Stannius, this hormone is probably involved with calcium homeostasis.

Urophysis

This is a neurosecretory organ found at the caudal end of the spinal cord. It is well vascularised, and blood drains into the renal portal system. The neurosecretory cell bodies lie within the spinal cord, and their non-myelinated axons end on the capillary walls of the vascular system — an arrangement similar to that seen in the hypothalamus of mammals.

Two urotensins have been identified and both are vasoactive, causing an increase in blood pressure. The main activity of this organ, however, may be involved with water and ionic balance.

Pancreas

The endocrine pancreas exists as the Islets of Langerhans which, in the lower teleosts such as salmonids and eels, are found scattered throughout the exocrine pancreas. In the higher teleosts some of the islets tend to be very large and are known as Brockman bodies.

The three cell types (α, β and δ) are contained within a fine fibrous capsule. Hormones secreted are glucagon, insulin and somatostatin respectively. The roles of these hormones are poorly understood, but they are probably similar to those in higher vertebrates. Insulin and glucagon are probably confined to a role concerning carbohydrate metabolism, although their action seems to be somewhat different to that in mammals. Somatostatin probably has a regulatory effect on the secretion of insulin and glucagon, as well as other, uncertain, distant effects.

Gastro-intestinal Hormones

Little is known about these hormones in fish. Gastrin is produced in the stomach and it stimulates the release of acid in the mucosa. Secretin, responsible for pancreatic secretion release in mammals, is probably also present.

Pseudobranch and Choroid Body

The pseudobranch is derived from the first gill arch in the embryo, but is not present in all species. Pseudobranch cells are similar in appearance to the chloride cells of the gills, and are located on a basal lamina close to an extensive network of capillaries. The capillaries are arranged in a parallel fashion supported by cartilage rods, and there is a direct vascular connection with the choroid of the eye. The choroid has a similar structure to the pseudobranch except that the capillaries alternate with rows of fibroblast-like cells.

This system is thought to be concerned with the supply of highly oxygenated blood to the eye, as well as having sensory and endocrine functions, but its role is not fully understood. The sensory involvement is suggested by the large afferent innervation by the glossopharyngeal nerve.

Gonads

Oestrogens and androgens are produced by the gonads under the control of gonadotrophins secreted by the pituitary. These hormones are produced by the interstitial tissue of the testes, and the follicular tissue of the ovary. They can have an effect on a wide range of tissues, and cause changes related to sexual development such as colour changes, development of kypes in salmonids, and swelling of the uro-genital area. They also have an effect on carbohydrate, protein and lipid metabolism. Androgens tend to increase protein retention, oestrogens tend to increase lipid reserves.

Reproductive System

There is a tremendous variety of breeding patterns in teleosts. Most species have male and female sexes although hermaphroditism, bisexuality, parthenogenesis (development from an unfertilised ovum) and gynogenesis (development from an ovum stimulated to divide by sperm which does not contribute genetic material) have all been known to occur. Sex reversal in adults is not uncommon.

The number of eggs produced by a particular species is usually determined by the amount of parental care given to them. A pelagic species, such as the cod, produces many millions of eggs each season and releases them into open water. Species which build complex nests and protect developing eggs and young, such as the stickleback, usually only produce a few tens of eggs. Some fish even brood their young within their mouths.

Fertilisation methods are variable, again usually related to the degree of care given. Eggs and sperm may simply be released into the water. In some species, copulation may take place resulting in the release of fertilised eggs or, alternatively, internal incubation followed by the release of live young (such as with the guppy).

Testes

These paired organs are suspended by a mesentery from the dorsal abdominal wall adjacent to the swim-bladder. They vary greatly in size according to the age of the fish and the season. From small strands of tissue in the juvenile, they can become very large and account for up to 12% of total body weight.

The testis lies within a thin tunica albuginea and is made up of a series of seminiferous tubules or blind-ending sacs, lined with spermatogenic epithelium either along their entire length, as in salmonids and cyprinids, or only at their distal ends. The caudal section of the testis in species such as the ictalurids and some cyprinids is lined with non-germinal secretory epithelial cells, which may be involved in sperm storage or nutrition, or may contribute to the ejaculate.

The spermatogenic epithelium gives rise to spermatocytes which eventually undergo meiotic division to produce spermatozoa. The spermatozoa are supplied with nourishment by the Sertoli cells until their release. In most species spermatozoa are carried from each testis by a vas deferens. The two ducts fuse caudally and the spermatozoa are conducted to the environment via a genital opening at the urinary papilla. These ducts are absent in some relatively primitive species, such as the salmonids, and the spermatozoa are released into the body cavity before leaving it via the genital opening.

The interstitial fibrous tissue contains hormone secreting cells. There is no lymphatic system of the type seen in mammals.

Ovaries

Ovarian structures vary from relatively simple to complex organs. Typically they are paired and suspended from the dorsal abdominal wall by a mesentery. Enclosed by a tunica albuginea containing fibrous tissue and smooth muscle, they usually appear as a small cluster of orange–white spheres in the immature fish. When mature they can account for as much as 70% of body weight.

In advanced species a short oviduct conducts eggs to the outside by means of a genital opening. Salmonids and other more primitive species do not have a complete oviduct, and the eggs are released into a fold of the mesentery which eventually releases them into the peritoneal cavity. They then gain access to the outside via the genital opening.

The parenchyma of the ovary consists of a well vascularised connective tissue stroma containing germinal and follicular epithelium. Hormones are produced by the follicular tissue. The primary ovarian cells line hollow cavities or potential cavities with complexly folded walls. Oogonia are shed into this cavity and gain a layer of small epithelial cells in the process. These are granulosa cells, which are responsible for yolk formation in the developing egg. This structure is the ovarian follicle, and as it grows a gradually thickening hyaline zone forms between the oocyte and the epithelial cells: this is the zona pellucida.

If an oocyte degenerates before ovulation, first the granulosa cells invade, and then macrophages. Eggs in all stages of development and degeneration may be seen on examination of the ovary.

Crustaceans — Anatomy and Physiology

Crustaceans belong to the largest of all the animal phyla, the Arthropoda. Members of this group are characterised by their hard outer body covering, or exoskeleton. The Crustacea are a large diverse group of invertebrates, but the most important commercial species all belong to the group Decapoda, which is further divided into two important sub-groups (in aquaculture terms): the Natantia (swimmers) such as the penaeid and caridean prawns, and the Reptantia (crawlers) such as lobsters, crayfish and crabs. For the purposes of this book only the former sub-group will be considered, although most features discussed are common to both. More detail of the biology of marine prawns is given in Chapter 16.

Body Structure

The exoskeleton is segmental (Fig. 1.9). The head and thoracic segments are fused together dorsally and laterally to form the carapace. The sides of the carapace hang down laterally and

FIG. 1.9 Normal anatomy of
a penaeid crustacean.

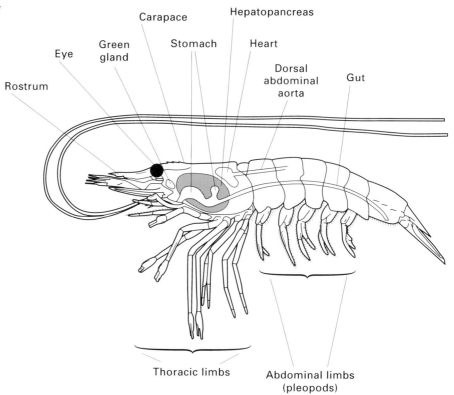

enclose the gills within well defined lateral branchial chambers. Bodies are often flattened from side to side.

In the Natantia, the first three pairs of thoracic limbs are modified for feeding and are called maxillipeds. Five other pairs of thoracic limbs are used for walking. Abdominal limbs (pleopods) are used for swimming. Limbs are made up of two basic sections forming the protopodite, and from this arises an inner and an outer branch, only one of which is obvious, but both of which may be made up of one or many sections. Different parts of the limb may carry highly developed processes, or appendages, developed for specific purposes. Damaged limbs can be shed in some species (the process of autotomy); regrowth of the limb then takes place.

Integument

The crustacean integument or cuticle is strong and flexible, and acts as a barrier to bacteria and osmotic effects. It is made up of the epicuticle and procuticle. The epicuticle consists of protein, lipid and calcium salts. Beneath this is the procuticle, characterised by the presence of chitin and divided into pre-ecdysial and post-ecdysial layers. The latter is further sub-divided into the principal layer and the membranous layer. The membranous layer overlays an epidermis, beneath which are tegmental glands which secrete part of the cuticle. The procuticle consists mainly of chitin, protein and calcium salts. Chitin is a polymer of 80–90% N-acetyl-glucosamine and 10–20% glucosamine. It is a very stable compound, insoluble in most solvents, and gives strength and flexibility to the cuticle.

Crustaceans are able to harden their cuticle by calcification. Calcium salts (calcium carbonate and calcium phosphate) are deposited within the organic matrix of the cuticle, filling the spaces which would otherwise be filled with protein. Calcium is absent from the membranous layer and the parts of the cuticle covering joints.

Crustacea, having an exoskeleton, need to moult in order to grow. The moult, or ecdysis, would involve considerable loss of body resources if the entire normal cuticle was shed, and certain processes occur to minimise this loss. In the pre-moult stage leading up to ecdysis, the inner layers of the old cuticle are digested and resorbed. The calcium from this process is stored in the digestive gland, the blood, or various other storage depots. During this process new cuticle is secreted beneath the old one. At ecdysis the remains of the old cuticle are shed; the new cuticle is then expanded by means of a large intake of water into the tissues, and finally the cuticle hardens. The new cuticle is then calcified with calcium obtained mostly from the diet or absorption from the water; the body stores supply only a small proportion. For this reason the availability of calcium in the water is particularly important. The water used to swell the new cuticle is then slowly replaced with new tissue.

Respiratory System

Crustacean gills are a vascularised sheet or sac-like outgrowth from the proximal section of the thoracic limbs. The surface of the gill consists of a very thin layer of chitin lined with epithelium. Water is drawn through the branchial chamber and thus over the gills by the beating of a specialised paddle-shaped projection of the second maxilla.

Circulatory System

Crustacea have a well developed heart and arterial system, the arteries containing valves. The degree of development of the arterial system depends on species. There are no veins, the blood returning to the heart by means of a series of sinuses.

Blood

Blood, or haemolymph, contains haemocytes of three types: small hyaline cells, large granulocytes, and semi-granulocytes between the two. These appear to be different stages of the same cell, with hyaline cells progressing to granulocytes with age. The hyaline cells tend to be entirely phagocytic, whereas the granular cells are more involved with wound repair and encapsulation. The respiratory

pigment, haemocyanin, is carried free in the plasma. This pigment is copper based and the blood appears blue when oxygenated, colourless when reduced. The number of haemocytes varies with age, nutritional status and proximity to ecdysis.

Agglutinins and lysins are carried by the blood as part of the humoral defence system; there are no antibodies, but there are antisomes.

Wound Repair

When the cuticle is breached, haemocytes migrate to the wound and granulocytes break down. Chemicals released in this process convert fibrin-ogen to fibrin, thus forming a clot which is then melanised. The melanin is produced by the action of phenyl oxidase on tyrosine, both chemicals being carried to the wound by the blood. The melanin is not part of the walling off process, but melanin, and some of the intermediate chemicals involved in its formation, is bactericidal and it is, therefore, part of the defence mechanisms.

Epidermal cells migrate beneath the melanised clot and secrete new cuticle. Eventually the melanised material is sloughed off. A similar process (encapsulation) occurs when the body is invaded by bacteria or other foreign bodies. The invading material is walled off by melanised material in an attempt to isolate it and prevent it doing harm.

Feeding and Digestion

Food is held by the maxillipeds and torn into small pieces before being pushed into the mouth by the mouth-parts.

The gut is divided into the fore-gut, mid-gut, and hind-gut. The first and last have a chitinous lining, the mid-gut does not. The fore-gut consists of a short oesophagus followed by a cardiac stomach and then a pyloric stomach. These two stomachs are dilations of the fore-gut divided by a constriction, and constitute the gastric mill.

Dorsal and lateral teeth are present on the walls of the gastric mill. The function of this organ is to grind up the food and mix it with enzymes, which are produced by the digestive gland (hepatopancreas) and secreted into the fore-gut. The degree of development of the gastric mill depends on how much the food is chewed before being swallowed, less grinding being necessary for well chewed food.

The digestive gland produces a protease, a lipase, and several carbohydrate splitting enzymes, all carried in a slightly acid medium. It also acts as a storage organ for glycogen, lipid and calcium, and is the primary organ of food absorption. Once the food particles are small enough, the muscular action of the gastric mill forces it into the digestive gland where absorption takes place. A little absorption also takes place in the mid-gut.

Excretory System

Urine is produced by the antennal or maxillary gland (green gland), and is excreted at the base of either the antennae or the maxillae. Ammonia is the principal nitrogenous waste product, but this can also be excreted through the gills.

Most crustaceans produce urine that is isotonic with the blood and therefore the green glands play little part in osmoregulation. Their role in ionic regulation is usually confined to conservation of potassium and calcium, and elimination of excess magnesium and sulphate. For most crustacea, the gills are the primary organs of osmoregulation.

Endocrinology and Reproduction

Hormones are produced by two endocrine glands and three neurohaemal glands which are adapted nerve cells. The most important gland for aquaculture purposes is the sinus gland found in the eye stalk. It produces, amongst other things, a moult-inhibiting hormone which also inhibits vitellogenesis. Removal of the gland (by removal of the eye stalk) can induce not only premature moulting but also reproduction. This process, known as eye stalk ablation, can be used to induce spawning.

The external genitalia of the penaeids are found at the thoraco-lumbar junction. Fertilisation takes place by the male placing sacs of sperm into the genital pouch of the female. Some types, such as the penaeids, shed many small fertilised eggs directly into the sea; others, such as the carideans, carry fewer large fertilised eggs on abdominal limbs.

Different species tend to hatch at different stages of development, but all crustacea pass through a series of developmental stages either inside or outside the egg: nauplius, zoea, post-larva, juvenile, adult.

Nervous System

The crustacean nervous system is well developed. The 'brain', or supraorbital ganglia, consists of three distinct adjacent regions. The ventral nerve and associated segmental ganglia arise from this 'brain'. Giant nerve fibres passing down the body are responsible for the tail flick response, an escape strategy. Sensory organs are well developed and include eyes, proprioceptors, tactile receptors and chemoreceptors.

2

Basic Husbandry on Fish Farms

ANDREW GRANT

The objectives of good husbandry and stockmanship are to produce a product of high quality, in a humane manner and with as little loss to disease as possible (and consequently with minimum need for medicines). These objectives must also be consistent with commercial return on capital.

The traditional principles of livestock husbandry cover, in general terms, handling of the stock with minimum stress, management of accommodation and environment, feeding, prevention of disease and harvesting. Record-keeping and the appropriate use of equipment are essential aids to good stockmanship.

The principles apply to fish farming as well as land-based agriculture, though the detail may differ. Farming in an aquatic environment presents unique challenges to the farmer and to the veterinarian but it will quickly be realised that most health problems have their origin in faulty management and the intensive nature of most commercial operations.

This chapter cannot describe good husbandry practices in great detail (these are covered for individual species in the specialist chapters of the second section of this book) but it will look first at the broad principles as they relate to the farming of salmonids at different stages in the life-cycle and will then outline specific practices for other species of fish.

Salmonids

General Management

Central to good husbandry in intensive livestock systems are the principles of rotational farming and the separation of the generations. In terms of fish farming, this means the ability to stock sites in such a way that the risk of disease transmission between generations is minimised, and also to allow for the fallowing of sites on a regular basis, preferably at the end of each production cycle. Both practices may be difficult to achieve when resources are limited and the grow-out period is long but there are great benefits to be gained by adopting them, especially where infectious disease is enzootic.

Water

Water quality, which is dealt with fully in Chapter 4, is crucial to fish health. Salmonids in particular are intolerant of low oxygen saturation and of waste accumulation, and good water exchange is a priority for these species.

The potential hazards of any water source should always be well understood and in this respect it is worth emphasising the importance of monitoring the hatchery water supply, which may be drawn from surface or ground water. Surface waters from rivers which experience large runs of wild salmonids are one of the most common sources of furunculosis (a serious bacterial infection caused by *Aeromonas salmonicida*) for salmonid hatcheries. Ground supplies are free from this risk but may be a more expensive source if water has to be pumped. Pumps may break down and back-up systems must always be available.

A problem with water under pressure is that it is frequently supersaturated with dissolved gases (oxygen, nitrogen, carbon dioxide) and this can lead to gas-bubble disease in hatched fish. On the other hand, oxygen saturation decreases as temperatures rise, to such an extent that at peak summer temperatures oxygen can become a limiting factor and may have to be supplemented.

Water-flow for fish at all stages of their life-cycle should be sufficient to meet oxygen requirements as well as to remove metabolic waste (e.g. faeces and surplus feed). However, fish may become exhausted trying to maintain their position in the water against a fast current.

Long-term health problems due to poor water quality are rare in areas of rapid flushing but sedimentary conditions on heavily used sea sites in areas of poor water exchange can deteriorate to the point where gas production poses a threat to the fish. In sea cages, net fouling must not be allowed to impede the passage of water. Blooms of harmful plankton are a regular problem on some fish farms. Simple monitoring methods can provide useful warnings of potential problems and in some cases prevent considerable stock losses. Environmental legislation may place a statutory obligation on the farmer to assess the impact of the farm's activities.

Light

In the hatchery, developing eggs and young fry should be maintained in dim light, or in darkness since exposure to strong light causes mortalities. Hatching troughs are usually covered and all rearing tanks must be shielded from strong sunlight (Fig. 2.1).

Photoperiod manipulation is one of the factors used to influence the process of smoltification. It should be noted that smolts reared in subdued lighting may burrow into the base of nets when transferred to sea cages, seriously damaging their heads and with significant loss of scales, which compromises osmotic regulation.

Tank hygiene

Tanks are cleaned daily to prevent the accumulation of organic material. Dead or dying fish must be removed at the same time, and a number of fish should be examined for parasites as part of this daily routine. Cleaning is manual but is assisted by water flushing. Some tanks are designed to generate self-cleaning flows; many tanks are circular for this reason, with a central drain. Care must be taken during cleaning to minimise disturbance; prolonged high water-flow rates stress the fish.

Stocking density

Stocking density is one of the imponderables of intensive farming; there is no 'correct' stocking density. The commercial need is to extract an acceptable return from the assets, which is fairly easy to calculate, while the biological need is to provide optimal conditions for the stock. It may be difficult to reconcile the two needs.

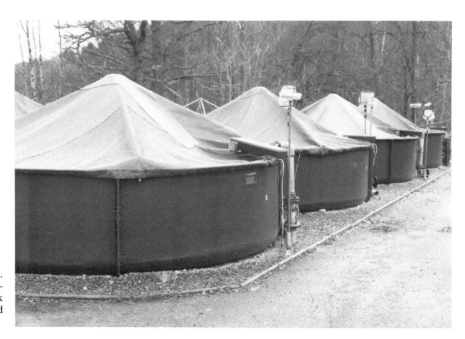

FIG. 2.1 Fibreglass fry tanks. Covers exclude strong sunlight. Note that each tank has its own hand net and cleaning equipment.

Physical conditions at the site will also be a factor.

From the point of view of husbandry and fish health, the following should be considered in relation to stocking density:

- Water quality and exchange rates.
- Current strength.
- Spread of infectious diseases.
- Total biomass on the farm.
- Peer competition at feeding.
- Available surface area in relation to the number of fish.
- Procedures which will involve crowding, e.g. treatments for sea lice, grading, etc.

Reducing stocking density will improve individual fish performance (all other things being equal) but, beyond a certain point, total yield will fall below commercially acceptable levels.

Grading

Grading is one of the most common procedures on a fish farm and is also one of the major stresses on fish. The reasons for grading are:

- To adjust peer groups into narrow weight ranges.
- To reject deformed or undersized fish.
- To reject fish which are unlikely to grow well.
- To thin stocks as biomass increases.
- To set up populations for transfer to on-growing facilities.
- To count fish into a new tank or cage.
- To control numbers.

Throughout the year, a population of growing fish may be graded several times, either by hand or, usually, by machine. Grading involves crowding the fish, often at high temperatures, and there can be large fish kills under these circumstances. Careful monitoring is essential and particular care must be taken when the fish are crowded for any length of time. In sea pens, for example, fish can be badly scaled by abrasion against nets and may experience periods of low oxygen, particularly if water temperatures are high. Where fish are removed from the water (perhaps for grilse grading), careful attention should be paid to the design of the equipment since damage can easily be caused by poor construction. The surfaces of all handling equipment should be smooth enough to offer minimum friction against the fish, in order to avoid abrasion and loss of scales.

Outbreaks of disease often follow grading, and should be anticipated. To minimise the need for repeated handling, the good stockman will try to incorporate several husbandry procedures (e.g. vaccination) at grading time.

Removal of mortalities

Throughout the growing period, there is an unavoidable natural wastage which may be impossible to attribute to a recognised fish pathogen. Frequent removal of mortalities is one of the most important measures in disease control in any intensive husbandry system, for the following reasons:

- Early detection of rising mortality.
- Removal of source of continuing challenge in an epizootic.
- Regular supply of fresh pathological material for disease diagnosis.
- Indication of the efficacy of disease control measures, e.g. antibacterials, vaccines.
- Reduction of self-pollution and the discharge of organic matter into the environment.
- More reliable assessment of stock numbers.

A special problem arises when fry are first introduced to floating pens: they all remain on the net floor, making the removal of dead fish difficult. As they grow and become stronger, they spend less time on the bottom and mortality removal becomes easier.

There are several ways of removing dead fish from pens. Ideally a system should make it possible to perform the procedure on a daily basis if necessary. Mechanical methods are all liable to systems failure and can be difficult to operate in poor weather. However, removal of dead fish is one of the key husbandry procedures and it merits investment in equipment and time. Typical methods are as follows:

Divers. Divers can guarantee that all the mortalities are removed, but there are doubts about the safety of frequent diving.

Raising net floors. The net floor may be raised so that dead fish can be lifted out in a hand-net. This

FIG. 2.2 Air lift system for removal of dead fish.

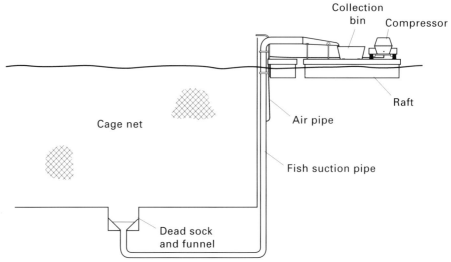

method is labour intensive and it crowds the fish. It is not always possible to reach all the fish.

Dead sock. The net floor may incorporate a central trap or 'dead sock', into which most of the dead fish should eventually roll. The floor is raised and the dead fish are removed from the sock with a hand-net. Tidal movements distort the net, so that mortalities may accumulate in the corners. Badly fouled nets can be extremely heavy, requiring mechanical lifting aids.

One variation of this method is the location of a removable keep-net within the dead sock. It can be winched to the surface by pulleys and replaced when empty.

Another adaptation is to incorporate the dead sock into an 'airlift' (Fig. 2.2). A funnel is fitted to the neck of the sock and is attached to a flexible plastic pipe, which runs along the outside of the net base and meets a rigid vertical pipe running to the surface. Compressed air is pumped to the base of the vertical pipe, displacing the water column upwards and creating suction in the funnel so that dead fish are delivered to the surface for disposal. The advantages of this system are:

- Minimum stress to the fish.
- Ease of use allowing at least daily mortality removal or more frequently in an epizootic.
- Relatively low cost.

Net management

Nets should be designed to anticipate husbandry procedures such as grading or chemical treatments. They should meet the following requirements:

- Durable, but light enough to permit handling.
- Mesh size appropriate to fish size, initially to prevent escape and thereafter to allow water exchange within the constraints of design.
- Non-abrasive net material.

As fish grow, nets are changed to a larger mesh size to maximise water exchange across the pen. Predator nets may be necessary to prevent attacks by seals, which can account for large losses. Double nets can be fitted on each pen, or curtain nets stretching to the sea bed can be deployed around a group of cages. Additional netting inevitably presents practical problems on a site but may be the only effective method of deterring seals.

Fouling of the nets can be a major problem. Fouled nets have to be removed and cleaned regularly during the summer, a procedure which inevitably crowds and stresses the fish and must be carried out with great care to avoid damaged fish and mortalities. The nets are cleaned by exposure to ultra-violet light and by drying. Fouling may be minimised by coating the mesh with anti-foulants, usually based on copper salts, to avoid (for a period) the need to remove nets for cleaning. Modern products are not toxic to fish but may make the mesh more abrasive, which results in descaling.

Feeding

Nutrition and feed formulation are dealt with fully in Chapter 8. Obviously the feed must meet the requirements of the fish for maintenance and growth, and at the most efficient food conversion ratio (FCR): feed is the most significant variable cost in farming and waste must be minimised. Feeding practices vary greatly but the following factors are important in determining a feeding strategy:

- Automatic and/or hand feeding.
- Meals or continuous feeding.
- Feeding frequency.
- Water temperature and appetite.
- Pellet size and sinking rate.
- Feed distribution over the pen area.
- Monitoring growth performance.
- Price of feed.

The 'best' way of feeding fish is by no means resolved. It is vital to assess performance at frequent intervals by weighing a statistically significant sample of fish in a population and adjusting feeding rates accordingly. Feeding behaviour in penned populations has received more attention recently and the interactions amongst individuals are more complex than has been generally realised. Small fish are intimidated by the presence of large individuals and it may be beneficial to grade a population to establish more evenly matched groups.

It is vital that fish are given the opportunity to feed to the calculated level with the minimum of waste. Overfeeding can be detected by suspending a trap on the net floor to catch uneaten feed. The number of pellets retrieved gives a guide in calculating the rate of overfeeding.

First feeders are ready to take artificial feed when they have absorbed their yolk-sacs (Fig. 2.3). The diet for first feeders must be of the highest quality and offered frequently. Fry denied access to food when they are willing to take it will quickly die. However, overfeeding carries the risk of fouling the water and increasing the Biological Oxygen Demand (BOD), as well as being wasteful. In reality, feeding at this stage is more or less continuous and most farms use automatic feeders.

Fry grow rapidly and expert stockmanship is essential during this critical phase. Feeding is adjusted as biomass increases and must be done carefully to avoid waste. Offering too large a pellet size will limit the growth of the fry.

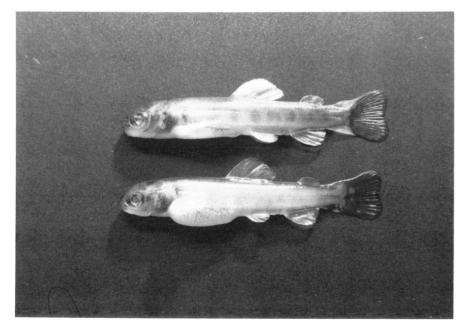

FIG. 2.3 Resorption of the yolk sac indicates readiness to take artificial feed.

Harvesting

Harvesting methods vary considerably and are usually determined by the scale of the operation. The need to produce large volumes quickly requires automation, although smaller operations can rely on manual methods. In either case the aim must be to maintain the quality of the final product through careful handling at harvest. There is evidence that excessive stress at harvesting can affect flesh quality and it is in the producers' interests to prevent this.

Increasingly buyers are demanding that fish are bled at harvesting. This requires some method of pre-stunning, which can be accomplished by a blow on the head, administered correctly, but the technique carries the risk of bruising if misjudged. Large numbers of fish may be rendered insensible by the proper use of carbon dioxide. Fish welfare must be considered when choosing a slaughter method.

Record keeping

Accurate and complete stock records are essential to good management and should include the following:

- Stock origin.
- Stock numbers.
- Mortalities and their causes.
- Disease investigation reports.
- Growth data and feeding details.
- Treatment records and medicine withdrawal periods.
- Medicine stock records.
- Environmental data, including water quality.

Records constitute a valuable history for the veterinary investigator who may not have frequent contact with the farm. By careful examination of records, it is possible to detect trends before problems become intractable and to target actions most effectively. Close familiarity with husbandry practices on a particular farm is essential if an effective veterinary service is to be provided. The efficacy of therapy should be monitored closely, to avoid unnecessary and wasteful use of medicines. There may be a statutory obligation to record use of medicines.

Husbandry of Salmonid Broodstock

Broodfish are selected for the qualities they impart to their progeny, such as growth rate, disease resistance, grilsing percentage and flesh quality. Sorting of potential broodstock, which is carried out from June or July of the year in which the fish will spawn, should take place as early as possible: stress can trigger disease, especially as water temperatures rise, and handling during sorting is inevitably stressful especially for large broodfish. Good husbandry aims to minimise the stress of handling.

The fish should be starved for 12–24 hours before they are to be handled as this will reduce the risk of stress and minimises faecal contamination of the water. It is unavoidably necessary to crowd the fish into a small space when they have to be removed from tanks or net pens but overcrowding must be kept to a minimum and should not be unduly prolonged, especially at temperatures in excess of 14°C. In sea conditions where there is a strong tidal flow, care must be taken to avoid the net being dragged under the flotation platform and 'bagging' the fish.

Handling broodfish for ripeness requires experience in recognising ovulated females as well as in minimising stress. Sedation and anaesthesia, which are often used when fish are examined individually, are covered in Chapter 9.

Hatchery Routines

The collection of milt from male salmon is simple with practice, although the greatest care must be taken to avoid contamination with urine, water or blood. Milt is fairly robust and its viability can be extended and preserved for later use or for transportation to fertilise eggs elsewhere.

The reproductive products of broodfish should be regarded as a potential route for the introduction of infection into a hatchery. In theory, it is possible for any pathogen present in the parent fish to be carried on the egg surface and true vertical transmission could occur. Strict hygiene must therefore be observed at all times.

Eggs which have been properly water-hardened may be disinfected by immersion for 10 minutes in an iodophor solution, e.g. 1% w/v diluted 1:100 and buffered, if necessary, to a pH value between

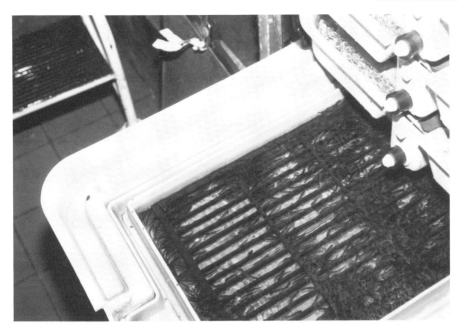

FIG. 2.4 Atlantic salmon alevins in a hatching tray with vertical supports. Egg debris falls through the grid.

6.5 and 7.5. The difference in temperature between the disinfecting solution and the transport water must not be more than 2–3°C. The eggs must not be allowed to dry.

Iodophor disinfectants are also satisfactory in simple footbaths for use by personnel before entering a unit, provided that the solution strength is maintained and that organic matter is not allowed to accumulate in the bath.

Incubation techniques vary greatly and are described in more detail in later chapters. The period from laying down eggs in the incubator to the eyed stage is crucial to survival and there must be minimal disturbance over this time. Particular attention is paid to water quality and cleanliness. Where incubating units are part of a flow-through water supply system, with water passing from one egg batch to the next, filters between the compartments will trap detritus and must be inspected and cleaned regularly, especially when hatching begins: a considerable amount of shell debris will pass out of each compartment, and blocked filters would restrict the water-flow. Many incubation facilities are designed so that newly hatched alevins fall through perforations in the base of the tray, leaving shell debris behind.

A substrate such as gravel or tufted nylon provides a suitably supportive surface for the alevins. Alternatively, the hatching tray has parallel slats for support (Fig. 2.4). The hatching tray is removed when all of the eggs have hatched.

It is not possible to remove dead eggs until the majority of the batch is eyed. To control fungal infections, hatcheries commonly flush eggs with a chemical such as malachite green, often every two days.

Transference

Transference of fry

The period of rapid growth of young fish may be completed in a land-based tank unit or in floating pens in fresh water. Figure 2.5 outlines the advantages and disadvantages of loch-rearing.

If fry are to be grown in lochs or lakes, they need to be transported at the appropriate time. This may be determined solely by existing tank capacity being exceeded, or due to inadequate water supply for the anticipated biomass. Fry are usually transported in insulated tanks at optimum stocking densities, with temperature and oxygen levels controlled. Temperature shock must be avoided. Prolonged transport results in the accumulation of metabolic waste, which can be dangerous. Disinfectants used to clean the tanks must be removed completely by rinsing.

ADVANTAGES AND DISADVANTAGES OF LOCH REARING	
Advantages	**Disadvantages**
Stable water quality Slow temperature changes Less risk of disease transmission from wild fish Water supply assured	Not easy to manipulate temperature and photoperiod Chemical treatments less well controlled

Smoltification

Smoltification is the process by which salmon parr undergo physiological changes which will allow them to adapt to a saltwater environment. Towards the end of the year of hatching there will be an obvious bimodal size distribution in a population, in which the larger fish are destined to become smolts the following spring (the S1 smolts).

There are several visible stages in smoltification which appear suddenly or over a period.

- Condition factor (a calculation which relates body length and weight) decreases progressively, producing a longer, thinner smolt.
- Parr marks are gradually lost as the characteristic silvery colour develops.
- From a bottom-living existence as parr, smolts come to the surface more often and tend to shoal.
- While parr swim against the current, smolts swim less actively and increasingly *with* the current.

To encourage adaptive changes, some producers gradually introduce sea water to smolts in tanks and incorporate salt in the feed. Stock selection, feeding strategies, photoperiod manipulation and the control of water temperature are used to influence the physiological changes in the young fish to the advantage of the farmer.

Handling of smolts inevitably leads to scale loss and every effort should be made to minimise it. In the months leading up to sea transfer, on-growers need to assure themselves of the health status of stock to be introduced to their farm. In particular they should seek satisfaction that smolts are free from specific pathogens — for example, by the use of stress testing for *Aeromonas salmonicida* (Chapters 12 and 13). However, no practical method

has been shown capable of the reliable elimination of the 'carrier' stage.

Transfer to sea

The transference of smolts to sea is a critical phase in the cycle. The optimum time is the subject of much debate: it is often said that there is a narrow 'window' for the operation. Fish transferred too early or too late will fail to thrive at sea.

There are advantages in early transfer. Sea temperature is usually several degrees higher than in fresh water at any given time, which increases the time available to grow out the fish and also releases fresh water facilities for the next generation. In fresh water, fungal growth increases as temperatures rise and smolts held back may become seriously affected.

Set against these benefits is the lower weight of the smolts at early transfer. Provided that fresh water grading has been thorough and weights are good at the point of transfer, then early losses in the sea should be within acceptable limits.

Method of transport. The smolts may be transferred in tanks by land, or by air or by well-boat. Sedation is unnecessary but, whatever the method of transport, certain constraints are important:

- Stocking density in transport tanks.
- Oxygen supply.
- Temperature shock.
- Length of transport.

Non-salmonids

The principles of good husbandry for non-salmonids do not differ from those already described but the biological requirements of each species will determine the relative importance of those principles.

Eels

Despite technological advances it is not yet possible to complete the eel's life-cycle in captivity. The eel farmer is dependent on wild-caught elvers for stocking and this obviously carries the risk of introducing disease.

The culture system is determined by the temperature range requirement of 18–25°C to reach marketable size. Extensive culture is possible where natural temperatures are not limiting but in temperate areas water recirculation systems are essential to conserve heat. The risk of disease is high at the elevated temperatures employed in eel culture and this is compounded by recirculation. Systems must therefore be designed so that there can be effective sterilisation of the supply and so that the tanks can be isolated if it becomes necessary to use treatment chemicals which might damage biofilters. The water reconditioning system must remove solids, reduce the circulating ammonia level, buffer pH, destroy pathogens and restore oxygen saturation.

Stocking densities can be up to 150 kg/m^2 at peak biomass. The introduction of artificial diets is one of the most demanding phases in eel culture and failure at this stage can result in high mortality. Elvers are olfactory feeders initially and the formulation must be presented in an attractive way until they can respond to the visual stimulation of floating or slowly sinking pelleted feed.

Growth rates vary widely between individuals within the same generation and can be easily checked by stress. Male and female eels have a parallel growth rate up to about 100 g. After which the males grow more slowly and rarely exceed 200 g. Females continue to grow without a check to the desired harvest weight range. Because of this size distribution in a population, frequent grading is carried out to reduce size disparity. As with other cultured species, handling introduces stress and can be a trigger for disease.

Channel Catfish

The most common system of cultivation for this warm-water fish is the earth pond though raceways, cages and tanks have been used. The ponds are usually shallow (1–2 m) with a large surface area. In terms of husbandry the factor of over-riding importance is water quality, and dissolved oxygen is the most important limiting factor in productivity.

Fish are spawned in ponds with little need for intervention. Egg batches are collected for hatching in troughs, where they are mechanically agitated to remove debris and dead eggs and to oxygenate the egg mass. After hatching sac fry (alevins) may be removed to a rearing facility where they are nourished by the yolk until they come off the bottom and swim up to the surface seeking food. As with salmonid fry, feed is offered frequently or continuously from automatic feeders. Stocking density, feed and water quality and temperature determine growth rate and mismanagement of any of these can lead to poor performance and losses to disease.

Organic waste (feed, faeces) increases the BOD in the system and the total load must not exceed the capacity of the system to remove or oxidise it. Nutrient enrichment can lead to dense plankton bloom which may elevate dissolved oxygen on bright days but at night total consumption in the ponds may reduce saturation to dangerous levels, although catfish are more tolerant of depressed oxygen than salmonids. For these reasons it is necessary to monitor oxygen continuously and to provide for emergency aeration.

As water quality declines, fish become stressed and vulnerable to infectious and environmentally associated disease. Of particular importance in catfish culture is the control of nitrite levels since this ion complexes with haemoglobin to produce methaemoglobin and clinical anaemia.

Handling operations such as grading and harvesting are best carried out at times when water temperature is lowest and thus oxygen saturation highest. Devices such as sedatives or cooling the holding water are used to lower metabolic activity during these operations. Antibiotics may be given prophylactically in the presence of infectious disease.

Carp

Several species of carp are farmed in a variety of culture systems, predominantly in Europe, Asia and Israel. The range is limited by the temperature requirements for economic growth rate and particularly for reproduction. In temperate climates carp are usually raised in shallow ponds with a large surface area and a low rate of water exchange to compensate for evaporation and seepage, so that temperature does not fall. In tropical conditions constant high ambient temperature allows a high rate of water exchange and more intensive stocking. Carp have a wide tolerance of cyclical fluctuations in water quality and can withstand dissolved oxygen levels down to 2 mg/l for short periods.

Spawning is temperature dependent and ponds must be managed to ensure the correct conditions for broodstock. Low temperature readily interferes with maturation and ripening and subsequent egg hatching. Ponds dedicated to spawning broodfish must be supplied with water of assured purity and only filled when the correct temperature range can be maintained.

Broodfish may be treated for ectoparasites before being moved to the spawning ponds to prevent the establishment of parasite populations in the pond, which would endanger the hatching fry. After spawning, broodfish are removed to prevent them cannibalising fry and damaging the pond structure. It may be necessary to lower the water level and dry parts of the pond for this purpose but eggs will not be damaged provided the operation is not unduly prolonged and is not carried out during periods of bright sunlight.

Fry are removed to nursery ponds, usually by netting; the procedure is made easier by lowering the water level and by netting in sunlight when fry will be on the surface. The spawning pond is emptied and disinfected and will remain dry until the next spawning.

Early fry are at greatest risk of parasitic infestation. Water quality management is crucial and the water source should be free of fish which could act as a source of infection. The water should be at a temperature which will allow rapid growth. Early carp fry will not take artificial food and depend upon natural sources; thus rearing ponds are fertilised before filling and stocking to encourage flora and fauna.

Fish may be moved through a succession of rearing ponds according to their size; generations may cohabit or be separated. Periodic emptying of ponds allows fallowing and disinfection to break disease cycles and reduce the parasite burden.

Fish overwintering in northern Europe must be protected from problems associated with low temperatures, i.e. ice formation, oxygen deprivation and depression in pH. Carp do not feed at temperatures below 5°C and should be in good condition before the onset of winter. To minimise icing, wintering ponds are usually deeper than rearing ponds and should be cleared of excess organic matter, which would increase BOD. Water exchange must be adequate to ensure sufficient oxygenation but at a flow rate which does not make demands on the fishes' energy reserves.

Turbot

Turbot require flowing water of high purity and oxygen saturation at all stages of the rearing cycle. In addition juvenile fish require live feed in the early stages of growth and this production process requires precise environmental control to ensure quality.

The general principles of hygiene, careful handling and maintenance of water quality that apply to salmon apply equally to turbot.

Broodfish are kept in conditions of controlled light to allow manipulation of spawning, which is also influenced by temperature. Turbot produce a large number of small eggs over the spawning season. These are disinfected after collection (as for salmon) and incubated in dedicated hatchery tanks where hatching into pelagic larvae occurs after 75 degree-days. Water supplying hatcheries and juvenile rearing units is filtered, sterilised and well oxygenated.

Larval turbot will start to take live feed a few days after hatching and will complete metamorphosis to become bottom-dwelling juvenile flatfish over the following month. Successful feeding of juveniles is one of the most demanding phases of turbot culture and the transition to inert food must be carefully managed. The need to use live food in the meantime carries with it the risk of microbial or fungal contamination, particularly in the elevated temperatures employed in turbot culture.

Juveniles are transferred to nursery tanks as they become capable of taking inert feed. Fish can be successfully transported in plastic bags, provided that an excess of oxygen is supplied; the journey time can be extended if the water is cooled. During the introduction of pelleted feed, overfeeding must be avoided to maintain tank hygiene. Turbot of all ages are repeatedly graded by hand to maintain an even population and this is made easier by the relatively placid nature of the species. Sedatives are rarely necessary.

On-growing in sea cages has not been successful to date and this phase is undertaken in shore-based tanks using pumped sea water. Quality and constancy of water supply are vital. Cleanliness of the tanks is essential: they must be kept clear of uneaten food since turbot spend long periods on the tank base. As with all intensive tank systems, it is necessary to monitor oxygen and to have back-up facilities available in case of system failure.

Further Reading

Huet, M. (Editor) (1979) *Textbook of Fish Culture*. pp. 436. Fishing News Books Ltd., Farnham, Surrey, England.
Shepherd, C. J. and Bromage, N. (1988) *Intensive Fish Farming*. BSP Professional Books. 404 pp.

3

Aquaculture Systems

JONATHAN SHEPHERD

Hatchery Systems

Egg Incubation

After fertilisation in a traditional salmon or trout hatchery, the eggs are poured onto hatchery trays (Fig. 3.1). These vary in size but are typically 50 cm square and 15 cm deep with a perforated aluminium base on which a single or double layer of eggs sits. The trays are usually arranged in series within a hatchery trough so that the water supply enters at the top end of the trough and has to pass upwards via the perforations in the tray and hence over the eggs before passing on to the next tray in the series. A common variation of this system uses vertically stacked trays, usually circular in design, with the water entering at the top of the stack before passing progressively down through each tray. Such vertical stacks save space and water and it is possible to slide each tray out for inspection and cleaning purposes. Both flat and vertical hatchery troughs are normally made of fibre glass and housed in a darkened hatchery building to protect the eggs.

An alternative form of egg incubator used by some larger salmonid hatcheries and by most marine fish hatcheries is the hatchery jar or vertical embryonator. This is a vertical incubation system in which water passes up through a solid column of eggs before overflowing at the top. The material is usually fibre glass or transparent perspex enclosing a flat, perforated screen at the base on which the entire egg mass rests. It is important to ensure uniform water distribution up through the stack, and the base has to be designed accordingly, often with a layer of gravel on the screen. Since it is impossible to 'pick' dead eggs using this system, there is usually a small valve on the inlet to each unit for adding a fungicide as required.

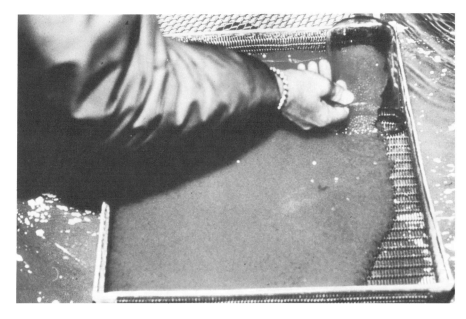

FIG. 3.1 Trout eggs being poured into a hatching tray. (Courtesy of N. R. Bromage.)

Certain fish, such as carp and freshwater catfish, spawn a gelatinous egg mass. Thus farmers of channel catfish commonly set out milk churns or a similar form of spawning chamber within spawning ponds or pens. The resulting egg masses are either left in the spawning chamber to hatch or they are transferred to hatching troughs. The latter are rectangular in shape, typically 1 m × 6 m × 25 cm deep, and the eggs are held in wire baskets. The catfish egg masses need to be continually rolled over during incubation, and each trough is equipped with paddles attached to a central shaft rotating at about 30 rpm.

Larval and Fry Rearing

Salmonids produce relatively few, large eggs and have a simple larval development. In a traditional hatchery tray, the newly hatched alevins drop down through the perforated bottom into the trough beneath and it is a straightforward procedure to take out all the trays after hatching, together with the eggshells and any dead eggs, leaving the alevins to develop on the trough floor. Some salmon farmers prefer to use a ridged aluminium floor or even an Astroturf substrate at this stage, in order to prevent undue movement by the developing alevins. In any event, first feeding of the alevins is normally undertaken in the hatchery troughs once they have almost used up the contents of their yolk sacs and this is more easily judged in trout ('swim-up fry') than in salmon. In the case of vertical egg incubation systems, it is of course necessary to transfer eggs or alevins to hatchery troughs in good time before this stage. Once the fry are feeding properly, they are normally transferred into specialist fry tanks or troughs.

Larval rearing of marine fish, such as bass, bream or turbot, is complicated by the small size of the larvae compared with salmonids. Larval feeding is still largely reliant on the use of live planktonic culture systems until the larvae are large enough to take artificially prepared diets. It is necessary to maintain close environmental control of such larval tanks with use of pumped filtered sea water at the optimum temperature, salinity and light intensity. Continuous aeration is necessary and tank hygiene is maintained using bottom siphons, skimming off any surface film,

as well as gradually increasing water exchange. Computer monitoring and alarm systems are commonplace in marine fish hatcheries to ensure the appropriate level of control.

Once marine larvae have metamorphosed into fry and are fully weaned onto artificial diets, they are normally transferred into fry tanks or directly into small net pens for on-growing outside. Trout fry are most commonly reared in hatchery tanks until they reach about 7 cm in length, when they can be transferred to earthen ponds outside without suffering clinical whirling disease. By this stage, trout fry cartilage has ossified so that whirling disease spores can no longer damage the cranial balance organs. Typical trout fry troughs are square fibre glass or rectangular concrete designs, usually built in a parallel block. Water-flow is controlled at each inlet by means of a manually operated tap valve. Water depth is controlled by means of a central adjustable stand-pipe or peripheral elbow joint, or alternatively via slatted wooden dam-boards (monks) at the outlet. Perforated aluminium outlet screens catch debris and mortalities for daily cleaning while preventing fish escapement. Automatic feeding systems are used routinely in most hatcheries for fry.

Fingerling and Smolt Production

Traditionally trout fry are known as fingerlings once they are large enough to be stocked in outside ponds, but this is a somewhat arbitrary distinction. Some trout hatcheries transfer fry out into tanks or raceways at about 0.5 g (unit weight), but if they wish to use earth ponds in a whirling disease area it is safer to wait somewhat longer. There is a diverse range of holding facilities, which are smaller-scale versions of the on-growing systems described in more detail below. Water-flow and therefore hydraulics of the rearing units are particularly important at this stage in order to maintain good water quality commensurate with the biomass and average weight of fish present without being excessive.

By contrast, the freshwater phase of Atlantic salmon production prior to seawater transfer (as 'smolts') is a discrete period in the growth cycle. The salmon 'parr' are usually reared in circular concrete or fibre glass tanks (Fig. 3.2) with peripheral inlet and a screened central outlet

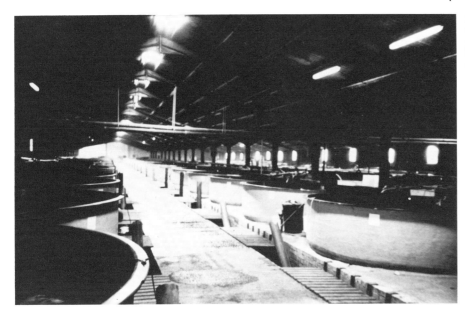

standpipe. Initially the tanks are approximately 4 m in diameter and 1 m deep, but once the fish reach about 10 g they are usually transferred to larger tanks (perhaps 10 m in diameter). Direct sunlight will harm the parr and the tanks are therefore shaded, often with horticultural fine-mesh netting which removes over 90% of ultra-violet radiation and also deters predators from entering the tanks.

An alternative means of rearing parr (up to smolt transfer) entails their transference to floating cages in freshwater lakes after grading out of hatchery tanks.

Ongrowing Systems

Static Pondfish Systems

Large earthen ponds with little, if any, water exchange are the principal means for growing channel catfish and other warm-water species through to market size. This industry is mainly centred in the south-east United States of America and the ponds are built either by damming natural basins to catch surface run-off water or by erecting dikes ('levees') on flat ground. The latter ponds vary in size, but are typically about 7 ha in area and 1–2 m deep. Water is pumped in to fill the ponds for stocking with fingerlings, after which the level is merely topped up (to compensate for evaporation) via a well drilled at the junction of adjacent ponds. Such ponds are usually equipped with a catch basin, together with a standpipe and outlet valve, in order to facilitate drainage and harvesting. The levees are wide and flat enough on top to allow feed trucks to travel all round the pond, blowing feed pellets out from a hopper. Water quality can become critical with high stocking rates during summer, particularly at night when oxygen levels fall due to consumption by plankton, and so emergency aerators such as paddlewheels are usually available.

Running Water Systems

Salmonids and other cold-water species require clean water with high oxygen levels, which means that static ponds are unsuitable under commercial stocking densities. Instead, freshwater salmonids are normally on-grown in ponds, raceways or tanks with continuous through-flow of water in order to maintain suitable water quality, i.e. running water systems. The only practical alternative offering sufficient water exchange is the use of floating cages within large bodies of water and this is the basis of marine farming systems. In theory water purification and re-use are possible but such 'recirculation' systems are not commercially

FIG. 3.3 Aerial view of Danish trout farm with excavated earth ponds.

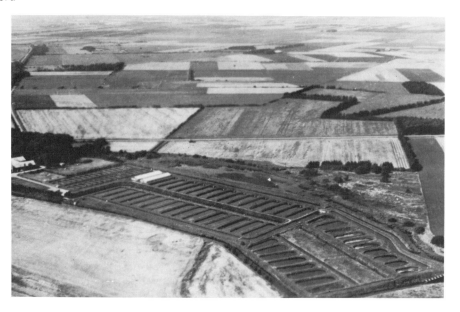

feasible for salmonids, except where small volumes of water are heated to speed up development in some hatcheries.

The traditional Danish system for rearing rainbow trout comprises excavated earth ponds in parallel, often arranged in herringbone fashion either side of a central outlet canal which also contains fish (Fig. 3.3). Such ponds commonly measure approximately 30 m × 10 m × 1.5 m deep and total water exchange rate is about three times per day, depending on fish size and stocking density. The pond bottoms may be compacted with clay, but the ponds are usually unlined. The water source is usually an adjacent stream, which is dammed and diverted into an inlet canal surrounding the pond area. The water then passes by gravity through wooden inlet monks into each pond. The ponds can be drained by means of outlet monks into the central canal, which goes back into the stream via a fish screen. Whereas marketable trout (200 g minimum weight) are normally seine-netted direct from the ponds, the wooden outlet monks are big enough for smaller fish to be flushed into holding pens within the outlet canal for grading purposes. It is normal for earth pond farms to have a concrete tank for holding fish immediately prior to marketing in order to allow for any earthy 'taint' to disappear. The relevant authorities are increasingly requiring freshwater farmers to install

sedimentation tanks in order to remove suspended solids from the farm effluent water before it is allowed back into the feeder stream or river.

Raceways and circular tanks represent a more intensive approach to running water systems for on-growing salmonids. As their name implies, raceways are long narrow channels with fast flow rates enabling very high stocking densities of fish to be held — up to tenfold that of Danish earth ponds (Fig. 3.4). They are normally made of concrete; their dimensions vary but typically each unit is 3–10 m wide with a total length of about 100 m divided by fish screens into three sub-units along its length. Depending on gradient, there may be a series of such units (e.g. each 30 m long) with a short drop and hence splashdown between each unit, which helps to re-aerate the water. Water depth is only 0.7–1 m and hydraulic design avoids dead areas or eddies so that water flows uniformly down the whole cross-section of the raceway. Raceways are often constructed in parallel blocks with common walls, preferably no more than two adjacent units wide to enable lorry access to each raceway.

Circular tanks for on-growing are made of concrete, fibre glass or corrugated iron, and may be lined with material such as butyl rubber. Such linings resist erosion on the walls of tanks due to the force of the inflowing water as well as

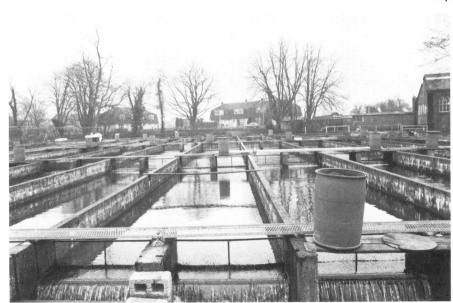

FIG. 3.4 Raceways for rearing trout. (Courtesy of N. R. Bromage.)

preventing algal accumulation. The same fast flows and exchange rates (three times per hour or more) may be produced in these tanks as in raceways. Operating typically at a water depth of 0.75 m, circular tanks vary in diameter from 4–5 m or more. Water supply to each tank is via a peripheral inlet, conveniently by means of PVC pipes with butterfly valves. The tank outlet comprises a central standpipe enclosed by a mesh screen. Water flows in a circular direction, creating something of a vortex effect with consequent self-cleaning, particularly if the tank bottom slopes down towards the central outlet.

Marine Farming and Floating Cages

An increasing range of truly marine species is now being farmed, particularly in Japan, and the on-growing phase is normally within floating pens or cages. A similar development is under way in southern Europe with sea-bass, gilthead bream and turbot and in northern Europe with cod and halibut. It has been necessary to use shore-based tanks with pumped sea water for flat fish farming of turbot or halibut, as these fish normally lie on the bottom and will not shoal within the water column inside a floating cage. However, cage farming in Europe has grown most rapidly with the marine on-growing of Atlantic salmon, and to

a lesser extent by sea water production of large rainbow trout.

There is a wide range of different technical solutions available to the marine farmer, including shore-based tanks, marine enclosures, submersible cages, etc. (Fig. 3.5). Floating cages are usually the most cost-effective and come in all shapes and sizes. The basic design involves a bag net suspended from a flotation collar. Nets are usually made from knotless nylon mesh and the mesh size is as large as possible without allowing the smallest fish to escape (e.g. 1.5 × 1.5 cm). Typical dimensions are 15 m × 15 m × 10 m deep and weights are attached to the bottom of the net to prevent it distorting and damaging the fish. For square cages the flotation collar is usually made from galvanised steel. Buoyancy is provided by polyethylene floats, etc. Walkways usually surround such cages, which are arranged in a linked group, often with an associated feed store. Anti-predator top nets may be fixed above the cage group to prevent heron and seagull attacks (Fig. 3.6), especially on salmon smolts soon after transfer to sea.

If underwater attacks by seals or diving birds are a problem, it is customary to deploy an underwater predator net like a skirt around the cages or even as an outer bag net enclosing the entire cage group. Storm damage is usually the greatest risk and so the most important features

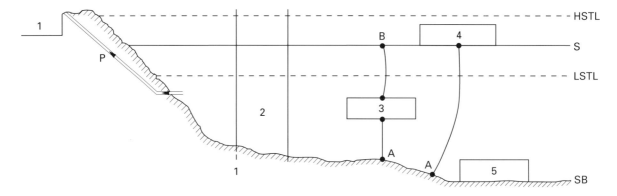

FIG. 3.5 Diagrammatic illustration of the different rearing systems used in marine farming (after P. H. Milne, 1972); key is as follows: A = Anchor, B = Buoy, P = Pumped sealine, HSTL = High water spring tide level, S = Sea level, SB = Sea bed, LSTL = Low water spring tide level. Systems: (1) Shore based facility using pumped water, (2) Fixed sublittoral sea enclosure, (3) Midwater facility, (4) Floating system, (5) Sea bed cage.

are strong brackets and couplings, together with a reliable mooring system. The latter is usually an anchor chain attached to 1-tonne concrete blocks dropped on to the sea floor at each end of the group (e.g. three chains fanning out to three separate blocks at each end, giving six in all). An alternative is to have a single point heavy-duty mooring with the whole group swinging through a 360° arc around it.

Rigid cage design predisposes to failure under storm or typhoon conditions unless the farm is moored at a well protected inshore site, which may not be available. More flexible systems are more suited to exposed sites — hence the increasing interest in large hexagonal or circular units of a diameter of up to 30 m or more, with a long flexible flotation collar which can bend with the wave action. Such systems need to be serviced by

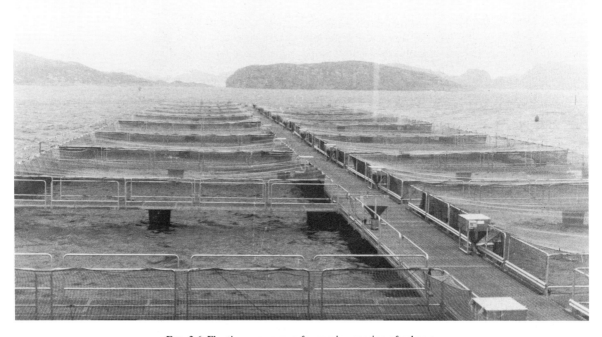

FIG. 3.6 Floating cage group for marine rearing of salmon.

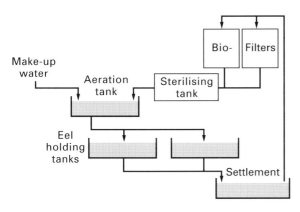

FIG. 3.7 Diagram of recirculation system for rearing eels (after J. K. Roberts, 1988).

specialised work boats and there are attempts to operate large barges incorporating cages, feed silos and staff living-quarters on an integrated basis for off-shore use.

Water Treatment Systems

Recirculation Systems

It is possible to purify water and therefore to grow fish in recirculation systems with 10% or less of new make-up water continuously introduced from outside. Given the cost and complexity, this is not commercially feasible for salmonids except where small volumes of heated water are used for egg incubation and fry rearing in some hatcheries. However, recirculation offers a controlled environment for eels and other species which can be reared in relatively less water. This means it is possible to rear eels at the optimum temperature of approximately 26°C even in cold climates, since only the make-up water needs to be heated in a closed loop. Reconditioning water in such a system involves adding air or oxygen, removing suspended solids (faeces and waste feed) and removing dissolved metabolites, particularly ammonia. Solids are removed by mechanical filtration or swirl separators, or in settlement tanks. The effluent is then passed through biological filters covered in nitrifying bacteria, which transform ammonia to nitrites and nitrates. Figure 3.7 shows a generalised recirculation system for eel culture which employs the additional step of water sterilisation before the cleaned water is re-aerated and returned to the rearing tanks.

The most sophisticated sterilisation units remove particulate matter by microfiltration before ozonisation, using electric arc discharge in order to oxidise

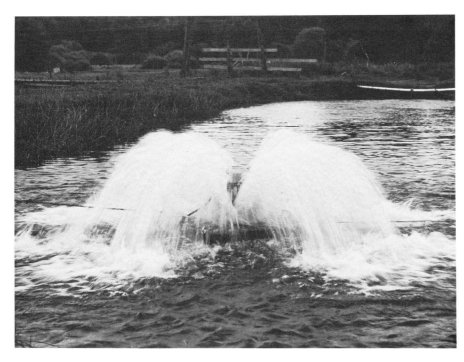

FIG. 3.8 Air-lift pump aerator (courtesy of Dansk Ørredfoder).

dissolved materials (e.g. humic acids) to their component elements. The toxic ozone then needs to be removed, preferably by a combination of ultraviolet radiation and contact with activated carbon. The sterilised water can then be released safely into the environment, but may need to be de-gassed before being used in a fish tank.

Aerators and Oxygenators

For salmonid rearing it is prudent to maintain the incoming water as close to full saturation with dissolved oxygen as possible, hence the use of splash-boards on trout pond inlets. On salmon farms artificial aeration is usually needed only during special procedures such as smolt transport or when giving bath treatments; in this case oxygen can be bled in from a gas bottle. If oxygen levels become critical during summer periods of low water flow, it is possible to install electrically driven or motorised aerators, such as paddle-wheels mounted on floats, or air lift pumps (Fig. 3.8). Such units are available for emergency use on many trout farms, but are essential on warm water catfish farms. The latter usually employ a combination of tractor-driven paddlewheels and electric surface agitators. Aeration of hatchery water is needed if there is any risk of supersaturation (e.g. from underground water) in order to blow off the excess nitrogen or other gas, which could otherwise give rise to 'gas bubble disease'.

Filtration and Sedimentation

Primary filtration of the large inflow to a commercial trout farm is normally restricted to coarse screening to keep out wild fish, as well as flotsam or leaves which could block pond inlets. Often these screens are equipped with electrically operated cleaning devices for use during danger periods, such as leaf-fall (Fig. 3.9). For smolt production units or marine fish hatcheries, mechanical self-cleaning filters may be used: these come with different sized filters, the smallest of which can remove particles of 10 microns or less. Otherwise water filtration is sometimes used to remove suspended solids from hatchery outlet water or in recirculation systems.

A more common form of treating fish farm effluent prior to release is by sedimentation in settlement lagoons. These are installed near the farm outlet and should be large enough to allow the suspended solids to sediment out, given the water-flow rates through the farm.

Feeding, Grading and Harvesting Systems

Feeding Equipment

Nearly all marine fish larvae are first fed on live planktonic organisms, such as rotifers and brine shrimp larvae (the nauplii of *Artemia*). Since rotifers have to be mass cultured, together with

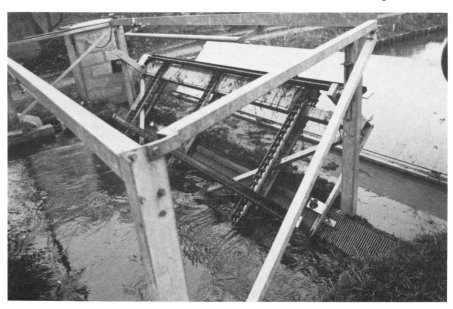

FIG. 3.9 Inlet screen with automatic cleaning device (courtesy of N. R. Bromage).

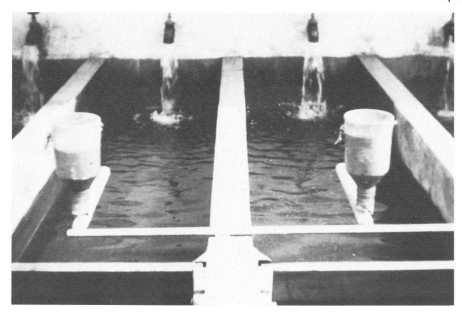

FIG. 3.10 Feed hoppers with compressed air-based feeding system mounted above concrete hatchery troughs for trout fry.

the marine algae on which they feed, this requires a rather complex integrated live feed production system with close control of water quality, temperature and other factors such as aeration and light intensity. The aim is to reach a stage where the larval fish can be reliably weaned on to inert diets as soon as possible.

Fortunately salmonid larvae have sufficiently large mouthparts that they can be first-fed on inert diets. Even the starter diets (particle size approximately 0.6 mm) can be readily dispensed by means of an automatic feeding system. These are operated usually by battery or mains electricity or by water power. Although there is a wide variety of designs, the commonest are a spinning disc, a vibrating plate or compressed air for projecting the feed further (e.g. along elongated fry troughs, as in Fig. 3.10). Time clocks are

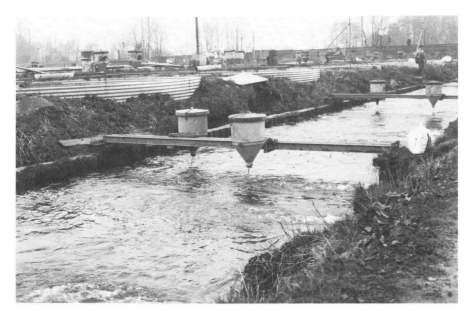

FIG. 3.11 Demand feeders mounted above outlet canal. Note use of circular tanks for on-growing trout in the background.

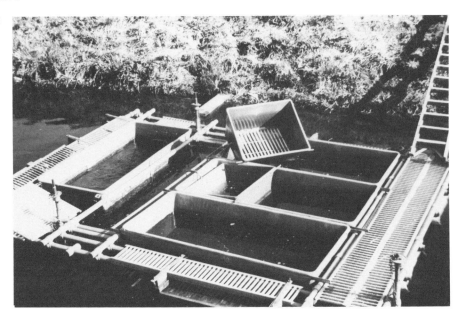

FIG. 3.12 Bar grading system in outlet canal of Danish earth pond trout farm. Trout fingerlings can be flushed from the adjacent pond via a wooden outlet monk directly into the holding bin on the left hand side.

used to control the frequency and duration of feeding.

For fingerlings and larger fish where continuous feeding is not needed, many farmers feed at least part of the daily ration by hand. Some trout farms use 'demand' feeders with a pendulum protruding from the hopper into the water (Fig. 3.11). The fish soon learn to nudge the pendulum in order to release feed pellets into the pond through a gate mechanism on the hopper. More commonly, larger farms use compressed air blowers mounted on a tractor or feed lorry: feed drops from the hopper into the air stream from a high-volume blower, to be distributed over the pond or raceway. Such farms frequently possess silos and can take feed deliveries in bulk instead of bags.

Floating cage farms use either hand or automated feeding, or a combination of both. Power packs are sometimes linked to small windmills. Larger versions of the hatchery disc or vibrator units are generally used, but some farms dispense feed from a silo via plastic pipes to each cage using either a water jet or compressed air, triggered by a time clock with manual override.

Grading Equipment

As fish grow they need to be size graded in order to equalise competition and give more uniformity for management and harvest. The basic system is to net fish from a pond and place them in a box with a slatted bottom, so that the smaller fish slip between the slats and the larger fish are retained (Fig. 3.12). It is quicker to lift the bar-grader out of the water and shake it for small fish. The same principle has been applied within raceways by crowding trout against slatted grills of variable dimensions positioned across the width of the raceway. Larger mechanised graders are now available with rotating rollers which can simultaneously divide fish into several different grades. Much of the manual labour in traditional trout farming is no longer necessary thanks to the use of fish pumps which rely on rounded impellers and wide-bore plastic pipes to move fish along in a slug of water with little stress. Fish can be pumped up from holding units via elevators into an automatic grader before passing along transfer pipes in to the on-growing unit more appropriate to their size (Fig. 3.13).

Salmon smolts are accurately counted into the transport tanks as they leave the hatchery for their sea farm destination; they can also be measured using a chute system with microprocessor technology. Thereafter they are not usually graded or counted until the grilse grade over a year later, when they may be passed over a Y-shaped fibre glass grader for manual splitting into two grades.

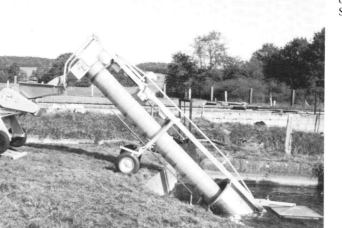

After lifting the nets to crowd the fish, salmon always used to be hand-netted on to the grader, but again there is increasing use of labour-saving elevator pumps.

Harvesting and Killing Systems

A seine net is dragged down the length of an excavated earth trout pond at harvest (Fig. 3.14) and the resulting mass of fish at the outlet is then hand netted or pumped out. On large catfish ponds a so-called 'mud line' sewn to the bottom edge of the seine keeps it on the pond bottom, while tractors or mechanical seine-haulers pull nylon ropes attached to the mud line; the net is usually put in using a boat. The large seine crowds the fish in one corner of the pond for a smaller seine to harvest them. Fish reared in earth ponds are usually transferred to concrete tanks just before harvest to remove any muddy taint. All fish are routinely starved for about 48 hours to empty the gut prior to slaughter.

Rainbow trout are either asphyxiated or electro-cuted in a killing tank before being placed promptly on ice. Salmon were formerly brailled directly out

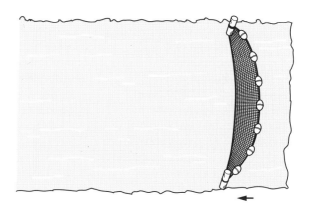

FIG. 3.14 Schematic diagram showing how to seine an excavated earth pond.

of the harvest cage to be killed by a blow on the head with a 'priest'. Many farms now transfer them (using mechanical hoists or live fish pumps) into well-boats so that they can be transported to onshore plants for killing and processing. Fish destined for smoking are usually killed by cutting across the gill arch so that they bleed to death via the branchial arteries, consequently improving final product appearance. Carbon dioxide may be added to the water before the fish are cut across the gill arches for more humane slaughter, although some argue it is not a true sedative.

Miscellaneous

Live Fish Transport

Many fish farms specialise in the production of fry and fingerlings, which are then sold to on-growers. Salmon hatcheries may be a long way from the sea farms, hence the need for smolt transport systems. There is, of course, a large international trade in eggs and in ornamental fish as well as in live shellfish for consumption. Sometimes fish are transported live from the farm to recreational fisheries (e.g. put-and-take lakes) as well as to rivers for restocking purposes. Finally, some restaurant outlets prefer to sell fish such as trout, live from holding tanks, whereas many salmon farms are remote from the killing station to which the harvested fish are brought live, usually by well-boat. Small numbers of fish are often transported in polythene bags to which are added a little water and plenty of oxygen before tying off securely; such bags may be boxed within polystyrene outers and surrounded by ice to lower metabolic rate during the journey. Purpose-built transport tanks are commonly made of fibre glass and may be insulated to minimise temperature changes. Oxygen is provided via aerators or gas bottles to maintain dissolved oxygen levels and to blow off excess carbon dioxide. The most sophisticated live fish transporters may have built-in refrigeration, an ammonia stripping system, and an in-cab console continually monitoring water quality parameters. In between these extremes lie the majority of smolt transport tanks, often modular units which can be carried on a lorry or even by helicopter, although an increasing proportion of smolts is now transported in specialised well-boats.

Health Equipment

The more capital-intensive farms maintain the necessary equipment to administer fish treatments on site. Hatcheries use a constant-volume delivery pump or a constant-head siphon to give a flowing-bath treatment. Floating cage units use a tarpaulin

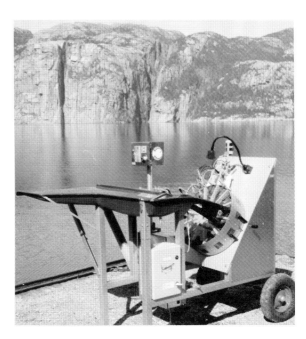

FIG. 3.15 Automatic fish vaccination machine (courtesy of Dansk Ørredfoder).

or plastic outer to enclose the bag net during treatment baths, together with oxygen bottles and diffusers to keep up oxygen levels while the tarpaulin is in place. In the case of in-feed medications, many farms possess mixing equipment, similar to large-scale concrete mixers, in order to coat feed pellets with medicaments.

For the prevention of bacterial diseases there is an increasing trend towards fish vaccination, including the use of specialised automatic multi-dose injection equipment (Fig. 3.15). Practical means of detecting health problems include the insertion of cone-shaped 'dead socks' into the base of bag nets, so that any fish mortalities can be readily checked simply by lifting the sock. Dead fish are hygienically disposed of in lime pits or by ensilement systems. Many farms monitor fish health using diagnostic kits, light microscopy and simple incubators for bacterial culture, particularly drug sensitivity testing. On a simpler level, hygienic rearing conditions require routine use of brushes to clean inlet and outlet screens, disinfectant foot baths, and in the case of marine cages the means for effective cleaning of fouled nets after net-changing.

Alarm Systems

It is necessary to install elaborate control systems in highly automated marine fish hatcheries. More conventional freshwater farms need float alarms at strategic locations in order to signal any dangerous alterations in flow rate. These usually sound a klaxon but can also be programmed to page staff by telephone, for example at night. Predators are a potential risk, especially to floating cage units. As an adjunct to predator nets, seal scarers are available which emit underwater sounds to deter seal attacks. Radar systems, with microprocessor control, can be powered by wind generator or solar panels to detect intruders approaching a farm.

4

Environmental Aspects of Aquaculture

EDWARD BRANSON

Most fish live their entire lives in water and in some ways they benefit from this arrangement. For example they do not need to expend energy in supporting their own weight; however, there are drawbacks. Water, as the universal solvent, makes prevention and control of physical and chemical contamination of water bodies much more difficult than in equivalent areas of land. Fish can be affected by such contaminants arriving from outside their normal habitats, and also arising from their own activities. Food they consume is carried within the water, and their waste products, such as faeces, are passed into it; their activities such as breeding and stirring up pond mud during feeding, all produce materials which move into the water column. These materials all come into intimate contact with the body surfaces of the fish, and they have to be 'breathed' and 'drunk'.

The quality of the water in which fish are contained is, therefore, very important to their livelihood. However, different species can tolerate different levels of contamination. For example, salmonids will grow only in conditions of good water quality, whereas species such as channel catfish can live in conditions where salmonids would have no hope of survival. Each species has a preferred set of water quality parameters, and at levels outside this range will suffer stress, probably with consequent disease, and eventually will be unable to survive. Despite this, fish can be adapted to survive at the limits of their range, as long as they approach these limits very slowly. In fact any changes in environmental parameters must be achieved very slowly in order to avoid stress.

Adverse environmental parameters can have direct or indirect effects on fish. Direct effects are where tissues are damaged directly by a water quality problem, such as ammonia causing gill damage. In some cases such effects can be mitigated by other parameters, for example the toxicity of ammonia is much reduced by low pH and low temperature.

The indirect effects of a less than ideal environment are high stress levels, and these lead to a reduced resistance to disease from other sources and reduced tolerance to other stress. In breeding populations, reproductive potential may also be reduced. One of the commonest causes of stress is rapid change in any environmental parameter. Other common stressors related to poor water quality are overstocking and disease treatments. Changes in the environment can also produce conditions under which disease-causing organisms, normally in balance with the fish, can multiply and precipitate disease. For example, a high organic loading can lead to bacterial gill disease.

For these reasons, the main objective in any fish holding system should be to create and maintain water quality within the tolerance limits of the species being held. In addition, it is probably equally important to maintain a stable environment.

In order to achieve these aims the water entering the aquaculture system should be within the required limits. Also, any materials introduced, either from external sources or by excretion, must be removed so that they do not become a problem. Such removal can be by processes within the system, such as filters, or by water replacement. The latter method is commonly used to keep the water quality of the system within acceptable limits, but moves the unwanted materials into the environment, so that some form of purification may be needed prior to discharge.

Discharges from some aquaculture systems may, therefore, have effects on the local environment. These include obvious and widely publicised effects such as the build-up of excess food and faeces beneath sea cages, and the release of chemicals associated with treatments. However, great advances have been, and continue to be, made in reducing environmental impact. Use of recirculated water in some systems helps to reduce the level of discharges. Modern foods are much more effective than in the past and give rise to much lower levels of effluent, most notably suspended solids, BOD, phosphates and ammonia. Improvements in husbandry and advances in vaccine technology are all aimed at reducing the need for chemotherapeutants.

In addition, controls on discharges from aquaculture facilities are applied in many areas (typically the UK) where the River Purification Board, National Rivers Authority or equivalent imposes restrictions on discharge of effluent, including chemicals, by requiring any aquaculture system to hold a discharge licence which specifically states what is allowed to be discharged into the water-course or body. This allowance is determined essentially by the harm likely to be caused by discharges and the capacity of the water body to withstand them. The discharges include not only normal waste products such as suspended solids, ammonia, etc., but also chemicals. These controls are significantly absent in some countries.

Although some local effects due to discharges are inevitable, they should be considered in relationship to the wider implications of aquaculture.

Wild fish stocks are a finite resource and, for ecological as well as commercial reasons, overfishing must be prevented. To some degree this may be achieved by aquaculture production satisfying some of the demand for fish which otherwise would be taken from wild fisheries.

It is possible to argue that aquaculture in fact contributes to overfishing in that most of the fish reared are carnivorous, and thus require fish meal in their diets. However, although significant, only a relatively small part (10–15%), of the world-wide production of fish meal is used in fish food, most being used for the production of food for other farmed animals.

Although no entirely adequate source of protein other than fish meal has yet been identified for these fish, upgraded vegetable protein is now beginning to be used as a partial replacement, and other protein sources are being evaluated. With these developments the need for fish meal should

decline. A move towards the production of more omnivorous species would also help.

With the balanced use of wild resources and non-animal protein sources, and the production of a good mix of fish types, aquaculture should therefore help to reduce the pressure on wild fish stocks. Some local environmental effects will inevitably occur, but these should be minimised by ever stricter discharge controls and advances in husbandry and nutrition.

Basic Requirements

Although water quality requirements vary with species, most parameters are relevant to all and can be considered under the main headings below.

Dissolved Gases

Oxygen

This is the most important dissolved gas for most species, although it is irrelevant for some air-breathing fish. Problems can be caused by deficiency or, in some cases, excess of dissolved oxygen (supersaturation). The main sources of oxygen are plant photosynthesis and diffusion from the atmosphere, although the latter occurs to a very limited degree. Because of the reliance on photosynthesis there is diurnal variation, with minimum levels occurring at night — especially just before dawn, before photosynthesis re-oxygenates the water.

The oxygen requirement of fish varies with species to a certain extent, but generally a minimum level of 5 mg/l is considered ideal. It may need to be higher for hatcheries.

Where oxygen levels are low they can be raised by bubbling air through the water — from air stones for example, or by mechanical agitation of the water, both methods increase the amount of oxygen entering the water by diffusion. However, the oxygen-carrying capacity of water is affected by temperature, salinity and atmospheric pressure, so that in certain circumstances it may not be possible to achieve required oxygen levels.

Symptoms of oxygen deficiency are, typically, 'gasping' at the surface and the gathering of fish at water inlets. This can be symptomatic of oxygen deficiency in the water, gill damage (which will impair oxygen uptake), or anaemia, which reduces oxygen bioavailability. High levels of carbon dioxide and ammonia can also interfere with oxygen uptake. In situations with marginal oxygen levels, signs of oxygen deficiency often appear after feeding or at times of high stress, when oxygen demand is greatest.

Oxygen deficiency in the water can arise from inadequate oxygenation or may be due to high rates of removal of the gas. Water at high temperatures or in conditions with high levels of dissolved solids, such as with high salinities, will naturally hold less oxygen than equivalent bodies of cooler, purer water due to the effect these factors have on gas solubility. De-oxygenation can result from a large biological oxygen demand (BOD); this will happen typically when large amounts of organic matter are being degraded aerobically, and can also be the result of the respiratory requirements of large quantities of water plants overnight.

Algal blooms in ponds are usually seen in the spring, when water nutrient levels are high due to the winter degradation of dead plants. They occur as soon as there is sufficient warmth and light for the algae to grow. These blooms typically produce night-time de-oxygenation and, to a certain extent, clogging of gills. Once the algae have used up the available nutrients they will die back and create a large BOD, again potentially causing de-oxygenation. Blooms can also occur to a lesser extent in the autumn, when algae are feeding on nutrients released by the decay of the spring bloom and other water plants. Thus the removal of dead organic matter is an important aspect of management.

Algal blooms may occur in the sea, where their effects are usually confined to overnight de-oxygenation and gill clogging. However, some algae can produce direct toxicity causing tissue damage, typically in the gill and liver. Some can cause mechanical gill damage by irritation related to their shape, usually in the form of silicaceous spines.

Supersaturation with oxygen can occur, usually associated with oxygen production by algal blooms, but this problem is more often due to atmospheric nitrogen, sucked into the water under pressure by faulty pumps. It can also occur when inflow water saturated with oxygen is heated, thus reducing the solubility of the gas.

Supersaturation produces a condition in fish which is similar to the bends seen in divers. Gas bubbles form within blood vessels and manifest themselves as gas-bubble disease. Small bubbles forming in superficial blood vessels can be seen, typically, on gills and fins and also behind the eye. If supersaturation is present, small bubbles will immediately form on any object placed in the water. The problem can be cured within the system by agitating, or just aerating, inflowing water in order to allow excess gas to escape, but nothing can be done to treat individual fish; those that recover will often be runts or more susceptible to disease. Young fish are especially susceptible. A chronic form of gas-bubble disease can occur due to low-level supersaturation, and may result in cataracts, fin rot and gill disease.

Carbon dioxide

This gas is essential for plant growth and is usually present as the free gas or in bicarbonates, carbonates and organic forms. The main sources of the gas are diffusion from the atmosphere, inflowing ground water, decomposition of organic matter and, of course, as a respiratory waste product of fish and other organisms. It is eliminated by chemical combination, diffusion into the atmosphere, and use in photosynthesis.

High levels of free carbon dioxide can cause problems and tend to occur at acid pH, due to the dissociation reaction of the gas in water:

$$H_2O + CO_2 \rightleftharpoons H^+ + HCO_3^- \rightleftharpoons 2H^+ + CO_4^{2-}$$

Levels of less than 6 mg/l of free carbon dioxide are usually recommended. High levels can interfere with oxygen uptake and can also cause nephrocalcinosis, a condition where calcium carbonate is deposited within the kidney tubules and for which there is no treatment.

In situations where water is constantly being replaced (such as sea cages), carbon dioxide is usually of no significance, but in situations where replacement water is rich in carbon dioxide (such as bore hole water) it may be very important.

Other gases

Chlorine may occur in tap water used for aquaria. It is extremely toxic to fish, causing acute gill damage consisting of epithelial hypertrophy and necrosis. Chronic exposure can result in epithelial hyperplasia with consequent respiratory distress. Toxicity will vary with species to a certain extent, and will be reduced if the organic loading of the water is high. All water from domestic supply to be used for fish should be allowed to stand for at least 24 hours, preferably with aeration, to allow any dissolved chlorine to dissipate. Alternatively the gas can be removed by use of an activated carbon filter.

Ammonia is usually a direct result of the metabolism of the fish and is discussed later. It can also arise from decomposition of organic matter.

Hydrogen sulphide and **methane** can be products of anaerobic breakdown of organic matter. These gases are directly toxic and can cause rapid death with few, if any, diagnostic signs. Unexplained deaths following pond or tank cleaning are often due to the release of these gases from sediment. They may also be released from anaerobic sediment beneath sea cages, usually in hot weather. Sub-lethal effects including gill, liver and spleen damage and poor growth can occur with very low levels of hydrogen sulphide.

Nitrogen, although occasionally associated with gas-bubble disease in small fish, is inert and non-toxic.

Metabolic Waste Products

The most important of these are ammonia and nitrites. Ammonia is probably the second most important water quality parameter after dissolved oxygen; nitrites are a by-product of the nitrification process. (Carbon dioxide also comes under this heading but has been considered above.)

Ammonia

Ammonia is the primary nitrogenous metabolic waste product of fish, but is also formed by the decay of organic matter. It may be present in inflowing water, especially where agricultural run-off is encountered, or high levels may simply indicate overstocking or overfeeding.

Un-ionised ammonia (the toxic form) will primarily cause direct gill epithelial damage with consequent hyperplasia and reduced ability to take up oxygen. Depending on species, there may also be liver, kidney and brain damage with reduced activity and growth. Low levels can produce chronic stress. The level will vary with pH and temperature, being minimised by low values of both these parameters:

$$NH_3 + H_2O \leftrightharpoons NH_4^+ + OH^-$$
$$\leftarrow \text{High pH, high temp} - \text{Low pH, low temp} \rightarrow$$

Ammonia is not usually a problem where plants are present, as it is used as a nitrogen source by the plants. This fact can be important for some freshwater fish farms as well as for pond fish. By passing effluent through large areas of vegetation, such as reed beds, the level of ammonia in the effluent can be significantly reduced. Ammonia may cause difficulties where there are too few plants, and where there is insufficient flow to carry away excess. Within such systems ammonia removal is necessary, and for this reason the natural path of conversion of ammonia back to nitrogen, the nitrogen cycle, is important (Fig. 4.1).

Biological filters incorporate the bacteria necessary for conversion of ammonia to nitrate. This type of filter consists of a large surface area, usually achieved by use of tanks full of specially designed plastic mouldings, which is put into the normal circulation of the water. Bacteria then grow up on the available surfaces. When such a system is new, time is required for the filter to mature because sufficient numbers of bacteria need to grow up in order to cope with the ammonia load. Once ammonia is introduced, levels stay high until enough *Nitrosomonas* sp. bacteria build up in order to convert it to nitrite. A nitrite peak will then occur until sufficient *Nitrobacter* sp. grow up to convert it to nitrate (Fig. 4.2). Oxygenation is important: both these nitrifying bacteria are aerobic and may die should the oxygen supply fail for any reason, for example due to the water-flow being interrupted. When flow is restored, large quantities of decaying bacteria will be flushed into the system.

Biological filters are quite common in aquaria

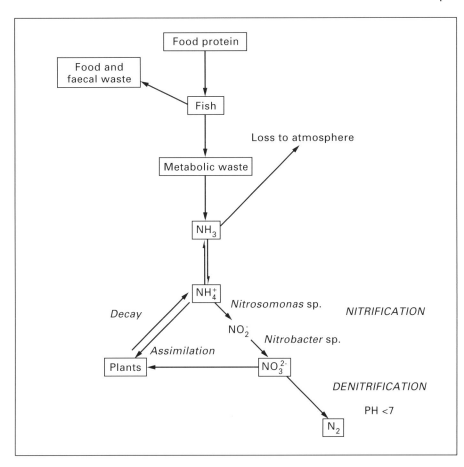

and ornamental ponds, and they are becoming less unusual in freshwater fish farms. Where levels of effluent ammonia are high, and where space constraints stop the use of plants, biological filters can be used to reduce effluent ammonia levels to acceptable levels. Ammonia removal may also be achieved by use of an ion exchange system.

Toxic effects of un-ionised ammonia on fish vary considerably with species and environmental conditions, but the following safe levels have been suggested:

Salmonids	< 0.002 mg/l
Non-salmonids	< 0.01 mg/l
Marine species	< 0.05 mg/l.

Nitrites and nitrates

Nitrates are generally considered to be non-toxic to fish, but nitrites are highly toxic. If present at sufficient levels, nitrites can cause the production of methaemoglobin with consequent hypoxia and cyanosis. It is not usually a problem in most natural waters but can reach toxic levels in closed systems. Toxicity is reduced to some extent by the presence of chloride ions as these will be taken up by the gills preferentially to nitrite ions; therefore the addition of sodium chloride may help to reduce toxicity in ponds. Minimum levels (mg/l of nitrite as nitrogen) generally regarded as safe are:

Chloride (mg/l)	Salmonid	Non-salmonid
1	0.01	0.02
5	0.05	0.10
10	0.09	0.18
20	0.12	0.24
40	0.15	0.30

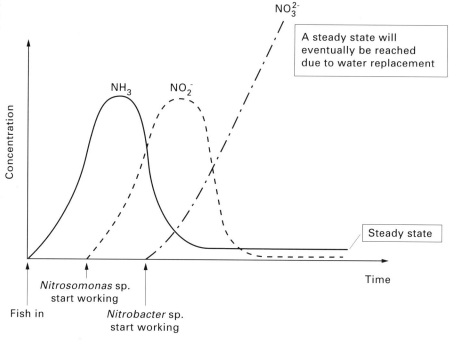

FIG. 4.2 The ammonia and nitrite peaks that occur with the establishment of a biological filter.

Faecal material

Faecal material can be significant because, along with waste food, it can cause de-oxygenation of the water if it is degraded aerobically. If degraded by anaerobic bacteria it can give rise to methane and hydrogen sulphide. In addition, faecal material will contribute to organic suspended solids which can lead to gill disease.

Other Important Parameters

pH

The pH of the water is a measurement of the level of hydrogen ions (H^+) present. It is related directly to the hardness and alkalinity or buffering capacity of the water and should be maintained within limits tolerable to the species in question. If it is allowed to vary significantly, stress-related problems may ensue. The optimum pH range for most species is between pH 6.5 and 8.5; outside this range direct toxic effects can occur and stress levels will be high.

In alkaline water, effects vary, but most species will die with a pH greater than 10. Sub-lethal

effects, such as gill damage and changes to the lens and cornea with consequent opacity, can occur if the pH approaches this level.

In acidic water, rising levels of hydrogen ions will cause direct gill and epidermal damage resulting in problems with oxygen uptake and osmoregulation. Generally a pH of less than 4 will kill most species, with sub-lethal effects occurring with pH values approaching this. Gill damage appears as an excess of mucus production and epithelial hypertrophy and necrosis, with epithelial hyperplasia if the damage is chronic.

If buffering capacity is low within a closed system, the pH will tend to fall with time due to the acidity of metabolic waste products (Fig. 4.3). Such systems therefore need periodic partial water changes, and problems can arise when this is carried out. If water changes are made using water with an appreciably higher pH than that in the system already, the sudden rise in pH will be extremely stressful to the fish. It is important to ensure that buffering capacity is sufficient to prevent this.

In ponds, acid rain may produce adverse conditions, and these can also occur in any aquaculture system supplied by natural water courses

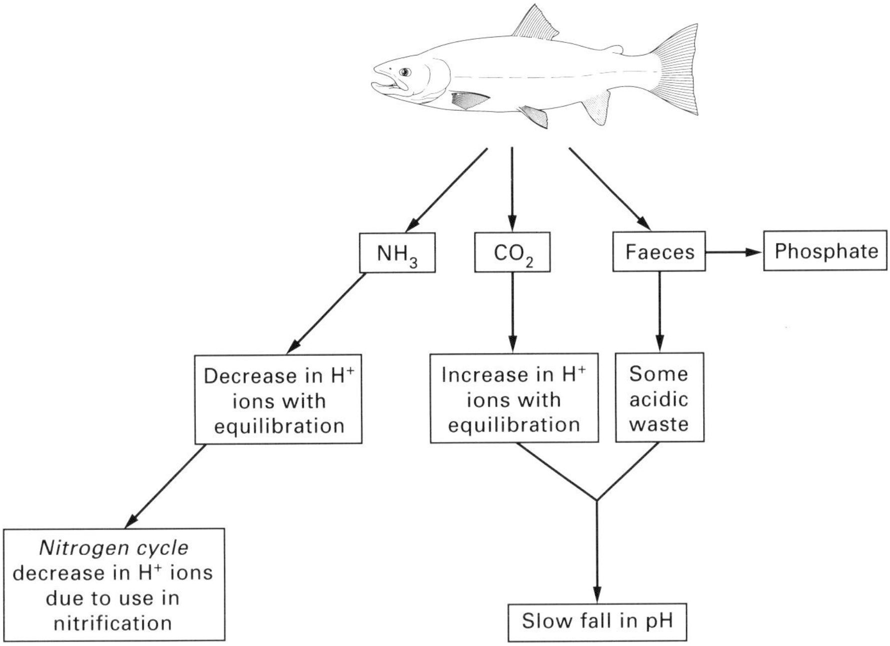

FIG. 4.3 The effect of fish waste on the environment.

which arise in acid areas. After rain, especially following a dry spell, acid flushes can occur in the streams. Heavy metals are more soluble in acid water, and consequently heavy metal toxicity can be associated with acidity problems.

Alkalinity

This parameter is a measurement of the total concentration of carbonate and bicarbonate ions, or bases, in the water, and reflects the buffering capacity, i.e. the resistance to pH change. It is also known as temporary hardness. It is not generally the cause of problems in sea water, as buffering capacity is usually very high, but it can be in fresh water and in some marine aquaria. Many artificial ocean mixtures used in marine aquaria rely on the buffering capacity of the fresh water used for mixing. If fresh water with a low alkalinity is used, then the final alkalinity of the artificial ocean will be inadequate. Levels of around 100 mg/l as calcium carbonate are generally regarded as desirable for freshwater fish culture, but levels above and below are regularly used.

Because of the influence of carbon dioxide on alkalinity, levels can vary on a daily and seasonal basis. Due to the respiration of pond plants carbon dioxide levels will be highest just before dawn, thus causing the pH to be at its lowest. Conversely, pH is at its highest in the afternoon due to photosynthesis. Water with high natural levels of bicarbonate or carbonate will be best protected against such fluctuations, but high buffering capacity may decrease the effectiveness of some disease and herbicide treatments. The addition of carbonate (in the form of, for example, calcium carbonate as lime) will help to increase the buffering capacity of the water.

Total hardness

This parameter is a measurement of the concentration of divalent metal ions and is expressed in terms of equivalence to mg/l of calcium carbonate. Total hardness is usually related to alkalinity because the divalent metal cations of total hardness and the anions of alkalinity are usually predominantly derived from the carbonate minerals (calcium and magnesium in particular).

Total hardness is important in that it tends to affect the toxicity of certain heavy metals: generally, the softer the water the more toxic any metal that is present. Calcium is also essential for crustacea and most of them will only thrive in hard water. Freshwater fish culture usually requires a total hardness of 20 mg/l as calcium carbonate or greater.

Conductivity

Conductivity is a measurement of the total ion content of water. It can cause stress if it is high or fluctuating. In aquaria where evaporation losses are replaced with anything other than distilled water, there will be a tendency for the ion concentration of the water to rise. Partial water changes should prevent this from happening.

Temperature

Water has a high specific heat so that it changes temperature relatively slowly. This is important, because fish can be very susceptible to rapid alterations. Ideally water temperature should be kept constant and any alterations introduced very slowly with, as a rule, changes of no more than 1°C every 2 minutes. When fish are moved there should not be a difference of more than 2–3°C. Rapid changes can result in temperature shock and consequent stress.

In large water bodies with little movement, stratification can occur and the temperature differences between layers can be quite considerable. Prolonged stratification can result in the lowest layers becoming de-oxygenated and laden with toxic gases due to aerobic breakdown of organic material followed by anaerobic breakdown. The result is that when the layers are disturbed and mixing occurs (due, for example, to strong winds) fish can be exposed to the released toxins with lethal results. In some sites with a tendency to stratification, it can be prevented to a certain extent by use of pumps or aeration to keep the water body moving and mixing.

In the sea it is not uncommon for algal blooms to occur where lower cool strata, rich in nutrients, mix with upper warmer strata. The resulting blooms can have serious effects, as mentioned earlier.

Suspended solids

Suspended solids are not usually a problem except in ponds or other aquaculture facility supplied with water from natural water courses, in which case occasional flushes of suspended solids should be expected. These can cause stress, gill clogging (with a possible increase in bacterial gill disease) and, if the material is irritant, actual gill damage. Such damage can result in excessive mucus production, 'coughing' and gill epithelial hypertrophy and hyperplasia, all resulting in reduced efficiency of oxygen uptake. This type of problem can also occur in cages where poor net cleaning has occurred and the debris from the net is released into the cage rather than outside it.

Some species are very tolerant of suspended solids, with carp and catfish able to cope with levels as high as 10,000 mg/l or more. Fish such as the salmonids can suffer problems with levels as low as 50 mg/l. High levels of suspended solids can coat eggs in hatcheries and interfere with oxygen uptake, and a level of less than 5 mg/l is usually recommended for salmonid hatcheries.

In addition to the direct effects on the fish, high levels can interfere with photosynthesis with consequent effects such as, for example, a reduction in oxygen production and clearance of ammonia.

Heavy metals

The most toxic heavy metals are mercury and cadmium, but many others are potentially harmful, typically aluminium, copper, iron, manganese, zinc and lead. Lead and zinc can be present in older domestic water supplies used for aquaria; copper may be present in newer ones. For this reason it is advisable to allow a certain amount of water to run to waste before collecting water for use. Spring and borehole water may contain high levels of heavy metals if the water arises from metal-bearing rocks, or if it is susceptible to industrial contamination.

Many factors may increase or decrease toxicity of the metal ions, including pH, hardness and the presence of organic materials. Generally a low pH increases the solubility of most metals and thus increases toxicity. There are exceptions to this, however. In water of pH greater than 7, iron will be present in the ferric (Fe^{3+}) form which produces a colloid that can precipitate on gills, cause gill clogging and consequently interfere with respiration. Aluminium, although at its most toxic at a pH of approximately 5, can also be toxic in its alumate form at a pH of 8 and above.

The increased solubility in acid waters can have implications in acid areas when heavy rains can produce flushes of heavy metals into the system.

Some metals such as aluminium may pass through a system as a flush causing no deaths, but leaving behind gill damage. A second flush a few days later can cause significant mortalities, as the damage is cumulative.

High levels of a metal tend to be tolerated better in hard water than soft. Toxicity due to heavy metals may be acute or chronic. There is, to a certain extent, some species variability in susceptibility to toxic effects, but generally young fish are more susceptible than old. Acute exposure usually results in sudden death with acute gill changes being the only clinical evidence: epithelial hypertrophy and necrosis. Chronic effects usually consist of gill epithelial hyperplasia with consequent respiratory distress and kidney and liver damage. Young fish may show developmental abnormalities. Levels generally considered toxic to most fish are given below in mg/l. Normally a level at least 100 times lower than this should be considered satisfactory.

Copper	3.0	Lead	1.0
Aluminium	0.3	Manganese	2.0
Cadmium	0.1	Chromium	5.0
Mercury	1.0	Zinc	1.0
Iron (variable)	0.3–10.0		

Other chemicals

Calcium and magnesium. High levels such as may be encountered in hard water may interfere with phosphate and iron uptake. They may also affect the action of several herbicides.

Potassium and sodium are not usually toxic.

Phosphate is not usually toxic. It is the limiting nutrient in fresh water, and is particularly important where fish are being held in nutrient-poor water bodies — for example salmon parr in Scottish lochs. Phosphate is a significant component of faecal waste. The role of limiting nutrient in sea water is usually taken by nitrate.

Sulphate is not usually significant.

Chloride is not toxic but can be important in reducing toxicity of other substances in certain circumstances, e.g. in reducing nitrite toxicity.

Water Contamination and Other Problems

Many other environmental factors can be relevant to aquaculture. Some involve materials introduced into the water supply, others are external influences such as weather, predators or human activities.

Toxic organic compounds

The number of organic compounds toxic to fish is huge and includes such chemicals as PCBs, detergents and hydrocarbons. Usually problems are due to accidental spillage or contamination of water supplies upstream. Clinical symptoms and toxic effects will vary with the type of compound, but tend to include distress, avoidance behaviour, respiratory failure and death. Sub-lethal effects may occur such as imbalance, blindness, anaemia, skin lesions, poor growth, tumours, etc.

Biocides

Most pesticides, herbicides and molluscicides are directly toxic to fish. Some may be used within fish holding systems, and in this case problems should occur only with overdosage. The most important source of these chemicals is agricultural run-off, and sometimes industrial waste, polluting water supplies. Toxic effects can be acute or chronic depending on the chemical and many of the compounds, such as the organochlorines, have a cumulative effect.

Most chemicals used for fish treatment purposes are biocidal and are consequently potentially toxic to fish. Many compounds used in bath treatments — such as formalin, malachite green, chloramine-T, etc. — have a direct damaging effect on the gills, and can induce respiratory distress if overdosage occurs. The effects of many can be cumulative. Toxicity of some compounds is variable with water chemistry; for example, chloramine-T and quaternary ammonium compounds are more toxic in soft water. Formalin will reduce water oxygen levels, and so its use in poorly oxygenated water can be dangerous.

Malicious poisoning, especially with cyanide, has been associated with poaching.

Weather conditions

Fish held in clear water, with no cover, and exposed to strong sunlight can suffer from sunburn with consequent skin lesions. Sudden falls in atmospheric pressure have been blamed for deaths in farmed rainbow trout.

Physical damage and stress

Violent spawning behaviour or reactions to parasitic invasion can cause self-inflicted damage; and vandals have been know to damage ornamental fish.

Poor husbandry can have adverse effects on the fish, for example, overfeeding can lead to poor water quality, and overstocking can be extremely stressful to some species.

Other factors can also cause stress, for example vibration due to heavy local traffic or explosions in the vicinity.

Other animals

Birds such as herons not only predate fish but can also introduce parasites such as eye-fluke. Snails may act as intermediate hosts for certain parasites, including eye flukes. Seals can kill large numbers of salmon in sea cages and cause significant stress to those not killed.

Disease and Environment

From the above it is clear that there is a complex interplay between environmental parameters. It is the function of good husbandry to maintain the balance and produce a good environment, and this begins with choice of site and control of water quality. In hatcheries on river systems or fish cages in the sea, for example, sites with consistent good water quality must be selected. In closed systems, good quality water must be used at the outset and then maintenance of water quality must be considered.

Whatever the system, an appropriate stocking density is very important. If it is too high, the fish will suffer however good the initial water quality and the rate of flow. The maximum stocking density is controlled by water-flow and tidal patterns in some sites, but the carrying capacity in other situations (such as aquaria) can often be increased by use of more sophisticated means of removing waste products.

Feeding is also important. Overfeeding will lead to a build up of excess food and large amounts of faecal waste, both of which can lead to a deterioration of water quality.

When a problem occurs within an aquaculture system environmental parameters must always be considered as a possible cause. In some cases the cause may be obvious, such as high levels of suspended solids causing gill damage; but in others it may be more subtle. For example, when fish in a pond are dying of infection with *Aeromonas hydrophila*, the infection may have been precipitated by stress caused by an environmental problem — perhaps pH fluctuations associated with heavy rainfall in a pond with low buffering capacity.

As a consequence, part of the history taken for any problem must include information about recent changes in environmental parameters, including heavy rains, recent pond cleaning, algal blooms, etc. Following this, measurement of certain basic water quality parameters (pH, alkalinity, levels of ammonia and nitrite, etc.) would probably be useful.

Treatments

When disease occurs within a group of captive fish, treatment materials introduce another factor into the environmental equation. Different chemicals, and the different methods by which they are applied, will have different effects on the environment, some insignificant, some less so. Because of this potential for producing environmental effects there is a constant effort to reduce the need for such chemicals. Taking the treatment of sea lice in salmon as an example, this effort can be seen in the use of wrasse as 'cleaner' fish within the salmon cage to eat the sea lice. This effective biological control method can reduce, if not eliminate, the need for other treatments. Research into an effective vaccine against these parasites is also being carried out.

The main methods of treatment are baths and oral medication. Dips are often used for applications of vaccines or other chemicals, but this process does not introduce a significant amount of material into the normal environment because the fish are taken to the medicament rather than vice versa. Injection is also used for some vaccinations, and is often the means by which drugs are administered to ornamental fish, but again there is little environmental impact except that some drugs may be excreted unchanged.

Generally, bath and oral treatments are of most importance. Baths are commonly used to treat parasitic or fungal problems, and sometimes to give antibiotics. Appropriate chemicals are added to the water containing the fish to be treated and then removed after a predetermined period of exposure, usually by changing the water. This method can involve the discharge of large volumes of contaminated water.

Most of the treatment chemicals are potentially toxic to fish, and this toxicity can vary considerably with certain water quality parameters. Softer water tends to increase the toxicity of some chemicals (for example, quaternary ammonium compounds) and pH values may also be important.

To a certain extent, the degradation of the chemicals will determine the environmental importance of the discharge. Different chemicals will react in different ways. Again taking the treatment of sea lice in Atlantic salmon as an example, chemicals currently being considered for use include hydrogen peroxide, organophosphates and avermectins. Hydrogen peroxide breaks down to water and oxygen, and has little, if any, harmful environmental effects as long as the chemical used is pure. The organophosphates have a short half-life in sea water, and the dilution effects of the sea, once outside the treatment cage, are said to make the impact minimal; however, there is some evidence to suggest that sub-lethal levels may have an adverse effect on invertebrate populations adjacent to fish farms. The avermectins have been shown to have detrimental effects on certain life forms at very low levels when used in a terrestrial

environment; their rate of breakdown in the sea and their consequent environmental effects are not known but it is possible that they could be serious, given the sensitivity of aquatic organisms to the drug and its probable persistence.

Antibiotics are usually given orally and the fact that they are used in farmed fish, could have implications at an environmental level. Inevitably, some of the medicated food is not eaten and the antibiotic contained within it will be released into the environment. Other antibiotic taken in by the fish may be excreted unchanged or as a metabolite, depending on the drug concerned. In recirculation systems which rely on biological filters, these filters can be adversely affected or even destroyed by antibiotics. The fate of antibiotics in systems such as sea cages is largely unknown, but there has been speculation that they may reduce the rate of sediment breakdown; also that contamination of mussels, for example, may increase the risk of human exposure to the drugs at low levels, and thus encourage the development of drug resistance in human pathogens.

Because of the possible risk of environmental effects, great effort is being made to minimise the use of antibiotics, most notably through improved husbandry. In addition, discharge licences applied to aquaculture facilities (where they exist), impose control on the use of all treatment chemicals.

From the above it is obvious that the use of therapeutic agents in aquatic systems may potentially affect the environment both locally and more widely. Improvements in husbandry and treatment methods can, and in some areas do, reduce the need for such use, and research is continuing in this area. Nevertheless the need for some treatment chemicals will inevitably continue, and any veterinary surgeon involved with aquaculture has an important role to play in ensuring that such therapeutic agents are used sensibly and with due regard for the environment.

5

Principles of Disease Diagnosis

RICHARD COLLINS

In comparison to traditional fields of veterinary medicine, the diagnosis of disease problems among fish is still in its relative infancy. While clinical and necropsy examinations are important, much emphasis must often be based upon a limited range of laboratory procedures. The eventual findings are not always very definitive, though the elimination of certain possibilities may still prove useful.

A meaningful diagnosis is most likely where the fish are under the closest supervision, and where the client is prepared to appreciate the cost involved. The veterinarian may be presented with fish from a variety of sources:

- Aquaculture, where fish are commercially reared for food.
- Ornamental fish, from professional importers, retailers, serious aquarists, and also pet fish owners.
- Fish reared for enhancement of wild stocks and sport fishing.
- Truly wild fish (these are less likely).

An important constraint on successful diagnosis is the rapid post-mortem autolysis that occurs in fish; one appearing in prime fresh condition for the table may be of very limited use for diagnostic purposes. Examinations are ideally undertaken on a representative sample of live but 'affected' fish; failing that, freshly killed sick fish may remain suitable for most diagnostic procedures for up to a few hours if maintained at 0–2°C on ice. Under no circumstances should fish be frozen unless examinations are to be limited to a gross appraisal or toxicology.

The local veterinarian may be in an advantageous position to examine and sample fish; however, diagnostic material will frequently need to be referred elsewhere. Specialist fish disease laboratories are few and far between, but establishment of a good rapport with one will prove worthwhile.

The approach to diagnosis follows a similar format to that applied among other animal species, but the emphasis will vary. A good history should be backed by personal observations before post-mortem examinations are undertaken. Following a gross appraisal, the most usual routines are parasitological examinations, bacteriology and histopathology, the latter two probably involving laboratory support. Other samplings and tests are included less frequently. The diagnostic procedures are represented schematically in Fig. 5.1.

History

It is important to obtain as full a history as possible, and useful information is likely to be gained by visiting the client. Fish farms usually have detailed records of stock numbers, movements, mortalities and management procedures. The following are just a few of the points to consider:

Previous history

Assess whether previous problems have been seasonal, or related to a particular age group. It is also possible that stock of a certain genetic origin are preferentially affected, or that problems focus on recent stock intakes.

Nature of problem

Fish may show poor appetite or ill thrift, or there may be unacceptable mortality. A rapid increase in mortality might suggest an infectious disease agent. With intermittent or low-grade mortality, it may be more difficult to define a cause. Mass fish kills might be attributable to an oxygen deficit or a toxic agent, and are sometimes

FIG. 5.1 Diagnostic procedures for fish.

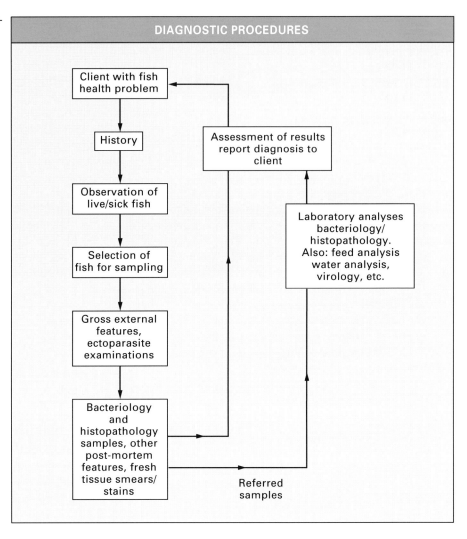

no longer a diagnostic proposition by the time they are recognised.

Management

Regular routines such as within-farm movements, gradings, sample weighings and anything liable to impose additional stress on the fish may predispose to problems. Besides the importation of fish of uncertain health status, stocking density is often a critical factor when infectious disease agents are present.

Hygiene

Inadequate removal of dead fish can aggravate infectious disease problems, as can the careless use of equipment between different groups of fish. Overfeeding and accumulation of faecal debris can lead to other non-infectious problems.

Environment

This can have a profound influence on disease in a variety of ways.

Temperature affects fish in their susceptibility to disease, and may also influence the appearance or disappearance of certain pathogens.

Adverse water quality can cause problems, particularly in fresh water when a prolonged dry period has been followed by heavy rainfall. Sudden changes in water chemistry must also be borne in mind when moving fish from one water source to another.

Long periods of bright sunshine can initiate problems, particularly in very clear water.

Storms may cause turbidity and lead to harmful levels of suspended solids. In cage culture they may cause physical damage to the body surfaces.

Damage to fish may not always be direct. The attempted avoidance of an unpleasant factor, within the confines of culture, can result in crowding, physical damage and stress-related problems.

Having gathered as much background information as possible, assess any relevance to the client's perceived problem.

Observation

Examination on-site allows fish to be viewed undisturbed within their captive environment. Subsequently, fish may be examined at close quarters when captured and held live in containers prior to sampling. (This also applies to fish submitted live to a practice or laboratory.) Both aspects of observation may yield useful information.

Examination On-site

This may not be easy if the holding facility is large, unless water clarity and lighting are favourable; polarising glasses can prove useful. Behaviour and some external features can be better appreciated in smaller systems, particularly aquaria. When observing the fish cause as little disturbance as possible, and on a farm pay particular attention to slack water areas, inflows and outflows, and down-current sides of cages. Attempts to collect suspect fish for sampling should be made after the inspection has been completed. Some of the points to watch for are as follows:

Swimming and Shoaling. The normal behaviour will vary according to species; any deviation from the normal should be noted. Sick fish are usually lethargic, lying apart from the shoal.

Abnormal movement. Ataxia, spiral swimming motions and spasmodic bursts of often uncoordinated activity may occur in a wide variety of conditions.

Side-swimming. Such fish may be otherwise co-ordinate and attempting to feed. Possible causes are previous 'cold-shock' or physical trauma. Conditions affecting the swim-bladder can present similar symptoms.

Jumping. This may be excessive if there is ecto-parasite irritation or perhaps environmental disturbance. A few irritated fish may cause other normal ones to start jumping. Self-inflicted trauma and other stress-related problems are possible sequelae.

Flashing. Fish rubbing on their surroundings may be parasitised and again there may be resulting self-inflicted trauma.

Respiratory activity. If fish are hyperventilating, either lying near the surface or crowding near inflows, suspect gill disease, anaemia, or low oxygen levels.

Colour. Sick fish often appear darker than usual, and may collect in slack-water areas. Under some circumstances such fish may become paler instead. Loss of colour is best observed in aquaria and again may suggest ill-health; however, colour changes may also be associated with the reproductive cycle.

Body surface abnormalities. Excess mucus and also superficial lesions are most easily seen when fish are in the water and may be less recognisable when they are later removed for sampling; therefore carefully note the distribution on the fish of any such abnormalities. Organic debris and algae may accumulate in surface lesions, altering their appearance.

Feed response. This is an important clue to the health of the fish, a fall-off in the response often being the earliest indication of a problem. Arrange that fish are not fed immediately prior to inspecting the stock, and offer feed once the inspection has been completed. In large holding facilities, this gives an opportunity to view normal stock at close quarters, though unfortunately disturbance (e.g. raising a cage-net) may be necessary to view and sample sick fish.

Examination in Containers

This gives a good opportunity to assess the extent of body surface abnormalities which may not be so obvious once fish are removed from the water. Sick fish may not be easily differentiated from healthy ones in the same group after euthanasia has been undertaken and therefore they should be clearly identified or moved to a separate container.

Fish will take on the tone of their container; for example they become quite dark when held in a black dustbin. They are almost impossible to see in black containers, and may become very agitated in white ones, so that a neutral tone is best.

Selecting Fish for Sampling

Four to six fish representative of a problem should be sufficient for diagnosis. As even a basic routine of samplings and examinations is time-consuming, much larger numbers should not be attempted in a single session. Separate groups of fish should be kept alive (aquarium aeration pumps are useful here) and attended to later.

Suitable fish are usually caught easily from aquaria and small tanks, but in large holding facilities it is often necessary to reduce the volume by partially draining a tank or by lifting a cagenet. Netting out fish which respond to a handful of feed is not generally useful for disease diagnosis. Patience is often required in capturing fish in the early stages of disease: they may still be able to evade a hand-net.

If live sick fish cannot be caught, then take the freshest dead ones for examination. If they have been dead for only one or two hours they are likely to provide more post-mortem clues than a random sample of healthy fish, though autolysis will be more rapid in warm conditions. Specific microbiological examinations (e.g. furunculosis) can sometimes still be performed on fish which have been dead for a day.

Live fish that are too large to be conveniently kept alive until examinations are undertaken should be killed immediately and kept on ice if the samplings cannot be undertaken promptly.

Euthanasia

The quantity of water in the container can be reduced to a minimum (the fish should still be able to swim, even if crowded) then an overdose of a suitable fish anaesthetic mixed in. Tricaine methanesulphonate (MS222) and benzocaine are virtually the same drug; the addition of either to the water at 100 mg/l should give at least a very deep anaesthesia (there are species variations). Add more if the effect is insufficient. If necessary, euthanasia of an unconscious fish can be completed by severing the spine just behind the cranium with a scalpel.

Large fish (> 1 kg) may be killed by an accurate sharp blow over the cranium, or by severing the spinal cord with a knife, or by placing the fish in a bag containing water with anaesthetic.

Some workers prefer not to use an anaesthetic prior to undertaking microscopic examinations for ectoparasites; however, a low dose giving light anaesthesia, followed by severing the spine, would seem unlikely to jeopardise results.

Work Space and Equipment

A work space with all necessary equipment immediately to hand should be arranged. When sampling on location, it is good practice to avoid operating near fish-holding areas. It is often necessary to adapt a makeshift area under conditions that are far from ideal. At all times, any refuse (which may contain material potentially dangerous to live fish) should be disposed of hygienically. Work undisturbed, and ensure that any assistant is fully conversant with the routine.

For a purpose-built laboratory area, consider the following features:

- At least 1.5 metres of clear bench space.
- A metal-topped draining area and large wash basin with lever-operated taps, adjacent to the work-bench.
- Good ventilation but no draughts; an extractor fan.
- Adequate diffuse lighting from the front.
- Space for bins containing fish and refuse bags.

As fish slide about on metal surfaces, use a wooden dissecting board for fish under 500 g. Those under 200 g should be secured at either end with stout pins (a cork surface is an advantage). Sampling equipment can be stored in a strong and generously proportioned waterproof case, and should include the following:

- Rat-toothed forceps or toothed tissue clasps.
- Blunt-ended forceps in medium and fine sizes.

- Straight, sharp-pointed scissors, a small pair for use with fingerlings and a larger size for other fish.
- Scalpel blade holder, medium-sized curved scalpel blades.
- Small butcher's knife.
- Dissection pins.
- Hand-lens and pen-torch.

Paper towels should be available. Iodophor disinfectant is suitable for washing down the work area, protective clothing and instruments. Consumable items such as fixative (e.g. 10% formalin), glass slides, coverslips and bacteriological requirements are discussed where appropriate below.

Microscopes

Many parasitological examinations and some bacteriological procedures demand the use of a good microscope. Binocular models are essential if viewing is likely to be prolonged; however, a good monocular model would be preferable to a cheap binocular one if the instrument is likely to be used only occasionally for short periods. For field use a monocular microscope with a mirror for reflecting an external light source should prove adequate. Objective lens powers are usually 'low', 'medium' and 'high', examples of magnification being 4×, 10× and 40× respectively. Combined with a 10× eyepiece lens, the final magnifications with such objectives will be 40×, 100× and 400×. There may be an additional higher powered lens for oil immersion use. Binocular microscopes in common use usually have a movable stage (for focusing and scanning), an adjustable condenser, and built-in electric illumination which can be varied.

Adjusting the microscope

With a binocular microscope the interpupillary distance must be accurately adjusted according to the distance between one's eyes, then each eyepiece should be adjusted to correct any focus discrepancy there may be between them. Both these adjustments are made exactly as when using a pair of binoculars.

Having focused the condenser lens on to a slide, the iris diaphragm should be closed to exclude around 30% of the light and thus improve definition (the adjustment is specific for the objective in use).

Examinations of fresh material usually entail use of the low and medium power objectives, in which case adjust the microscope for the medium one. Use of high power and oil immersion objectives (e.g. for examining bacteriological stained smears) may require further adjustment of the iris diaphragm and also an increase in illumination.

If the microscope is to be used by others, keep a record of the preferred settings.

Gross External Features

Sick fish often present little in the way of distinctive features. The general body condition and any abnormal coloration should be noted.

Skin Lesions

These may give clues regarding environmental insults and also some specific conditions.

Raised or proliferative lesions are suggestive of a response to an insult, and may include pox virus lesions or neoplasia.

Localised swellings may result from a subcutaneous lesion, or from an abnormality much deeper within the muscle.

Ulcerative lesions are varied in origin and appearance. They are frequently caused by physical trauma, and may initially be shallow, though there will be an even progression outwards and also into deeper tissue if there is secondary bacterial establishment. Consistently localised ulcerations often point to a behavioural and environmental origin. Some lesions may have a primary infectious origin.

In any ulcerative condition, the extent to which the white stratum compactum has been disrupted will be of ultimate importance to the individual fish. Old, repaired lesions of this type acquire melanin depositions, and may also result in physical malformation due to contraction.

Fin Lesions

Fins may suffer erosion as a result of the confines of culture. Decide whether such abnormalities are likely to have any deleterious health implications.

The Eye

Corneal damage may be traumatic in origin, in which case there may be other skin and fin erosions. Mild focal corneal opacity may appear very rapidly following capture for sampling, and should be differentiated from lens cataracts (use an ophthalmoscope). If lens lesions are apparent, further dissection and examination under magnification should be undertaken.

Haemorrhage within the anterior chamber may indicate a generalised condition, or may occur following bodily trauma.

True bilateral exophthalmos may occur in a wide variety of infectious or debilitating conditions; a unilateral protrusion is more likely to represent a localised lesion.

Other External Signs

Fungus infection, bacterial colonisation or mucus accumulation may be visible, with or without any obvious underlying lesion. Capillary congestion or cutaneous haemorrhage may be associated with a generalised condition such as septicaemia. A swollen, inflamed vent, with trailing faecal casts, may merely indicate a non-feeding fish. Terminal oedematous changes encountered in fresh water, particularly among cyprinid fish, may include exophthalmos, ascites and 'ruffed out' scales.

Fresh Gill Preparations and Parasite Examinations

These examinations must be undertaken promptly after the fish has been killed, therefore the person on the spot (which may include the veterinarian) is likely to be involved. Furthermore, they are a particularly important part of the diagnostic routine. Ideally, ectoparasite examinations should be undertaken on fish removed directly from their water of origin.

Gill

Small fish may be those most susceptible to gill disease problems, and dexterity is required in undertaking microscopy when fish weigh much less than 5 g. The thickness of gill tissue becomes a problem with fish over 100 g.

Use large rectangular coverslips and glass slides frosted at one end — these can be identified by pencil.

Remove the operculum, then cut out all (small fish) or part (larger fish) of a gill arch. An appraisal of gill condition should include areas of the second or third arch slightly away from the central (posterior) part, also avoiding the dorsal and ventral extremities.

Use forceps to grasp a portion of gill by the cartilage and lay it in a drop of water on the slide.

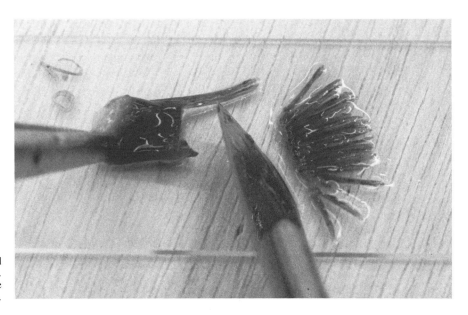

FIG. 5.2 Preparing fresh gill tissue for direct microscopy. The primary filaments are separated from the cartilage.

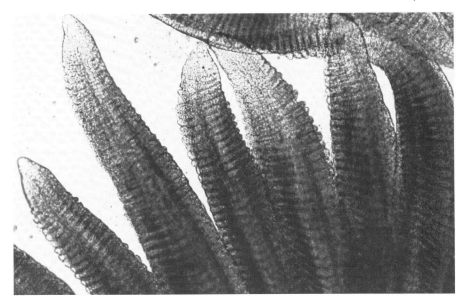

Fɪɢ. 5.3 Healthy gill tissue from a 30 g salmonid seen under a high-power objective. The secondary filaments should be well defined.

Cut free the primary filaments by gently rolling a curved scalpel blade over the material (Fig. 5.2) and discard the cartilage. Gently lay a coverslip over the material; a further drop of water can be added from a pipette at the edge if necessary. Very slight pressure can be applied to the coverslip to encourage the filaments to spread out, but the material should not be squashed. Gill material from three or four fish may be included on the same slide if desired.

All the tissue is first examined at low power then scanned through again at medium power. At 100× magnification, healthy gill from a salmonid of around 30 g should appear similar to that in Fig. 5.3. The distal ends of the primary filaments should be tapered; the individual secondary lamellae, with blood capillary sinuses running across the primary filaments, will be visible unless there are extensive pathological changes. Excess mucus accumulations and also the larger protozoan parasites may be detected. Further high power examinations of selected areas are necessary to check for small protozoans such as *Costia* and bacterial colonisations. The use of the oil immersion objective is usually impractical due to the thickness of the preparation.

Body Surface Smears

A scalpel blade is scraped over suspect areas or behind pectoral fins, beside the dorsal fin, and the base of the tail, and smeared onto a slide with a drop of water. A coverslip is added, and examinations for microscopic parasites undertaken as described for gill.

Other Parasite Examinations

Larger parasites (e.g. crustaceans) should be self-evident, though examinations with a hand lens may be necessary for the juvenile stages. Internal helminth parasites may be noted later on during the dissection. Examinations for alimentary tract protozoans may be undertaken on faecal material squeezed from the anus of small fish, or on intestinal mucosa smears after dissections and other samplings have been completed.

Sampling Live Fish

With extreme care, a small ENT swab can be inserted very gently under the operculum or over the body surface to collect any excess mucus accumulations, and examined on a slide as described. The use of an anaesthetic may be necessary.

Identification and Preservation of Parasites

Check the characteristics of the types of parasite most likely to be encountered before undertaking examinations. The fish red blood cell (7–12 μ) is a useful size marker when present. Preservation of microscopic parasites is difficult unless they remain firmly attached to tissues and are thus recognisable during histological examinations. Visible helminth and crustacean parasites may be preserved for subsequent identification: place them in water, then slowly add an equal volume of 10% formalin (histology fixative) to give 5%.

Live helminths can be immobilised in an extended position if they are placed in Berland's fluid (19 parts glacial acetic acid, one part concentrated formaldehyde) for one minute, and then transferring to 70% ethanol. The alcohol solution can be used directly with small helminth parasites.

Assessment

Histological examination (described below) is necessary for a critical appraisal of gill condition.

Although low numbers of parasites do not necessarily indicate a problem, remember that fish debilitated for any reason may become preferentially parasitised.

Some parasites depart rapidly following the death of their host; other firmly attached types remain detectable for longer. The haptors (attachment hooks) of monogenean gill flukes may still remain visible among gill microscopy preparations after other structures have become unrecognisable through autolysis.

Dissection Procedure

Further dissection is undertaken for the purpose of pathological sampling and also for the appraisal of gross internal post-mortem features.

The operculum may have been removed already for examinations of gill. Place the fish on its side on a dissection board. For a right-handed person, it is more convenient to lay the fish with the head to the left. Grasp the abdomen in the region of the uppermost ventral (pelvic) fin with rat-toothed forceps. Use a scalpel with a curved blade to cut through the ventral abdominal wall (Fig. 5.4) from between the ventral fins in an anterior direction as far as the pericardial cavity. Open the remaining part of the abdominal cavity by cutting in the reverse direction, taking care not to incise the rectum.

Bacteriological sampling of internal organs is undertaken immediately the body cavity has been opened (see below). Acquire a basic familiarity of the fish's anatomy before proceeding with the dissection: the positions of the main organs of a salmonid (Fig. 5.5) are relatively straightforward but cyprinids and cichlids have complex swim-bladders and it is best to cut away the whole of one side of the abdominal wall.

Gross Necropsy Features

Visible abnormalities of gill and internal organs should be noted while proceeding through pathological samplings. Gross lesions, when present,

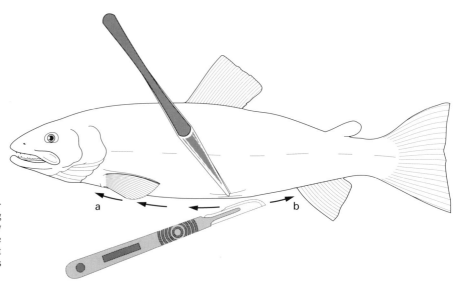

FIG. 5.4 Opening the abdominal cavity. Holding the scalpel at a shallow angle, first cut from the ventral fin area to the throat (a) then cut similarly towards the vent (b).

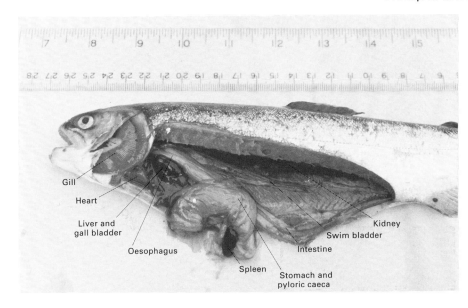

Fig. 5.5 A partly dissected salmonid with viscera *in situ*.

are often non-specific but may enable likely looking individuals to be selected for detailed examinations.

It is good practice to adopt a routine — for example starting with the gills, followed by heart, liver, gut/pancreas, spleen, kidney, the remainder of the digestive tract and finally the carcass.

Disease conditions may show varied manifestations, and the normal may vary greatly both within and between species. It is only possible to generalise on a few points:

Gill

- *Consistently pale gills* among fresh specimens may indicate anaemia (kidneys are likely to be similarly pale).
- *Focal haemorrhages* may represent parasite damage or septicaemia.
- *A swollen appearance* with mucus accumulation may occur in environmental gill disease.
- *Fibrotic ragged edges* (often present in older fish) may harbour adequate amounts of healthy tissue beneath.

Viscera

- *Terminal congestion* may result in an enlarged, dark kidney and spleen, and also gills, with patchy 'haemorrhages' over liver and other viscera, and sometimes serosanguinous abdominal fluid.
- *Septicaemia* is likely to give more well defined petechial and ecchymotic haemorrhages.
- *Clear, straw-coloured fluid* within the peritoneal cavity may represent serum effusion from any of the adjacent viscera, due to disease of an individual organ or a generalised condition; a primary peritonitis with fibrinous adhesions may also occur. Pericardial fluid accumulations, or pericarditis, may have a similar aetiology.
- *Liver size and colour* may vary greatly. A very reduced, dark liver may occur in prolonged anorexia and ill-thrift. A large pale or yellow liver with soft consistency may indicate excessive fatty accumulation and possibly degenerative change.
- A markedly distended *gall-bladder* is commonly present in the earlier stages of anorexia.
- *Abdominal fat* may sometimes be minimal during rapid growth.
- Localised, often nodular, *lesions* may occur in the kidney and other organs. Appropriate samplings (described below) should assist in the differential diagnosis.
- *Parasitic cysts* or *free helminths* are often present within the abdominal cavity, and may cause pathological changes if very numerous. Similar cysts may be easily overlooked when within the pericardial cavity.

Gastro-intestinal Tract

- Note whether the fish has fed recently. The presence of *feed in the stomach* of sick fish usually indicates an acute problem, less so if digesta are only present in the lower intestine.
- *Yellow–white mucoid accumulations* within the tract may occur in longer-term anorexia.
- A *marked congestion of the terminal tract* often occurs in moribund fish and need not represent a significant abnormality.
- Examinations for alimentary tract *helminths and protozoans* may be undertaken after other pathological samplings have been completed.

Carcass

The fish should be laid on the other side in order to check that no gross lesions have been overlooked. A few deep cuts may then be made through the flesh, checking for lesions within the muscle, and any suspected spinal lesions may be examined.

Histopathology

Histological examinations may yield much useful information that cannot be gained by either direct microscopy or gross examinations. Any person on-site at the time of a problem can be instructed to collect samples into a fixative solution, after which distance from a diagnostic facility becomes less of a problem. The veterinarian attempting a diagnosis is almost certain to be reliant on pathological expertise elsewhere; results may require a few days, and the service may be quite expensive. However, histopathology is often an essential routine in the diagnosis of fish disease.

Tissue Fixation

Fish tissues autolyse rapidly. Only freshly killed specimens should be sampled, and the thickness of the tissue samples should not exceed 0.5 cm. In hot weather, the fixative solution should be kept cool at sampling and for a few hours thereafter.

An adequate fixative is 10% formol saline (38% W/V formaldehyde diluted with 9 parts by volume of water, including 0.9% W/V NaCl) but 10% phosphate buffered formalin is preferred for fish tissues:

Concentrated formaldehyde 38% W/V	100 ml
Water	900 ml
Sodium dihydrogen phosphate (NaH$_2$PO$_4$·H$_2$O)	4 g
Disodium hydrogen phosphate (Na$_2$HPO$_4$)	6 g

The volume of fixative should be 30 times that of the tissue; alternatively use a smaller volume (10×) and change it after 4–6 hours. After 24 hours the solution can be replaced by a smaller amount of fresh fixative to facilitate packing and dispatch to a laboratory, but at all times tissues must be covered by fluid and never allowed to become dry.

Procedure

Post-mortem change affects gills most rapidly and therefore they should be sampled first, before opening the fish. Bacteriological sampling from viscera should be done immediately after the fish is opened, after which internal organs may be sampled for histology, avoiding any areas just sampled for bacteriology.

The six tissues described below can be considered routine for most purposes, though it is often useful to include others such as eye, swim-bladder, lower intestine or skin and lateral muscle. Figure 5.6 illustrates suitable samples from a salmonid of around 500 g.

Gill

Select a portion of gill including about 0.5 cm of the cartilage, from the second or third gill arch, avoiding the middle posterior area and also the attachment extremities. With small fish of 30 g or less, include the whole gill arch.

Heart

Include the whole organ from fish up to 100 g, or just one side from larger individuals (proportionally less if they are much larger).

Liver

Cut out a portion with one broad flat surface of approximately 1 cm. This will include pancreas in some species.

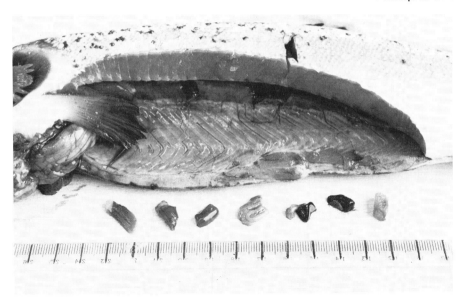

FIG. 5.6 Tissue portions suitable for histopathology. From left: gill, heart, liver, pancreas/caeca, spleen (+ fat), kidney and skin/lateral muscle. The rule is marked in centimetres.

Pancreas and gastro-intestinal tract

With smaller fish, sample a 0.5 cm transverse section of gut including the attached pyloric caecae, discarding the caecal extremities. With fish of 500 g or more, cut out a flat section of the proximal 1 cm of four or five caecae at their attachment to the gut wall. A portion of upper tract with attached adipose tissue may be sampled from species which lack caecae, and this may also include some liver.

Spleen

Include the whole organ from small fish, or a flat section (as described for liver) from larger fish. A portion of the attached fat body may usefully be included.

Kidney

In salmonids, the sample site is at, or just posterior to, a level with the dorsal fin. Use four separate cuts to isolate an area 1 cm × 0.5 cm and gently ease out the portion with a scalpel. With small fish, make two transverse cuts and ease out the whole of the organ between them. The structure and position of the kidney varies in non-salmonid species. In cyprinids it is bilobed, lying above the anterior part of the swim-bladder.

Small Fish

Very small fry should be killed by anaesthetic and preserved whole, with cuts made behind the cranium and into the abdominal wall as they become larger. Fingerlings may be dealt with in two ways. In each case remove one operculum to assist fixation of gill tissue. Then either slit open the ventral body surface from vent to pericardial cavity, teasing out the viscera (including swim-bladder) and removing one side of the abdominal wall (Fig. 5.7a); or sample the head and two transverse body sections (Fig. 5.7b).

Sample Transport

Tops of containers should be secured firmly but not too tight, and fixed with adhesive tape. Each pot should be identified clearly with a reference in indelible marker, and well wrapped in plenty of absorbent material. Finally all the samples should be packed into at least two watertight bags. All relevant data should be written clearly on a separate sheet (outside the bags containing the samples) with further protective material to guard it against damage in transit.

Fish preserved whole (already adequately fixed) may be wrapped in paper tissues saturated in fixative, and enclosed by several watertight layers, with adequate absorbent and protective material outside in much the same way.

FIG. 5.7 Sampling small fish for histopathology. Either (a) slit open ventrally to expose the viscera or (b) sample the head and two transverse body sections. The operculum should be removed.

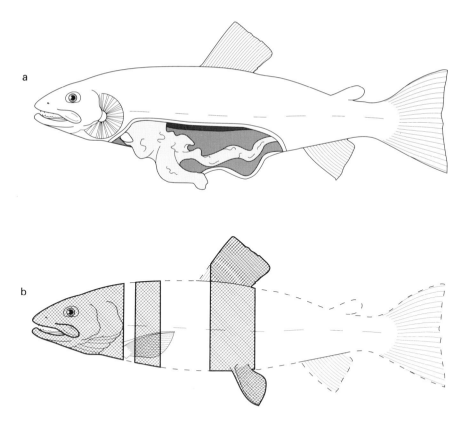

If bacteriological samples are to be included within the same package as histopathology samples, they must be completely isolated from each other since spillage of formalin will effectively kill off bacterial cultures.

Bacteriology

Without a fully equipped laboratory, bacteriology is likely to be limited to the collection of samples, a basic characterisation of organisms, and the undertaking of drug sensitivity tests; samples being referred elsewhere for definitive results. In addition to equipment already mentioned, the following will be required:

- A gas burner (a spirit one may suffice).
- Platinum sampling and inoculation loops and holders; alternatively, swabs and sterile plastic loops may be used.
- An incubator or other clean area with a stable temperature of around 20°C.
- A supply of recently prepared culture media.

Sampling Technique

Clean the body surface of the fish with a damp paper towel, and have all equipment immediately within reach. Cut open the abdomen, as already described for dissection. Routine bacteriological samples are frequently taken from the kidney. The whole of one side of the abdominal wall may be cut away, but sampling is quicker and less prone to contamination if this is omitted. Hold the flap of the abdominal wall with forceps or clasps, in a raised position, until the sample has been taken. With a scalpel or blunt forceps in the other hand, push the viscera aside out of the abdominal cavity, then strip away the swim-bladder from the posterior end until the more anterior part of the kidney is exposed (Fig. 5.8). Hold the platinum sampling loop in the burner flame until red hot; insert it into the mid to anterior region of the kidney (Fig. 5.9 illustrates the technique, though with a sterile plastic loop), then hold it still for a few seconds to allow it to cool. The loop should finally be pushed forward to the anterior kidney before

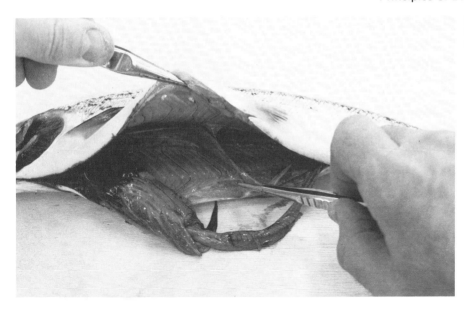

FIG. 5.8 Bacteriological sampling: stripping away the swim-bladder.

withdrawing it. At no stage should the loop touch anything other than the kidney between flaming and inoculation.

Swabs

When these are used to obtain samples, a sterile blade or hot sear may first be required to break the kidney membrane. The swab, within a sterile sheath, may be kept for two or three hours before inoculating onto growth media, though normally such delay should be avoided.

Sterile plastic loops

These may be used when a burner is not available, though again it may be necessary to break the kidney membrane in a sterile manner first. Further fresh loops should be used when streaking the inoculum over the agar.

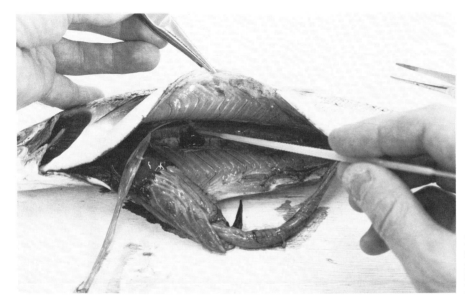

FIG. 5.9 Bacteriological sampling: using a sterile plastic loop to obtain an inoculum from the anterior kidney.

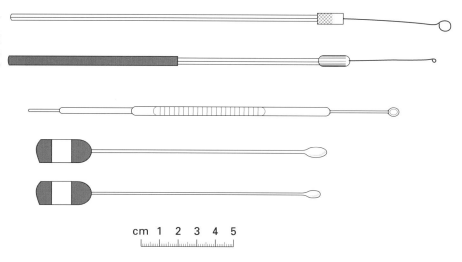

FIG. 5.10 Sampling equipment for bacteriology. From top: large and small platinum loops, disposable plastic loop, sterile swab and ENT swab.

cm 1 2 3 4 5

Plastic loops and sterile swabs may be used in different sizes, as appropriate to the fish being sampled (Fig. 5.10).

Sampling other tissues

The exterior body surface or organs such as liver should first be seared with an almost red-hot blade held flat on the tissue. Sampling is then undertaken through the resulting sterilised area, and must extend to tissue away from that influenced by the heat. Open body surface lesions or small focal lesions may be sampled directly but the cultures are likely to include contaminant organisms.

Inoculation of Media

Pick up the base of an agar plate containing the medium (it should be lying uppermost). Streak the loop back and forth near (but just away from) one edge of the medium to create a primary inoculation well. Reflame the loop, allow it to cool for a few seconds, and make four or five streaks from the well out across one side of the plate. Reflame again, and repeat the process but cross over these streaks onto fresh agar. Only the very slightest pressure — just the weight of the loop — is required during the inoculation. The aim is to dilute out bacteria over the surface of the agar so that individual colonies may later be picked off. The final inoculation pattern should be similar to that in Fig. 5.11. Identify the outside of the base of the plate with an indelible marker, taking care not to obscure the inoculated areas.

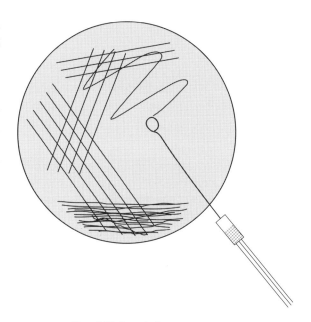

FIG. 5.11 Inoculating an agar plate.

Culture Media

Tryptone soya agar (TSA) is used routinely in culture for organisms derived from freshwater fish. Where organisms of marine origin are likely 'salt TSA' (which includes NaCl at 2%) may be used. Both these media are commercially available as ready-to-use plates. Duplicate culture on both media is sometimes useful: preferential growth on one rather than the other may be a clue to the origin of an organism.

Blood agar may be used if neither of these TSA

media are available. Some fish pathogens are very fastidious, requiring special media and culture conditions; if such organisms are suspected it is better to arrange for fish to be forwarded to a specialist laboratory.

Contamination of Media

This is the main problem for the inexperienced operator. Possible causes include:

- Poor sampling technique.
- Sampling in dusty, draughty conditions.
- Improper storage of media. Plates should be kept media-side uppermost in their sealed packs in a refrigerator, and discarded if not used within a few weeks.
- Condensation. Before use, allow plates to attain room temperature, then gently shake out any water droplets present within the lid. Condensation can seriously aggravate any contamination problem; if inoculated plates are posted elsewhere, they should be sealed around the sides with masking tape and protected by clean packing material.

Incubation

Agar plates should be maintained under aerobic conditions, media-side uppermost, between 18 and 22°C. Any area or receptacle may be used provided the atmosphere is clean and the temperature never exceeds 25°C. (Note that in tropical conditions, or for tropical aquaria, a more appropriate incubation range is perhaps 25°C to 30°C.) Temperatures much lower than 18°C will merely delay bacterial growth. Some of the commoner pathogens should show substantial growth within 48–72 hours if present in significant numbers; individual colonies can then be selected for further tests. Cultures should be maintained for a week to be sure of a negative result.

Consistently similar bacterial colonies along the lines of inoculation should be considered of possible significance. Varied types, there and elsewhere on the media, are usually contaminants.

Identification of Bacteria

Many of the more common fish pathogens are Gram-negative rods. Further classification is by biochemical tests, initially for oxidase activity, and for oxidation and fermentation of glucose. Such tests, and subsequent definition using the API system of biochemical tests, are likely to be beyond the scope of many veterinary practices but a few basic characterisation techniques may be undertaken.

Stained smear

A bacterial colony is picked off with a loop, and mixed with a drop of clean water on a slide. The emulsified drop is evenly spread over an area of approximately 1.5 cm diameter, and allowed to air-dry. Heat-fix by passing the slide through a flame two or three times, then stain by Gram's method:

(1) Flood slide with 0.5% crystal violet for 30 seconds.
(2) Drain slide, then flood for 30 seconds with Lugol's iodine (1 g iodine, 2 g potassium iodide, 100 ml water).
(3) Decolorise with absolute alcohol or acetone until no more violet emanates from the smear (this should take not much more than a few seconds) then wash with water.
(4) Stain for 30 seconds with 1:10 carbol fuchsin (stock solution: 1 g basic fuchsin, 10 ml absolute alcohol, and 100 ml 5% phenol in water). Alternatively, stain for 2 minutes with a safranin solution (0.25 g safranin dissolved in 10 ml 95% ethanol, 90 ml water added).
(5) Wash with water, blot gently, and allow to dry completely by air. Examine first under medium and high power microscope objectives to locate an area where numbers of organisms may be present, then under oil immersion. Gram-positive organisms stain violet-blue, Gram-negative ones pink–red. The morphology should also be noted.

Motility

Make a ring of vaseline on a glass slide. Then make a wet preparation with a bacterial colony and a drop of water on a coverslip, and place on the ring of vaseline with the drop suspended beneath, clear of the glass slide. Allow to stand for a minute, then examine under medium and high powers of the microscope. Motile bacteria show obvious movements which should not be confused with Brownian motion.

Vibrostat 0/129 test

Although not definitive, this may assist differentiation between *Vibrio* species and other Gram-negative rods such as *Aeromonas* species. The technique is exactly as for an antibiotic sensitivity test (described below) but using either blood agar or TSA media. Two discs are used, containing 150 µg and 10 µg respectively of the vibriostat 0/129. If there are clear zones of inhibited bacterial growth around both discs after incubation, a *Vibrio* species may be suspected. A zone of inhibited growth around only the stronger disc indicates a partially sensitive organism, while no inhibition around either disc indicates a resistant organism such as *Aeromonas hydrophila*.

Serological tests

Slide agglutination tests are available for some of the commoner fish pathogens, and are useful when there is already good reason to suspect a particular organism. However, there may be false negatives or non-specific reactions. A drop of reagent containing antibody is placed on a dark grey card, and a bacterial colony picked off the culture with an inoculation loop and mixed with the reagent. The card is tilted gently a few times, and compared with a positive control for signs of agglutination (clumping).

Antibiotic Sensitivity Tests

Having cultured a suspected pathogen, these tests are undertaken if drug therapy is to be implemented. If the primary culture is not pure, then preliminary subculturing of the colonies onto fresh media may be necessary. The test should be undertaken only when a pure colony can be picked off the medium.

'Definitive' method

(1) Suspend a single bacterial colony in 0.5 ml sterile peptone water.
(2) Dilute six times with more peptone water.
(3) Transfer 0.1 ml (3 drops) by sterile pipette onto either Müeller–Hinton or 'Sensitest' agar.
(4) Use a spreader (e.g. right-angled glass rod) to distribute the suspension evenly over the surface of the agar; first immerse the rod in spirit, pass it through a flame to burn off the spirit and then allow it to cool before use.
(5) Allow the plate to stand for two minutes to absorb the suspension.
(6) Using fine forceps, place 'sensidiscs' (containing appropriate drugs) at even intervals on the surface of the agar, briefly flaming the tips of the forceps after each disc has been firmly placed down.
(7) Place the lid on the agar and allow to stand for a while to ensure the discs adhere. Then carefully invert the plate and incubate at 20°C.

'Multodiscs', attached to a single circular strip of paper, or pre-loaded automatic dispensers which distribute discs in a similar way, may alternatively be used.

Depending upon the bacterium, the plate may be ready for examination in 24–48 hours, when there should be an even growth of organisms other than where inhibited by drug diffusing from the discs. A zone of inhibited bacterial growth of total diameter 13 mm or less is indicative of resistance to the drug in question. With fish pathogens, zones of inhibition well in excess of 20 mm in total diameter may be taken as an indicator of sensitivity.

Drugs which have commonly been used in this test for fish pathogens include, among others, oxolinic acid impregnated into the disc at 2 µg (OA–2), oxytetracycline at 30 µg (OT–30) and trimethoprim–sulphadiazine at 25 µg (SXT-25).

Simplified method

TSA may be used if special test media are not available.

(1) Dampen the tip of a sterile swab in the condensation water in the lid of the test-media plate.
(2) Pick off a single bacterial colony with the tip of the swab, and spread it as evenly as possible across the whole surface of the test media.
(3) Place sensidiscs on the surface of the agar; then continue as already described.

Figure 5.12 shows sensitivity to oxolinic acid, resistance to oxytetracycline, and an intermediate result for trimethoprim–sulphadiazine. Outright *in vitro* resistance is a contraindication for therapeutic use, otherwise these tests should be only a basic guide. If possible, they should be undertaken on three or four isolates from any one population of fish. Problems with these tests may occur through the use of too heavy an inoculum, or of one containing more than one type of organism. In the latter case, there may be apparent zones of inhibition with additional growths within.

Direct Tissue Smears

When suitably stained, direct tissue smears may enable a prompt diagnosis without the need to refer samples elsewhere. The procedure for wet-mounted preparations is as already described for skin smears. If fungal bodies are present, their

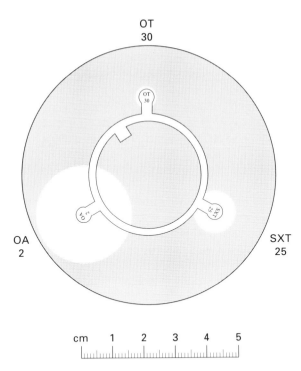

OT
30

OA
2

SXT
25

cm 1 2 3 4 5

FIG. 5.12 Antibacterial sensitivity test, showing sensitivity to oxolinic acid (OA), resistance to oxytetracycline (OT), and reduced sensitivity to trimethoprim–sulphadiazine (SXT).

definition may be improved by the addition of a drop of lactophenol cotton blue (20 g phenol, 10 ml lactic acid, 40 ml glycerol, 20 ml distilled water, 0.075 g cotton blue). Place a drop of this solution with a trace of alcohol at the edge of the wet-mount, and allow it to spread under the coverslip.

Impression Smears

These may be made from kidney, spleen or any visceral lesion. A small portion of organ is held in forceps and blotted gently on clean tissue paper. Lightly press its freshly cut surface onto a glass slide, making several repeated adjacent impressions. Identify the correct side of the slide, and allow it to air-dry. If staining by Gram's method, heat-fix the preparation as already described; avoid heat in other staining methods where the integrity of cells must be maintained. The Giemsa stain is useful for a variety of purposes, including the identification of internal protozoans. The May–Grünwald–Giemsa stain is recommended for

the rapid diagnosis of proliferative kidney disease (PKD) in young salmonid fish.

Giemsa stain

(1) Air dry the smear or blood film.
(2) Fix in absolute methanol for 2 minutes.
(3) Stain for 5 minutes with Giemsa stock solution diluted with twice its volume of distilled water.
(4) Irrigate with distilled water from a wash bottle until the film (if blood) appears pink.
(5) Blot and dry.

May–Grünwald–Giemsa stain

(1) Fix smear or film in absolute methanol for 2–10 minutes.
(2) Stain for 15 minutes in a 1:1 mixture of May–Grünwald stock solution and pH 7.2 phosphate buffer.
(3) Stain for 30 minutes in a mixture of 1 part Giemsa stock solution and 9 parts pH 7.2 phosphate buffer (available in tablet form for dissolution in distilled water).
(4) Rinse with phosphate buffer, blot and dry. Cytoplasmic granules are well stained by this method.

Where lesions are more solid or granulomatous, a smear may be made by crushing a small portion of material between two glass slides. Such lesions may be caused by various organisms, or they may represent mineralisation. Diagnosis of *Mycobacterium* species infection, which is fairly common among tropical aquarium fish, is best made on the basis of histological examination as the granulomata may not be visible to the naked eye.

Aquatic Invertebrates

The examination of wet mounts, stained smears, bacteriological sampling and histopathology may also be applied in the case of invertebrates. Euthanasia with MS222 or benzocaine may be attempted prior to post-mortem examination, but this may need to be supplemented by chilling or decapitation.

Bacteriology

Samples may be taken from the flesh of molluscs after first searing the surface with heat. Crustacea may be sampled from the haemolymph, along the midline, after first partially severing the body behind the cephalothorax (Fig. 5.13a).

Histopathology

With molluscs, a steak of tissue 3–5 mm in width should be cut out from the visceral mass. Samples

Fɪɢ. 5.13 (a) Site for bacteriological sampling from
the haemolymph of a crus-
tacean. (b) Suitable histopathology samples from a
crustacean to demonstrate
(1) midline, (2) outer areas
of cephalothorax and (3)
midline or other sections of
upper abdomen.

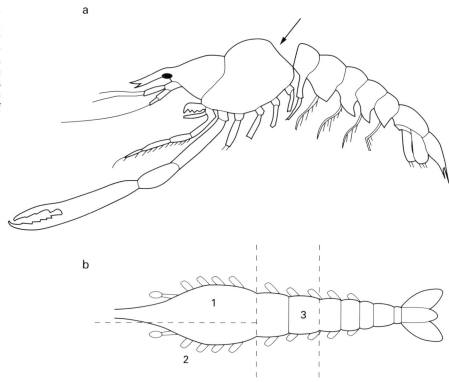

from crustaceans should be taken in such a way
that the final preparations will demonstrate a
section along the midline of the cephalothorax,
another sagittal one showing outer areas, and a
third one in the same plane along the midline of
the upper abdomen. First cut off the appendages
near their attachments, then cut the cephalothorax
apart from the abdomen, and split it in two just off-
centre of the mid-line. Remove the gill covers.
The two portions of cephalothorax and a portion
of upper abdomen (Fig. 5.13b) are then placed in
fixative. Small shrimps and larval forms may be
sampled whole.

Fixative solution

Davidson's fixative is preferred for invertebrates.
The formula is:-

95% Ethyl alcohol	330 ml
38% W/V Formaldehyde	220 ml
Glacial acetic acid	115 ml
Water	335 ml

After 12 hours (small specimens) to 2 days (large
ones), transfer the material to 70% alcohol.

Haematoxylin and eosin staining (as used

routinely for fish histology preparations) frequently
needs to be supplemented by special staining
techniques.

Other Procedures

A number of other procedures may be undertaken. Some are used only for specific circumstances; others are not yet established for regular
use in fish disease diagnosis.

Blood

A wide range of biochemical analyses, and also
basic haematological examinations, may be made
once appropriate samples have been obtained.
The results with some parameters often tend to
be variable in fish.

The caudal vein is a preferred sampling site,
though it may be difficult with fish weighing less
than 60 g. The fish should be adequately sedated
and held absolutely still. If the individual is from
a population of farmed fish where latent infection
is known to be present, it is advisable to kill the
specimen afterwards.

Equipment

Equipment should be scaled to the size of the fish and also to the expected sample volume, which should adequately fill the collecting tube.

- Plastic disposable syringes: 2 ml or 5 ml.
- Needles: 21 gauge (0.8 mm) or 20 gauge (0.9 mm), from 19 mm to 25 mm in length.
- Sample tubes: 3–10 ml.

Plain tubes, with no additive, are used for clotted samples (serum is suitable for most biochemical analyses). Potassium EDTA tubes are used for haematological analyses; lithium heparin ones are also suitable for some haematological parameters and certain biochemical tests. Vacutainer systems are not suitable for withdrawing blood samples unless fish are very large, but they are ideal for sample collection.

Blood sampling

Hold the fish firmly, ventral surface uppermost. Take the sample from a point on the midline just anterior to the caudal peduncle, behind the anal fin, aiming downwards and slightly forwards until the needle just touches the vertebral column (Fig. 5.14). It may be necessary to rotate the needle slightly before slowly and steadily withdrawing the sample.

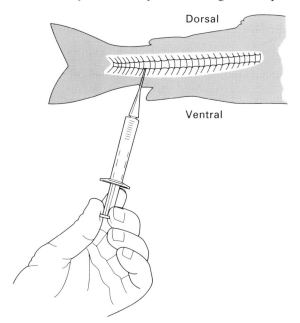

Dorsal

Ventral

FIG. 5.14 Withdrawing a blood sample from the caudal vein.

Remove the needle and tube stopper, decant the sample into the tube, replace the stopper and pierce it with the needle to release any pressure. Anticoagulant treated tubes should then be gently tilted back and forth for a minute. Clotted samples should be allowed to stand upright in a cool place; it is preferable to separate the serum for despatch by post, and also for freezing and storage.

If there is difficulty in sampling from the caudal vein, an alternative site is the heart. Insert the needle at a point on the ventral midline level with the most anterior parts of the pectoral fins.

The only practical way of sampling from small fish is to cut off the caudal peduncle, immediately following euthanasia, collecting directly into an open tube.

Packed cell volume (haematocrit value)

The sample is collected into a heparinised capillary tube, either directly from the fish (the severed caudal peduncle) or from an EDTA or heparinised sample. When 80% filled, one end of the tube is sealed with plasticine or a flame; seal both ends if the tube is to be transported.

The tube is centrifuged for 4 minutes at 12,000 g. The length of the red cell column compared to that of the whole blood column gives the PCV, expressed as l/l or as a percentage.

Blood films

A capillary tube is used to place a very small drop of blood (either very fresh or treated with anticoagulent) near the end of a glass slide. Another slide with a corner broken off (to make it narrower) is used as a spreader: hold it over the blood drop at an acute angle, then move steadily towards the other end of the slide. The blood, carried within the angle behind the spreader, should be deposited as an even film. The slide is then air-dried. A standard Giemsa stain should allow an estimate of the proportions of cell types, and any unusual morphology can be noted.

Virology

A definitive diagnosis of virus disease frequently depends upon obtaining growth on tissue culture. Very few laboratories undertake this work, which is time-consuming and expensive. Sampling for virology should be a totally separate exercise from other diagnostic samplings, and extreme care must be taken to avoid cross-contamination between different sample groups. The sampling procedure is as advised by the laboratory.

Internal organs are sampled into sterile containers which should be maintained and despatched on ice, to arrive at the laboratory within 24 hours of the fish being killed. With small fry, heads and posterior abdomens are discarded and the remaining bodies of a number of individuals are grouped together.

Immunostaining techniques allow virus particles to be detected in histological preparations when clinical disease is present, but their use in routine fish diagnostic work is not widely established.

Electron Microscopy

Viruses may be detected by EM when clinical disease is present. However, this technique has limitations. A very small area of tissue must be targeted for examination, and the work is likely to be expensive.

Sampling for EM involves smaller tissue portions (3–4 mm) than those taken for histopathology and usually a different fixative, such as glutaraldehyde (this should be discussed with the recipient laboratory). Immediately before use, the required volume of 25% EM grade glutaraldehyde should be diluted with an 8 × volume of phosphate buffer (tablets are available). Once fixed, samples should be stable for a long time.

ELISA Tests

Enzyme-linked immunosorbent assay tests have been developed for some of the commoner bacterial fish pathogens and there may also be potential for their use in the identification of virus disease. The availability of test kits has been uncertain. Those intended for rapid 'pond-side' use directly on fresh fish tissue should be useful in assisting an initial tentative diagnosis.

Digestive Function

The trypsin digest test, used to assess exocrine pancreas function in domestic pet animals, may

be used on digesta from the intestine of fish. There may be difficulty in obtaining the one gramme of material, in which case the dilution method (below) may have to be adapted, starting from a higher dilution.

(1) Add 1 g faeces to 4 ml water and mix well.
(2) With 10 tubes in a rack, add 1 ml of water to each of tubes 2–10.
(3) To tube 10, add a very small quantity of trypsin powder. (This is the positive control.)
(4) Add 1 ml of the faecal suspension to each of tubes 1 and 2.
(5) Mix tube 2 well; transfer 1 ml (half the contents) to tube 3.
(6) Repeat the process up to tube 8, but discard 1 ml from this tube after mixing.
(7) Tube 9 remains as a negative control.
(8) Add 1 ml 5% sodium hydrogen carbonate solution to each tube.
(9) Add 2 ml 7.5% gelatin, preheated to 37°C, to each tube.
(10) Incubate all tubes at 37°C for 30 minutes, then refrigerate at 4°C for 20 minutes.

The result should be read while the positive control (tube 10) is still in a liquid state. Dilutions from tubes 1–8 successively double from 20× to 2560× respectively, the test result being the maximum dilution at which the gelatin has liquified.

This test is sometimes used to assess exocrine pancreas activity in farmed salmon, but it is at best crude and interpretation should be guarded. Healthy fish may give a value of 640 or more; those with chronic digestive inactivity usually give 40 or less. Fish undergoing active pancreas damage may give an elevated value. Only fresh faeces or intestinal content should be used for this test.

Tissue Analysis

Tissue analysis may give more accurate results than serum samples for some biochemical analyses, trace elements and vitamins. For each analysis, collect 5 g liver into a clean 8 ml polypropylene tube or wrap in aluminium foil. Other toxicological examinations may require larger amounts of liver or muscle, and possibly also specially prepared containers. This should be as agreed with the recipient laboratory.

Feed Analysis

Suspicion of a nutritional problem may require the analysis of feed for oxidation products of unsaturated fatty acids, and also for antioxidant (vitamin E) and for other parameters on occasions. Feed samples for such analyses should be well wrapped, with air excluded as far as possible, and stored frozen until required.

Old or incorrectly stored feed may also be subject to fungal contamination and subsequent problems among fish, in which case examinations for mycotoxins and fungal counts should be arranged.

Water Analysis

Adverse water quality factors frequently contribute to gill disease. Their recognition may be difficult, particularly if they are transient or intermittent. Suspended particulate matter may be readily identified, but account must be taken of the nature of the solids. Peaty material is relatively innocuous, while even small amounts of fine sand may be very damaging.

Any worthwhile examination for a range of basic water quality parameters involves a substantial investment in equipment, and in practice samples are referred to a specialist water analysis laboratory. Polypropylene bottles of 100 ml are suitable for collection of samples; they should be absolutely clean, and rinsed out several times with the water to be sampled before they are finally filled. If samples cannot be tested promptly, they should be refrigerated.

Sudden changes in water chemistry may cause problems among fish, even though analyses fail to detect any adverse factor.

Packaging Live Fish

When transporting live fish for examination at a laboratory, special attention must be given to ensure that they arrive at their destination in a reasonable state. At least two layers of stout, clean polythene bags should be used to contain the fish, filled to one-third of their capacity with water. The volume of the water should be ample in proportion to the total biomass of the fish. For example, to transport fish for two or three hours, a bag measuring 60×180 cm is adequate for a maximum of perhaps four 200–300 g fish.

The inner bag should be inflated with oxygen, the open ends closed securely, and the whole package protected by a rigid water-tight container to which ice may be added in hot weather.

Summary

There is a limit to the number of investigative routes that can be pursued at one time. With a sample group of six fish, the following routine is suggested:

(1) Make fresh gill and skin-smear preparations from three of them.
(2) Sample further portions of gill into fixative solution.
(3) Examine the fresh preparations under a microscope. (This should not be allowed to take too long.)
(4) Open abdominal cavities, take bacteriological samples.
(5) Sample internal viscera for histopathology.
(6) Take impression smears from internal viscera when gross lesions suggest this may be worthwhile.

If more extensive examinations for any purpose are intended, further fresh specimens should be obtained.

The number of times a diagnosis can be based upon clinical and gross features is likely to be limited. However, when a number of fish are available, initial gross post-mortem examinations may enable more selective pathological samplings.

Where fish appear clinically similar, histopathology samples from up to six fish may be included together. Fish displaying unusual features should be sampled and identified individually.

Samples submitted for analysis elsewhere should be clearly labelled and packing should comply with regulations applicable to the particular method of despatch. Information should not be written on sample bottles; a clear reference identification is essential, with full details given on a separate note.

Finally, results must be reported. Even in the absence of anything obviously noteworthy, a preliminary report to the client will be appreciated and will at least indicate that work is in progress.

Acknowledgements — To Jim Turnbull for assistance with the section on invertebrates, to Geoff Foster and Bob Reid for guidance with some of the laboratory methods, and to Audrey Cameron for typing the manuscript.

References

Clifton-Hadley R. and Richards R. H. (1983) Method for the rapid diagnosis of proliferative kidney disease in salmonids. *Veterinary Record*, **112** (26), 609.

Frerichs, G. N. (1984) *Isolation and Identification of Fish Bacterial Pathogens*. Institute of Aquaculture, University of Stirling, Scotland.

6

Disease in Aquaculture

PETE SOUTHGATE

As with all animal production systems, disease is a considerable constraint on production, development and expansion in the aquaculture industry. The control of disease is particularly difficult in that the fish are often farmed in systems where production is dependent on natural environmental conditions, in contrast to all other intensive animal production where environmental parameters can be very closely controlled. Several of the major disease conditions encountered are caused specifically by changes, or deterioration, in the aquatic environment and many other conditions are precipitated or exacerbated by environmental effects.

A second major constraint on disease control is the relative paucity of therapeutic agents and preventive measures available for the control of infectious agents. Even when suitable therapies are available, their application to animals in the aquatic environment is often very difficult in practice — and sometimes impossible.

The majority of disease conditions in aquaculture will be significantly reduced if proper attention is paid to good husbandry and to the maintenance of optimum environmental conditions, especially water quality.

All classes of infectious and non-infectious disease occur in cultured fish but the knowledge of these diseases varies enormously depending upon the species in question. Research into disease in salmonids and catfish is extensive, for example, whereas at present very little is known about halibut or sturgeon. The main categories of disease and the principal presenting signs are outlined below. Description is necessarily superficial but there is more detail in the species chapters (Chapters 12–24). More specific texts are suggested in Further Reading at the end of this chapter.

The gross clinical picture presented by diseased fish is common to very many conditions, so that detailed laboratory examination is frequently necessary to identify specifically the condition or combination of conditions present. Common signs of disease include inappetence, lethargic swimming near the surface of the water, colour changes (frequently darkening), swelling of the abdomen and eyes and the presence of grossly detectable lesions such as skin ulceration. Figure 6.1 gives a general guide to the major presenting signs, with some of their common causes.

Disease conditions can be broadly split into two categories: non-infectious and infectious.

Non-infectious Disease

Non-infectious disease includes the direct effect of all environmental factors on the health of the fish. It must be remembered that outbreaks of infectious disease may be precipitated by adverse environmental effects, which include any 'stress' acting upon the fish either from change in the physical environment or from management of the fish themselves, including handling, grading, crowding and even the administration of treatment compounds.

Direct Environmental Effects

Temperature

A sudden rise or fall in water temperature is a direct stress: survival rate and the ability to combat disease are much lower outside the optimum temperature range of the fish. High temperatures also result in a fall in dissolved oxygen in the water which may cause respiratory distress, particularly if the respiratory capabilities of the fish are already compromised by the presence of established gill disease. This situation can lead to acute mortalities

FIG. 6.1 The major presenting signs of disease in fish and some of their common causes. Several disease symptoms (inappetence, lethargy, darkening) are common to a great many diseases; they are of little use in differential diagnosis and are not included here. The list is not exhaustive and should only be considered as a guide to possible causes.

CLINICAL SIGNS AND COMMON CAUSES

Clinical signs	Common causes
Sudden death of many fish with few preceeding symptoms	Low dissolved oxygen Exogenous toxins Peracute bacterial disease Malicious poisoning
Respiratory distress (gasping, crowding at inlets)	Low dissolved oxygen Gill parasites Environmental gill disease Bacterial gill disease Gill mycosis Water borne toxins Anaemia
Irritation (jumping, flashing, rubbing)	Ectoparasites Environmental irritants/toxins
Overproduction of gill and/or skin mucus (blue slime disease)	Ectoparasites Environmental irritants/toxins
White spots in skin	*Ichthyophthirius*
White or discoloured 'cotton-wool' patches on skin	*Saprolegnia* infection *Cytophaga* infection
Swellings of the skin	Parasitic cysts Physical damage Tumours
Growths on the skin	Tumours or viral infection (papilloma, pox, lymphocystis)
Haemorrhages of the scales, fins	Bacterial infection Viral infection
Skin lesions/ulcers	Nutritional imbalance Physical damage Predation Cannibalism Ectoparasitism (often with secondary infection of damaged areas) Systematic bacterial disease Sunburn
Fin rot	Physical damage Overstocking Cannibalism *Cytophaga* infection *Saprolegnia* infection Ectoparasites Nutritional imbalance
Corneal opacity	Gas-bubble trauma Physical damage Poor water quality Nutritional imbalance Gas-bubble trauma
Cataract	Eye fluke Eye fluke
Skeletal deformities	Nutritional imbalance Genetic abnormalities Nutritional imbalance Toxins Incubation temperature shock
Exophthalmus/ascites	Viral/bacterial infection Exogenous toxins Abdominal granulomata/tumours
Visceral haemorrhages Swelling within internal organs	Bacterial/viral infections Parasitic cysts Granulomata Tumours

continued

FIG. 6.1 *continued*.

CLINICAL SIGNS AND COMMON CAUSES	
Clinical signs	**Common causes**
White/grey swellings within kidney	BKD PKD Fungal, bacterial granulomata Nephrocalcinosis

and highlights the complex relationship between the environment and the manifestation of disease.

A sudden temperature change can precipitate outbreaks of infectious disease, perhaps because the pathogen adapts more rapidly than the immune system of the fish to the changes in temperature. Sudden temperature changes during egg incubation (temperature shock) can result in developmental abnormalities in the fish.

pH

There is an optimum pH range outside which most fish will be stressed. There will be a degree of adaptation to abnormal pH values, however, and it is not unusual to find fish populations surviving at values far outside the optimum, especially at higher pH. The most damaging situation is a sudden change in pH and this can occur particularly in areas affected by acid rain where a flush of low-pH water can enter the aquaculture facility. This is illustrated dramatically in areas where accumulated acid snow melts and there is a sudden flush of acid water through the system. The principal effect is acute gill damage with respiratory distress and death; there may also be damage to the skin, fins and cornea and possibly long-term effects on physiology and growth in surviving fish.

The severity of the effect of acid water is frequently increased by the presence of aluminium and possibly other metal ions which have been brought into solution by the acid water. The aluminium ion is at its most toxic at the pH values encountered during these episodes and greatly exacerbates the effect on the fish.

Because of the great buffering capabilities of sea water, there are no significant problems with changes in pH in marine culture.

Gas-bubble Trauma

Gas-bubble trauma occurs when fish are exposed to water which has become supersaturated with air (atmospheric nitrogen). This can occur when air is forced into the water under pressure (e.g. when air is sucked into a system through cracked or leaking pipes), when water is heated and becomes supersaturated, or when fish are transported in tanks with strong aeration and no means of escape for excess gas. Small nitrogen bubbles form within the tissues of the fish and these can often be observed under the skin, in the eyes or in the fins. Depending upon the severity of the supersaturation, there may be acute mortalities through gas embolism or, at lower levels of supersaturation, chronic damage to the gill, eyes and other tissues.

Suspended Solids

The presence of particulate matter in the water can cause irritation to the gill epithelium and result in significant pathological changes and respiratory problems. The severity of the pathology varies with the nature and quantity of the particles involved. The most damaging are hard, angular or needle-shaped particles which may be introduced by heavy rainfall, rivers in spate etc. Overfeeding and high levels of fish faeces in the water will cause a general deterioration in water quality and also contribute to the suspended solids.

Gill Problems

The gill is vulnerable to attack from a large number of agents and gill disease is a very common

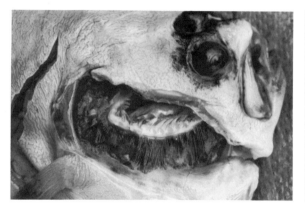

FIG. 6.2 Gill necrosis in turbot due to exposure to chlorine.

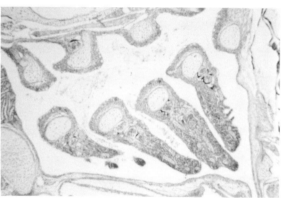

FIG. 6.3 Environmental gill disease of Atlantic salmon parr, showing accumulted debris and myxobacteria within the gill cavity and chronic proliferative change of the gill epithelium (H + E × 40).

cause of losses in aquaculture, particularly in the early stages of a fish's life-cycle.

The majority of the insults to the gill, whether environmental, parasitic or bacterial, give rise to very similar pathology and hence a similar clinical picture. This ranges from sudden high levels of mortality from a severe acute insult (e.g. a flush of chlorine through the system; Fig. 6.2) to long-standing reduction in respiratory capacity due to chronic, low level damage causing low grade losses (e.g. persistent poor water quality due to high levels of suspended solids).

In acute cases the pathology is limited to an increase in mucus production (which may be noted grossly) with necrosis and swelling (hypertrophy) of the gill epithelium. In surviving fish this pathology is reversible when the insult is removed but if the damaging element persists chronic, hyperplastic pathology of the gill epithelium develops which can result in extreme thickening of the gill tissue and severe reduction in the ability of the fish to carry out gaseous exchange (Fig. 6.3).

The skin is subject to similar attacks and responds in a very similar way to the gill.

Endogenous Toxins

This refers to the toxic effect that the waste from the fish themselves can have on their health. The principal concern here is with nitrogous waste products — ammonia and nitrite — which will lead to death or chronic gill pathology unless they are maintained at acceptable levels appropriate water treatment. High levels of carbon dioxide in the water can lead to nephrocalcinosis, a condition in which insoluble calcium salts are deposited in the kidney causing extensive kidney damage and failure.

Exogenous Toxins

These are the countless compounds which may be introduced into the water and have a toxic effect. Many have been described, but the short-term and long-term effects on fish are poorly understood. In general there are acute mortalities from high levels of the toxin, either as a direct effect or because the toxin causes an acute reduction of dissolved oxygen. The most frequently encountered pathology is gill and skin damage, as described above, along with acute or chronic liver and, to a lesser extent, kidney pathology. Several categories of compounds are toxic to fish.

Effluents. Industrial, agricultural and domestic wastes often cause problems by depleting oxygen.

Metals. High levels of metals may be found naturally in some waters or are present in industrial and agricultural wastes; they can cause extreme acute or chronic gill and liver damage.

Organic toxins and industrial wastes. (Petrochemicals etc.) A large number of these can cause a wide variety of pathological changes. This category also includes the toxins produced by algal blooms which can cause complete 'fish kills'.

Gases. Chlorine, hydrogen sulphide etc. mainly cause gill pathology.

Biocides. Pesticides, algicides etc. are extremely toxic to fish. Malicious poisoning with agents such as cyanide is not unknown.

Therapeutic agents. Treatments used for fish are frequently toxic themselves.

Sunburn

Ultraviolet radiation has been implicated in skin damage and ulceration in a number of species. This damage makes the fish more susceptible to secondary bacterial and fungal infection. Sunburn is thought to be a significant contributor to summer lesion syndrome (SLS) in salmon — a severe ulcerative skin disease with bacterial (*Vibrio*) infection, which can be very refractory to treatment.

Predation

Most fish farms are susceptible to predation by many species of animal and bird. This can result in very large losses of fish from direct damage and also from the stress caused by the attack. Seal attacks in caged salmon cause high numbers of fish to be lost from bite wounds and also from consequent outbreaks of bacterial disease. Many predators carry the larval or adult stages of fish parasites and may also act as mechanical vectors of disease.

Physical Damage

Fish are very susceptible to damage caused by a variety of management procedures such as netting, handling, grading and injecting. The epidermis and scales are easily removed during these procedures, leaving areas open to invasion by secondary bacterial and fungal infection and causing a breach in the 'waterproof' protection of the skin. This can lead to the development of deep ulcerated areas and a failure of osmoregulatory control. Similar damage can occur with storms, floods and overcrowding.

It is important that handling is minimised and appropriate prophylactic measures are considered when carrying out essential management procedures.

Nutritional Disease

There can be a wide variation in the quality of the diet received by farmed fish. Factors include the poor availability of suitable constituents, poor formulation and processing, lack of knowledge and understanding of dietary requirements, or inappropriate storage. The formulation, quality and consistency of some fish diets (especially those for salmonids) are probably much better than for species whose aquaculture is in the early stages of development or in countries where appropriate constituents are not available. However, problems can still occur with well established diets.

Starvation

Starvation can occur for a number of reasons other than obvious underfeeding (which is usually due to an incorrect assessment of the weight of fish receiving the food). It may result from the presentation of a feed of inappropriate physical characteristics — usually when the size of the individual particle (pellet or crumb) is too large for the size of fish, or possibly if the feed is too hard or sinks too quickly through the water. Signs of starvation are easy to spot and include loss of condition and weight, 'ill-thrift' and a failure to reproduce. There may be an increase in cannibalism, ranging from fin nipping to attempts to swallow whole fish (particularly very young ones). If the 'wrong' feed is being given, it may be taken by the fish but then rapidly 'spat out', so that there is a build-up of uneaten feed on the bottom of the tank.

Starvation may affect only a proportion of fish in a group if there is a significant size disparity within the population; there is a strong feeding hierarchy which becomes more emphasised as size differences increase. The dominant fish receive more feed than those lower in the 'pecking order' and, consequently, the size difference increases. Again this can lead to aggressive behaviour and cannibalism by the larger fish in the group. The problem can be corrected by grading the fish into groups of similar size and by attention to feeding technique, ensuring that all fish have access to the feed.

Imbalances of Specific Dietary Constituents

Signs of starvation will also be seen if there is a deficiency of certain essential nutrients, e.g. an essential amino acid or vitamin. The nutritional value of the diet will be limited by the level of the specific nutrient.

Protein

The natural feeds of fish are normally protein-rich, although this varies greatly with the species. Deficiency of protein or essential amino acids (of which ten have been identified in fish) will normally result in retarded growth and symptoms similar to those seen in starvation.

Imbalances may occur when formulating diets using constituents deficient in, or containing an excess of, one or more amino acids. A small number of pathologies have been linked with a specific amino acid deficiency (e.g. cataract in methionine and/or tryptophan deficiency, and spinal deformity also associated with tryptophan deficiency and possibly other amino acids such as lysine); however, it would be very difficult to identify these deficiencies precisely in normal farming conditions.

Lipids

The feeding of excess fat, diets deficient in essential fatty acids and diets containing oxidised fat can all result in pathological conditions. The ability of a fish to store and metabolise excess dietary fats varies greatly with species: it is limited in salmonids and an excess can lead to fatty infiltration of the liver with the possible consequences of liver, kidney and blood disorders, and an increased susceptibility to stress and disease. Diets deficient in essential fatty acids can result in retarded growth, fatty livers and fin erosion.

The most important pathology associated with

lipids is that caused by an intake of rancid (oxidised) fat. Fish diets contain a very high level of unsaturated fatty acids and these are very prone to oxidation, which can occur when there is insufficient anti-oxidant in the diet (vitamins E and C are important anti-oxidants) or when the diet is stored in damp, warm conditions. Lipid oxidation results in the production of compounds such as peroxides and free radicals, which are toxic to the fish and also reduce the nutritional value of other dietary constituents. The toxins cause liver and kidney pathology and extreme anaemia. Symptoms associated with this 'liver lipoid disease' include pallor of the gills, darkening of the skin, the presence of a swollen, fatty, pale liver and often ascites and popeye. Mortalities can be high in severe cases.

Minerals

Experimentally induced mineral deficiencies have caused several pathological conditions in a number of species but under natural conditions very few diseases have been linked to specific mineral imbalances. Those which have been recognised include zinc-deficiency cataracts in trout and carp (cataracts can also be caused by an excess of calcium and phosphorus), goitre in various salmonids caused by iodine deficiency and iron-deficient anaemias. Other mineral deficiencies have been said to cause anorexia, poor growth and other relatively non-specific symptoms.

Vitamins

Figure 6.4 shows the problems associated with vitamin deficiencies.

Dietary Toxicity

Many toxic components of fish diets have been identified. Calcium, in addition to cataract production, can cause the formation of mineralised granulomata within tissues and has been implicated in nephrocalcinosis (see Endogenous Toxins, above). Organic compounds include mycotoxins (e.g. aflatoxins — see Neoplasia below), algal and bacterial toxins (e.g. botulinum toxin). Intentional additives which are potentially toxic include binders and therapeutic compounds. Contaminating toxins

FIG. 6.4 Problems of vitamin deficiency.

PROBLEMS OF VITAMIN DEFICIENCY	
Vitamin	**Symptoms of deficiency**
Water-soluble	
Ascorbic acid (vitamin C)	'Brittle bones' and skeletal deformities
	Poor wound healing
Thiamine (vitamin B$_1$)	Poor growth and nervous symptoms
Riboflavin (vitamin B$_2$)	Cataract and corneal opacity
	Pigmentation abnormalities
	Poor growth
	Fin erosion
Pantothenic acid	'Clubbing' of gill filaments (nutritional gill disease)
Pyridoxine	Nervous symptoms
	Poor growth
Vitamin B$_{12}$	Blood dyscrasias
Folic acid	Blood dyscrasias.
The conditions reported to be caused by deficiencies of other water-soluble vitamins are too non-specific (poor growth, haemorrhages etc.) to indicate precise causes. Water-soluble vitamins can be readily leached from the diet in the water — vitamin C is particularly susceptible — and substantial amounts can be lost before the diet is taken by the fish. This is usually anticipated by the manufacturers, who incorporate high levels of the vitamins in the diet.	
Fat-soluble	
Vitamin A	Blindness
	Pigmentation abnormalities
Vitamin D	Few specific deficiency signs reported
	Fatty liver
Vitamin E	Muscular dystrophy
	Steatitis
	Possibly associated with pancreas disease in Atlantic salmon
Vitamin K	Haemorrhage

may include petrochemicals, heavy metals and pesticides.

Neoplasia

All cell types are capable of neoplastic transformation and tumours of the majority of fish tissues have been described. As neoplasms occur more frequently with the increasing age of the individual and usually affect very small numbers in a population, they are generally of little concern when dealing with farmed fish involving large numbers of relatively young animals. There are, however, a few neoplastic conditions which are of importance in aquaculture.

Papillomata

Skin neoplasms (ranging from benign epidermal hyperplasia to very invasive carcinomata) are the most frequently reported fish neoplasms, probably because they are easy to see. Atlantic salmon and carp can be affected by epizootics of papillomata, frequently called salmon pox and carp pox (Fig. 6.5), which can affect a large proportion of the population.

Salmon papilloma usually affects freshwater parr and can be carried over when the fish are transferred to sea. The problem appears in the

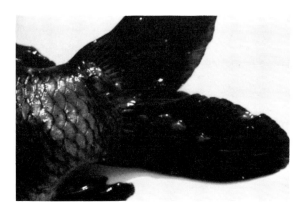

FIG. 6.5 Carp papilloma (carp pox).

summer as off-white warts, which usually disappear in the winter; ulceration is frequent and, although not considered a serious condition, secondary infection with fungus and bacteria increase the severity of the lesions and could result in losses.

Carp papillomata often appear like blobs of jelly or candle wax on the skin of the fish. They too, usually develop in the summer and regress as water temperatures fall; ulceration and secondary infection can sometimes be severe. Recurrence of the condition the following year is not uncommon.

Flatfish and eels also suffer epizootics of papillomata. Eels frequently develop the lesions around the mouth (cauliflower disease), which can prevent feeding. Viruses are implicated as causes in all these cases and with the eel and flatfish there is strong evidence that pollution is a significant contributory factor.

Hepatoma

Outbreaks of liver neoplasia have been experienced in rainbow trout culture due to the ingestion

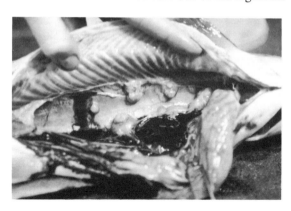

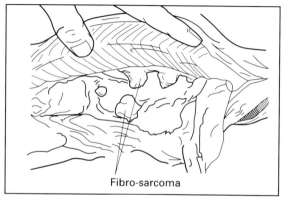

Fibro-sarcoma

FIG. 6.6 Swim-bladder fibro-sarcoma in Atlantic salmon.

of aflatoxin cause by the contamination of feed by the fungus *Aspergillus flavus*. Rainbow trout are particularly susceptible to the toxin but other species are also affected. The resulting neoplasm (strictly a hepatocarcinoma) causes extreme enlargement of the liver, which becomes very friable and haemorrhagic; the tumour is very invasive and metastases can occur. The condition is rare where attention is paid to the quality and storage of food but is a problem with some cultured species such as tilapia, in which aflatoxins are thought to cause neoplasia of a variety of tissues.

Swim-bladder fibroma

Outbreaks of tumours of the swim-bladder in Atlantic salmon (Fig. 6.6) have caused loss of condition and swimming ability (see viruses).

Infectious Disease

Virus Diseases

Dozens of different viruses and viral-like particles have been identified in fish, not all associated with disease conditions. There are several conditions where virus involvement is suspected but, as yet, unproven — including several of the neoplasms and pancreas disease in Atlantic salmon.

Some of the virus infections are of great economic importance in aquaculture. A number are notifiable diseases and a great effort is made to prevent the spread of these viruses into other countries, farms or fish stocks. The source of infection is usually from farmed or wild asymptomatic carriers in the watercourse: virus shedding and clinical disease may not be seen until the fish become stressed by movement, crowding, temperature rise, etc. Viruses can be carried by non-susceptible species of fish and probably by other aquatic animals and birds; and the movement of these, along with movement of susceptible species between different watercourses, plays an important part in the epizootiology of infection.

Transmission can be horizontal between fish where the principal routes of infection are skin abrasions, the gill and the gut; or vertical through the egg from infected broodstock to their offspring.

The most economically important virus diseases

are detailed below, categorised by the principal species affected.

Salmonid Viruses

Infectious pancreatic necrosis (IPN)

Classically a serious disease of first-feeding trout fry, IPN can occur when asymptomatic carriers become stressed from crowding, transportation etc. (stress-mediated IPN). The virus has a worldwide distribution and can be carried in many freshwater and marine fish other than salmonids and also in invertebrates.

Outbreaks of disease in rainbow trout growers in the sea and post-smolt Atlantic salmon have been attributed to IPN but the involvement of the virus in clinical disease in salmon and its relationship to pancreas disease is still very unclear. The virus has several serotypes and the severity of the disease will vary with the serotype involved, the age and species of fish concerned and the environmental conditions.

Clinical signs include inappetence, darkening, ascites and exophthalmia, loss of equilibrium and trailing faecal casts. On post-mortem, ascitic fluid is present and the gut is usually filled with a white exudate; there may occasionally be haemorrhages over the viscera. Mortality levels can be very high — up to 90% in very young first feeders — but the disease becomes less severe with the increasing age of the fish.

Pathology is restricted to necrosis and inflammation of the exocrine pancreas accompanied by necrosis of the gut mucosa. Diagnosis is based on clinical signs, typical pancreatic pathology and isolation of the virus. Control relies on the use of disease-free fish for stocking and broodstock (the virus can be carried on, and probably within, the egg) and rearing of young in water uncontaminated by other farmed or wild fish.

Infectious haematopoietic necrosis (IHN)

A disease affecting several Pacific salmon and trout species in North America, IHN has also been isolated in Europe (but not the UK). It is usually confined to very young fish, in which mortality levels can approach 100%. Temperature has a marked effect on the progress of IHN: at 10°C the disease is acute, with the highest losses experienced; below 10°C the disease is more chronic, with fewer losses.

Clinical signs include very erratic swimming, darkening, ascites and exophthalmos. Haemorrhages of the fins and head tissues may be seen; the fish may appear anaemic. On post-mortem there is frequently ascitic fluid which may be haemorrhagic, the liver is often pale, the kidney may appear swollen and there may be visceral haemorrhages. Histopathology shows a necrosis of the haematopoietic tissues of the kidney and spleen and focal necrosis of other tissues. Destruction of the eosinophilic granular layer of the intestine is a specific finding.

Transmission of the virus can be horizontal and also vertical within the egg. Control relies on detecting and avoiding infected potential broodstock and avoiding contaminated water sources.

Viral haemorrhagic septicaemia (VHS)

This is an acute to chronic disease of rainbow trout throughout several countries of Europe, though not the UK. Chronically infected farmed and wild trout are the most common source of infection; other wild fish species may act as reservoirs of the virus.

The clinical appearance of the disease varies considerably. There is an acute haemorrhagic condition with gross signs of high mortality, darkening, exophthalmia and anaemia; internally haemorrhages are seen in the muscle and viscera which, along with some tissue necrosis, is the main histological finding. In a chronic form, with lower mortality, the fish are usually extremely dark with pronounced ascites and exophthalmia; internally the kidney and spleen appear very swollen and the liver pale. Outbreaks will show a clinical picture varying between these two conditions. The disease is most severe in trout up to six months of age; it can occur in older fish but mortalities are much lower.

Transmission is thought to be horizontal from asymptomatic carriers in the water course; there is no evidence for vertical transmission and control relies upon the use of uninfected stock, avoiding infected water sources and regular testing.

Atlantic salmon fibrosarcoma virus

A small number of cases of fibrosarcoma of the swim-bladder in Atlantic salmon have been recorded in Scotland. Outbreaks occur in growers in sea cages and affect a high percentage of the population. Large multiple growths appear to affect the function of the swim-bladder and cause difficulties with swimming ability and loss of condition; there is evidence to suggest that there is a greater susceptibility to stress and bath treatments against sea lice. Outbreaks of the condition seem to occur almost spontaneously in sites which have not experienced the problem for several years. Electron miscrocopy and transmission studies indicate a viral aetiology but isolation of the virus has yet to be recorded.

Atlantic salmon papilloma virus

This condition is described under Neoplasia.

Erythrocytic inclusion body syndrome (EIBS)

Virus infections causing the formation of inclusion bodies in erythrocytes have been recorded in several countries including California (Coho salmon), Norway, Ireland and Scotland (Atlantic salmon). The condition was thought to cause anaemia in Coho salmon but erythrocytic inclusions are quite commonly seen on examination of Giemsa-stained blood films from salmon and it is difficult to correlate their presence with clinical disease.

Carp Viruses

Virus infections are involved in a group of conditions affecting carp which are collectively known as the carp dropsy syndrome. The syndrome is complex and involves both viral and bacterial infection (see *Aeromonas*: carp erythrodermatitis) but two specific viral conditions have been identified: spring viraemia or carp (SVC) and swim-bladder inflammation (SBI).

Spring viraemia of carp

SVC affects a number of species of wild, farmed and ornamental carp in several European countries.

Serious outbreaks of the infection occurred in stocks of carp in the UK in the late 1980s due to the importation of infected ornamental fish, which emphasises the need for strict control, testing and quarantine of imported fish destined both for aquaculture and for ornamental purposes.

The condition is characterised by extreme abdominal distension with exophthalmos and swelling of the vent. There is usually a loss in swimming ability, skin darkening, and haemorrhage of the gills, skin and vent. Internally there is marked ascites and peritonitis with petechial haemorrhages of the internal organs. Secondary bacterial infection is common. The condition is usually seen as water temperatures begin to rise in the spring and is most severe when fish are crowded and suffer any physical damage.

Control lies in excluding infected fish from the water course; antibiotic treatment may be of value in controlling secondary bacterial infection.

Swim-bladder inflammation

SBI shares the same gross signs as SVC but there is an obvious inflammation of the swim-bladder with congestion of its blood vessels, haemorrhage and pathology and sloughing of the swim-bladder wall. The condition affects a range of carp species throughout Europe.

Carp papilloma (carp pox)

This condition has already been described under Neoplasia.

Catfish Viruses

Channel catfish virus (CCV)

This disease affects fry and fingerling catfish during the summer throughout the southern United States. The virus appears to affect only ictalurid species, primarily the channel catfish. Fish are thought to be infected by older carriers shedding virus into the water; fry are probably also infected through the egg from infected broodstock.

Clinical signs include erratic swimming, nervous signs and hanging vertically and motionless in the water. There are usually haemorrhages of the fins and the skin of the ventral surface, with abdominal distension and exophthalmos. Internally the viscera are very haemorrhagic and the abdomen is filled with a yellow exudate. Secondary bacterial or fungal infection is common.

Control rests with avoidance of contaminated stocks and water but vaccination could be a future possibility.

Other Virus Diseases

Lymphocystis disease virus (LDV)

This virus causes the formation of multiple nodular skin and fin lesions (Fig. 6.7) on many species of marine and freshwater fish. The pearl-like lesions — lymphocysts — are giant cells formed from virus-infected fibroblasts. Where lymphocysts are seen on mesentery and peritoneum, there can also be systemic infection as the nodules eventually slough and the lesions heal. Although mortality from the disease is generally low, it can cause significant problems in marine aquaculture (e.g. sea-bream cage culture) where a large number of fish can suffer high levels of infection with a consequent loss in performance, unsightly appearance, the possibility of secondary bacterial infection and mortalities. As the disease is thought to be transmitted through skin abrasions, relatively high stocking density and more frequent handling predisposes these fish to infection. The only control available is the isolation and restriction of movement of infected fish.

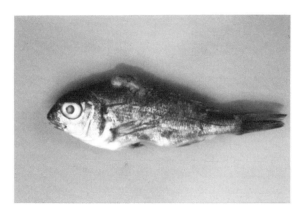

FIG. 6.7 Epitheliocystis lesions on dorsum of gilthead sea-bream.

Turbot herpes virus

This causes giant cell formation on the skin and gills of young turbot, resulting in gill pathology and high mortalities.

Oncorhynchus masou virus

This causes severe liver pathology in Masou salmon in Japan.

Snakehead rhabdovirus

This is thought to contribute to severe epizootics of ulcerative disease in a number of south-east Asian fish species, including striped snakehead.

Bacterial Diseases

The majority of bacteria causing disease are normal saprophytes of the fish and its environment. Several may be found on the surface or in the gut of the fish but only cause clinical disease when the fish is compromised by 'stress' or the presence of other disease. One or two species can be regarded as true obligate pathogens relying on the presence of fish for long-term survival but even with these, outbreaks of clinical disease usually occur only when the fish is stressed in some way. Overcrowding, temperature change, handling, grading and predator attack are some of the stressful conditions that can result in an outbreak of bacterial disease.

A large number of pathogenic bacteria are Gram-negative rods giving rise to very similar clinical disease — invariably a haemorrhagic septi-caemia with or without skin ulcers. It is often necessary, therefore, to carry out detailed laboratory analysis to identify the precise cause of the disease.

A small number of Gram-positive bacteria cause significant disease in some fish species. Acid-fasts have occasionally been identified as the cause of chronic granulomatous disease and some disease conditions have been shown to be caused by rickettsia and chlamydia.

Figure 6.8 gives a basic classification of the families of bacteria pathogenic to farmed fish.

FIG. 6.8 Bacteria pathogenic to farmed fish.

BACTERIA PATHOGENIC TO FARMED FISH		
Family	**Genus**	**Example of disease condition commonly caused by the genus**
Gram-negative		
Vibrionaceae	*Aeromonas, Vibrio*	Furunculosis, vibriosis
Pseudomonadaceae	*Pseudomonas*	Pseudomonad septicaemia
Enterobacteriaceae	*Yersinia, Edwardsiella*	Enteric red mouth
Pasteurellaceae	*Pasteurella*	Pseudotuberculosis
Cytophagaceae	*Cytophaga*	Cold-water disease
		Bacterial gill disease
Gram-positive		
Coryneform group	*Renibacterium*	Bacterial kidney disease
Streptococcaceae	*Streptococcus*	
Mycobacteriaceae	*Mycobacterium*	Piscine TB
Bacillaceae	*Clostridium*	

Aeromonas

This genus contains one of the most important salmonid pathogens: *Aeromonas salmonicida*, the causative agent of furunculosis (Figs 6.9 and 6.10).

A. salmonicida is a non-motile obligate pathogen. (Other pathogenic aeromonads are motile.) It can survive for several weeks outside the host, particularly in association with remnants of fish tissue and other organic material. The infection is usually introduced by the movement of infected fish into a culture facility or by wild carriers shedding bacteria into the watercourse, but fish tissue, equipment and 'escapees' moving from infected sites may also be important in transmitting the disease.

All salmonids are susceptible to furunculosis but the Atlantic salmon is the most susceptible and rainbow trout the most resistant species. The disease has a virtually world-wide distribution, although Australasia has so far maintained a furunculosis-free status.

Clinical manifestation of the disease varies from acute to chronic depending on the age and species of fish concerned, the strain of bacterium involved and the environmental conditions. Younger fish are more likely to suffer the acute form of the disease when there may be few clinical signs other than a rapid loss of appetite, darkening and acute mortality. Less acute cases show signs typical of haemorrhagic septicaemia: internal organs are haemorrhagic, and haemorrhages are frequently seen at the bases of fins, at the vent and beneath scales. Small, haemorrhagic skin lesions may be seen, but classic 'furuncles' (swollen, boil-like skin lesions which rupture to release bloody, bacteria-rich fluid) are usually seen only in older fish suffering more chronic infection.

Histopathology in acute cases may show little more than limited necrosis of tissues, while sub-acute and chronic cases typically show the presence of accumulations of bacteria in many tissues with accompanying necrosis but little inflammatory response.

Diagnosis of furunculosis is based on clinical signs, histopathology and the laboratory isolation of *A. salmonicida* from affected specimens. The isolation of the bacterium and an assessment of its antibiotic sensitivity pattern is extremely important if effective therapy is to be achieved. Control of the disease relies partly on preventing the movement of infected fish into non-infected

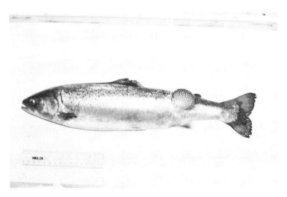

FIG. 6.9 Furunculosis — Atlantic salmon showing classic 'furuncle'.

(a)

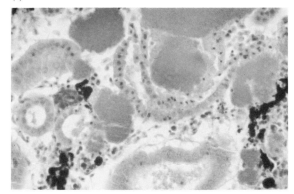

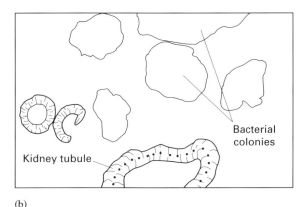

(b)

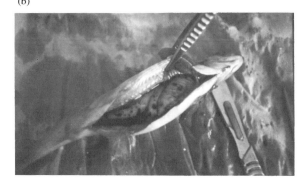

FIG. 6.10 (a) Furunculosis—colonies of *Aeromonas salmonicida* in kidney (H + E × 100). (b) Visceral haemorrhages in acute furunculosis Atlantic salmon.

sites (the stocking of infected smolts in the sea has led to major outbreaks of furunculosis in salmon sea cage sites) although this does not avoid the possibility of wild carriers introducing infection into the watershed. Separating stocks and reducing handling stress also helps in control.

The existence of asymptomatic carrier fish in infected populations makes control more difficult

as there is no 100% effective means of detecting these carriers. The stress-induced furunculosis test (SIF test) will, however, give an indication of furunculosis status and helps in assessing the risk of moving and stocking the fish into a clean site. The test involves administering cortisone to the fish and subjecting them to heat stress; this procedure 'uncovers' latent infection and, although not foolproof, does give some idea of the level of infection in the fish.

The disease is usually treated with oral administration of antibiotics but the emergence of resistance to available antibiotics is an increasing problem. Antibiotic therapy will not rid a population of carriers and a site must be considered endemically infected once the infection has established. Removal of all stocks and fallowing a site significantly reduces the risk of subsequent disease outbreaks. Vaccines against furunculosis have been available for a number of years; their effectiveness continues to improve and their use should play an important role in the control of this disease in the future.

A. salmonicida has been isolated from many non-salmonid species, both freshwater and marine, and has caused outbreaks of disease in some of these species. Atypical strains of the organism have been isolated from outbreaks of ulcerative disease (Fig. 6.11) in salmonids and non-salmonids and are responsible for so-called ulcer disease in brook trout and rainbow trout in the USA and carp erythrodermatitis in Europe.

Ulcer disease. Originally attributed to infection with *Haemophilus piscium* but now recognised as

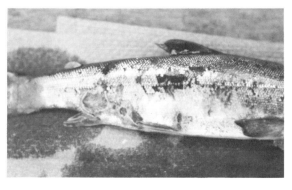

FIG. 6.11 Skin ulceration in atypical furunculosis due to achromogenic *Aeromonas salmonicida*.

an atypical *A. salmonicida*. The condition is characterised by the development of shallow ulcers, typically with a white rim and a dark centre, over the body of the fish. The fins, tail and mouth may also become ulcerated and there may be an accompanying haemorrhagic septicaemia.

Carp erythrodermatitis (CE) has been included in the carp dropsy syndrome (see Viruses) but should really be considered as a separate bacterial disease. It is an important condition of European carp culture, occurring in early summer, and is usually restricted to the skin, although systemic disease can occur which may result in mortalities. Crowding and traumatic damage predispose to the disease. Superficial infection with atypical *A. salmonicida* (probably through minor skin damage) causes small, haemorrhagic lesions which gradually develop into large skin ulcers, usually over the flanks of the fish. Secondary bacterial and fungal infection of the lesions is common. Although mortality levels are usually low, the ulcers heal as unsightly scars and may cause severe deformity which reduces the value of the fish.

Aeromonas hydrophila is a motile bacterium responsible for significant outbreaks of haemorrhagic septicaemia in freshwater fish. A typical opportunist pathogen, it is ubiquitous in the aquatic environment, particularly in water with high organic loading, but only causes outbreaks of disease in fish suffering stress, damage or primary infection. Control involves improving water quality, removal of stress, and antibiotic treatment.

Vibrio

Several species of *Vibrio* are responsible for haemorrhagic septicaemias in marine fish. They have also been reported in fresh water in some countries (e.g. in rainbow trout in Italy). *Vibrio anguillarum* (and its various serotypes) is a primary fish pathogen responsible for serious epizootics (vibriosis) in many farmed and wild marine species including eels, salmon, turbot and cod. The bacterium may be found extensively in marine and brackish water and is likely to be carried in the gut of wild fish; outbreaks of vibriosis may be associated with the shedding of the bacterium from wild fish in the vicinity of fish farms.

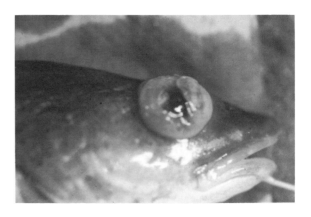

FIG. 6.12 Vibriosis in cod showing exophthalmos.

Other *Vibrio* species frequently act as opportunistic pathogens causing disease in fish which are stressed in some way — most frequently infecting fish which have been damaged by storms, handling etc.

Vibriosis (Fig. 6.12) can be acute or chronic in nature. The acute condition in young fish often shows little, if any, clinical signs other than darkening and anorexia. Older fish will usually exhibit typical haemorrhagic septicaemia accompanied by deep, haemorrhagic skin/muscle lesions and destruction of internal tissues due to toxin production by the bacterium. Secondary infections of damaged areas with *Vibrio* spp. usually result in the development of extensive ulcerative lesions with subsequent bacteraemia and osmotic imbalance due to the resulting skin deficit. Secondary *Vibrio* infections have been implicated in the development of severe ulcerations in newly-transferred Atlantic salmon smolts. The lesions are frequently seen adjacent to the pectoral fin and it is thought that the action of the fin (possibly already eroded) causes erosion of the skin surface allowing a *Vibrio* infection to establish. Consequent lesions frequently penetrate the abdominal cavity.

'Winter sore' is a condition seen in salmon growers in Norway and some parts of Scotland. The condition is seen at low water temperatures and results in extensive skin loss, most frequently in the area of the caudal peduncle. A primary cause has yet to be established but *Vibrio* infection is probably a significant contributory factor.

Diagnosis of vibriosis is based on the clinical appearance of the disease, histopathology showing the tissue necrosis typical of a septicaemia, and the laboratory isolation and identification of the bacterium.

In Norway, *Vibrio salmonicida* is thought to be a major contributing factor in Hitra disease, a condition causing high losses in Atlantic salmon stocks. The disease is usually seen at low water temperatures and frequently following periods of rough weather when disturbance of the sea bed may occur with a consequent fall in water quality. Affected fish are dark and anorexic with distinct haemorrhages of the viscera, and accompanying ascites and anaemia.

Because of the ubiquity of *Vibrio* species, control of infection is difficult, although there are effective commercial vaccines available. Antibiotic therapy may be successful although in the case of secondary *Vibrio* infections following traumatic damage it is unlikely that the badly damaged fish will consume medicated feed to control infection.

Pseudomonas

Infection with *Pseudomonas fluorescens* usually occurs in conditions of poor water quality, crowding, physical damage or other 'stresses' and results in a haemorrhagic septicaemia identical to that seen with *Aeromonas* septicaemias. The bacterium has a world-wide distribution in fresh and salt water and it is likely that all fish species are susceptible, although it is most frequently seen in pond culture when fish are stressed by poor environmental conditions. The disease can have an acute or chronic course with large, haemorrhagic skin lesions and haemorrhages of internal tissues being the most frequently encountered clinical signs.

Diagnosis is based on the clinical appearance of haemorrhagic septicaemia and the specific identification of the causative agent in the laboratory. Antibiotic therapy may be used, but the most effective form of control is to improve environmental conditions, and reduce crowding and physical damage to the fish.

P. anguilliseptica is a significant pathogen of Japanese eels causing ulcerative haemorrhagic septicaemia.

Yersinia

Yersinia ruckeri is the causative agent of enteric redmouth (ERM), a serious haemorrhagic septi-caemia found in most areas where rainbow trout are cultured. Although infection is most severe and widespread in rainbow trout, other salmonids are susceptible and outbreaks of the disease have been seen in Atlantic salmon culture. The bacterium is present as part of the gut flora in carrier fish and non-salmonid carriers are likely to be important in the epizootiology of the disease. The condition is typical of a Gram-negative septicaemia with skin, fin and internal haemorrhages but skin ulceration is not a principal feature. The classic 'redmouth' — congestion, haemorrhage and ulceration of the mouth — is often *not* seen. More chronic cases may show extreme darkening, exophthalmia and blindness.

Diagnosis is based on clinical signs, histopathology typical of haemorrhagic septicaemia and the isolation of *Y. ruckeri* from affected fish. Antibiotic therapy is usually successful and effective commercial vaccines are available.

Edwardsiella

Edwardsiella tarda is the cause of serious disease epizootics in Japanese eels, American catfish and several other cultured fish species including seabream and tilapia. The bacterium is particularly associated with polluted waters. Clinically the fish exhibit small skin lesions which penetrate deep into the underlying muscle. There is rapid necrosis of the affected tissue resulting in the formation of cavities in the muscle which are filled with foul-smelling gas. Internally there is necrosis of the viscera and an accompanying pronounced peritonitis. Epizootics usually occur when water temperatures are relatively high (e.g. 30°C).

Edwardsiella ictaluri is a specific pathogen of channel catfish in southern USA causing severe haemorrhagic septicaemia with affected fish showing small haemorrhagic skin lesions or ulcerations and a loss in swimming ability. The disease is diagnosed from the gross clinical appearance, histopathology of necrotic skin lesions and peritonitis, and the laboratory isolation of the bacterium. Control relies on the use of antibiotic therapy, improving water quality and the isolation or destruction of affected individuals.

Pasteurella

Pasteurella piscicida has been responsible for severe epizootics causing rapid and heavy mortalities in cultured and wild marine fish species in America and Japan. Species affected have included yellow-tail, sea-bream, striped bass and white perch and it is likely that other cultured marine fish will be susceptible. The clinical appearance is of a haemorrhagic septicaemia with the formation of granulomata in the tissues (the condition has been called pseudotuberculosis). Diagnosis is based on clinical signs, histopathology and the isolation of *Pasteurella* in the laboratory. The condition is responsive to antibiotic therapy.

Cytophaga (Flexibacter)

The old name *Flexibacter* is still in common usage: for example, *Cytophaga columnaris = Flexibacter columnaris*. The *Cytophaga* species pathogenic to fish belong to the family Cyto-phagaceae. These bacteria are frequently, but erroneously called the Myxobacteria and are responsible for a wide range of conditions of the external (and occasionally internal) tissues of the fish including columnaris disease, cold-water or peduncle disease, and bacterial gill disease. They contribute significantly to fin and tail rot.

Cytophaga spp. are difficult to culture in the laboratory and diagnosis is usually based on the microscopic examination of fresh material from skin and gill lesions. Control of infections lies in improving environmental conditions, removing primary causes of damage and using surfactant treatments to remove bacteria and damaged tissue.

Cytophaga columnaris is the causative agent of columnaris disease affecting all species of fish in fresh water throughout the world. The bacterium is part of the natural environmental flora and is found associated with the skin and gill mucus in clinically unaffected fish. High levels of organic material and harder, alkaline water favour the bacterium. The disease usually occurs only at high water temperatures (above 20°C) but may occur at lower temperatures with a more virulent strain or more susceptible host. Nutritional deficiencies such as fatty acid deficiency may be predisposing factors.

Disease often occurs in fish which have been damaged in some way by handling, crowding, grading, etc. Small de-scaled or eroded areas become colonised rapidly by the bacteria, forming raised off-white bacterial plaques (frequently looking like cotton wool) which often develop into ulcers. Predilection sites for infection are around the base of the dorsal fin (saddleback lesions), around the mouth and head tissues. There can be a subsequent and fatal septicaemia.

C. columnaris may infect the gill, resulting in severe tissue destruction and high mortality levels.

Cytophaga psychrophila is the most common cause of bacterial fin and tail rot and peduncle disease in the USA. (Other species may be responsible for these conditions in other temperate countries.) It commonly causes disease at water temperatures below 10°C and is sometimes known as cold-water disease. The bacteria usually only invade previously damaged tissue — typically an area of erosion on the edge of the fins or tail. Infection then progresses to involve the complete fin or tail and caudal peduncle. The lesion com-prises high levels of bacteria along with proliferated epithelial tissue and mucus which sloughs to leave significant tissue deficit.

Infection with *Cytophaga* is only a part of the complex syndrome of fin and tail rot. Many environmental, behavioural, nutritional and hus-bandry factors contribute to the initiation and development of these lesions; bacterial involve-ment is usually only a secondary factor and all aspects of the husbandry and management of the fish must be examined if this is identified as a problem.

Other *Cytophaga* infections. *Bacterial (environ-mental) gill disease.* It is also associated with *Cytophaga* species and occurs as a secondary infection of gills previously damaged by an irritant in the water. The irritant may be ammonia produced by the fish themselves or possibly sus-pended solids in the water. The irritant results in initial gill pathology which then becomes colonised by a mixed *Cytophaga* infection resulting in the destruction of gill tissue and the formation of a huge bacterial mass which can be seen grossly on the gill and protruding from the gill cavity.

Marine species, e.g. *Cytophaga maritimus*, have been responsible for skin and fin lesions in several species of marine fish and severe mouth erosion in cage reared sea-bream. Again infection usually only occurs in fish which have suffered physical damage.

Rainbow trout fingerling syndrome (RTFS) seen

in the UK, France and Denmark is thought to be caused by *Cytophaga psychrophila*, at least in part. The condition causes heavy losses of young trout in spring and early summer. Affected fish become dark and anorexic, with exophthalmos, ascites and anaemia. Although *C. psychrophila* is frequently identified as a systemic infection, the aetiology of the condition is still uncertain. There is usually a response to high levels of antibiotic.

Renibacterium

Renibacterium salmoninarum is the causative agent of bacterial kidney disease (BKD) in all salmonid species. It occurs throughout Europe, USA, Canada and Japan usually as a chronic disease but also as an acute infection. The disease is seasonal, increasing as water temperatures rise in spring, becoming less severe at peak temperatures and increasing again as temperatures fall. The bacterium is an obligate intracellular pathogen and vertical transmission within the egg is important in the epizootiology of the disease.

Losses are usually low but prolonged; affected fish are dark and lethargic, frequently with exophthalmus. There are often small ulcerating skin lesions over the flanks. Internally the kidney is usually swollen and grey; multiple small, white miliary lesions may be seen in the kidney, liver, spleen and heart. There may be peritonitis and pericarditis. Pacific salmon may have large muscle cavitation.

Renibacterium salmoninarum is slow growing and fastidious in laboratory culture. Diagnosis is based initially on clinical signs, on the examination of Gram-stained kidney smears for the presence of typical small Gram-positive rods, and histopathology showing distinct cellular (macrophage) response, peritonitis and pericarditis. (It should be noted that this is one of the few Gram-positive organisms seen in aquacultural diseases.) Diagnosis will be confirmed by the laboratory isolation of the bacterium following extended incubation.

Antibiotic therapy is usually unrewarding, although some success has been achieved in administering antibiotic to broodstock prior to spawning. At present, the only realistic method of control is avoidance.

Streptococcus

Streptococcus spp. have been responsible for serious losses in cultured marine (and some freshwater) fish in Japan. Epizootics have occurred in yellowtails, rainbow trout and eels. The clinical appearance is similar to Gram-negative haemorrhagic septicaemias and definitive diagnosis relies on the isolation of the causative agent. There is usually a good response to antibiotic therapy.

Mycobacterium

Mycobacterium spp. have in the past caused significant disease in cultured fish, particularly Pacific salmon. This was principally a result of feeding infected trash fish and the condition has declined dramatically since the cessation of this practice. Occasional *Mycobacterium* granulomata may be identified but this condition (piscine TB) is of far more importance in the ornamental fish industry than in aquaculture.

Clostridium

Clostridium botulinum has been responsible for severe losses of trout reared in earth ponds in Denmark (bankruptcy disease) and very occasionally in other countries. The condition results from fish ingesting the toxin of the bacterium which has formed in the bodies of decaying fish on the bottom of the ponds or from contaminated feed. The condition is extremely rare but emphasises the need for the maintenance of good husbandry standards and hygiene.

Chlamydia and Rickettsia infections

Very few pathogenic chlamydia or rickettsia have ben identified in fish.

Epitheliocystis. Chlamydia are thought to be responsible for the formation of multiple small swellings on the gills and skin of several marine and freshwater species including sea-bream, sea-bass, carp and salmon. The swellings are caused by individual epithelial cells becoming distended by masses of organisms. Infection can be so heavy that there is interference with normal gill function and losses may be high in young fish. There is no known method of control.

The Coho syndrome. High mortalities of up to 70% in stocks of Coho salmon reared in sea cages in Chile have been experienced since the late 1980s. The causative agent of the condition, known as the Coho syndrome, is thought to be a rickettsia, *Piscirickettsia salmonis*. Affected fish are dark and lethargic, and frequently exhibit raised or ulcerated skin lesions. There is often severe anaemia, internal haemorrhages and peritonitis. Attempts at control using antibiotics have had little success.

Fungal Diseases

Only a small number of fungal species are pathogenic to fish. Frequently these are common saprophytes which act as opportunist pathogens in poor environmental conditions, or take advantage of damaged tissues etc.

Saprolegnia

This is the most important freshwater fungal pathogen in fish culture. The fungus is ubiquitous and may affect all fish species, usually acting as a secondary invader of damaged fish or fish which have been compromised by the presence of other disease, malnutrition etc. Predisposing factors include high organic loading in the water, the presence of a large biomass of fish or eggs, and any dead or decaying fish or eggs in which the fungus thrives, greatly increasing the fungal load in the water. *Saprolegnia* infection is usually worse at lower temperatures, probably because the ability of the fish to resist infection is lower and the healing response of damaged areas is slower. Sexually mature fish appear to be more susceptible to skin infection with *Saprolegnia*, possibly due to the hormonally-controlled skin changes at that time.

It is a common infection of egg incubation — the fungus invades any dead eggs and spreads to suffocate and kill adjacent eggs, which can then become invaded by the fungus. *Saprolegnia* can invade any small injury on the fish and commonly occurs after handling or grading. It will also contribute to fin and tail rot and infect ulcerated

areas caused by the presence of other diseases such as furunculosis. The resulting mycelial growth spreads over the surface of the body, causing erosion and ulceration of the underlying tissue. There may be deeper invasion of the underlying tissues, particularly in yolk-sac fry and small fish where spread of the fungus deep into the body can occur. The fungus can invade the gills and may contribute to bacterial/environmental gill disease.

The infection appears as raised white plaques with a 'cotton-wool' appearance. The plaques may be coloured by trapped organic matter and sediment. A frequent finding is fungal infection of dorsal fin rot lesions, spreading down the fin and over the back of the fish around the base of the dorsal fin as a classic saddleback lesion.

Internal *Saprolegnia* has been described in small fish probably as a result of ingesting fungal spores. These germinate in the gut, and the mycelium invades the viscera.

Control relies on good husbandry, the removal of dead fish and eggs and the use of topical fungicides such as malachite green.

Branchiomyces

Species of *Branchiomyces* are responsible for gill rot, an economically important disease of European freshwater fish culture. Although most freshwater fish are susceptible, the disease is most important in carp culture. Branchiomycosis has also been identified in Japan, India and USA.

Organic pollution and poor water quality favour the infection, which is most severe at high water temperatures (20–30°C). Spores attach to gill tissue and the developing mycelium spreads into the gill tissue and capillaries, resulting in necrosis and sloughing of the tissue. The gills take on a marbled and ragged appearance. Affected fish become very lethargic and exhibit respiratory distress. Treatment is impossible and control relies on stocking with uninfected fish, improving water quality and the frequent removal of dead fish.

Ichthyophonus hoferi

This is an important fungal infection of wild marine fish, causing epizootics of granulomatous disease. The infection has occurred in cultured fish following the feeding of infected trash fish but incidence of the disease is now rare.

Other fungal infections

Several other fungal species have been identified as a cause of disease in fish but generally the incidence is low. Systemic infections have been reported with *Aspergillus* spp. (aflatoxin is also responsible for hepatoma formation — see Neoplasia), *Phialophora, Exophiala* and *Phoma* (these occasionally occur as swim-bladder infections in small fish). Occasional granulomata identified as having a fungal cause suggest that the fish has ingested spores in the feed or water. They are not economically significant unless found in high numbers.

Mycotoxins

Apart from aflatoxicosis, very little investigation of the effect of mycotoxins in food or water has been carried out.

Parasitic Diseases

A great number and diversity of animal species are capable of parasitising fish, ranging from microscopic protozoans to grossly visible crustaceans and annelids. A basic classification of fish parasites is presented in Fig. 6.13.

In the wild, there is a large range of parasites but they are usually only present in small numbers; they can be considered a normal finding and rarely cause disease problems. There is a stable relationship between the parasite and the fish host in the wild and regulating systems have evolved to ensure that parasitic burdens do not increase to threaten the life of the host. It is only if these regulating systems become disturbed, often by the action of man, that parasitic disease in the wild may be seen. It must be borne in mind, however, that outbreaks of parasitism in the wild may go unnoticed.

In cultured fish, there is a more limited range of parasites but they are often present in much larger numbers than seen in the wild. There is always a risk of parasitic epizootics in farmed fish and this increases with the intensification of the farm system. Many factors in fish culture will favour parasitic disease; an awareness of these factors will allow remedial or preventative action to be attempted.

CLASSIFICATION OF FISH PARASITES

Ectoparasites

Protozoa
Flagellates: *Oodinium*
 Cryptobia
 Ichthyobodo
Amoebae: *Thecamoeba*
Ciliates: peritrichous (cilia restricted to specific areas of the body)
 Trichodinids
 Scyphidians
 holotrichous (cilia distributed regularly over the body or arranged in rows)
 Ichthyophthirius
 Chilodonella

Metazoa
Monogenean trematodes (flukes):
 Gyrodactylus
 Dactylogyrus
Crustacea:
 Copepoda: *Lernaea*
 Lepeophtheirus
 Branchiura: *Argulus*
 Annelida: *Piscicola*
 Mollusca: glochidia

Endoparasites

Protozoa
Flagellates: *Trypanoplasma*
 Hexamita
Coccidia: *Eimeria*
Microsporidia: *Glugea*

Myxosporidia: *Myxosoma*
 Ceratomyxa

Metazoa
Digenetic trematodes (flukes):
 Diplostomum
 Cryptocotyle
Cestodes (tapeworms):
 Ligula
 Diphyllobothrium
Nematodes (roundworms):
 Contracaecum
 Anisakis
Acanthocephala (thorny-headed worms): *Pomphorhynchus*

FIG. 6.13 This greatly simplified table gives details of the major groups of organisms containing species which are obligate or opportunist parasites of fish. Common examples of parasites from each group are given but this table should be considered as a guide only: for more detailed classification, specialist texts should be consulted.

(1) Stocking density is usually high in fish culture systems and the propinquity of the host fish favours the transmission of parasites. This is particularly the case with parasites having a direct life-cycle, such as the ectoparasitic protozoa, which always have substantial reproductive capabilities to ensure that some offspring locate a suitable host. Hosts are readily available in a farm environment and overwhelming parasitic infestation can occur.

(2) Farmed fish are more prone to physical trauma due to handling, grading, storms etc. and this gives an opportunity for parasites to colonise and feed on damaged tissue.

(3) Water in a fish farming facility is frequently sub-optimal in quality and quantity. Low flow rates allow the accumulation of infective stages within the system. High levels of ammonia irritate the gills and skin, causing an increase in mucus production and an increase in surface bacteria and organic material — producing a very favourable environment in which protozoan parasites can flourish and cause further damage to the surface of the fish. At the same time high levels of nutrients from waste feed and faeces will increase the local populations of bacteria and free-living protozoa, again providing food for the parasites. In this situation many free-living protozoa will use the fish as a convenient feeding platform and, while not directly parasitic to the host, may cause problems due to the sheer numbers of protozoa present. Some of the crustaceans and molluscs feeding on the waste organic material may act as intermediate hosts to some of the parasites with indirect life-cycles. Increased nutrient levels in the water may also irritate the gills and skin of the fish, again favouring parasitic invasion.

(4) Fish are often selectively bred for qualities other than disease resistance and some strains may be particularly susceptible to disease.

(5) The introduction of exotic species of fish may introduce new parasites to existing (often highly susceptible) fish stocks and expose the introduced fish to parasites already present in the facility and to which the resident fish are more resistant. *Any* introduction of new stock may precipitate disease in either the existing stock or the introduced stock.

(6) Fish stocks will attract predators (e.g. piscivorous birds), which may act as intermediate hosts to some parasites.

(7) The health status of the fish may be poor due to the presence of other disease, poor nutritional status, poor water quality, stress etc., so that they are more susceptible to parasitic infestation. There are several 'debility' parasites which take advantage of fish compromised by other factors but cause no problems in healthy individuals. Certain husbandry practices (e.g. transportation) may cause stress and render the fish more susceptible to disease — it is possible to anticipate some of these procedures and consider prophylactic treatment.

(8) Environmental changes, such as a sudden rise in temperature, may favour the parasite but stress the host. Outbreaks of parasitic disease are common in overwintered fish whose disease resistance may be poor, making them very susceptible to the increase in parasite numbers that occurs when water temperatures start to rise in spring. Any change in water quality may also stress the host while favouring the parasite.

(9) The system of husbandry may be more likely to expose fish to parasites. Earth pond systems favour the completion of the life-cycle of some parasites, particularly the sporozoans, and also favour the presence of intermediate hosts. Concrete systems reduce these risks but may cause more physical damage. Cage systems expose the fish directly to the parasitic fauna of the wild fish and allow the fish to feed easily on invertebrate intermediate hosts. The husbandry system also dictates the ease with which treatment and control may be administered; tank systems are more easy to treat than sea cages.

(10) The parasites to which the fish are exposed vary with the source of water. River and lake sources will carry a much wider range and higher numbers of parasites than bore-hole water.

Control of Parasitic Disease

There are very few effective parasiticides available for use in fish and control should be based on an appreciation of the above factors along with an understanding of the biology and life-cycle of the parasite. By understanding life-cycles and the conditions under which parasites flourish, it may be possible to improve or change these conditions and interrupt certain stages in the life of the parasite so that their impact on the fish is greatly reduced. The basic, and simplified, life-cycles of the major groups of fish parasites are shown in the accompanying diagrams. Control measures aimed at breaking the life-cycle of specific parasites are outlined in the text.

Fish parasites can be divided broadly into ectoparasites (those infesting the superficial tissues of the skin, fins and gills) and endoparasites (those infesting internal organs, including the gastro-intestinal tract). For the purposes of this book, however, gut parasites are considered separately from other endoparasites.

Ectoparasites: Protozoa

There are three main groups of protozoa para-sitising the external tissues of fish: flagellates, ciliates and amoebae. They have a direct life-cycle, mostly reproducing by binary fission; some species have cyst forms, off the host. The general effect of these parasites is to irritate the epithelial surfaces causing an increase in mucus production, which may be seen as a blue slime on the skin or as trailing mucus from the gills. Eventually mucus cells may become exhausted and the fish will be dry to the touch. Gill damage and 'blockage' due to the numbers of parasites present may cause respiratory distress and signs of oxygen starvation, while skin irritation may cause the fish to 'flash' in the water or rub itself on objects in an attempt to relieve the irritation. There may be thickening of the epidermis of the skin, sloughing and ulcer formation, fin rot and self-inflicted trauma. Damaged areas may be invaded by secondary bacteria or fungi. The fish are usually lethargic and inappetent.

The majority of the ectoparasitic protozoa can be seen by microscopic examination of fresh skin and gill preparations. Examples are shown in Fig. 6.14.

Ichthyobodo *spp.*

Also commonly known as *Costia*, these flagel-lates are obligate parasites with a direct life-cycle on the host (although cyst forms have been described). They affect all species of freshwater fish worldwide and are found in a free-swimming form on the host or attached to, and feeding on, the epithelial cells. The free-swimming form is kidney-shaped (10–20 μ long) with two pairs of flagellae; the attached form is pear-shaped and attaches to the gills and skin, often in areas sheltered by the fins and covered by the opercular flap.

The disease is typical of ectoparasites, with increased mucus, gills and skin hyperplasia, epi-dermal sloughing, ulceration, ragged fins, signs of irritation and respiratory distress. It is frequently a disease of salmonid fry, causing a rapid mortality,

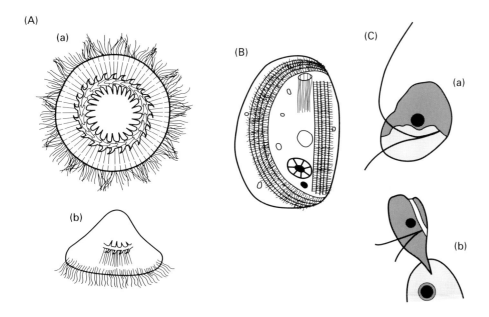

FIG. 6.14 Examples of ectoparasitic protozoa. (A) Trichodinid (a) dorsal view, (b) side view; (B) *Chilodonella* and (C) *Ichthyobodo* (a) unattached, (b) attached.

and can also be carried to sea with smolt transfer where it may cause significant gill damage and poor performance. There may also be truly marine species of *Ichthyobodo*. The parasite responds to standard fish ectoparasiticides.

Cryptobia *spp.*

Confusingly similar to *Ichthyobodo*, *Cryptobia* (12–22 µ) has two flagellae and is found in fresh and salt water. It does not attach so strongly to the epithelial cells as *Ichthyobodo* and feeds on nutrients in the water rather than the host cells.

The disease has been implicated in mortalities in young European and Chinese carp but there is no evidence of direct pathology. It is probably a commensal but its presence may indicate poor water quality. *Cryptobia* are thought to occur in the blood as trypanoplasms.

Oodinium *spp.*

These dinoflagellates are found in warm waters (*Oodinium* spp. in fresh water, *Amyloodinium* spp. in salt water). The trophont is the parasitic stage (50–100 µ), usually containing brown/gold chlorophyll, which attaches to the cells of the gill or skin; it eventually detaches and divides to produce many dinospores which are actively host-seeking.

Serious disease outbreaks have been experienced in sea-bream, sea-bass, mullet and tilapia. Affected areas include the Mediterranean, Red Sea, Gulf of Mexico etc. The parasite causes severe pathology at the point of attachment on the skin and gill resulting in haemorrhage, inflammation and extensive epithelial hyperplasia. It responds to few chemical treatments, although copper sulphate may be effective.

Ichthyophthirius multifiliis

This ciliate, up to 1 mm in diameter, causes white spot or 'Ich' in most species of freshwater fish world-wide; a marine equivalent is *Cryptocaryon*. The parasite is a sphere, covered in short cilia, which has a characteristic slow, rolling movement in fresh gill and skin preparations. The mature form of the parasite, the trophont, has dark cytoplasm within which a paler, horseshoe shaped nucleus can usually be seen. The life-cycle (Fig. 6.15) is direct but spent partly off the host. The trophont is found within the epidermis of the host, where it consumes cellular material and is seen grossly as a white spot. The mature parasite leaves the fish, encysts and divides to produce many host-seeking tomites. The tomites penetrate the skin and gills of the fish to complete the life-cycle.

When the mature trophonts digest their way out of the skin they irritate the fish and produce lesions, which are open to secondary infection. If there are many parasites they will cause large skin lesions, and this results in osmoregulatory disturbance. On the gill, there is epithelial hyperplasia and disturbance of gill function. Affected fish are restless and inappetent, and show signs of irritation. Eventually there is skin sloughing with ragged fins and evidence of white spots.

Chemical treatments are only effective against the free-swimming stages of the parasite. Repeat treatments are therefore necessary to eliminate the free-swimming stages as they occur. As the life-cycle is temperature dependent, the period between treatments varies with temperature; for example, three treatments at 5-day intervals at 16°C and three treatments at 14-day intervals at 10°C.

Chilodonella *spp.*

The *Chilodonella* spp. have a dorso-ventrally flattened kidney-bean shape; they are up to 80 µ in length, with cilia arranged in rows along the body. A distinguishing feature is the cytopharyngeal basket made of stiffened cilia around the cytostome, and this is usually readily visible on microscopic examination. The organism has a characteristic gliding and flipping motion and is found world-wide, affecting all species of freshwater fish. *Brooklynella* is the marine equivalent of *Chilodonella*.

This is an example of a debility parasite taking advantage of fish in poor condition. It rarely causes problems in healthy stocks of fish but is classically a problem of overwintering fish in temperate and sub-tropical climates which are in relatively poor condition. Carp, salmonids and catfish are the species most commonly affected. The parasite feeds on organic material in the water, plankton, and cellular debris on the epidermis of the fish.

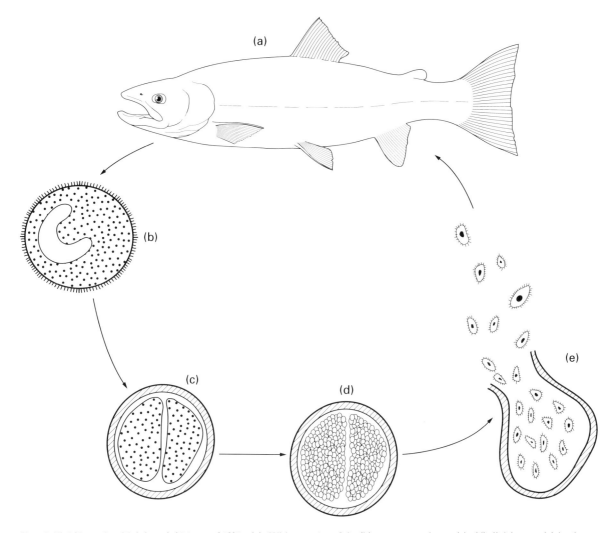

FIG. 6.15 Life-cycle of *Ichthyophthirius multifiliis*. (a) 'White spot' on fish, (b) mature trophont, (c), (d) divisions and (e) release of ciliated tomites.

Clinical signs are typical of external parasitism. The parasite is often found associated with bacterial gill disease. Control is by general environmental improvement and standard ectoparasite treatments.

Tetrahymena

This is a normal free-living freshwater ciliate, very similar in appearance to *Chilodonella* but without the cyto-pharyngeal basket. If there is a high loading of organic material in the water there can be an explosive increase in numbers of ciliates, which can invade fish. *Uronema* is a marine equivalent.

The ciliate penetrates under the scales and can invade the underlying muscle causing localised swelling, necrosis and ulceration. Large numbers could cause extensive damage. Control is by environmental improvement. Chemical treatment may kill the ciliates off the host.

Trichodinia *spp.*

Three genera form the Trichodina complex: *Trichodina, Trichodonella* and *Tripartiella*. They are up to 100 μ in diameter and all have a basic saucer-shape with a fringe of cilia around the perimeter. A circular arrangement of tooth-like structures within the body gives them a characteristic appearance in fresh gill and skin preparations. They browse over the surface of the gills and skin with a spinning motion, damaging the host tissues and consuming the resulting tissue debris. The parasite has a world-wide distribution and affects most freshwater and marine fish species.

The disease shows typical signs of ectoparasitism with excess mucus production, frayed fins and skin erosion. Outbreaks are often associated with poor water quality and stress. Control is by standard ectoparasiticides and environmental improvement.

Scyphidia *spp.*

Several species of these flask-shaped ciliates (up to 100 μ long) are found world-wide in fresh and salt water. The body shape varies with the species but they all have a spiral of cilia at one end. The other end attaches to the surface of the fish, frequently by way of a stalk (Fig. 6.16). They are commensals, feeding on organic material in the

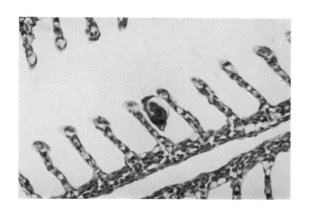

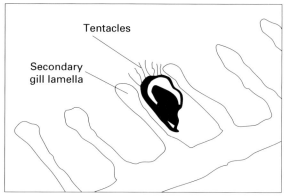

FIG. 6.17 Trichophyra — showing extended tentacles (H + E × 100).

water, and use the fish merely as a feeding platform.

It is unlikely that *Scyphidia* cause significant pathology but they can cause skin irritation or disturbance to normal gill function when present in large numbers. They will colonise damaged and ulcerated areas of the skin. Their presence tends to indicate high levels of organic matter in the water. Control is by improving water quality and flows; chemical treatment can be used.

Trichophyra

This is another ectocommensal (up to 100 μ) found in water with high organic load (Fig. 6.17). It occurs world-wide but most reports are temperate freshwater fish, e.g. eels and salmonids. On microscopic examination, they appear like small blobs of jelly from which rod-like tentacles are extended periodically to trap organic material in the water.

Like the Scyphidians, they are unlikely to cause

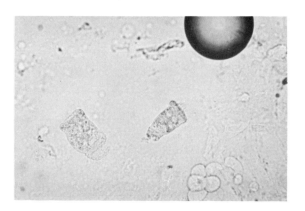

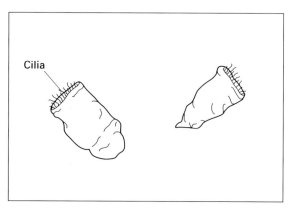

FIG. 6.16 *Scyphidia* — fresh gill preparation × 100.

significant pathology but in large numbers may cause minor skin irritation or interfere with gill function. Their presence again tends to indicate poor water quality: control is by improving water quality and flow rates; chemical treatment can be used if necessary.

Amoebae

Several species of amoeba (e.g. *Thecamoeba* spp.) have been implicated in gill disease in salmonids. They are probably feeding on bacteria on the surface of the fish and may multiply rapidly, particularly when water temperatures are high, resulting in severe gill damage. Heavy salmonid losses due to gill amoebae have been reported in England and Australasia.

Ectoparasites: Metazoa

Fish parasites are represented in several metazoan groups including monogenean trematodes (the gill and skin flukes), crustaceans (lice, gill maggots,

anchor worm), annelids (leeches) and molluscs (larval mussels). All have direct life-cycles but the period of their life-cycle during which they act as fish parasites varies considerably with the species concerned.

Monogenean trematodes

These gill and skin flukes (Fig. 6.18) have a world-wide distribution and are found in fresh and salt water. They appear like microscopic worms up to 2 mm in length attached to the surface of the fish by a posterior hooked attachment organ. Damage is caused to the host by the penetration of the attachment organ and by the browsing action of the mouth at the free end. The two most common representatives of this group are *Gyrodactylus* and *Dactylogyrus*.

***Gyrodactylus* spp.** Commonly known as skin flukes and are found all over the surface of the body, including the fins and occasionally the gills. They are up to 1 mm in length and may just be

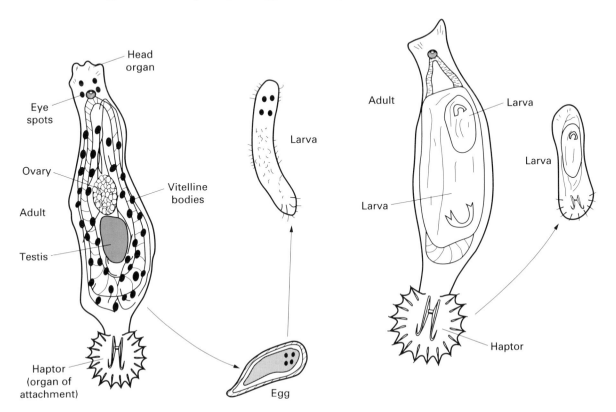

Fig. 6.18 Monogenetic trematodes.

visible to the naked eye. *Gyrodactylus* species are viviparous: on microscopic examination of fresh skin preparations it is possible to see an embryo, with its hooked attachment organ, within the body of the adult. *Another* embryo may be seen developing within the embryo. The life-cycle is completed entirely on the host and parasite burdens can build up extremely rapidly. They move by a characteristic looping action, and small puncture wounds occur each time the hooks penetrate the host.

Explosive epizootics can occur, often associated with high stocking densities and poor general husbandry. There is frequently a concomitant protozoan infestation. Extensive skin and fin damage occurs due to the action of the hooks and the feeding activity of the parasite. Affected fish are restless and inappetent and may 'flash' in the water. The skin is often grey due to excess mucus production and epidermal damage, and the fins are frequently frayed.

It is believed that *Gyrodactylus salaris* has

recently been introduced into Norwegian rivers, where it has been implicated in causing widespread loss of Atlantic salmon parr.

Control is by improvement in husbandry and environmental conditions. All stages of the parasite are susceptible to chemical treatment.

***Dactylogyrus* spp.** Known as gill flukes (Fig. 6.19), although they are not exclusively restricted to the gills. They are viviparous and the golden-brown vitelline (egg-forming) bodies can be seen easily under the microscope. The adult parasite produces eggs which are disseminated into the environment; they hatch to produce a host-seeking oncomiracidium.

Localised gill damage occurs due to the action of the hooked attachment and the feeding activity of the fluke. Heavy infestations may cause interference with gill function and respiratory incapacity, particularly when water temperatures are high. Some species cause serious losses in European carp culture; overwintering eggs hatch to produce larvae which heavily infest juvenile fish.

Repeated chemical treatments are necessary to eliminate parasites produced from newly-hatched eggs. Cleaning and sterilising the facility, where practical, will eliminate those eggs.

Other pathogenic monogeneans. These include *Axine* spp. on mullet, *Entobdella* spp. on soles and halibut and *Benedenia* spp. on mullet and yellowtail.

Crustaceans

Three groups of crustacea contain important fish parasites: the *Branchiura*, the *Copepoda* and the *Isopoda*.

Copepoda

This group contains the most important ectoparasitic crustaceans. These have a complex life-cycle, usually direct although some may require intermediate hosts. There are several larval stages which increase in size between moults. Newly-hatched nauplii larvae moult through a series of stages to become copepodids. In some species the copepodids are parasitic, in others they are free-living. The final copepodid stage is usually when

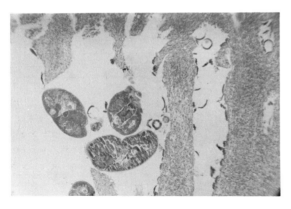

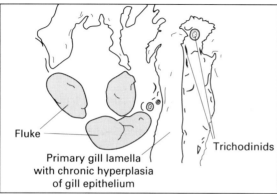

Fluke

Primary gill lamella
with chronic hyperplasia
of gill epithelium

Trichodinids

FIG. 6.19 Gill infestation with flukes and trichodinids showing chronic hyperplastic change of gill epithelium (H + E × 100).

fertilisation occurs, after which the male usually dies. The adult female, parasitising the host fish, produces paired egg sacs which release eggs into the water to complete the cycle.

Lernaea **spp.** The most important in this genus is *L. cyprinacea*, the anchor worm found in fresh water in Europe, North America and Asia. Although normally associated with carp, they are not host-specific. Other *Lernaea* spp. are encountered on other fish species in both fresh and salt water. The stage usually seen is the adult female, up to 22 mm long, attached to the surface of the fish. This is a highly adapted crustacean whose head takes the form of an 'anchor' which penetrates the host's skin to form an extremely strong and damaging attachment. The body of the parasite resembles a worm, with vestigial appendages and paired egg sacs trailing from the posterior end (Fig. 6.20). There are three nauplii stages followed

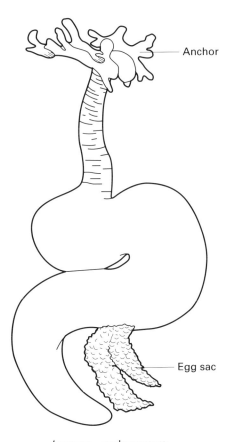

Lernaea – anchor worm

Fig. 6.20 *Lernaea* — anchor worm.

by five copepodid stages: parasitic attachment to the host occurs at stage three, when fertilisation occurs. The male dies while the female metamorphoses and penetrates the host tissue. The parasite does not survive well at low temperatures and cannot reproduce below 15°C. It is therefore more of a problem in warm water and during the summer months in temperate regions.

The anchor worm actively feeds on the tissues of the host, eventually causing a large granuloma to form around the feeding site. Where the parasite enters the skin, there is often inflammation and haemorrhage. In small fish the damage can be deep and death can be rapid if vital organs are penetrated. Even in large fish, small numbers can be very damaging and cause spoilage so that the fish has no market value. Affected fish show signs of irritation, lethargy and loss of condition. Wounds caused by the parasite are prone to secondary infections. *Lernaea* is a serious problem of Indian polyculture systems.

Repeated treatments with organophosphorous will destroy the juvenile stages but not the adults. Draining and drying will kill all stages, including eggs.

Salmonicola **spp. and** ***Ergasilus*** **spp.** are the gill maggots of fresh and salt water in Europe and North America. They are large — up to 3 mm long — and are adapted to clasp the primary gill lamellae of a wide range of host species. The clasping attachment causes severe gill damage and interference with gill function. There have been reports of serious losses in salmon hatcheries, in brook trout and in mullet.

Lepeophtheirus **spp.** *Lepeophtheirus salmonis* is the 'sea louse' or 'salmon louse' and is the most important parasite of the marine culture of Atlantic salmon (Figs 6.21 and 6.22). Infestation with the closely-related *Caligus* spp. may also be seen. Other *Lepeophtheirus* spp. may be found on other marine fish species. There are ten stages in the life-cycle. The first copepodid stage attaches to the skin and fins of the host by a frontal filament and moults through four so-called chalimus stages. The parasite then loses the filamentous attachment, becomes attached to the host by suction and is free to move over the surface of the fish. Two pre-adult stages are followed by the adult stage.

FIG. 6.21 Life-cycle of the sea louse *Lepeophtheirus salmonis*. (a) Adult, (b) nauplius I and II, (c) copepodid, (d) chalimus I–IV and (e) pre-adult I and II.

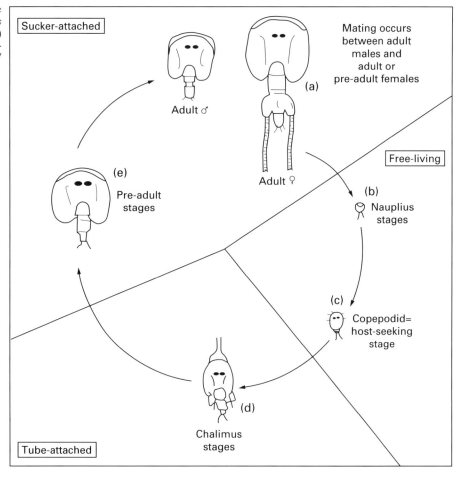

Mating occurs during the last pre-adult and adult stages and the female produces paired trailing egg sacs which release eggs into the water. These hatch to produce free-swimming nauplii and complete the cycle.

The suction-attached stages are the most damaging; the parasites browse on the epidermis of the fish, gradually eroding the skin and causing extensive ulcerative lesions. A predilection site is the dorsal surface of the head, where the skin can be eroded down to the bone, but damage can occur all over the body surface. Many hundreds of parasites may be found on each fish; fish in poor condition or suffering other diseases (e.g. pancreas disease) are particularly vulnerable to attack. The early stages, when attachment is by the frontal filament, are not so damaging but can cause punctate haemorrhagic lesions, particularly on the ventral surface of the fish.

Although *Caligus* spp. are not thought to be as damaging as *L. salmonis* there can be epizootics of these lice, probably brought into the site on wild fish (*Caligus* appears to be able to transfer between hosts more freely than *Lepeophtheirus*). They can rapidly and severely damage farmed stocks.

Several husbandry methods help in the control of sea lice infestation, including the separation of year classes and the fallowing of sites between stocking. Organophosphorus baths are the traditional treatment but there are problems associated with this, including practical difficulties in administering the bath, resistance of the lice to organophosphorus, only the suction-attached stages being susceptible to treatment and unexplained fish deaths during treatment. Alternative treatments are being developed including in-feed parasiticides, hydrogen peroxide and pyrethroid

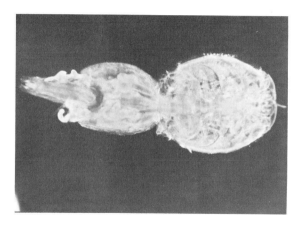

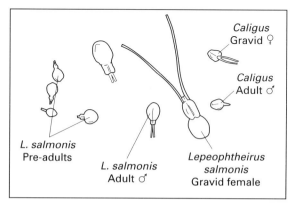

FIG. 6.22 Sea lice. Photo of *Lepeophtheirus*. © British Crown Copyright reserved.

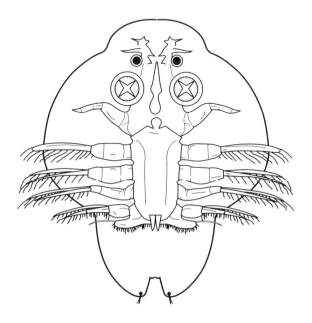

FIG. 6.23 *Argulus* (ventral view).

baths, biological control using cleaner fish (wrasse) and chemical repellents including onions and garlic.

Branchiura

The most important member of this group is *Argulus*, the freshwater fish louse (Figs 6.23 and 6.24).

Argulus spp. are large, dorso-ventrally flattened crustaceans up to 1 cm long. They have a world-wide distribution and are found on many host species. They are very motile and are frequently found on the head of the fish or in sheltered areas behind the fins. Fish-to-fish movement is common and they can survive for extended periods off the host. Mating takes place on the host; the female leaves the fish to lay eggs on vegetation, which hatch to release actively host-seeking larvae.

The parasite feeds by piercing the epidermis with a stylet and digesting skin tissue, causing haemorrhagic ulcers which are prone to secondary infections. Attachment hooks on the underside of the parasite also cause mechanical damage. Heavy infestations can cause high losses, particularly in small fish. Mortalities can also occur due to secondary bacterial infections. Affected fish show signs of irritation, lethargy and loss of condition; there are obvious parasites and lesions, often with secondary fungal infection. There is evidence that *Argulus* can transmit virus infections. *Argulus* infestation is a serious problem of pond culture in Europe, Africa, Asia and the Far East.

Organophosphorus treatments are effective.

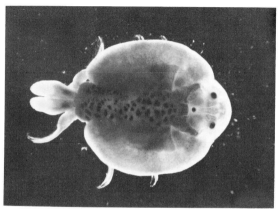

FIG. 6.24 *Argulus* (dorsal view).

Draining and drying will kill all stages of the parasite and the periodic removal of vegetation with attached eggs will help to reduce parasite numbers.

Isopoda

A number of isopods have been implicated in fish disease in fresh and salt water. They are more important in warm water and there are reports of serious problems in Israeli cage culture. Many are nocturnal blood feeders.

Annelida

Several species of leech parasitise fish in fresh and salt water. Typical infestation occurs in earth ponds and gravel pits, where water-flows are slow.

Piscicola and *Hemilepsis* spp. are common in fresh water, while *Hemibdella* spp. have caused problems in cultured marine flatfish. They are segmented worms up to 2 cm long and browse over the fish taking periodic blood meals, leaving the fish only to reproduce.

In small numbers they are tolerated but heavy burdens can cause anaemia and severe skin damage which is prone to secondary infections. Leeches will transmit blood flagellates and possibly viruses. Control is by draining, drying and liming ponds.

Mollusca

The larval stages of some freshwater mussels undergo an obligatory parasitic phase on the gills of fish (also sometimes skin and fins). The larvae are called glochidia (Fig. 6.25): they encyst within the host tissue and very heavy burdens may interfere with gill function or damage the tissue when they finally leave the host.

Endoparasites of the Viscera, Musculature, Skeleton and Eye: Protozoa

All endoparasitic protozoans (excluding those found in the gut) belong to the Sporozoa. Fish parasites are found in the classes Myxosporidia and Microsporidia (Fig. 6.26).

Myxosporidia

Many species of myxosporidians are found world-wide in a wide variety of fish hosts. Only a few cause significant disease. These are spore-forming parasites, the spore consists of two or more valves within which is sporoplasm containing two or more polar capsules (Fig. 6.27).

Myxosoma cerebralis is the causative agent of whirling disease in salmonids, a serious disease in the rainbow trout industry in Europe and America which, due to changes in husbandry, has become less of a problem in recent years. Spores measure 10 µ in diameter and consist of two valves with two polar capsules. The spores need a period of maturation (possibly within a tubificid worm intermediate host) before they are infective. The spore is probably ingested by the fish; polar filaments are extruded from the polar capsules, which allows attachment to the gut wall, and the parasite migrates to the target organ — the head cartilages of young fish. Spores can be detected by the microscopic examination of Giemsa-stained head

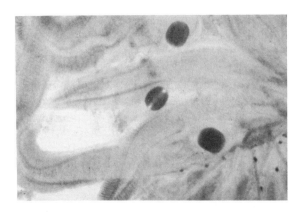

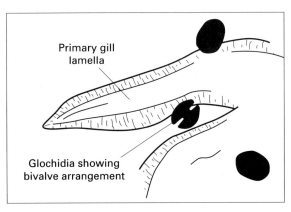

Fig. 6.25 Mussel glochidia — fresh gill preparation × 100.

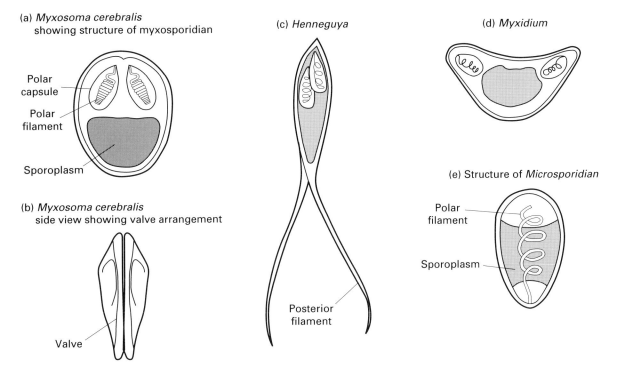

(a) *Myxosoma cerebralis*
   showing structure of myxosporidian

Polar
capsule

Polar
filament

Sporoplasm

(b) *Myxosoma cerebralis*
   side view showing valve arrangement

Valve

(c) *Henneguya*

Posterior
filament

(d) *Myxidium*

(e) Structure of *Microsporidian*

Polar
filament

Sporoplasm

Fig. 6.26 Examples of endoparasitic protozoa. (a)–(d) Examples of myxosporidian spores: (a) *Myxosoma cerebralis* — showing structure of myxosporidian, (b) side view showing valve arrangement, (c) *Henneguya* and (d) *Myxidium*, (e) Structure of microsporidian.

tissue, and various digestion/concentration techniques facilitate diagnosis.

Whirling disease is classically a disease of young fish in earth pond systems. Spores liberated from dead infected fish or asymptomatic carriers (possibly brown trout in the watercourse) mature in bottom sediments or tubificid worms in the mud, and young fish ingest infected material before ossification of the head cartilages occurs. The presence of the parasite in the cartilages causes skeletal deformities and problems with balance and pigmentation. Affected fish classically display vertebral deformity, darkening of the tail and a whirling swimming action. Older fish are far less susceptible to the disease because ossification of the cartilages has already taken place.

The disease is controlled by rearing young fish away from earth ponds until they are not susceptible to the disease. Draining, drying and liming of ponds helps to eliminate the parasite.

Myxobolus cyprini is an important parasite of East European carp culture, causing pernicious anaemia. The spore has a very similar appearance to Myxosoma; it is 10–16 μ long with two pear-shaped polar capsules. Spores can be detected in cysts in many tissues; when mature, the cysts burst and the spores are released into the water.

Typically, young carp are infected in their first summer by spores of this parasite overwintering from the previous year's stock. The most severe pathology occurs in the kidney and gills, causing mass mortalities. Affected fish are anaemic, suffer osmoregulatory disturbance and lose condition. Control is by separation of year classes, and by drying and liming of ponds. Other *Myxobolus* spp. cause cyst formation on the gills, skin and in the muscle of carp throughout the world and are a cause of serious fish losses in some countries.

***Henneguya* spp.** (Fig. 6.28) are elongated myxozoans with posterior filaments. They are widespread but cause little pathology in the majority of cases. They are often seen as white cysts on the skin, gills and fins. An interlamellar gill form in channel catfish causes severe pathology and losses,

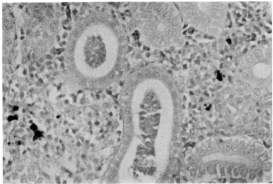

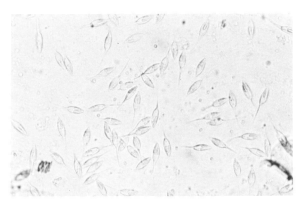

FIG. 6.28 *Henneguya* — fresh gill preparation × 40.

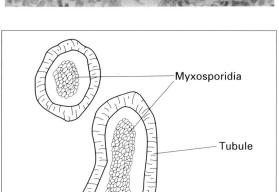

FIG. 6.27 Myxosporidia within kidney tubules of Atlantic salmon (H + E × 100).

but an intra-lamellar form is relatively innocuous. *Henneguya* spp. also cause cyst formation ('boil disease') in the muscle of Pacific salmon.

Myxidium spp. *M. giardi* is an important parasite of eels world-wide. The spore is crescent-shaped with polar capsules at either end. Cysts occur in many tissues: they are not particularly damaging to the fish but can be very unsightly. *Myxidium* spp. may be found in the biliary system of salmonids but do not appear to be pathogenic.

Proliferative kidney disease (PKD) is one of the most economically important diseases of rainbow trout culture in Europe and North America. The causative agent — the 'PKX' cell — remains to be identified but is likely to be a myxosporidian, possibly a *Sphaerospora* species. The organism can infect most tissues but those principally involved are the spleen and the kidney, where the PKX cell can be demonstrated in histological section or in

Giemsa-stained kidney smears. Secondary and tertiary daughter cells can be seen within the cell.

PKD affects fish in their first summer. Freshwater rainbow trout are the major species involved although other salmonids and rainbow trout in sea cages may also be affected. Infected fish exhibit grey, swollen kidneys with ascites and anaemia. On histological examination there is a tremendous cellular proliferation, mainly in the kidney, within which the PKX cells are scattered. Morbidity and mortality can be extremely high, the fish suffering mainly from an anaemia which renders them extremely vulnerable to stress and low oxygen levels.

As the life-cycle of the parasite is poorly understood control is difficult. Water quality and oxygen levels must be good and stressful procedures avoided if possible, particularly at times of high temperatures and low oxygen. Malachite green has been shown to have some action against the organism.

Ceratomyxa shasta. An important parasite of the liver and kidney of North American salmonids, causing high losses in juvenile fish.

Sphaerospora spp. Commonly found in the kidney and swim-bladder of carp and are seen in freshwater salmonid culture. They are of questionable significance.

Microsporidia

The microsporidians are obligate intra-cellular parasites. The spores are much smaller than

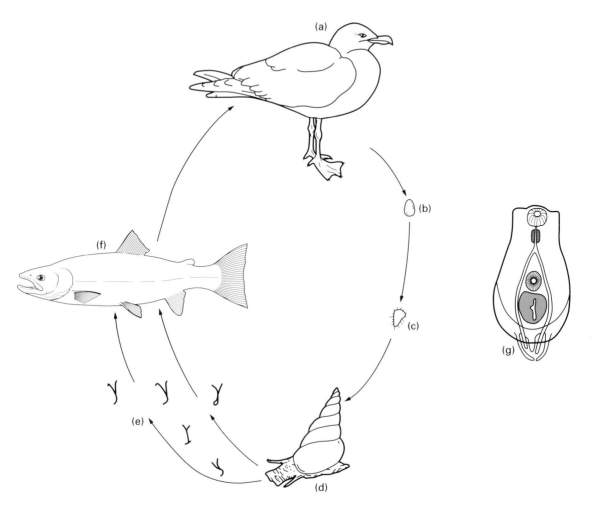

FIG. 6.29 Life-cycle of the eye fluke *Diplostomum*. (a) Adult in intestine of final host, (b) egg, (c) miracidium, (d) snail — 1st intermediate host, (e) cercariae, (f) metacercariae in eye of fish — 2nd intermediate host, (g) structure of metacercaria.

the myxosporidia and have no valves or polar capsules, although they do contain a single polar filament. The microsporidia are usually parasites of warm water and marine fish. Depending on the species, there may be a diffuse infiltration of the muscle and viscera or cyst formation. Many species have been identified, some causing significant pathology (e.g. *Glugea* spp. in cultured flatfish) and they are seen periodically in salmonid culture. However, microsporidians are not considered particularly important parasites in fish culture.

Endoparasites of the Viscera, Musculature and Eye: Metazoa

Endoparasitic metazoans infesting the viscera, muscle and eye include species of digenetic trematodes, cestodes and nematodes.

Digenetic trematodes

These have a complicated indirect life-cycle with at least one intermediate host (Fig. 6.29). The stage most commonly encountered in fish is the larval metacercaria which may be found in the tissues within a cyst or unencysted, depending on species. The most common first intermediate host is a snail (winkle in marine species) and the final host is usually a piscivorous bird. Damage can occur to the fish when the cercarial larvae first invade through the skin of the fish — a heavy invasion can result in significant, haemorrhagic lesions which, particularly in small fish, may result in heavy losses. Some metacercaria are extremely damaging to their target organ while others cause very little harm, although their presence may be aesthetically unappealing.

***Diplostomum* spp.** These eye flukes invade the lens of many freshwater fish species in Europe and America. (Several other digenetic genera also parasitise various sites in the eyes of fish.) The metacercariae in the lens cause cataract formation and eventual blindness so that the fish is unable to feed and loses condition. It also becomes more susceptible to predation by piscivorous birds, in which the adult parasite is found. Although affecting many species of fish, this parasite is particularly important in freshwater salmonid culture, with significant economic loss. Massive invasion by metacercariae has caused heavy losses in young rainbow trout. Control is by elimination of the snail intermediate host by the use of molluscicides, filtration and removal of vegetation. Affected fish may be treated with a suitable parasiticide.

***Cotylurus* spp.** Encyst within the pericardium of a number of fish species. There is little evidence that they cause harm but there may be a loss in condition or an increased susceptibility to other disease.

***Nanophyetus* spp.** These cause considerable damage to many tissues of farmed salmonids in America.

***Clinostomum* spp.** Also known as the 'yellow grub' is found in many species of (mainly) warm-water fish throughout the world. They are very large, producing cysts up to 5 mm in diameter which, when present in sufficient quantity, can cause considerable damage to the viscera and muscles.

Cryptocotyle. A marine digenean which encysts within the muscle, skin and gill of many fish

species. Although it has little pathological effect, it evokes a strong melanin response in the form of black spots, which may render the fish unacceptable at market.

Cestodes

All the cestodes have an indirect life-cycle with at least one intermediate host. The plerocercoid stage is that most commonly found in the viscera and musculature of fish. The first intermediate host is an invertebrate in the zooplankton (e.g. *Cyclops*). The final host may be a piscivorous bird or predatory fish.

***Ligula* spp.** (Fig. 6.30) One of the most common and widespread cestodes and a parasite of Cyprinid fish found in fresh water world-wide. The tapeworm can attain a length of 25 cm in the abdominal cavity and causes pressure atrophy of the viscera (gonadal atrophy leads to sterility) and fibrinous adhesions. There is evidence to suggest that the parasite causes changes in behaviour, making the fish more susceptible to predation. There seems to be no effective control available apart from deterring the final hosts. Some parasiticides may be of use.

***Triaenophorus* spp.** These are important parasites of salmonids in Europe and North America. Plerocercoids encyst in the liver and other viscera, causing extensive damage. The final host is the pike and the parasite is a particular problem when the two fish species are in close proximity.

***Diphyllobothrium* spp.** A large number of *Diphyllobothrium* spp. occur world-wide, *D. latum*, the broad tapeworm in humans (not in the UK), is found in a wide variety of fish. *D. dentriticum* and *D. ditremum* (in the UK) are most commonly found in salmonids and they encyst on the connective tissue of the viscera, where they cause little damage unless the parasitic burden is extremely heavy. In small fish, large numbers of parasites may cause damage to viscera, condition loss and an increased susceptibility to other diseases. There have been reports of migration of these parasites into the muscle causing rejection of carcases. The parasites are most commonly found in freshwater cage culture. No treatment has been found to be

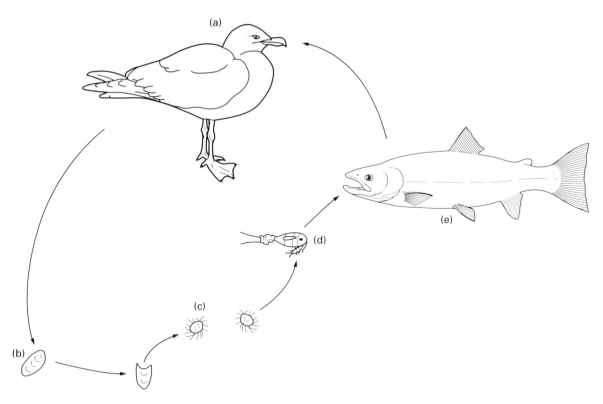

FIG. 6.30 Life-cycle of *Ligula intestinalis*. (a) Adult tapeworm in intestine of bird, (b) egg, (c) coracidium (d) coracidium is eaten by 1st intermediate host to form procercoid, (e) plerocercoid in 2nd intermediate host — fish.

effective but it may be possible to treat the final hosts with parasiticides.

Nematodes

The life-cycle of the nematodes is very similar to that of the cestodes. The first intermediate host is an invertebrate; fish act as second intermediate host and the larval parasite is present in the viscera or muscle. The final host is a piscivorous bird or predatory fish.

Only a few species are of any significance. *Eustrongyloides* spp. encyst in the viscera and muscle of salmonids; they are long (10 cm) and red and, although relatively harmless to the host, their presence will cause rejection of the fish. *Contracaecum* spp. encyst in viscera and muscle; their migration through tissues may cause minor damage. *Philometra* is an adult nematode found in the muscle of carp; it is viviparous and penetrates the skin to release larvae into the water. Carp fry may be killed by the migration of these parasites.

Anisakis spp. encyst in the muscle of many marine species: they may infest man but the larvae will be destroyed by cooking or by freezing below −20°C.

Parasites of the Blood–Vascular System

Trypanosoma *and* Trypanoplasma

Many species of these blood flagellates are found. They are of questionable pathogenicity, although *Trypanoplasma* spp. have been implicated in disease and are said to render the fish more susceptible to stress. They can be transmitted by leeches and *Trypanoplasma* may be found on the external surface of fish as *Cryptobia*.

Sanguinicola *spp.*

This blood fluke is a digenean, with the adult living in the blood system of the fish. The parasite is found in European carp culture and salmonids in America. In young fish, eggs released by the parasite block capillary networks, particularly in the gill, causing ischaemic necrosis. Larvae from the hatching eggs can also cause severe gill damage in small fish. In older fish, eggs lodging in other organs such as the kidney can cause chronic damage.

Protozoan Parasites of the Gastro-intestinal Tract

Although many protozoans may be found in the gut of fish, few are considered to be significantly pathogenic.

Hexamita *spp.*

Also known as *Octomitis*, this small (10 μ) flagellate is frequently found in the intestine of many cultured species, typically eels and salmonids. It is debatable whether it is a significant pathogen, though it has been linked to a catarrhal enteritis and improvements in the condition of fish are reported if treatments are carried out. *Hexamita* may be another example of a debility parasite, taking advantage of fish weakened by other factors. Some in-feed antiprotozoal agents are effective.

Coccidians

Many coccidians have been found in fish — the majority in the gut. (Visceral coccidiosis does occur but is of little importance in farmed fish.) Two of the most important gut coccidians are found in European carp culture: *Eimeria carpelli* and *Eimeria subepithelialis*. The very complex development of the coccidia occurs in the gut wall of the host and infective sporocysts are released into the water. Sporozoites from the sporocysts are ingested by a susceptible host to complete the life-cycle.

E. carpelli causes coccidial enteritis, a severe condition of carp in their first summer which may result in significant losses in young fish. Affected fish suffer a haemorrhagic enteritis, abdominal swelling, lethargy and inappetence.

E. subepithelialis causes a nodular coccidiosis in the sub-mucosa of the gut. Although less serious than *E. carpelli*, the disease can cause loss of

condition and mortalities in fish during their first year.

Control is by separation of year classes, draining and liming ponds, and the use of coccidiostats.

Intestinal helminths

Many intestinal helminths are found but few are considered to be significantly pathogenic.

Cestodes

Caryophyllaeus spp. are common in carp, causing a mucoid enteritis, reduced growth and inappetence. This tapeworm has a tubificid worm as an intermediate host and can be controlled by drying and liming ponds.

Eubothrium spp. are found in European and American salmonid culture. They are relatively innocuous but when present in large numbers may cause blockage of the intestine, particularly in small fish, and may make the fish more susceptible to stress and other diseases.

Bothriocephalus acheilognathi, the 'Asian tapeworm', is probably the most harmful of all carp gut tapeworms. It is a large (up to 20 cm) native parasite of Chinese carp which has been introduced into Europe and North America. The tapeworm causes blockage of the intestine in young carp resulting in loss of condition, inappetence, atrophy of internal tissues, localised haemorrhage and death.

Nematodes

Many species of nematodes are found in the intestine of fish; none are of much pathological significance.

Acanthocephala

These thorny-headed worms, found world-wide, have a characteristic anterior proboscis which carries numerous backwardly-directed hooks. The life-cycle is indirect, involving an invertebrate intermediate host. The adult worm is found in the gut of the fish.

The hooked proboscis is embedded in the intestinal wall of the host; there is local damage and the worm sometimes penetrates the gut wall.

However, they are not considered to be particularly pathogenic. Some, such as *Acanthocephalus* spp. and *Pomphorynchus* spp. have been implicated in causing significant ulceration of the gut mucosa when present in large numbers but there is little evidence that this has any effect on performance or mortality levels.

Miscellaneous Diseases

A number of disease 'syndromes' have been identified in Atlantic salmon culture whose aetiology has still to be fully understood. They include pancreas disease, infectious salmon anaemia and the 'fading smolt syndrome'.

Pancreas disease

Pancreas disease (PD) is one of the major problems of the marine phase in Atlantic salmon culture. It causes a large loss of production in Scotland, Norway and Ireland and has been identified in France, Spain and North America.

PD usually affects post-smolts in their first summer. Affected fish show a rapid reduction in feeding response, becoming lethargic and hanging at the surface of the water at the sides and corners of cages. There may be evidence of mucoid 'casts' — plugs of mucus and degenerate cellular material ejected from the gut following cessation of feeding — attached to the sides and bottom of cages. Affected fish are very prone to infestation by sea lice.

The course of the disease can be relatively acute with rapid recovery within 2–3 weeks, or prolonged with inappetent, emaciated fish present for several months. Most fish will recover but, particularly in prolonged episodes, a proportion (up to 10%) may never come back to feeding and are usually culled.

In general the earlier in the summer the fish become affected, the more rapid is recovery. In late summer and autumn the disease often has a more prolonged course, with some very poor fish present throughout the winter showing no sign of recovery. Mortalities from PD are usually low unless it occurs in combination with other disease or parasitism but significant economic loss occurs due to the check in performance of affected fish.

Stocks of fish which have suffered an episode of PD appear 'immune' to further outbreaks but it is possible for the disease to occur in one-sea-winter fish which have been previously unaffected. Outbreaks are frequently precipitated by stressful management procedures including changes in feeding, lice treatments and grading.

The principal pathology is of pancreatic necrosis and fibrosis but there is frequently a myopathy of the cardiac and red muscle. There is a great deal of debate over the relationship of the myopathies to PD — they are not seen in all cases and some authorities believe they are secondary to the pancreatic pathology, although they have occurred synchronously with acute pancreatic pathology and occasionally prior to pancreatic lesions.

A related 'sudden death syndrome' has been seen in Ireland and Scotland: fish which have been through an episode of PD suffer sudden mortalities with few preceding symptoms (though nervous behaviour is seen occasionally). It is thought that the cause of the death is heart failure due to residual cardiac lesions.

In Norway cardiac myopathy syndrome (CMS) has been linked to PD. It occurs mostly in one-sea-winter fish although it has also been seen in post-smolts. Degenerative lesions of the heart muscle lead to a weakening of the ventricle and atrium, resulting in dilatation and occasionally in rupture.

The aetiology of PD remains to be identified. There is strong experimental and epidemiological evidence for a primary, probably viral, cause. Unaffected fish are more likely to suffer if stocked near affected fish; there is less risk of PD if sites are fallowed, and fish appear to develop a resistance to the disease. Laboratory transmission of the disease has been reported but attempts at virus isolation have so far been unsuccessful. Various nutritional parameters (particularly in relation to vitamin E) have been proposed as primary or contributory factors in the aetiology of the disease.

It is believed that if IPN occurs in combination with PD there can be a synergistic effect resulting in significant mortalities.

Control of PD relies on limiting stressful procedures and strictly controlling feeding regimes following smolt transfer. It is thought that overfeeding and increasing pellet sizes too rapidly may predispose to PD and carefully controlled feeding policies restricting the amount of feed taken do appear to reduce the occurrence of the disease. At present, the preferred management procedure in reducing the severity of the disease is to starve the fish for a few days and then gradually introduce feed with a smaller pellet, using fish oil as an attractant.

The fading (or failed) smolt syndrome

In recent years a phenomenon has been recognised in Atlantic salmon culture where a proportion (up to 30%) of smolts have failed to thrive. These fish become apparent some eight weeks after sea transfer and are usually lost through physical damage, parasitism or failure in osmoregulation. It must be borne in mind that there is always a certain proportion of smolts which fail to thrive following transfer — fish which are too small or have not sufficiently smolted, or are possibly over-smolted.

Failed smolts appear to be unable to survive physiologically in the marine environment. This could be because, although they appear to have smolted, certain conditions and feeding in the freshwater phase have encouraged them to survive and possibly mature in freshwater rather than adapting physiologically to the marine environment. Hierarchical feeding behaviour within populations of fish may also have an effect on the ability of some fish to thrive.

Infectious salmon anaemia (ISA)

ISA, also known as infectious lax anaemia (ILA), is an important condition in the marine phase of farmed Atlantic salmon in Norway. The disease occurs in localised geographic areas in western and northern Norway. There is probably a viral aetiology and there appears to be an association between ISA and intra-erythrocytic virus particles which have been demonstrated on electron microscopes. However, virus isolation has been unsuccessful. Affected fish develop a severe anaemia, ascites and characteristic necrotic/haemorrhagic lesions in the liver. Death occurs due to anaemia and circulatory failure.

Problems of yolk-sac fry

Various abnormalities of the yolk-sac have been identified in salmonid fry. Blue-sac disease is the

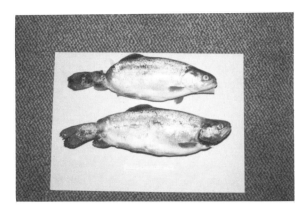

FIG. 6.31 Congenital vertebral deformity in rainbow trout.

term given to a condition where the yolk-sac becomes swollen, apparently oedematous and discoloured; the cause is not known but is thought to be a water quality problem (high levels of metabolites, changes in pH etc.). White spots or patches in the yolk-sac ('coagulated yolk-sac') are also thought to be due to a problem with water quality, and salt baths are sometimes beneficial in these conditions. Deformed or pinched yolk-sac, where the sac becomes divided into a 'dumb-bell' shape, is thought to be caused by excessive flows or lack of substrate in hatchery trays. The posterior portion of the sac frequently sloughs off.

Genetic abnormalities

Several developmental abnormalities and deformities in cultured fish are presumed to have a genetic origin. They include defects in newly hatched fry, vertebral foreshortening in rainbow trout (Fig. 6.31) and jaw deformities in salmon. There is a danger that the relatively small gene pool used in some fish culture may lead to an increased occurrence of genetic abnormalities; selection pressure for certain characteristics such as fast growth may cause a concomitant increase in some undesirable characteristics such as a greater susceptibility to disease.

Further Reading

Austin, B. and Austin, D. A. (1987). *Bacterial Fish Pathogens — Disease in Farmed and Wild Fish*. Ellis Harwood.

Ferguson, H. (1989) *Systemic Pathology of Fish*. Iowa State University Press.

Hoffman, G. L. and Meyer, F. P. (1974) *Parasites of Freshwater Fishes*. T. F. H. Publications, New York.

Post, G. (1987) *Textbook of Fish Health*. T. F. H. Publications, New York.

Roberts, R. J. (Ed.) (1989) *Fish Pathology*. Baillière Tindall.

Roberts, R. J. and Shepherd, C. J. (1989) *Handbook of Trout and Salmon Diseases*. Fishing News Books Ltd.

Sinderman, C. J. (1970) *Principal Diseases of Marine Fish and Shellfish*. Academic Press, New York and London.

7

Therapy in Aquaculture

PETER SCOTT

Circumstances on fish farms vary considerably according to the species farmed, the holding facilities, water quality and composition, water-flows, temperature and other factors, so that treatment regimes used for fish diseases need to be adaptable. The treatments themselves may either be supplied by the veterinarian on prescription or be available to the client direct on general sale. In either case, the veterinarian should be responsible for all fish treatments.

Depending on the type of disease, sick fish should be either removed and treated separately, in isolation, or kept with the rest of the fish and all treated collectively. Outbreaks of contagious disease are best dealt with *en masse*, but high value fish affected with certain bacterial diseases may be treated individually. Fish affected with large, visible parasites such as anchor worm (*Lernaea* spp.) and fish lice (*Argulus* spp.) may require individual treatment.

Treatment via the Water

The normal procedure is as follows.

- Make a diagnosis of the problem.
- Decide on a course of action. This will usually include:
  - Elimination of the initiating/predisposing factor.
  - Formulation of a regime which includes symptomatic treatment for the fish and elimination/control treatments against any pathogens.
- Check legal requirements. Potential therapeutants likely to enter watercourses may need to be notified to a local authority.
- Assess the condition of the fish, especially the gills, with regard to the use of any potential treatments.
- When appropriate, starve the fish for 24 hours.

This may be necessary for treatments regarded as stressful.
- If the treatment is new to the facility, consider the use of a test dose on a few fish in a separate container.
- Whenever possible, treat fish with the water level reduced. This offers the option of quickly raising the water level to dilute the treatment in the event of an adverse reaction.
- Consider the possibility of adverse reactions to treatment and anticipate the action which could be taken to correct this:
  - Stop the treatments.
  - Flush out the treatment.
  - Have aeration available. (Aeration already fitted and in use may be insufficient, as farmers have often stocked to take advantage of the additional oxygen available.)
- Consider the effect on fish downstream, either receiving the full dose (as in an in-series raceway) or receiving the dose into part of their water-flow (as in an outlet channel receiving water from many tanks or ponds). The former need the same precautions as those taken for the fish being treated. All fish being exposed to the treatment at any level may need to be withdrawn from sale, depending on statutory guidelines.
- Treat at the least stressful time of day, usually in the early morning when temperatures are lowest, bearing in mind that oxygen levels on some rivers will also be low at such times.
- Watch the fish throughout treatment and be ready to take any necessary emergency action.
- Record everything in the farm daybook, and in the medicines record book.

Methods of Treatment for Different Holding Systems

Where possible, fish should be held in tanks designed to allow easy and safe dosing during the period where such dosing may be necessary. This means that fry are held in troughs or small raceways, or in small circular tanks where everything is controllable. To avoid affecting fish downstream, the water should not be recycled.

Similarly, fish which may need dosing with malachite green against proliferative kidney disease (PKD) are best dosed in circular tanks where the long retention time and homogeneity of the water ensure an even dosing. These tanks should not discharge into systems containing fish which are to be marketed within the statutory withdrawal period. Residues may persist for 500 degree-days or more.

Fry troughs

Fry troughs are 'controlled' systems with a relatively short turnover time. A common technique is to treat them as static systems and then restore flow to flush out the treatment. To achieve this:

- Have aeration available, and be prepared to use it.
- Lower the water to half the normal level. With trout, a common approximation is to allow 15 cm of water depth per 200–250 kg of fish.
- Mix the treatment chemical with as large a volume of water as is practicable.
- Add the diluted chemical to the tank using a watering can. Avoid pouring it directly onto masses of fish.
- At the end of the treatment period (usually 30–60 minutes) turn on the flow and restore the water level, allowing the tank to flush out the treatment chemical.
- Be ready at any stage to terminate the treatment by restoring the flow.

If the flow cannot be turned off for some reason, then constant-head siphons or continuous dosing systems can be used (see Raceways).

Raceways

Raceways often present somewhat different problems to those for troughs. They usually accommodate bigger fish; they are often arranged in series with no bypass system; and the water-flows are often so high that they would flush out

treatment chemicals. This means that treating one batch may entail treating all of the raceways in a particular 'run'. When a series of raceways is involved, aeration can be a problem if the treatment chemicals (e.g. formalin) either stress the fish or lower the oxygen levels. It may be necesary to move batches of fish which are downstream of those to be treated.

Raceways which can be turned off can be treated as if they are troughs. Those which cannot be turned off may be treated by other methods.

If the water-flow cannot be altered, then a continuous siphon (Fig. 7.1) or its human equivalent is needed, the administration rate being adjusted

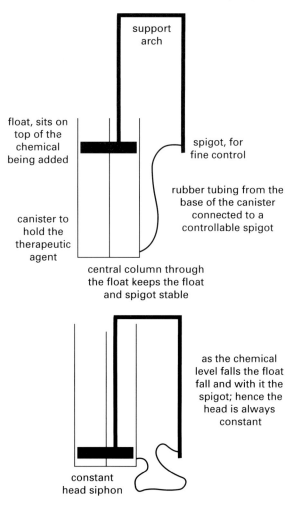

FIG. 7.1 The constant head siphon is a useful device which can be home-made. Various pumps are available which pump at a set rate and so give the opportunity to make up a stock solution to suit the flow rate. Siphons, however, are cheap and less prone to mechanical failure.

to dose the incoming water at the chosen concentration. Pumps are available which deliver constant flows; once calibrated by measuring the delivery rate, a stock tank can be prepared to give the desired effect. Veterinary 'giving' or drip sets and spigot controlled delivery can be used but they are subject to changes in pressure as the head varies, and for critical use their delivery rate needs constant monitoring. The human equivalent sits at the head of the raceway and adds a measured amount at a regular interval from an appropriate container. This manual method is easier to operate if the water-flow can be reduced at all.

Rapid flushes are used in raceways which cannot be adjusted and, again, if the water level can be dropped this will speed the flow through. Normally the treatment chemical is diluted into a few litres of water and is added at the head of the raceway over a period of 1–2 minutes. Fish are able to retreat from the flow and then rush through it when they can go no further, which results in a reduced dose rate; consequently rapid flushes use higher levels of chemical. The problem of fish escaping the treatment can be reduced by crowding them at the downstream end of the raceway, where mixing of the treatment will be most thorough and fish cannot escape.

It is safer to use a reduced flow for a high-dose flush, so that the treatment chemical can be flushed through even more quickly if a problem is seen.

More than most methods, this calls for careful record keeping. Initial treatments at low levels are carefully increased, depending on the effect. The hydrodynamics of individual raceways call for treatments tailored to the situation.

Circular tanks

Circular tanks are highly controlled, normally with a fully adjustable flow and the option to change the depth of water by means of the central overflow pipe. The hydrodynamics of circular tanks are intended to produce a homogeneous body of water as a doughnut around the central drain with a self-cleaning action on the tank bottom. This intention is often theoretical: flow rates influence what actually happens, or unstable systems are constructed. Circular tanks tend to retain treatments far longer than do raceways, so that there is mixing and maximum use of the water.

The tanks, like fry troughs, can be treated as static systems, the flow subsequently being restored to flush out the treatment. This system is particularly useful in the medication of trout affected with PKD, where the aim is to achieve a long exposure of fish to malachite green.

Ponds

Ponds can be difficult to treat because the turnover rate is often slow. The dose rate of any chemical needs to be adjusted for the longer retention time. A common compromise is to lower water levels and add treatment chemicals to the inlet over a period of 20 minutes. After all the treatment has been added, the pond is allowed to refill and normal flow is resumed. Constant dosing can be used, adding the treatment at a low dose over many hours.

With large ponds or lakes it may be necessary to add chemicals with a backpack spray or even to add them into the wake of a boat's outboard motor. The latter method is used in the treatment of lakes for problems with *Argulus* spp. The lake

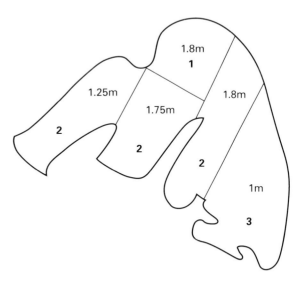

FIG. 7.2 By dividing a known area into arbitrary units (bold) based on the smallest area of the lake and extracting the known surveyed area of the lake (which may be available from estate records), the surface area of each 'unit' can be determined. The average depth in each area is assessed by a man in a boat taking readings with a measuring stick or similar. Thus the volume of each 'unit' and that of the whole lake can be determined. The alternative is to have the lake metered when it is filled, but this is generally impossible with large lakes or those fed by springs.

is divided up on paper and the quantities needed for each section are worked out theoretically (Fig. 7.2). The calculations are put into practice by placing pegs or other markers on the banks of the lake and adding the appropriate amount to each lake section by pouring it into the wake of the outboard motor.

Dip treatment

This is frequently used where fish are being handled routinely or if they are held in a system where they cannot be dosed *in situ*. The method is best suited to small numbers of fish which can be handled easily. Fish are dipped for a short time in a relatively high concentration of the treatment chemical. The dip should always be aerated, since the method is highly stressful. It is not suitable for fish with gill disease.

Cages

The salmon industry has been under serious pressure to achieve effective treatment methods for fish in cages. The methods vary considerably in sophistication and according to the therapeutant to be used.

In one method, the active ingredient is suspended in an oil layer which stays within the cage for 5 days while fish jump through the oil, exposing sea lice on their skins to the treatment. In practice this has not been very satisfactory. Despite the use of a retaining skirt, the treatment can be affected by factors such as photodegradation, storms, intercurrent disease and reduced jumping frequency.

This 'passing through a film' method has been modified by the use of a tube in which a thicker column of compound can be used. The fish can then be anaesthetised and passed through the column back to the cage. In practice there may be secondary disease problems as a result of the extra handling. However, compounds with increased activity could make the technique applicable to non-anaesthetised fish.

There is a bath technique which involves the raising of the centre of the cage bottom to a known depth (say, 2 m) to reduce the amount of treatment chemical required and also to crowd the fish so that all of them are more likely to be exposed to the treatment. A tarpaulin is placed around and under the net, totally enclosing it. Alternatively, a weighted tarpaulin skirt at least double the

reduced net depth is used to surround the sides of the cage, without covering the base. Aeration/oxygenation is essential in both systems as fish are undoubtedly somewhat stressed by the change in the net, even before the use of the chemical. The water movement caused by aeration or oxygenation also ensures that the chemical is well mixed.

Calculating Doses

When working out the dose of a new chemical for a new holding tank, it is sensible to write down every step.

- Calculate the volume of the tank, as shown in Fig. 7.3.

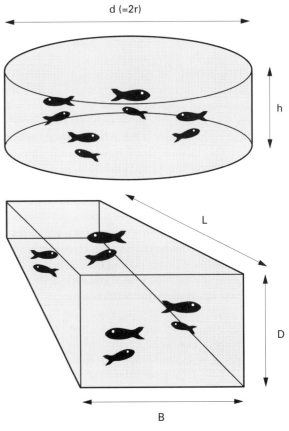

FIG. 7.3 *Round tanks*: volume = $\pi r^2 h$. Example: tank 3 m in diameter and 0.75 m deep — Volume = $3.142 \times 1.5 \times 1.5 \times 0.75 = 5300$ litres. *Troughs and Raceways*: volume = $L \times B \times D$. *Note*: Where the sides are tapering (trapezoidal), take the average breadth. For example, if the top is 3 m wide and the bottom 2 m wide, use the average of 2.5 m. To calcuate the volume of an irregular shape (pond or lake): divide it into smaller units based on these patterns, estimate the volume of each unit and then add them together.

- Calculate the dose required for the chemical being used. Write down every step of the calculation (even when simple changes in the unit and position of the decimal point are made) so that it can easily and quickly be checked for accuracy and remains simple to understand after considerable time has passed.
- Keep the records of the calculation *and* record the effect.

Compounds Used for Treatment via the Water

The various dose rates suggested in the following detailed sections should be applied carefully with an appreciation of the situation being treated. Consideration of the principles already discussed is important.

Benzalkonium chloride

This is a blend of quaternary ammonium compounds specially selected for the treatment of fish. The chemicals in this family are powerful disinfectants with an additional detergent action. The chain length of the molecule is important: in general, shorter chain lengths around 10–14 are safer and more effective for the treatment of fish than are longer ones of 16–18.

Uses. The additional detergent action of these disinfectants is very important in the treatment of fish disease. They are particularly useful in treating external bacterial infections such as Bacterial Gill Disease (BGD) where myxobacteria are multiplying within a film of mucus on the gills. The dual action of benzalkonium chloride inhibits bacterial growth and lifts off the mucus. In this instance the treatment is used as a true symptomatic treatment, to make 'breathing' easier. In many cases the use of benzalkonium chloride can be used as part of a treatment regime to ease the fish's respiration and strip off mucus which may protect pathogens.

Benzalkonium chloride also has a role, concurrently with specific oral antibacterial treatment, in generally reducing the bacterial loading in the water containing fish with bacterial diseases such as enteric redmouth, furunculosis or rainbow trout fingerling syndrome (RTFS). Other potential uses are as a net disinfectant where baths of other chemicals might be dangerous, and as a potential substitute for malachite green in the treatment of broodstock, since it has mild antifungal properties. Compounds related to benzalkonium chloride with much more powerful antifungal properties are being investigated as replacements for malachite green.

Dosage and administration. In rapid turnover systems (5–10 minutes) up to 10 ppm benzalkonium chloride may be needed. With slower turnover systems (30 minutes) up to 5 ppm may be used. For bath treatment in a static system, 1 ppm is used for 1 hour. Doses of 0.1–0.5 ppm (mg/litre) have been used in domestic ponds.

It is particularly important to err on the side of caution with this compound. A tiny amount does an excellent job: use low or very low doses frequently when treating stressed fish, in preference to higher ones looking for an immediate cure. In general, a lower dose is preferred on the grounds of safety; it is also generally non-stressful and fish may not need to be starved before treatment.

Warnings. The toxicity of benzalkonium chloride is increased in soft water, in which treatment levels should be at least halved. If in doubt, try lower doses first and increase as circumstances permit. It is reported that salmon intended for release should not be treated since the chemical inhibits the sense of smell and so can affect the ability of the salmon to return to its home river.

Summary

Benzalkonium chloride
By bath: 10 mg/l for 5–10 minutes.
5 mg/l for 30 minutes.
2 mg/l for 60 minutes.
1 mg/l for several hours.
By prolonged immersion: Doses of 0.1–0.5 mg/l have been used in domestic ponds. In general the lower dose is preferred.

Chloramine T

Chloramine T is one of the most useful chemicals available to the fish farmer. It has an effect against myxobacteria, *Costia, Trichodina*, white spot

THERAPEUTIC DOSE (mg/l)		
pH	Soft water	Hard water
6.0	2.5	7.0
6.5	5.0	10
7.0	10	15
7.5	18	18
8.0	20	20

FIG. 7.4 Therapeutic doses (mg/l).

and *Gyrodactylus* and all their various related pathogens. Its use can be something of an art but the results which can be obtained certainly merit some application. As with all treatments, the low doses can be extremely effective and it is worth starting with low doses and working up if necessary. This approach will save money on purchase of the chemical and is often more effective than using the higher published doses. Low-dose treatments are generally non-stressful and fish may not need preliminary starvation.

Dosage and administration. In general, again always err on the side of caution: start with 2 ppm and increase carefully as necessary. The table of doses in Fig. 7.4 was suggested for treatment of rainbow trout suffering from white spot in a circular tank system with a 4-hour turnover. Where appropriate, the doses can be repeated three times at 4-hour intervals to achieve a 12-hour exposure. Whilst it is certainly not necessary to use these doses for all conditions, they give a broad idea of the way the compound can be used.

Chloramine T can be a very useful part of a treatment regime with benzalkonium chloride; it has a broader spectrum than the latter but lacks any detergent effects. However, it should not be used in the same body of water at the same time as benzalkonium chloride or indeed any other chemical. Treatments should be allowed to flow through before others are used.

Warnings. Care needs to be taken with the source of the chloramine T since the less pure industrial grades may contain impurities such as sulphonic acid which, particularly at higher doses, could form toxic compounds with metal surfaces. Care should be taken to avoid contact between chloramine T and bare metal surfaces. It is also important to avoid contact with the human skin or eyes, and a mask and gloves should be used.

The action of chloramine T is based on a slow breakdown to hypochlorous acid, releasing oxygen and chlorine. Because of this, it should not be used at the same time as other chemicals such as formalin or benzalkonium chloride.

Do not use chloramine T as a high-dose dip: its chemical action will cause serious gill damage.

Chloramine B has been used for treatment of fish diseases when chloramine T has been unavailable. In general its potency appears to be lower, so that slightly higher dosage levels are used.

Summary

Chloramine T
By bath: Range 50–200 mg/100 l.
   The dose is dependent on pH and water hardness:
      In soft water < pH7 — use lower dose.
      In hard water < pH7.5 — use high dose.

Copper sulphate

Copper sulphate is used in the treatment of ectoparasitic infections, especially in marine aquaria. Dip and bath treatments have been used in fish farming in the past but are generally not now recommended. Copper used in this way has been shown to have a serious astringent effect and is certainly effective at removing mucus from gills by literally shrinking the cells off the mucus; it also has an effect on the cells of the liver. This profound astringent effect on gill and liver lasts some 5 days after dip or bath treatments and may take 3 weeks to repair if repeated during this time.

Dose. For long-term exposure in marine systems, a copper concentration of 0.1 mg/l is generally recommended. This is achieved by first preparing a stock solution of 400 mg $CuSO_4 \cdot 5H_2O$ dissolved in 1 litre of water. This is then used at a dose of 1 ml/l. Water changes should be carried out if the level of copper becomes too high. Daily tests should be carried out to maintain a level of 0.1–0.2 mg/l for at least 10 days. Care needs to be taken in fresh water since the dose depends on hardness.

Warnings. Copper sulphate is potentially very toxic in soft water systems with low pH values: it kills marine invertebrates and elasmobranchs. Copper can be removed from the system by water changes, although this takes time. For a more rapid effect, use a large amount of activated carbon (approximately 3 g for every litre of water being treated).

Dichlorvos and trichlorphon

Dichlorvos has become the salmon industry's standard treatment for *Lepeophtheirus salmonis* and *Caligus* spp. sea lice and is still used frequently despite serious resistance problems on some sites. It will probably supercede the long-established compound, trichlorphon, for use in freshwater systems as well as in the sea — for example against *Argulus* spp. in ponds and lakes, and against larval *Lernaea* spp.

Trichlorphon has also been used for many years as a treatment against skin and gill monogenea such as *Dactylogyrus* spp. and *Gyrodactylus* spp. but the latter are now showing resistance to treatment at levels of trichlorphon which are safe for fish: the dose required to kill them has risen in some cases from 0.25 mg/l to 25 mg/l, which is toxic for the fish. A combined treatment of trichlorphon with mebendazole is used by goldfish farmers in the United States; mebendazole has been found effective against *G. elegans* at doses of 0.1 mg/l but has no effect on *Dactylogyrus vastator* at up to 2 mg/l, though fortunately resistance in the latter is not as widespread. Because trichlorphon appears to reduce the efficacy of mebendazole, a final dose rate of 0.4 mg/l mebendazole and 1.8 mg/l trichlorphon has been suggested; the minimum exposure time is 24 hours and no adverse effects have been reported on a range of ornamental fish except perhaps catfish. Successful trials have been reported in goldfish (*Carassius auratus*), oscar (*Astronotus ocellatus*), angel fish (*Pterophyllum scalare*), molly (*Poecilia velifera*) and gourami (*Trichogaster trichopterus*).

Trichlorphon is unavailable in some countries due to medicine licensing procedures. It breaks down over a variable period (depending on water chemistry, pH and hardness) to release dichlorvos, taking up to 3 weeks in acid water, for example. The half-life at 20–23°C is 21 days for a pH value of 7 but only 1 day for a pH value of 9. It is likely that the breakdown of dichlorvos follows a similar pattern.

In fresh water, the normal level of treatment with trichlorphon is 0.2 ppm of active agent. Although as yet no dose titration has been done for dichlorvos in fresh water (and it is unlikely that this will be done by manufacturers), a dose of 0.1 ppm dichlorvos might be a starting point in fresh water. It should be noted that this is only one tenth of marine doses for dichlorvos, but prolonged exposure will be the routine, rather than the 1 hour marine dose.

Dosage and administration of dichlorvos. Against sea lice, dichlorvos is usually used at a dose of 1 ppm active (2 ppm of product) for up to 60 minutes. If used above this dose, the withdrawal period for the treated fish is extended to 500 degree-days. Because dichlorvos does not affect juvenile sea lice, a population survey needs to be carried out to assess the population dynamics (the relative proportions of juvenile chalimus stages attached by frontal filaments, and pre-adults and adults attached by suction) to judge the best time for treatment. Surviving juveniles mature in a further 10–20 days, at which stage a second treatment should be carried out if there are sufficient numbers, and repeated if necessary after another 10–20 days. Vigorous oxygenation of the water helps to ensure good mixing of the treatment and minimises stress on the fish. The active agent is normally diluted at a rate of 1 in 16 at the net side before being added to the tank at the oxygenation points.

The method of administration of dichlorvos is as described earlier. Sea cages may be either enclosed or skirted by tarpaulins (see page 134). Additional oxygenation must, of course, be provided. Complete enclosure is the most effective but can be very stressful to fish because they tend to burrow to the bottom of the cage. The use of a skirt around the cage, while potentially less stressful, leads to inaccurate dosing in the cage so that more active agent tends to be used.

Cage fish must be starved for 24 hours before treatment. Once the tarpaulin is in place, additional aeration should be initiated before the dichlorvos is added. Dissolved oxygen concentrations in the water should not be allowed to fall at any stage. The fish should be observed continuously throughout the treatment and it should be aborted if the fish start burrowing into the tarpaulin or appear sluggish and narcotised. After 15–20 minutes they will start to jump and appear excitable. Most lice should fall off the fish after 1 hour.

Treatment should not be initiated on very sunny days, when the fish will swim 'deep' and may appear to be burrowing. In practice one may count juveniles, adults and nauplii to determine when treatment should be initiated, and the success of a treatment can be determined by examination of live, anaesthetised fish for numbers and stages of sea lice remaining on them.

Warnings. In freshwater, repeat treatments need to be based on water chemistry (as above). Weekly treatments in hard water areas appear to be the norm, whilst in soft water these may be too frequent.

When treating 'new' species, do so with caution as there appear to be certain aspects which are highly susceptible to the chemical's toxic effects. Both trichlorphon and dichlorvos are toxic to characins in general, and problems have been noted in orfe (*Leuciscus idus*), chubb (*L. cephalus*), rudd (*Scardinius erythrophthalmus*) and possibly in golden tench (*Tinca tinca*), although green tench (also *T. tinca*) do not seem to be affected. Toxicity to other fish and higher animals is relatively low; its highest toxicity is towards invertebrates, especially crustacea. Problems of mortalities and fish narcotisation have been ascribed to a solvent used with dichlorvos in a commercial preparation.

There are environmental considerations when using this compound. In the UK, consent from the appropriate water authority must be sought prior to its use. Conditions of poor water movement should mitigate against its use in the sea; the normal flushing action of sea lochs is important. As with all chemicals, care should be taken not to contaminate ponds, streams, waterways, ditches etc. with the product or used containers.

Dichlorvos therapy can be dangerous to operators and great care needs to be taken with operator safety. Instructions from manufacturers must be followed carefully and all safety precautions given on data sheets should be recorded.

Note: Dichlorvos is licensed in the UK by Ciba Geigy Agrochemicals as Aquagard®. Trichlorphon has been widely available from Bayer as Dipterex® and Masoten®.

Formalin

Formaldehyde Solution BP is widely available as a 34–38% w/w solution with methyl alcohol as a stabilising agent to delay polymerisation. This is loosely referred to as 'formalin'. It is used for the treatment of ectoparasitic infections of fish, particularly the protozoa — *Costia (Ichthyobodo)*, *Trichodina* and *Chilodonella* — and is also effective against monogenetic skin and gill flukes such as *Dactylogyrus* and *Gyrodactylus*.

Dosage and administration. The normal treatment level is 1:6000–1:4000 (167–250 ppm) for up to 1 hour, i.e. 17–25 ml/100 l for 30–60 minutes. There is often confusion about the calculation of this dose. It should be made clear that the dose refers to formalin, not formaldehyde, so that a recommended dose of 1:4000 is the same as 1 ml of formalin in 4 litres of water.

In most cases the lower level is preferred, although the high dose may be necessary against *Epistylis*, particularly if temperatures are low.

Formalin is also used as a dip (200 ppm) which should be aerated during use, or as a low-dose long-exposure treatment in closed systems such as ponds and tanks at 2 ml/100 l for 12 hours.

Formalin has been used successfully to reduce the levels of peritrichous ciliates on cultured marine shrimp (*Penaeus stylirostris*). In earth ponds, 25 ppm for 4 hours gave the lowest 'effective' result, although the actual dose may be lower due to organic contamination. Rates of 25–50 ppm would leave enough parasites for recolonisation after 48 hours; better results are obtained at 50–100 ppm.

Warnings. Formalin has a deoxygenating effect and toxicity may be seen during the course of treatment or for up to 24 hours afterwards. Fish with gill disease or anaemia should only be treated with great caution because they may not be able to get sufficient oxygen. Any white deposit of *para-formaldehyde* should be filtered out or the formalin disposed since it is extremely toxic to fish.

Operators should avoid contact with skin and inhalation of formaldehyde fumes.

Summary

Formalin
By bath: 17–25 ml/100 l for 30–60 minutes.
By prolonged immersion: 2 ml/100 l for 12 hours.

Leteux–Meyer mixture

There are several variations on the basic combination of formalin and malachite green which aim to give a treatment dose in the region of 25 ppm formalin and 0.05–0.1 ppm malachite green. One common formulation adds 3.68 g malachite green to 1 l formalin. This is used at 25 ppm for 1 hour, i.e. 2.5 ml/100 l for 1 hour.

In static ponds a weaker mixture of 3.3 g malachite green in 1 l formalin can be used at 15 ppm, i.e. 1.5 ml/100 l. If necessary, providing that dissolved oxygen levels remain above 5 ppm and the temperature below 28°C, it may be used at intervals of 3–4 days.

Summary

Leteux–Meyer mixture
By bath: 2.5 ml/100 l for 1 hour.
By prolonged immersion: 1.5 ml/100 l as 3
   treatments at intervals of 3–4 days when
   appropriate.

Malachite green

Malachite green is $C_{23}H_{12}N_2$ and it contains no copper. The most commonly available form is industrial, precipitated by the addition of $ZnCl_2$ and produced as a double zinc salt. Malachite green oxalate is never produced in this way: it is free from zinc and is the form which is generally recommended.

The strength of malachite green is referred to as a percentage of the dyeing ability of the same manufacturer's dry dye. The strength of a saturated aqueous solution is only 7.6%. Aqueous solutions greater than 30% solution can be made using acetic and hydrochloric acids.

Malachite green exists as two ionic forms (Fig.

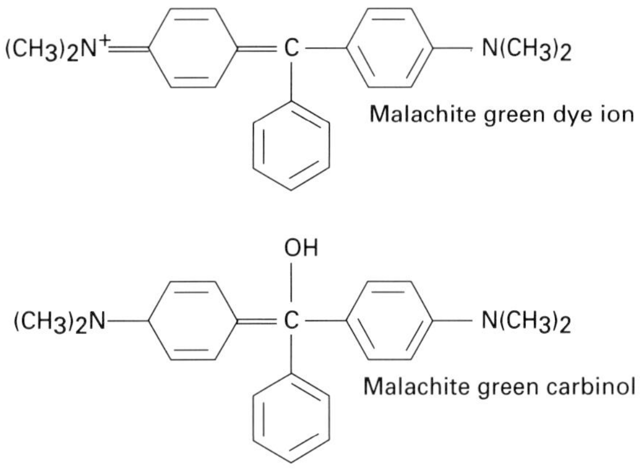

FIG. 7.5 At pH 4.0, 100% of malachite green is ionised; at 6.9 only 50% is ionised (hence 6.9 = pKa); at 7.4, 25% is ionised at 10.1, 0% is ionised. Equilibrium for this ionisation is reached within 5 hours.

7.5). The coloured dye salt reacts slowly with –OH to produce a colourless, non-ionised carbinol (also called pseudobase or colour base). The carbinol is more liposoluble and this may be the form which enters cells; it is less soluble in water. When malachite green is added to water it will gradually form the carbinol, which will come out of solution as a greenish-white deposit (although not in a flowing situation).

This whole family of dyes is known to have an affinity for organic material and so, in the fish farm situation, malachite green will probably become attached to this type of material and then become oxidised in the presence of air and light. There does not seem to be any published work on the ultimate fate of the carbinol; it probably forms *p*-dimethylbenzophenone.

Uses. Malachite green is used prophylactically and for treatment of fungal infections. Mixed with formalin it is used to treat protozoal infections (see Leteux–Meyer mixture).

Until recently it was not fully appreciated how deeply malachite green penetrated the tissues of the fish being treated. But it is now apparent that malachite green can be used very successfully against Proliferative Kidney Disease (PKD) in salmonids. It is possible that it could also be used against similar disease processes such as *Mitraspora cyprini* in goldfish. It has also been used as a 'general systemic disinfectant'.

Dosage and administration. When treating fish eggs against fungal infections, use a 2 ppm flowing treatment for 30–60 minutes. For broodstock with infected skin lesions a 50–60 ppm dip may be used for 30 seconds (this is often used prophylactically after handling fish during stripping). In soft water it is advisable to halve the dose.

Malachite green may be sold as a powder or as 2%, 10% or 50% solutions. These solutions are considered as w/v although strictly speaking they are not — as explained earlier they refer to dying capability, and so

$$10\% = 10 \text{ g}/100 \text{ ml}$$
$$= 0.1 \text{ g/ml}$$
$$= 100 \text{ mg/ml}.$$

As an example, if a fry trough requires a total of 0.6 g (600 mg) for treatment:

10% (at 0.1 g/ml) needs 0.6/0.1 = 6 ml
50% (at 0.5 g/ml) needs 0.6/0.5 = 1.2 ml.

Determining doses of malachite green for treatment against Proliferative Kidney Disease requires precise calculation which is easier in circular tanks. The aim is to achieve a dose exposure of some 100 ppm minutes over a 4 hour period. Computer spreadsheets modelling of the flow rates and necessary dose rate allows a dose to be computed which gives this exposure. A section of a typical spreadsheet is shown in Fig. 7.6.

The sensitivity of juvenile lobsters (*Homarus americanus*) to different concentrations of malachite green during various states of the intermoult cycle has been investigated. Malachite green was found to be an effective treatment for lobsters during the intermoult state C4 at about 700–800 mg/l for 6 minutes. Juveniles are sensitive during the intermoult state A–B.

Warnings. Toxicity in ponds or other slow turnover systems may be apparent as respiratory

EXAMPLE OF DOSAGE CALCULATIONS		
Tank diameter:	9m	
Tank depth:	1m	
Flow rate:	50 m^3/hour (833.33 l/minute)	
Tank volume:	63.63 m^3 (63,625.50 l)	
Turnover time:	76.35 minutes (1.27 hours)	
Dose of malachite required:	1.5 ppm	
Total amount added:	95.44 g	
Total dose:	**191** (ml of 50%)	
Cumulative dose after 4 hours:	109.03 ppm minutes	
Remaining concentration:	0.0625	

minutes	ppm	ppm minutes
0	1.5	
1	1.48	1.49
2	1.46	2.9608
3	1.44	4.4122
4	1.42	5.8446
5	1.40	7.2582
6	1.39	8.6534
7	1.37	10.03
8	1.35	11.389
9	1.33	12.73
10	1.31	14.053
11	1.30	15.36
12	1.28	16.649
13	1.26	17.921
14	1.25	19.176
15	1.23	20.415
16	1.21	21.638
17	1.20	22.845
18	1.18	24.036

FIG. 7.6 An example of a dosage calculation.

distress — usually immediate rather than delayed. The effect of malachite green is dependent on its action as a respiratory poison, blocking thiol-containing enzymes and the cytochrome oxidase system in the mitochondria.

Some American work suggests possible carcinogenic risks associated with malachite green. This issue has, to some extent, been answered but there is a possibility of teratogenicity. It is quite likely that the compound will be outlawed as a fish treatment over the next 5–10 years.

Summary

Malachite green
By dip: 5–6 g/100 l for 10–30 seconds.
By bath: 100–200 mg/100 l for 30–60 minutes.
   The higher dose should only be used for large fish in hard water.
By prolonged immersion: 10 mg/100 l for 30–96 hours.
Eggs, by bath: 50 mg/100 l for 1 hour.
   TAKE CARE — SERIOUS RESPIRATORY POISON

Methylene blue

This has been in use for many years as an antiprotozoal treatment but rarely on fish farms for this purpose. Its major use now is as a treatment for nitrite toxicity to convert methaemoglobin back to haemoglobin.

Dose. 1 mg/litre.

Warnings etc. This chemical is extremely harmful to biological filter systems and for this reason should not be used in recirculation systems without taking precautions for treatment off-circuit or stripping down and re-establishing the filter.

Summary

Methylene blue
Stock solution: 10 g/l.
By prolonged immersion: 20–40 ml/100 l stock solution. Dose may be doubled.
   TOXIC TO SCALELESS FISH
   HARMFUL TO BIOFILTERS

Potassium permanganate

This treatment for protozoal and monogenean parasites, Bacterial Gill Disease (BGD) and oxygen depletion is also used with formalin to generate formaldehyde gas as a fumigant for buildings.

Dosage and administration. The use of potassium permanganate requires careful observation and effort to devise regimes which are both safe and effective. It has been used at 2 ppm in ponds against various ectoparasites. For the treatment of BGD in tanks and troughs it is used at 1–5 ppm for 1 hour, repeating as necessary for 2–3 days. An alternative means of administration is by short duration (10–40 seconds) dip treatment in a 1,000 ppm solution. As an emergency procedure in static ponds it has been used for treatment of oxygen depletion at a dose of 2 ppm.

Summary

Potassium permanganate
By bath: 500 mg/100 l for 1 hour.
By dip: 100 g/100 l for 10–40 seconds.
   If organic load is high, repeat treatment after 24 hours.
      EMERGENCY OXYGENATION:
      200 mg/100 l
      or 300–400 mg/100 l if high organic load present.

Warnings. In muddy water the compound may be neutralised totally and rendered ineffective; it may lead to toxic effects due to the deposition of manganese dioxide on the gills. Care needs to be taken in warm water and with scaleless fish such as eels.

Sodium chloride (salt)

Sodium chloride has a variety of uses and has justifiably been a fish farmers' standby for a great many years. It has been used for the treatment of ectoparasitic infestations such as *Costia* and *Chilodonella*, particularly in fry, and for the treatment of alevins with coagulated yolks. It is a safe treatment for use along with reduced feeding in alevins and fry suffering from bacterial gill disease: the salt has a mild astringent effect and so 'lifts' mucus off the gills.

Salt can also be used for cleaning the muddy flavour from otherwise marketable fish and for reducing osmotic stress on individual high value fish. In these situations it is used for longer periods.

Dosage and administration. Alevins and small fry can be treated with 0.5% (5,000 ppm) for 30 minutes, or 1% (10,000 ppm) for 6–10 minutes. Larger fish may be given progressively larger doses such that portion-sized fish (8–10 oz) can be treated with 3% salt (30,000 ppm) until they show signs of distress.

For treatment of high value fish such as koi to reduce osmotic stress, a level of 0.15% (1,500 ppm) on day 1 can be built up to 0.5% (5,000 ppm) over 3 days. If any signs of distress are seen the solution should be diluted. In emergencies the fish can be placed straight into 0.5% (5,000 ppm) but may show signs of stress for a few hours.

Fry in troughs and fish in large and otherwise untreatable ponds can be very usefully medicated by placing a pile or bag of salt on the bottom of the trough or pond. Bags should be secured with a rope so that they do not drift off when empty and block the screens. Under these circumstances fish will often follow the salt concentration and virtually swim into the bag, dosing themselves to effect before swimming away.

Warnings. As a general rule it is recommended that alevins and fry under 5 g (or 100 fish per pound) should not be exposed to over 1% (10,000 ppm) sodium chloride, and that fish under 100 g (5 fish/lb) should not be exposed to levels greater than 2% (20,000 ppm).

Summary

Sodium chloride
By bath: 1.0–1.5 kg/100 l for 20 minutes.
By dip: 2–3 kg/100 l until fish show signs of stress.
By permanent bath (for supportive purposes): 500 g/100 l.

Iodine compounds

These are used for the disinfection of fish eggs and are generally available in solutions giving 1.6% available iodine.

Dose. By bath, 3 ml/l for 10 minutes. Rinse ova thoroughly in clean water.

Warnings. This type of treatment can be toxic to unfertilised ova and to live fish.

Antibiotics given via the water

These should not be used with bacterial filtration.

Oxytetracycline	13–120 mg/l (chelated by hard water)
Oxolinic acid	10 mg/l
Doxycycline and Minocycline	2–3 mg/l
Chloramphenicol	20–50 mg/l
Co-trimazine (80 mg trimethoprim and 400 mg sulphadiazine per ml)	1 ml/100–120 l
Nifurpirinol	0.1 mg/l
Metronidazole	7 mg/l (double for *Oodinium*)
Dimetridazole	5 mg/l (said to inhibit spawning)
Neomycin	50 mg/kg (used in sea water)
Gentamycin	4–5 mg/kg (used in sea water)
Kanamycin	50–100 mg/l

The fish farm situation is rarely appropriate for the application of antibiotics by immersion, although they may be used this way with ornamental fish. Hard water in particular tends to cause problems since it chelates tetracyclines and renders them useless except in very high doses. When used at lower doses the micro-organisms living in the aquarium are exposed to levels which tend to cause resistance, with its consequences.

Other UK licensed compounds

Praziquantel. Used at 27.4–34.25 mg/kg bodyweight in a successful trial to eliminate *Bothriocephalus acheilognathi* from carp (*Cyprinus carpio*), grass carp (*Ctenopharyngodon idella*), tench (*Tinca tinca*) and wels (*Silurus glanis*). It has also been used at 35–100 mg/kg (given by stomach tube) effectively and safely in grass carp infected with *B. acheilognathi*. A dose of 125 mg/kg body-weight fed over a three day period by top-dressing pelleted food has also proved effective.

Ivermectin has been used in goldfish by injection at a dose of 200 µg/kg (first diluted 1:125 with physiological saline, this is then used at 0.1 ml/50 g by intramuscular injection at the base of the dorsal fin). It has been reported that the parasite dies and healing occurs rapidly. It is uncertain whether this treatment eliminates the larvae on the gills. Ivermectin at 100 µg/kg however, may affect the fish before it affects the parasites.

Antimalarials. These agents (e.g. chloroquine) have been used very successfully against protozoan infections in ornamental marine fish. Experience suggests that these drugs may have disastrous effects used this way in the newer 'complete ecosystem' tanks which are dependent on the interaction between fish, invertebrates, algae and bacteria.

Levamisole. It has been used for a number of years with apparent success at 10 mg/l against nematodes in fish, such as live-bearers infected with *Camallanus* spp. or discus (*Symphysodon discus*) infected with *Capillaria* spp. No adverse effects have been reported and fish have bred afterwards.

Vaccination

When a fish is immersed in vaccine, the vaccine is picked up by macrophages in the gill and delivered via the blood system to melanomacrophage centres in the spleen, kidney and epicardium. In small fish, some goes to the thymus.

Lymphocytes are then exposed to the antigen to begin production of a cell-mediated (T cell) or antibody-mediated (B cell) response. The primary response is T cell from the thymus, which in trout

is active over 4°C and which persists for longer. The thymus is probably the source of both T and B cells. Fish seem to have only one class of agglutinating antibodies, corresponding to a four sub-unit IgM.

Commercial vaccines which can be administered by dip, spray or injection are currently available for salmonids, carp, and lobsters (Fig. 7.7).

The evidence indicates that fish weighing less than 1 g should not be vaccinated: below this size, salmonids are probably not immunocompetent. A better response is seen in fish weighing more than 2.5 g; for routine purposes 5 g is suggested as the most suitable size. Smaller fish have been vaccinated successfully with oral vaccines but these are not yet available commercially.

In the USA, where larger fish are vaccinated because of the presence of other fish pathogens, certain farms encounter problems in vaccinating fry because the stress caused by the handling required for vaccination triggers outbreaks of infectious pancreatic necrosis (IPN) or infectious haematopoetic necrosis (IHN).

The response to vaccination is considered to be more a function of size than age, and the time taken to reach protective levels of antibodies after vaccination is temperature dependent. For example, after a 5-second immersion in vaccine, protection is effective in 10 days for fish held at 10°C, whereas at 18°C the period is 5 days. It is generally recommended that 14 days be allowed to build up immunity.

Duration of immunity appears to be size dependent. In fish vaccinated at a weight of 1 g, immunity lasts approximately 120 days; the duration

COMMERCIAL VACCINES CURRENTLY AVAILABLE IN THE UK			
Disease	**Agent**	**Fish species**	**Treatment**
Furunculosis	*Aeromonas salmonicida*	Atlantic salmon	Injection/dip
Enteric redmouth	*Yersinia ruckeri*	Rainbow trout	Dip/injection
Vibriosis	*Vibrio anguillarum*	Rainbow trout	Dip
Carp erythrodermatitis	*A. salmonicida*	Carp	Dip
Divalent and trivalent combination vaccines are also available, as are vaccines against diseases occuring outside the UK:			
Gaffkaemia	*A. viridans*	Lobster	Dip
Hitra disease	*Vibrio* spp.	Atlantic salmon	Dip

FIG. 7.7 Commercial vaccines currently available in the UK.

increases to 180 days if vaccination is at 2 g, and to over a year for fish weighing more than 4 g at vaccination.

The duration is also dependent on the route of administration. At an experimental level, the route producing the best overall results is i/p injection, although in most cases direct immersion is more cost effective because of the labour involved.

It is important to note that vaccination has no effect on chronic carriers of ERM and vibriosis. The method should be used to protect healthy fish before they leave a 'clean' site to come to an infected farm, rather than give false reassurances about possibly infected and hence carrier fish. Vaccination against ERM seems to produce a cell-mediated response rather than one dependent on antibodies.

There has been speculation about immunosuppression associated with vaccination. Logically this would be nonsense since exactly the opposite is demonstrated by the licensed use, i.e. to produce protective immunity. There appears to be no evidence for this although the same phenomenon seen when vaccinating other animals may be seen, i.e. the vaccine 'mops up' any circulating antibodies and potentially leaves the fish temporarily open to infection or to the stress-induced triggering of an existing infection.

Commercial use of vaccination generally gives better than a 60% protection rate, although in practice a much better rate is expected.

Intraperitoneal injection gives a rapid and more solid protection with a smaller amount of vaccine; it is, however, more costly in manpower. An experienced operator is said to be able to vaccinate 600–700 fish per hour but this requires support teams and a strong constitution.

Immersion is a much more cost effective technique for the average farm. Initially this was a two stage method: the fish were immersed in a hyperosmotic bath and then transferred to the vaccine bath which was stressful to the fish. It was shown to be unnecessary because fish can take up sufficient vaccine for an adequate 'take' by simple dipping. Adjuvants have been developed which potentiate the effect. Most commercial vaccines are formulated so that fish are sprayed or dipped in a 1-in-10 dilution of the vaccine for 5–30 seconds.

Oral vaccination would be the ideal route for farmers to use: it would be non-stressful and require no extra staff time. The areas of the fish intestine likely to respond to vaccine uptake are the distal ones, which presents problems of delivery. Certainly the acid digestion of the salmonid stomach tends to inactivate antigen as it passes through.

Treatment via the Food: Antibacterials/Antibiotics

Antibacterials, as their name implies, are only truly effective against bacterial diseases. Some cross the borders and are effective against other groups of pathogens, for example, furazolidone is effective against *Hexamita*. In many cases their use will be required even if the bacterial disease is secondary.

There are certain general principles for the use of antibacterials:

- Use antibacterials only when there is a strong likelihood of a bacterial infection.
- Start treatment as early as possible, having taken samples for bacteriological examination.
- Use an antibacterial of as narrow a spectrum as possible in order to conserve normal bacterial ecology.
- Avoid prophylactic antibacterial therapy.
- Give the correct dose for the correct length of time to ensure proper tissue levels.
- Adopt a policy of restriction or rotation in the type of antibacterial agent used.

The choice of antibacterial agents is often suggested initially by experience and modified later as information from sensitivity tests becomes available. This process can be helped by routine sampling to build up a picture of the 'normal' sensitivity profile of the farm. Various factors influence the veterinarian in selecting the first antibacterial to use in a given situation. In general the 'best practice' or even 'the only legal recourse' will be to use licensed products in a particular country. Other factors are:

- Experience of the disease.
- Information on the pathogen.
- Previous use on the farm.
- Previous use of antibacterials locally.
- Sensitivity profile.

FIG. 7.8 Administration of oral antibacterials.

ADMINISTRATION OF ORAL ANTIBACTERIALS

Feeding rate
  Sick fish generally have reduced appetites and so the batch should be fed at a low
  level of food — say 1%
  At a 1% body-weight feed rate:
  50 kg fish require 500g food/day = 5kg in 10 days

Treatment: Furazolidone at 75 mg/kg fish/day
  Medicate 5 kg food with (75 mg x 50 kg fish x 10 days)
    = 37500 mg
    = 37.5g furazolidone/5 kg food

Application
  To encourage the medication to stick to the food, use up to
  1l corn oil/25 kg food = 200 ml corn oil/5 kg food
  Alternatively use 5% gelatine or agar

- The need to rotate drugs.
- Withdrawal periods when the fish are to be marketed.
- Cost.
- Legal status of using the drug in fish.

Efficacy of the antibacterial agent is always governed by the sensitivity of the pathogen. It is not a straightforward matter to give concentrations of drug which exceed the MIC in plasma for survival in the face of disease since other factors play a part, such as the severity of the initial impact of the disease and any predisposing factors. These,

and speed of diagnosis and treatment, will govern the proportion of fish which are likely to be well enough to eat sufficient food and antibiotic to recover.

Administration of Oral Antibacterials

A sample treatment regime is given in Fig. 7.8. As a general rule, fish are medicated by mixing antibacterials with food (Fig. 7.9). The fish are most commonly given approximately 1% of their body-weight per day as medicated food; any additional food is given unmedicated. Occasionally

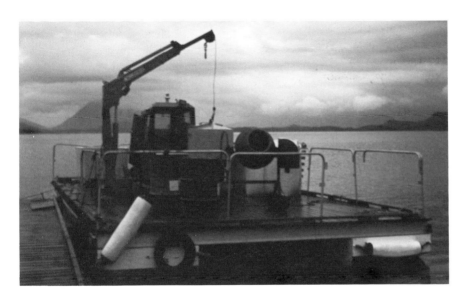

FIG. 7.9 On larger farms, medicated feed may be mixed by the side of the sea cage requiring medication.

(a) QUANTITIES OF COMMON ANTIBACTERIALS USED PER 25KG FEED				
	Percentage body-weight to be fed			
	0.5%	1.0%	2.0%	3.0%
25kg of food feeds	**5000 kg**	**2500 kg**	**1250 kg**	**833 kg**
Oxytetracycline at 75 mg/kg : pure	375 g	187.5 g	93 g	62.5 g
Furazolidone at 75 mg/kg : pure	375 g	187.5 g	93 g	62.5 g
: 20%	1.9 kg	938 g	465 g	313 g
Co-trimazine at 30 mg/kg : pure	150 g	75 g	37.5 g	25 g
: 40%	375 g	187.5 g	93 g	62.5 g
: susp	313 ml	157 ml	79 ml	52 ml
Oxolinic acid at 10 mg/kg : pure	50 g	25 g	12.5 g	8.3 g
: 20%	250 g	125 g	62.5 g	41.5 g
Amoxycillin at 80 mg/kg : pure	400 g	200 g	100 g	66.5 g

(b) QUANTITIES OF COMMON ANTIBACTERIALS USED PER TONNE FEED			
	Percentage body-weight to be fed		
	0.5%	1.0%	2.0%
1000kg of food feeds	**200,000 kg** **200 tonnes**	**100,000 kg** **100 tonnes**	**50,000 kg** **50 tonnes**
Furazolidone at 75 mg/kg : pure	15 kg	7.5 kg	3.75 kg
Oxytetracycline at 75 mg/kg : pure	15 kg	7.5 kg	3.75 kg
Co-trimazine at 30 mg/kg : 40%	15 kg	7.5 kg	3.75 kg
Oxolinic acid at 10 mg/kg : pure	2 kg	1 kg	0.5 kg
: 50%	4 kg	2 kg	1 kg
: 20%	10 kg	5 kg	2.5 kg
Amoxycillin at 80 mg/kg : pure	16 kg	8 kg	4 kg

FIG. 7.10 Quantities of common bacterials used (a) per 25 kg feed, (b) per tonne of feed.

the food rate will be different, but for general purposes the 1% level is standard.

Fish are cold-blooded (poikilothermic), and their activity and required feeding rate are temperature dependent. Accordingly, each feed manufacturer issues a chart which relates fish weight or size to water temperature and gives recommended feeding levels in terms of percentage body-weight. These charts are intended only as guidelines; the fish farm management will establish suitable feeding regimes and modify the feed chart to suit its own facility (Fig. 7.10a).

The oral dose of antibacterials is administered to the fish by taking into account the feeding rate and incorporating the drug at an appropriate level. It is also affected by the presence of disease in a batch of fish. By knowing the percentage feeding rate and the total weight of the batch, the amount of food needed in a day can be easily worked out. In practice the feeding rate used will often be 0.5% or 1%. Knowing the amount of food to be eaten per day and the total weight of fish enables the veterinary surgeon to advise on the amount of drug to be added per kilogram of food.

DRUGS USED AGAINST BACTERIAL FISH DISEASE				
Generic name	Those holding UK product licences	Species	Dose (mg/kg)	Withdrawal period (degree-days)
Oxytetracycline	Tetraplex (PH Pharmaceuticals)	AS	75	400
	Microtet (Microbiologicals)	AS, RT, AC	75	RT & AS 350
				AC 500
Oxolinic acid	Aquinox (PH Pharmaceuticals)	AS	10	500
	Aqualinic powder (Parke Davis)	AS, RT, BT	10	500
Co-trimazine	Tribrissen (Pitman-Moore)	AS, RT	30	RT 350, AS 500
	Sulphatrim (PH Pharmaceuticals)	AS	30	500
Amoxycillin	Micromox (Microbiologicals)	AS	80	150
	Aquacil (PH Pharmaceuticals)	AS	40	50
	Vetremox (Vetrepharm)	AS	80	40
Furazolidone	Not licensed for fish	AS, RT	75	500
Erythromycin	Not licensed for fish	AS, RT	25–100	500
Flumequine	Not licensed for fish in the UK	AS, RT	12–50	–
Ormetoprim: sulphadimethoxide	Licensed for fish in the USA	AS, RT	50	–
AS = Atlantic salmon; RT = Rainbow trout; AC = Arctic char; BT = Brown trout				

FIG. 7.11 Drugs used against bacterial diseases in fish.

Pharmaceutical companies can provide tables to give guidance in this calculation (Fig. 7.11). The drug may either be 'incorporated' in the feed at the feed mill or else top dressed onto the pellet by the fish farmer on the farm (Fig. 7.10b). Duration of therapy varies from country to country but is usually in the range of 5–14 days.

Antibiotic Types and Products

The array of antibacterials available for use in fish is relatively restricted and only a few are licensed in the majority of countries. Those in common use are shown in Fig. 7.11, for which much of the information is based on products licensed for use in fish in the UK.

Amoxycillin

Amoxycillin is a synthetic penicillin in its own right rather than simply an ester of ampicillin, with which it shares many properties. It is modified to be acid resistant and suitable for oral use; food does not interfere with absorption. It shows low protein binding and a susceptibility to penicillinase, and operates by interfering with cell wall production. In mammals, 50% is excreted via the kidneys as an active metabolite.

Resistance to amoxycillin is likely to be R-plasmid mediated with bacteria acquiring the ability to produce β-lactamase. It is possible that this will develop relatively rapidly where the use of amoxycillin is forced on those farms which already suffer from multiple resistant strains of bacteria.

MIC data recorded in the literature

Species	µg/ml
Aeromonas hydrophila	0.2
A. salmonida	0.78
Pasteurella piscida	0.2
Streptococcus spp.	0.39–0.78
Edwardsiella tarda	0.39–1.56
Vibrio anguillarum	25–100

The product, as demonstrated in the clinical trials, is palatable at 80 mg/kg. No adverse effects have been reported in yellowtail in terms of palatability or toxicity at inclusion rates of 5× the recommended level (i.e. 400 mg/kg).

Summary

Amoxycillin
Oral therapy: 40–80 mg/kg for 10 days.

Co-trimazine

This and other related combinations of trimethoprim and a sulphadrug (in this case sulphadiazine) have been used in fish. Trimethoprim was developed to be part of a sequential blockade, supporting and improving the action of sulphadrugs.

Although not particularly useful against *Pseudomonas* spp. it has proved effective against *Aeromonas* spp. and *Yersinia ruckeri*. The bulk of the absorbed drug is excreted through the kidneys. In sea water, where fish naturally excrete concentrated urine, there is a danger of causing crystalluria by overdose.

The recommended dose rate per kilogram is 30 mg of the combined ingredients. Current UK withdrawal periods are 350 degree-days for Atlantic salmon and 500 degree-days for rainbow trout.

Summary

> **Co-trimazine**
> *Oral therapy:* 30 mg/kg for 5–7 days.
> *Palatable* at high inclusion rates.
> *Sensitive:* Aeromonads etc.

Erythromycin

Erythromycin has been used in salmonids to help control Bacterial Kidney Disease (BKD). Erythromycin thiocyanate has been used orally in pre-smolting salmon and trout at a dose of 100 mg/kg body-weight for periods exceeding 21 days, and by sub-cutaneous injection at a dose of 11 mg/kg into wild salmon as they enter trapping facilities and at 21–30 day intervals thereafter. No injections are given within 30 days prior to spawning. Some fish are reported to 'bronze' following this treatment which is believed to be an icteric response.

A bath technique using erythromycin phosphate showed some effect but only when fish were 'prepared' by a hyperosmotic treatment (in 5.5% NaCl) prior to 3 minutes in the erythromycin phosphate. Serum levels of 22.19 μg/ml were achieved. Some work was also done using surfactants in combination with erythromycin phosphate dips, which also helped with the absorption of therapeutic levels.

Water hardening in erythromycin phosphate at 2 mg/litre has been used to control egg transmission of *Renibacterium salmoninarum* but detailed studies indicated that this was not successful.

Fumagillin DCH

Workers in the USA, and more recently in the UK, have considered the potential use of fumagillin against Proliferative Kidney Disease (PKD) in salmonids. Prior to this its use was against the parasite *Nosema* in honey bees.

Nitrofurans

This group has contributed two useful compounds: nifurpirinol and furazolidone. The former is particularly well absorbed via the skin, to the extent that it has gained a place as a water treatment as much as an oral treatment, widely used for ornamental fish and certain farmed species, especially eels.

Summary

> **Nifurpirinol**
> *Long-term bath:* (3–5 days): 0.05–0.1 ppm.
> *Short-term bath:* (5–10 minutes): 1–2 ppm.
> *Oral therapy:* 2–4 mg/kg.

Furazolidone has been used for 20–25 years. Although poorly absorbed through the gut in mammals, it appears effective against septicaemic diseases in fish. The standard dose in freshwater species is 75–100 mg/kg. Palatability is poor with salmonids but toxicity is low. It has been reported that rainbow trout have been seen to 'vomit' some time after feeding if dose rates are high. It has been widely used as an antiprotozoal in salmonid fry affected with *Hexamita* (*Octomitis*).

Summary

> **Furazolidone**
> *Oral therapy:* 75–100 mg/kg.
> *Not palatable* at high inclusion rates.
> *Sensitive:* Aeromonads, *Hexamita* etc.

Oxolinic acid

A dose rate of 10 mg/kg body-weight is recommended for routine use in fresh water. Although oxolinic acid is licensed for use in some countries at this rate, in practice many veterinarians find they must prescribe 30 mg/kg in marine environments to obtain efficacy.

The mode of bactericidal effect of oxolinic acid is by interference with the action of bacterial DNA-gyrase. This controls supercoiling DNA during cell replication, which is consequently prevented by the interference. Strangely, at high concentrations this effect appears to be altered and the compound becomes bacteriostatic. It is apparent, then, that oxolinic acid is only active against bacteria which are dividing.

Resistance is not mediated via plasmids and arises through mutation. *In vitro*, it is possible to induce resistance rapidly and increase the organisms' MIC to very high levels over a number of generations. Resistance may also decrease, although more slowly *in vitro* than it develops. This is also seen in the clinical situation.

MIC data recorded in the literature

Species	µg/ml
Aeromonas salmonicida,	
A. liquefaciens,	
Vibrio anguillarum and	0.02–0.09
Flexibacter (Chondrococcus) columnaris	
Pasteurella piscida (from yellowtail — Seriola quinqueradiata)	2.66
Yersinia ruckeri	1 (bacteriostasis — 25/25 isolates)
Yersinia ruckeri	5 (bacteriodical — 23/25 isolates)
A. salmonicida	0.8–20

Because oxolinic acid has relatively low solubility, a micronised ultra-fine preparation has been developed to increase bioavailability.

Summary

Oxolinic acid
Oral therapy: 10–30 mg/kg for 10 days.
Palatable at high inclusion rates.
Sensitive: Aeromonads, etc.

The dosage may have to be increased for infections occurring in marine fish (30 mg/kg × 10 days).

At the time of writing no maximum residue limit (MRL) is being set in the UK and so statutory withdrawal periods apply (currently 500 degree-days).

Oxytetracycline

Oxytetracycline is probably the most widely used antibacterial for fish therapy. It was the first antibiotic to be the subject of any quantitative work on absorption. This was in comparison with chlortetracycline, which was found to be ineffective. Oxytetracycline is licensed in the USA for both salmonids and lobsters.

Dose rates which have been recommended are:

Dose (mg/kg)	Species	Indication
75	brook trout	Ulcer disease — *Haemophilus piscium*
50–75	rainbow trout	*Aeromonas salmonicida* and *H. piscium*
25–35	rainbow trout	Ulcer disease
50–80	rainbow trout	Enteric redmouth, furunculosis; vibriosis. Columnaris disease

In practice, this range of doses has narrowed down generally to 75 mg/kg and the drug is still used widely for all these conditions.

Response times in clinical situations seem to be within 3–5 days in the majority of cases. Once a disease has broken out, there will always be a lag phase for response if the mortalities have escalated rapidly. Those fish which are already sufficiently affected by the disease to be off their food or only accepting very reduced amounts will either die or recover.

Various clinical reports show that high inclusion rates of up to 24 g/kg are still palatable. It is this very acceptability which makes 100% formulations so valuable, being able to achieve high levels of inclusion without various binders etc. which may adversely affect palatability.

It has been suggested that the humoral immune response of the fish might be susceptible to low levels of oxytetracycline, although the cellular response remains unaffected. This effect is not observed clinically at the dose rates used normally in rainbow trout.

The extensive use of the drug for approximately

35 years and its wide range of efficacy make oxytetracycline essential to the fish veterinarian. Pure material is probably the most useful since it permits the high inclusion rates necessary for the treatment of disease in the Atlantic salmon industry, which must deal regularly with low temperatures and feed rates. It is also of great value to the trout farmer who may have sick fish eating very little, again requiring high inclusion rates.

MIC data recorded in the literature

Species	µg/ml
Vibrio anguillarum	
Aeromonas salmonicida }	1.56
Yersinia ruckeri	3–12
A. salmonicida	0.25
A. liquefaciens	0.5
Pseudomonas fluorescens	5.0
Flexibacter (Chondrococcus)	8.0, 10.0
columnaris	

A cost-saving technique which has been used in Scotland involves increasing the daily dose to 120 mg/kg or even to 240 mg/kg and feeding the medicated feed at intervals of 4 days. Acceptable serum levels are apparently achieved and maintained with this regime.

Summary

> **Oxytetracycline**
> *Oral therapy:* 75 mg/kg for 10 days.
> *Palatable* at high inclusion rates.
> *Sensitive:* Aeromonads, Myxobacteria etc.

Current UK withdrawal periods for licensed products are:
    Microtet – 350 degree-days for rainbow trout and Arctic chair; 500 degree-days for Atlantic salmon.
    Tetraplex – 400 degree days for Atlantic salmon.

Sarafloxacin hydrochloride

This new drug, a bactericidal aryl-fluoroquinolone, is related to oxolinic acid, an earlier generation quinolone. The data for sarafloxacin seems to indicate that, for strains of *Aeromonas*

spp. resistant to oxolinic acid, the MIC is approximately a quarter that of oxolinic acid. This means that some strains of bacteria which are resistant to oxolinic acid may be sensitive to sarafloxacin. As with other quinolones, any resistance will not be plasmid mediated and so spread is unlikely; a major benefit over the earlier compounds is the reduced likelihood of developing resistance.

Recommended dose rates are not yet available but the data suggests that 6–14 mg/kg is effective against *Yersinia ruckeri* in rainbow trout, or 10–14 mg/kg against *Vibrio anguillarum* and *Aeromonas salmonicida*. The dose rate for sarafloxacin hydrochloride is therefore likely to be in the region of 10 mg/kg fish for 5 days. The withdrawal period is likely to be very short, approximately 75 degree-days.

Other products

Enrofloxacin has also shown some promise. An injectable form is licensed in the UK for use in dogs while a 10% liquid for oral use is available in other European countries.

Compounds structurally related to chloramphenicol are being investigated, including thiampenicol and its fluorinated analogue florfenicol. The latter has shown considerable promise in trials with Atlantic salmon at doses up to 20 mg/kg. Toxicity and palatability trials indicate no problems at 100 mg/kg.

Romet 30 is a potentiated sulphonamide (ormetoprim and sulphadimethoxine) which is licensed for use in channel catfish, trout and salmon in the USA. The recommended dose is 50 mg active drug/kg body-weight of fish for 5 days. It is active against *Aeromonas salmonicida*, *Cytophaga psychrophila*, *Chondrococcus (Flexibacter) columnaris*, *Yersinia ruckeri*, *Vibrio anguillarum*, *Aeromonas hydrophila*, *Edwardsiella ictaluri*, *Aeromonas liquefaciens* and *Pseudomonas liquefaciens*.

Bacterial Resistance

Over the years, as in other forms of disease treatment in other species, bacterial resistance has appeared and in many cases this is R-plasmid mediated and so spreads rapidly.

For *Vibrio anguillarum* the quinolones (including oxolinic acid) are the most effective drugs with

CONCENTRATIONS OF VARIOUS ANTIBIOTICS REPORTED IN FISH SERUM				
Fish species	**Antibacterial**	**Dose rate (mg/kg)**	**Fresh or sea water**	**Serum level (µg/ml)**
Rainbow trout (Oncorhynchus mykiss)	Oxolinic acid	10	Fresh	1.2
Atlantic salmon (Salmo salar)	Oxolinic acid (20% preparation)	10	Sea	0.9 ± 0.3
		30	Sea	2.1 ± 0.77
		50	Sea	5.7 ± 2.0
Red sea bream (Sparus auratus)	Oxolinic acid: Standard preparation	30	Sea	1.53
	Ultra-fine preparation			4.24
	Oxytetracycline	20	Sea	2.5 ± 0.8
		80	Sea	1.4 ± 0.1
		80	Fresh	2.0 ± 0.25
		240	Fresh	3.4 ± 0.75
	Amoxycillin	80	Fresh	0.97

FIG. 7.12 Concentrations of various antibiotics reported in fish serum.

MICs between <0.075 µg/ml and 0.3 µg/ml. Oxytetracycline is also quite low at <1.56 µg/ml. *Aeromonas salmonicida* and *Yersinia ruckeri* give similar results, with an increased resistance to oxytetracycline.

Resistance profiles vary from site to site and from year to year. It has been reported that resistance to oxolinic acid by both *Aeromonas salmonicida* and *Yersinia ruckeri* has built up reasonably quickly in Scotland but this has not been the case generally in southern England, although there is evidence of an increase in the MIC of strains of *Aeromonas hydrophila* on certain farms. Recent surveys of *A. salmonicida* from Atlantic salmon in Scotland have shown that 55% were resistant to oxytetracycline and 37% resistant to oxolinic acid. Retrospective surveys by MAFF and DAFS since 1982 have shown increased MICs in isolates over the period, indicating increased resistance to oxolinic acid. It is generally accepted that there is a degree of cross resistance between oxolinic acid and other quinolones.

Reported concentrations of various antibiotics in fish serum, selected from the literature, are shown in Fig. 7.12. It is important to 'rotate' drugs to reduce the development of resistance and it goes without saying that antibiotics are only one part of the treatment of fish diseases: good husbandry and vaccination procedures should help reduce the use of antibiotics.

Immuno-stimulants

Yeast and algal derivatives are entering the field as immuno-stimulants. This area was investigated to a minor degree with levamisole some years ago but serious claims are now made for glucans extracted from the cell walls of *Saccharomyces* spp. Glucans have been used as adjuvants for vaccines and as feed additives, and in both roles it is claimed that they increase resistance/response. The mechanism is believed to be due to increased activity of lysozyme and complement.

Management Aspects of Therapeutics

Various management practices are used with diseases. The system with proliferative kidney disease in rainbow trout shown in Fig. 7.13 serves as a useful model.

There is a typical sequence in which some sub-clinical problem, or a change in circumstances such as water temperature or oxygen levels, causes fry or larvae to eat more slowly than normal. This allows water-soluble vitamins to leach from the food and leads to low-grade deficiencies, perhaps of the B vitamins, which will compound the

MANAGEMENT PRACTICES WITH PKD	
Fact	**Action**
There is a strong indication of seasonality in PKD. Fish become infected at any time from May until the end of July	Introduce fish to infected water as late in the PKD season as possible (i.e. during July) Avoid early introduction
The pathology of the disease is such that the fish are profoundly anaemic. PCV is reduced from 45% to 10%: fish therefore have problems transporting oxygen	Consider installing aeration Minimise stress of affected batches during July–September, i.e. grade and thin out in May/June Shade netting to reduce stress
The act of feeding may increase oxygen demand three-fold; also the specific dynamic action of the food imposes an oxygen demand for digestion	Reduce feeding levels Use food of high digestibility Stop feeding at least 4 hours prior to falls in oxygen levels
Fish are generally compromised by the disease	Treat promptly any other diseases which may occur, such as ERM, furunculosis, external parasitic problems Use vaccines against possible bacterial diseases
The disease can be treated with malachite green, and perhaps in the future with fumagillin	Use strategic medication regimes to reduce quantities of drug used

FIG. 7.13 Management practices with PKD.

original problem by causing poorer feeding, raising the level of uneaten food and ammonia, and perhaps inducing skin and gill damage. In such circumstances, the food can be top-dressed with vitamin additives (using oil) to correct existing deficiencies and prevent further ones. The additives also provide extra vitamins which may be of importance in healing or responding to disease.

Further Reading

Michel, C. and Alderman, D. J. (1992) *Chemotherapy in Aquaculture: From Theory to Reality*. Office International des Épizooties, Paris, 567 pp.

Herwig, N. (1979) *Handbook of Drugs and Chemicals Used in the Treatment of Fish Diseases*. Charles C. Thomas, Springfield, Illinois, 272 pp.

Roberts, R. J. (1988). *Recent Advances in Aquaculture*. **3**, Croom Helm, London.

8

Nutrition in Aquaculture

AUD SKRUDLAND

The subject of nutrition needs to be considered during the diagnosis of a clinical problem. Unfortunately too little is known about the relationships between nutrition and health, growth and welfare in fish.

Companies who develop fish feeds aim to produce better, cheaper products which enhance fish health and growth, improve farm economics and consumer quality, and ensure a better environment in and around the fish farm. However, the science of nutrition for farmed fish has only developed since the 1960s and the level of knowledge is not as high as for mammalian livestock.

Fish farmers also need to know how much feed their livestock have actually consumed but this can be difficult to judge. For example, on a cage site it is hard to estimate how much feed is actually eaten by the fish and how much passes directly through the water column and falls to the sea bed. Behavioural strategies in feeding (e.g. hierarchical structures in a fish population) must be taken into consideration as well.

Practical Feeding

Manual Feeding

There is no doubt that the best way of feeding fish is by hand, using observation of appetite to complement the use of feeding tables in calculating feeding rates according to fish size, species and water temperature. (Figures 8.1 and 8.2 give examples of feed charts for Atlantic salmon and channel catfish respectively.) Visual assessment at feeding gives maximum evidence of appetite, behaviour and early signs of diseases. The person responsible for feeding will be aware of sudden drops in appetite due to strong sunlight or water temperature changes and will also notice when fish fail to feed for no apparent reason.

Automatic Feeders

In intensive fish farming, where large quantities of fish are produced on a single site and labour costs are expensive, it often becomes necessary to use automatic feeders. These may vary from

EXAMPLE OF A FEEDING TABLE RELATED TO EXPECTED DAILY GROWTH FOR ATLANTIC SALMON IN SEA WATER (Value in % daily growth of biomass)				
	Fish size			
Water temp (°C)	30–150 g	150–600 g	600–2000 g	>2000 g
2		0.2	0.2	0.1
4		0.5	0.3	0.2
6		0.7	0.5	0.3
8	1.3	1.0	0.6	0.4
10	1.6	1.2	0.8	0.5
12	1.9	1.4	1.0	0.6
14	2.2	1.7	1.1	0.7

FIG. 8.1 To calculate the daily feeding from a growth table, the feed conversion rate for the actual feed must be multiplied by the growth rate. This will give a recommended daily feeding rate as the percentage of biomass/day. This table clearly shows the relatively high rate of growth of smaller fish and the temperature dependent effect on growth. After Akvaforsk, Norway.

EXAMPLE OF A FEEDING TABLE FOR CHANNEL CATFISH				
	Fry and fingerlings		Food-size fish	
Water temp (°C)	Feeding frequency/day	Feeding rate (% body-weight day)	Feeding frequency/day	Feeding rate (% body-weight day)
>30	2 times	2	1 time	1
26–30	4 times	6	2 times	3
20–25	2 times	3	1 time	2
15–19	1 time	2	1 time	2
10–14	Every 2nd day	2	Every 2nd day	1
<10	Every 3rd–4th day	1	Every 3rd–4th day	0.5

FIG. 8.2 This clearly shows the drop in feeding rate with higher summer water temperatures, due to the low oxygen content of the water.

simple ones which give a certain amount of feed every hour to sophisticated computerised feeders which take into account the hour of the day, water temperature, growth rate of the fish and so on. In either case, 15–25% of the calculated feed demand each day should be fed manually so that the stockman may observe the fish. Figure 8.3 shows the combined use of automatic and manual feeding.

Control of Feeding

Good records are essential to establish whether or not fish are feeding well. This involves sample weighing of a group of fish to calculate the rate of growth since the last sample weighing. Feed conversion rates may then be calculated. If growth rates are low (and conversion rates therefore higher than expected) the feeding needs to be adjusted (Fig. 8.4).

Unfortunately many fish farmers do not have accurate information on biomass or the number of fish per cage or tank. This is obviously a problem when deciding how much feed should be offered and is even more of a problem for the veterinarian prescribing in-feed therapeutants when treatments are necessary. Fish veterinarians should always emphasise the importance of accurate records of biomass, numbers and mean weights of fish on any

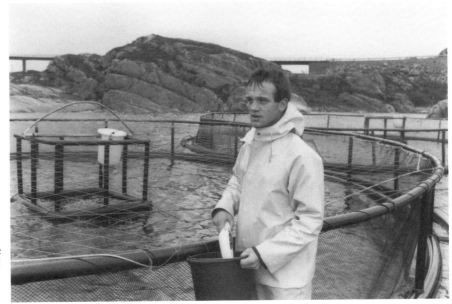

FIG. 8.3 Feeding of Atlantic salmon by combination of automatic and hand feeding. (Photograph by R. Sevaldsen.)

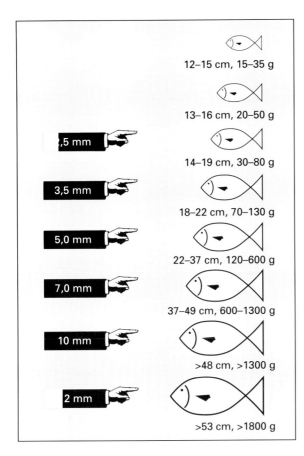

12–15 cm, 15–35 g

13–16 cm, 20–50 g

2,5 mm

14–19 cm, 30–80 g

3,5 mm

18–22 cm, 70–130 g

5,0 mm

22–37 cm, 120–600 g

7,0 mm

37–49 cm, 600–1300 g

10 mm

>48 cm, >1300 g

12 mm

>53 cm, >1800 g

FIG. 8.4 Recommended feedsize/fishsize by T. Skretting for Atlantic salmon in sea water.

site. It is helpful to attend sample weighing on a fish farm (when no disease problems are present) to observe at first hand how the stock records are produced.

Cost of Feed

It is not unusual for more than 50% of the production expenses in intensive fish farming to be related to feed. Thus fish food must be as economic as possible while still providing good growth. On the other hand, a more expensive diet giving better growth in a shorter time might prove more economical in the long run.

Types of Fish Feeds

Starter Feeds

In the production of some species it is necessary to use algae or rotifers as starter feeds. These are

deliberately grown on site, and may be enriched by additives such as vitamins before they are fed to the fish larvae. In some hatcheries the growth of these starter diets is as much of a problem as the growth of the fish larvae themselves. Naturally occurring plankton may also be filtered from water as a starter feed. In species such as salmonids, artificial dry diets (usually crumbs of pelletised feed) show good results.

Grower Feeds

In some farms, it is still the practice to feed some species with whole fish. This may easily give an unbalanced diet, producing vitamin and mineral deficiencies. Occasional supplementation of this 'wet' diet with dry pellets may produce inappetence, since fish are creatures of habit and have taste preferences for wet diets rather than dry (and possibly dull) commercial feed pellets. However, the majority of fish are fed with dry pelletised feed.

Dry Pellets

Dry pellets are usually processed in sophisticated feed mills and contain up to 90–95% dry matter in a formulation designed to meet all energy and nutritional demands.

Dry feed may either be pelleted or extruded. In the extrusion process the pellet is put under high pressure and temperature, which improves the digestibility of some raw materials and enhances the physical quality of the pellet. By changing the expansion in the extruder it is possible to produce pellets which sink in the water at a varying rate. Some pellets are designed to float so that feeding can be observed more carefully. Some fish species will more readily accept a floating particle than a sinking one. For artificial starter feeds, pellets are crumbled into smaller particles that are acceptable to the fry. The composition of dry pellets from feed-mills is usually in accordance with the nutritional needs of the fish.

Moist Feeds

Moist feeds are usually produced on or close to a specific fish farm. The material consists of fresh or frozen trash fish, or perhaps fish-processing industry waste, which is grained and mixed with vitamin and mineral enriched binders. It is also possible to mix trash fish with organic acids to produce a stable silage which can be stored for a time before the production of moist feed is anticipated. In this way it is possible for fish farms to use waste which may otherwise be a problem to the fishing industry and fishing vessels, and turn it into high value fish. Moist feed producers must carefully adjust mixing time and the concentration of binders to make a feed with good consistency. If the feed falls apart when being handled or on contact with water, it will present an unacceptably high risk of environmental pollution.

The nutrient composition of moist feed varies considerably. Trash fish and fish waste vary according to season and to the production process, and the quality is also affected by storage of the raw materials.

Broodstock Feeds

Broodstock feeding aims to give the fish optimal levels of vitamins, minerals and protein to support the growth of the developing gonads. For species like salmonids, which stop eating as they mature, it is important to start the brookstock feeding as much as 6–9 months before spawning.

Maintenance Diets

Sometimes it becomes important to maintain fish at a constant weight for a specified period. This may be done either by a pattern of starving the fish at intervals (i.e. two weeks without feed followed by one week of feeding) for some time, or by using a low energy feed with an appropriate content of vitamins and minerals. Merely reducing the quantity of food is not recommended: it causes stress and leads to aggressive behaviour among the fish, which creates feeding hierarchies and all the associated problems of increasing size differentiation within the population.

Shrimp Feeds

Shrimp are omnivorous detritus feeders which live on the algal mat growing in farm ponds, or else on added vegetable and/or animal feed. It is probable that a high proportion of the added feed acts as a pond fertiliser and not as a direct food for the shrimp.

Nutritional Demands

The energy and nutrition requirements of fish vary according to species, age and size, maturation grade and water temperature.

Protein

Fish have no real demand for protein as such but rather a demand for a balanced composition of amino acids in amounts which are adequate to sustain growth. In all fish species which have been investigated, the same 10 amino acids are essential for life as for mammals. They are: arginine, histidine, isoleucine, leucine, lysine, methionine, phenylalanine, threonine, tryptophan and valine. Among these, tyrosine may partly substitute the demand for phenylalanine, and cysteine may reduce the demand for methionine. Diets insufficient in essential amino acids may give well defined deficiency diseases. The amino acid requirements will usually be covered by using processed fish meal as the major protein source in fish feed. the use of mainly vegetable proteins in a diet may make additional amino acid supplementation necessary.

For the healthy maintenance of most fish species, 1.0–1.5 g protein/kg body-weight/day is required. Protein is also required for muscle growth. The required concentration of protein in the feed will vary with fish species, size, age, water temperature, energy levels in the diet, and the quality of the protein (digestibility, amino acid content) being incorporated into the diet.

Protein is the most expensive ingredient in fish feed, and it may be tempting to economise on this. Too little protein in the diet will retard or inhibit growth and may also reduce resistance to disease. Surplus protein which is not utilised for growth will be used as an energy source which might be supplied from more economical sources.

Lipids

Lipids supply the fish with essential fatty acids which are necessary structural components of all cell membranes and are of great importance for physiological processes. Lipids are also necessary for absorption of some vitamins and they are a relatively cheap energy source. Up to a certain point a higher lipid content in the diet will give better utilisation of the protein in the diet, and the ratio between protein and lipid is important.

Essential fatty acid demands are not known in detail for all species but they are known to be very variable. Linolenic acid (18:3 *n*-3) is essential for rainbow trout, while Pacific salmon need both linoleic (18:2 *n*-6) and linolenic acid. Halibut and shrimps require the very long-chained omega 3 fatty acids (20:5 *n*-3, 22:6 *n*-3).

In general essential fatty acid deficiency produces poor growth, erosions of the base of the fins and an enlarged, pale liver. In rainbow trout deficiencies are known to produce a loss of consciousness during sudden activity — the so-called shock syndrome.

The high level of polyunsaturated fatty acids in fish will be more and more important to the fish farming industry as the positive properties of these with respect to human nutrition are better known. It is possible, to some degree, to elevate the level of these in fish by increasing their proportion in the feed. The quality of the lipids used in the diet is very important. Polyunsaturated fatty acids are easily oxidised under storage, and rancid lipids are known to induce for lipoid liver disease.

Optimal requirements for lipids in the diet vary from species to species. Most consumers disapprove of eating 'overfat' fish with an excessive lipid content. In rainbow trout and salmon diets the lipid content may be as high as 30% with a satisfactory result, while commercial catfish feed do not usually contain more than 5–6% lipids.

Carbohydrates

In nature most fish species are close to the top of the nutritional pyramid, and they are therefore carnivores, especially in a marine environment. Carbohydrates may be used as an energy supply by some species, but up to a certain level, most species have a limited ability to metabolise them and have no nutritional demands for them. However, carbohydrates are important as binders in commercial fish feed production.

A general rule is that simple carbohydrates are better utilised by fish than complex ones and that the digestibility of the complete ration is reduced by larger amounts of complex carbohydrates in the diet.

Since carbohydrates are poorly utilised by fish, they are eliminated in the faeces and cause pollution concerns on fish farm sites. It is also thought that their presence in fish feed may adversely affect fish health.

Vitamins

Fish are dependent on having almost the same vitamins supplied in the feed as for mammalian species (Fig. 8.5). There are some differences among species regarding levels of vitamins; for

VITAMIN REQUIREMENTS OF SOME FISH SPECIES			
	Requirements (mg/kg or IU/kg dry diet)		
Vitamin	Salmon	Carp	Channel catfish
Thiamin	0–15	3	1
Riboflavin	0–25	10	9
Pyridoxine	5–20	10	3
Pantothenic acid	40	40	15
Niacin	200	50	14
Choline	800	1500	R
Biotin	1.5	1.5	R
Ascorbate	150	50	60
Vitamin A (IU)	2500	2000	2000
Vitamin D (IU)	2400	N	1000
Vitamin E	30	100	30
Vitamin K	10	R	R

R = Required, but level not known
NR = No requirement known

FIG. 8.5 This table demonstrates the large inter-species variation often seen in aquaculture and also points to the lack of basic knowledge in fish nutrition.

FIG. 8.6 Mineral requirements of some fish species.

MINERAL REQUIREMENTS OF SOME FISH SPECIES (per kg feed)					
	Salmon	Carp	Channel catfish	Sea-bream	Eel
Calcium (%)	0.03	0.03	0.03	0.34	0.27
Phosphorus (%)	0.6	0.7	0.4	0.6	0.3
Magnesium (%)	R	0.05	0.04	NR	0.04
Iron (mg)	60	20	20	?	170
Copper (mg)	5	3	3	?	?
Manganese (mg)	20	13	2.4	?	?
Zinc (mg)	30	15–30	20	?	?
Iodine (g)	R	?	?	?	–
Selenium (g)	0.15	R	0.25	R	R

NR = No requirement known
? = Requirement not known
R = Required, but level not known

example, it is known that warm-water species are capable of synthesising vitamin B_{12} in the intestine provided that a sufficient level of cobalt is included in the diet.

Some of these vitamins are unstable in storage, including ascorbic acid, which is why more stabilised ascorbic acid has been added to the diet by some manufacturers. Some of the vitamins are also heat labile and must be added in excess before feed processing — for example, vitamin K. Thiamine will be destroyed by thiaminases found in fresh herring and this must be taken in account when producing and storing moist feed pellets. Vitamin E is often added as an antioxidant to fish oils to prevent their degradation, and will be consumed by oxidising processes during storage.

Vitamin deficiencies with specific symptoms are seldom seen in modern fish farming due to the increasing knowledge of nutritional needs and the quality of the feed. However, it is possible that more rapid growth and better feed conversion ratios may induce higher metabolic demands than are reported as optimal for protection against diseases and growth. It is also possible that endoparasites can induce poor absorption of vitamins.

Minerals

Fish have basically the same mineral demands for metabolism and skeletal structure as mammalian species (Fig. 8.6). They require additional minerals for maintenance of osmotic balance between body fluids and their environment.

Mineral deficiencies are seldom seen in farmed fish, compared with mammalian species. Fish are able, to some extent, to absorb minerals from the surrounding water and in fact more disease conditions are due to excess mineral in the diet than to mineral deficiencies *per se*.

Symptoms of mineral deficiency usually occur due to a reduced bioavailability of minerals in the diet. This may be due either to mineral imbalance or interaction between minerals and other dietary components. It is well known that phytic acid (found in vegetables) may reduce availability of several minerals — for example calcium, magnesium and zinc — and that high levels of calcium may reduce absorption of iron, copper and zinc. This may be a problem if the diet includes large quantities of fish-processing waste which contains high amounts of bones. A problem with excessive minerals can arise from zinc accumulation in the feather meal which is used to a variable degree in fish diets. High levels of iron in the diet induce heavier losses due to bacterial diseases in salmonids. Urolithiasis and nephrocalcinosis are both seen clinically with high levels of carbon dioxide.

Pigments

To achieve an attractive red flesh colour in salmonids, pigments must be added to the feed. Quite large levels of shrimp meal in the diet can achieve good results, but usually synthetic analogues of the naturally occurring pigments astaxanthin or canthaxanthin are used as additives. These pigments may also be produced from yeast preparations. There has been some controversy on the use of canthaxanthin, as it does not occur naturally in the marine environment. A level of 40–50 ppm is sufficient if it is included in the diet for most of the growing period. However, inclusion rates of pigments vary from country to country and from species to species according to consumer preference.

Corn contains a pigment called xanthophylls, which will impart an undesirable yellow colour to the flesh of catfish if fed at levels exceeding 11 ppm in the feed.

Further Reading

Halver, J. E. (Editor) (1989) *Fish Nutrition*, 2nd edn. Academic Press.

Cowey, C. B., Mackie, A. M. and Bell, J. G. (Editors) (1986) *Nutrition and Feeding in Fish*. Academic Press.

9

Anaesthesia

MICHAEL STOSKOPF

Derived from the Greek word *anaisthesia*, meaning insensibility, anaesthesia is usually associated with the relief of pain. To be technically precise, however, anaesthesia is considered to provide immobilisation, relaxation, unconsciousness and freedom from reflex response, as well as relief from pain. Certainly each of these components of general anaesthesia provides important advantages to the veterinarian, fish handler and fish producer.

Anyone with practical experience knows that fish respond to noxious stimuli, often violently, making handling and manipulation of the animal a challenge. If for no other reason, anaesthesia is important in fish medicine to provide immobilisation and release from reflex responses. An immobile, non-reactive patient allows faster, more precise and less traumatic intervention in any procedure performed on a live fish. Muscle relaxation and neuromuscular blocking agents solve many of the immediate needs for handling fish, but they do not prevent other physiological responses and are inappropriate used alone for stressful or invasive procedures.

No one experienced with fish would deny their ability to perceive and react to their environment. The effects of stressors on fish and their pituitary and adrenergic responses to disease conditions, disease treatments, water pollutants and husbandry procedures (including transport) have all been described and investigated in considerable detail. The general conclusion is that any procedure is stressful to fish, and they exhibit most, if not all, of the physiological and biochemical responses to stressors which are seen in mammals. Their stress reactions involve catecholamine and adrenergic cascades similar to those known in mammals. Immunosuppression, osmoregulatory derangement, reproductive failure and metabolic aberration are all important results of inadequate stress manage-

ment in a fish facility. Stress responses are generally considered adaptive in natural situations and a total lack of stress would be an impossible and perhaps deleterious goal; nevertheless, prolonged or severe acute stressors can result in increased susceptibility to disease, poor growth and even direct mortality.

Tranquillisation or sedation (the behavioural state in which a patient is calm and unconcerned about surroundings) can reduce the physiological impact of environmental changes and is an important tool in fish management. Light tranquillisation has its place in a continuum ranging from acute awareness to the unconsciousness obtained in properly applied general or surgical anaesthesia.

Analgesia, or relief from pain, remains a viable objective of fish anaesthesia, although scientists still debate whether or not fish perceive pain. No spinal thalamic tract analogous to that found in primates has been identified in fish but pain perception in non-primate animals is served by a more diffuse fibre system. Spinocervical, spinoreticular and spinotectal tracts may carry nociceptive (pain) signals in various species and no particular tract seems to be essential to pain transmission. It is, therefore, a mistake to make assumptions of pain perception in fish based on human anatomy, physiology or experience. Specific stimuli painful to most humans may not cause pain perception at the same levels in fish but, conversely, stimuli not perceived as painful by humans may indeed elicit pain in fish. Physiological changes associated with pain perception in other animals, such as increased respiratory rate, are readily observed in fish subjected to mechanical trauma. Although such observations can in no way confirm the perception of pain in fish, neither can it be ruled out by the lack of behavioural responses such as vocalisation or anorexia.

Characteristics of an Ideal Anaesthetic

The ideal anaesthetic agent for fish:

- renders them insensible to pain
- provides good immobilisation and muscular relaxation
- induces unconsciousness, tranquillisation or sedation in a predictable manner related to dose
- is easily administered
- induces anaesthesia quickly
- provides a rapid, predictable and uncomplicated recovery
- has a wide margin of safety — the dose that will cause irreparable harm or the death of the fish should be much greater than the dose required to achieve suitable anaeshesia
- is inexpensive — leaves no tissue residues and requires no withdrawal times before the anaesthetised fish can be brought to market
- uses chemicals which are stable, have a long shelf life and break down rapidly in the environment to safe and physiologically inactive metabolites.

No agent or combination of agents can be considered ideal. However, the consideration of these properties provides valuable guidance in selecting and evaluating anaesthetics.

Administering and Monitoring Anaesthesia

All of the major methods of inducing chemical anaesthesia in fish involve immersion in a solution of the agent. Regardless of the drug being used, all possible steps should be taken to reduce additional stresses on the fish being anaesthetised. Responses to stress will increase the dose needed for effective anaesthesia and will therefore reduce the margin of safety.

Immersion is usually accomplished in induction tanks or bags. These should be prepared in advance and filled with water that closely matches the habitat of the fish with regard to pH, temperature, salinity or hardness. Recovery tanks or water should also be prepared in advance to match the habitat water.

Fish should be handled as little as possible and it is important to avoid damaging their epithelium. When anaesthetising only a few, place the fish in the induction tank and slowly add the anaesthetic. When more fish are being processed, they can be added directly to anaesthetic-laden water. In the case of a new species, or fish held under unusual conditions, it is good practice to anaesthetise a few individuals first, to observe induction and recovery closely before anaesthetising larger numbers. It is usually sensible to start with a relatively low induction dose, except with very fast-swimming fish such as tuna. For these, a low induction dose can be more risky than a carefully observed high dose which gives a rapid induction and reduces damage from struggling. The anaesthetised fish can then be transferred to lower maintenance dose solutions if more time is required.

As fish undergo induction, observe them closely. They will generally pass through planes of anaesthesia very similar to those encountered in mammals (Fig. 9.1). As with mammals, there is considerable individual and species variation in response to anaesthetics. Individual susceptibility can be the result of differences in metabolic rate (including those due to water temperature) or physical condition (particularly related to the amount of body fat). In general, fish in poor condition or suffering from disease require much lower doses to achieve a given plane of anaesthesia. These variations affect how rapidly the fish pass through the various planes of anaesthesia and in some cases it may well appear that stages and planes are completely bypassed because the individual or species progresses through them so rapidly.

Hypoxia is a significant problem when inducing anaesthesia by immersion, and it is important to aerate the induction solutions. This becomes even more critical as more fish are passed through the same induction water. It is important to have a recovery tank or bag available, to which the fish can be transferred rapidly if the level of anaesthesia becomes too deep.

During recovery, it is important to observe the opercular movements carefully. If they are extremely weak or absent, remedial methods must be employed. Check for tone by opening the fish's mouth to see whether the animal responds to this action. Jaw tone will return before opercular movements in recovery. Alternately opening the mouth and propelling the fish forward in the water can help pass water over the gills of a fish which is too deeply anaesthetised. This helps to exchange

STAGES OF ANAESTHESIA IN FISH			
Stage	Plan	Category	Behavioural response of fish
0		Normal	Swimming actively Reactive to external stimuli Equilibrium normal Muscle tone normal
I	1	Light sedation	Voluntary swimming continues Slight loss of reactivity to visual and tactile stimuli Respiratory rate normal Equilibrium normal Muscle tone normal
I	1	Light narcosis	Excitement phase may precede increase in respiratory rate Loss of equilibrium Efforts to right itself Muscle tone decreased Still responds to positional changes weakly
II	2	Deep narcosis	Ceases to respond to positional changes Decrease in respiratory rate to near normal Total loss of equilibrium No effort to right itself Muscle tone decreased Some reactivity to strong tactile and vibrational stimuli Suitable for external sampling, fin and gill biopsies
III	1	Light anaesthesia	Total loss of muscle tone Responds to deep pressure Further decrease in respiratory rate Suitable for minor surgery
III	2	Surgical anaesthesia	Total loss of reactivity Respiratory rate very low Heart rate slow
IV		Medullary collapse	Total loss of gill movement followed in several minutes by cardiac arrest

Fig. 9.1 Stages of anaesthesia in fish.

the drug and keep the fish oxygenated. When jaw tone returns, however, and the fish begins to breathe on its own, it is usually best to leave it alone unless it is at risk of predator damage. The rate and strength of opercular movement are good indicators of whether a fish is continuing to recover or has relapsed into a deeper stage. After recovery, the fish should be observed periodically for the first 4 hours and again 24 hours later for long-term effects.

When fish are sedated for transportation, much lower doses of drug are used and the fish are immersed throughout the transport with little or no opportunity for careful observation. Remember that sedation will not compensate for poor transport methods. Tranquillised or sedated fish may have reduced responses to stressors, but they are not oblivious or anaesthetised, nor have they been rendered physically immune to environmental influences.

Commonly Used Chemical Anaesthesia Agents

Benzocaine

Benzocaine (MW = 165.2) (also called ethyl aminobenzoate) is a colourless crystal or white odourless crystalline powder which has been used for years as a fish anaesthetic. However, it is almost insoluble in water and although it does not require buffering to counter acidity, stock solutions are usually prepared in ethanol or acetone, which are themselves irritating to fish. The salt of the drug, benzocaine hydrochloride, is much more expensive but it is more water soluble and is used frequently in place of benzocaine. Stock solutions made with the salt should be buffered. Because the drug and its salt break down in sunlight, stock solutions should be stored in dark or opaque airtight containers.

Benzocaine is usually administered as an immersion bath. A standard stock solution is 100 g benzocaine per litre of ethanol or acetone. Anaesthetic doses vary considerably according to species: a useful dose range for trout and salmon is 25–45 mg/l but northern pike require 100–200 mg/l to induce anaesthesia.

Benzocaine has a reasonably wide margin of safety, but at routine salmonid water temperatures a dose that is safe for induction in 5 minutes will be lethal if the fish is exposed for more than 15 minutes. It is also important to remember that benzocaine is hydrolysed to *para*-aminobenzoic acid, and caution should be exercised when administering this anaesthetic to patients being treated with sulphonamides.

Benzocaine appears to have hypoxic effects on fish similar to those described below for tricaine. Strong aeration of the induction solutions throughout induction and anaesthesia is important. Higher doses of benzocaine are required in warmer water, presumably because of the metabolism of the drug by fish; however, benzocaine is also more toxic in warmer water, a fact which greatly narrows the margin of safety. The efficacy of benzocaine is not affected by water hardness, alkalinity or pH.

Benzocaine is not toxic to mammals in a topical exposure at concentrations used in fish anaesthesia. It is highly soluble in fat and its retention in body tissues is directly related to their fat levels. The drug accumulates in mature, older fish and gravid females, which can result in prolonged recovery times and the need for longer withdrawal times. Otherwise a withdrawal time of only 24 hours is necessary for trout and large-mouth bass, but salmon require longer.

Tricaine

Tricaine methane sulphonate (MW = 261.3) is sometimes better known as MS-222, its experimental designation when it was developed by Merck as a sulphonated analogue of benzocaine with high solubility in water. It is more than 250 times as soluble in water as benzocaine. Tricaine is the most commonly employed anaesthetic in North America and is widely used world-wide.

Tricaine is supplied as a crystalline powder, which is stable when kept cool and dry. Standard stock solutions are made by adding 10 g tricaine to a litre of water, and these must be stored in dark or opaque containers because solutions of tricaine are unstable in sunlight. Photodegradation of the drug forms methylsulphate, turning solutions dark; little activity is lost due to this process but it is advisable to change stock solutions once a month. The shelf life of stock solutions can be extended by refrigeration or freezing.

Solutions of tricaine are acidic, due to methane sulphonic acid formation, and require buffering prior to administration to freshwater fish. Many practitioners buffer their stock solutions by adding sodium bicarbonate to saturation, which effectively stabilises the pH of a 10 g/l stock solution between 7 and 7.5. Buffering highly concentrated stock solutions can result in excessive desulphonation, forming aminobenzoate ethyl ester that comes out of solution and forms oil droplets on the surface, reducing potency. If necessary 1 g/l solutions of tricaine can be autoclaved without loss of anaesthetic properties or increase in toxicity. Topical exposure to tricaine stock and induction solutions is not toxic to mammals, and tricaine is not mutagenic.

Although tricaine is considered to be a relatively safe drug, its toxicity varies considerably, depending upon fish species, fish size, water temperature and water hardness. It has a narrow margin of safety for some species and particularly for young fish. It is more toxic in warm, soft waters.

A good starting concentration for tricaine anaesthesia of adult fish of an unfamiliar species in unknown water conditions is 50–100 mg/l. This can be achieved by adding 5–10 ml of a 10 g/l stock solution to every litre of water being used for the immersion bath. More drug is required to anaesthetise salmonids in colder water, and induction times are longer; however, safety tends to increase. This cold water effect does not seem to hold across all species and is not seen with channel catfish.

When working with young fish or fish in relatively warm water, it may be advisable to begin with a 50 mg/l induction solution.

It is important to remember that when high densities of fish are exposed to tricaine solutions, drug is absorbed and actual exposure concentrations are reduced. Induction solutions need to be replenished when induction times become prolonged.

Blood lactate levels tend to increase throughout tricaine anaesthesia, supporting the view that the drug may have asphyxiant properties, forcing increased dependence on anaerobic metabolism. It is not clear that this is a function of direct drug effect or due to decreased opercular activity in the anaesthetised fish, but aeration of induction and anaesthesia solutions should be practised. Blood lactate levels increase to much higher levels in fish which have been fed up to 24 hours prior to anaesthesia. Blood glucose levels remain stable throughout routine tricaine anaesthesia.

Tricaine diffuses rapidly across the gills, providing fast recovery times that vary according to the concentration used and the duration of exposure. Recovery times longer than 10 minutes generally indicate that too high a final concentration of drug is being used, or that the exposure time is too long, and doses should be adjusted downward.

Absorbed tricaine is excreted in the urine for about 24 hours after exposure. In rainbow trout, 77–96% of the drug excreted through this route is acetylated. Blood levels of free drug reach about 75% of the concentration of the immersion solution, and are cleared in about 8 hours. Tissue residues decline to less than detectable limits (0.1 mg/kg in fish flesh) in about 24 hours, but regulatory withdrawal times in the USA are 21 days because of a lack of mammalian safety data.

Quinaldine Sulphate

Quinaldine sulphate (MW = 241) is also referred to as Quinate, or 2-methylquinoline sulphate. This drug is increasingly used in fish anaesthesia, despite being more costly than tricaine. It is usually supplied as a light yellow crystalline powder, which is highly water soluble.

Quinaldine stock solutions are acidic and should be buffered and sodium bicarbonate can be used as described for tricaine. Stock solutions should be protected from light and kept in tightly sealed containers. A stock solution of 10 g/l is most frequently used.

Quinaldine sulphate is sometimes combined with tricaine in a ratio of 10:1 tricaine to quinaldine.

This mixture achieves faster induction than either drug alone. A common induction solution for the mixture is 25–30 mg/l tricaine and 2.5–3.0 mg/l quinaldine sulphate.

When used alone, quinaldine sulphate offers the advantages of rapid induction and recovery. Anaesthetised fish retain a strong touch response after losing equilibrium, but this response seems to extinguish after about 20 seconds of contact. Most procedures are readily performed after the touch response extinguishes. The avoidance and coughing responses seen when the nonsulphated form of quinaldine is administered in alcohol or acetone are not seen with the water soluble quinaldine sulphate.

An induction dose of 25 mg/l quinaldine sulphate for salmonids will result in loss of equilibrium in less than 4 minutes with recovery times between 1 and 13 minutes. In warm water species, induction solutions of 15–60 mg/l are usually employed. Species vary in susceptibility to the drug. Large-mouth bass are particularly sensitive, while carp are relatively insensitive. The 96 hour LC_{50} for quinaldine sulphate in large-mouth bass is 6.8 mg/l, while in carp it is 72.5 mg/l.

Quinaldine sulphate is less toxic in very soft water than in hard water because decreased pH reduces the concentration of active un-ionised drug. Warm water increases the toxicity of quinaldine sulphate, probably by driving the equilibrium toward the ionised form.

Quinaldine sulphate is apparently not metabolised by fish but is excreted entirely unchanged. Muscle residues are essentially nil at 24 hours post-exposure. There is no evidence that quinaldine sulphate has any carcinogenic properties.

Metomidate

Metomidate (MW = 266.7), also known as azaperone, has been used successfully for anaesthesia of fish. It is an imidazole-based nonbarbiturate hypnotic closely related to etomidate (a human sedative that has also been used as a fish anaesthetic). Metomidate received considerable attention in the 1980s because fish anaesthetised with it were found not to have the spikes in serum cortisol seen when other anaesthetic agents were employed. The drug was described as the 'stressless' anaesthetic. Unfortunately, it is more likely that the lack of a cortisol peak is related to a metabolic blockade of cortisol synthesis through the suppression of 11-β-hydroxylation of cholesterol, rather than a lack of stress. Similar findings in etomidate have resulted in its removal from the human pharmacopeia in the UK.

Nevertheless, metomidate does serve well as a fish anaesthetic. The dose commonly employed with salmonids is 5 mg/l; however, lower doses of 1–2.5 mg/l are used in channel catfish. Muscle fasciculation is common in catfish anaesthetised with this drug at these doses. Marine tropical fish and sharks are readily anaesthetised with metomidate solutions of 2.5–5 mg/l. Very low doses of 0.06–0.20 mg/l are used for transport sedation of various species, including salmonids.

Long recovery times from metomidate anaesthesia reported by some workers are related to prolonged exposure times. Induction with this drug is rapid, and fish should be removed and processed soon after losing equilibrium. This may be within a minute or two of exposure. If this is done, recovery times will be more rapid than when tricaine is employed. However, if the fish are allowed to remain in induction solutions after loss of equilibrium, recovery times can be very prolonged, with the duration of recovery directly related to how long fish were in the induction solutions.

Some species and individuals will turn very dark when anaesthetised with metomidate. This is thought to be related to the metabolic blockade of cortisol production, which also effectively blocks the negative feedback loop of ACTH production. Since ACTH and melanocyte-stimulating hormone synthesis are linked, the lack of cortisol causes melanophore responses.

Non-chemical Methods

In addition to chemical anaesthesia, non-chemical means have been used historically for fish. They are attractive because they do not leave chemical residues in the fish flesh and, therefore, are not subject to withdrawal time regulations. However, they are *not* preferred methods.

Hypothermia

The exploitation of hypothermia depends on the fact that fish become torpid and immobile when rapidly cooled from their acclimation temperature. Sensitivity to stimuli also decreases as chilled fish lose equilibrium and co-ordination. Commonly, hypothermia has been achieved by putting fish directly into crushed ice or snow for 10–15 minutes. Fish have also been cooled for transport by dramatically reducing water temperatures, and the technique has been combined with chemical anaesthesia in a number of species and applications. The degree of torpor and immobilisation is more profound when the technique is used on fish acclimated to warm water. Although the technique is inexpensive, avoids residues and is environmentally safe, the degree of analgesia is not well controlled, and thermal injuries can occur. A recognised syndrome called 'cold shock' can result in death. Major osmoregulatory alteration during generalised hypothermia results in dramatic shifts in ionic balance, as well as haematological perturbations, including increased clotting times.

Electroanaesthesia

Electroanaesthesia methods have been investigated for applications where drug withdrawal times preclude the use of chemical anaesthesia or where minor procedures such as tagging require immobilisation primarily to facilitate short fish-processing times. This translates into a need for rapid induction and recovery times. Electrical anaesthesia provides instantaneous induction and nearly as rapid recovery. It does not leave any chemical residues. Mortality is negligible when the technique is applied correctly, but complications can include vertebral dislocation, internal haemorrhage and cardiac fibrillation.

Early trials with electronarcosis in mammals had problems with hyperthermia, convulsions and respiratory depression. Individual adjustments of electrode current were needed to avoid electro-tetany of muscles and to maintain narcosis and similar considerations appear to be important when using the method on fish. In mammals, electroanaesthesia is accompanied by increased blood pressure and plasma corticoid, epinephrine and norepinephrine levels.

A variety of current forms have been used to immobilise fish. Continuous direct current (12-volt) using two electrodes, and varying amperage to effect, induces immobilisation without loss of equilibrium, with the fish aligned to the anode. This method is effective for tagging salmonids in low salinity waters (up to 18 ppt), but a six-electrode, alternating-polarity unit needs only deliver 150 mA to provide more reliable immobilisation in sea water. Unrectified alternating current (50 Hz sine wave at 60 Vrms for 30 seconds) has been used to induce electroanaesthesia, but half-wave, rectified current pulsed with a 200 V peak is less damaging.

Summary

Anaesthesia in fish is a very useful tool either for stress-free manipulation of individuals or groups of fish or for tranquilising fish which are to be transported.

Since fish species vary in their sensitivity it is best to find one or two anaesthetic agents which work well in the species under the veterinarian's care. Practice is essential to ensure safe anaesthesia and recovery. Always anaesthetise one, or a few, fish initially before applying the technique to a large population. Be aware that fish which have been starved of food before anaesthesia make better patients and allow for the effects of water quality (including temperature) when choosing an anaesthetic agent.

Further Reading

Brown, L. (1992) Anesthesia and restraint. In: *Fish Medicine*, (Editor Stoskopf, M.), pp. 79–90. W. B. Saunders, Philadelphia.
Lumb, W. V. and Jones, E. W. (1984) *Veterinary Anesthesia* (2nd edn) pp. 693. Lea & Febiger, Philadelphia.
Pickering, A. D. (1981) *Stress and Fish*. Academic Press, London.
Summerfelt, R. C. and Smith, L. S. (1990) Anesthesia, Surgery and Related Techniques. In: *Methods for Fish Biology*. (Editors Schreck, C. B. and Moyle, P. B.), pp. 213–272. American Fisheries Society, Bethesda, Maryland.

10

Welfare Aspects of Aquatic Veterinary Medicine

GRAHAM CAWLEY

There has been a considerable volume of work, research and law aimed at the welfare of farmed mammalian and avian species but relatively little on the welfare of farmed fish. This is probably a reflection of the historical size of the aquaculture and 'terraculture' industries, particularly in the western world where concern for animals assumes a higher position on the political agenda. It may also be related to the greater likelihood of anthropomorphism towards mammals or towards birds than towards fish.

This relative lack of investigation does not mean that it is impossible to make general recommendations about the welfare of farmed fish. As with all stock management, satisfactory welfare and economic production need good husbandry, and good husbandry demands that the various needs of the stock be adequately understood and supplied. It is necessary to bear in mind the differences in anatomy, physiology, ethology etc. between fish and the higher vertebrates. In particular, as fish are fully aquatic poikilotherms they are even more dependent on the quality and constancy of their environment than homeothermic terrestrial animals.

Good welfare practice (and good husbandry) recognises the importance of social balance. The majority of the farmed species are aggressive predators and will eat carnivorously if the opportunity arises. Therefore it is important that all the fish within one holding unit are of a similar size; if not, they will eat each other.

The provision of enough space for each fish is complex. Fish are naturally shoaling animals and the available evidence suggests that they are content to live in very high density systems as long as there is an adequate supply of good quality water passing over them. Rather than a simple measure of available space, a calculation which also takes into account the volume and quality of the incoming water is required, though as yet there are no definitive values for this parameter. A good stockman will recognise when the situation is not correct as the fish will be stressed.

In general, it is appropriate to consider the welfare of fish under the five headings or freedoms defined by the Brambell Committee (1965) and used by the Farm Animal Welfare Council. To these should be added a further two, recently proposed by Seamer (1992):

(1) Freedom from thirst, hunger or malnutrition.
(2) Freedom from thermal or physical discomfort.
(3) Freedom from pain, injury or disease.
(4) Freedom from fear and distress.
(5) Freedom to express normal patterns of behaviour.
(6) Freedom from stress or suffering when transported.
(7) Freedom from stress or suffering when slaughtered.

This list may also be used as an assessment guide when considering the suitability of a management system.

Freedom from Thirst, Hunger or Malnutrition

The appetites of fish vary considerably with water temperature and with the stage of their life-cycle. Because of the nature of poikilothermic existence, the provision of food should *not* be constant: at lower water temperatures (and hence lower body temperatures) appetite is reduced and feeding less at such temperatures would not be cruelty but good husbandry. Provision of more food would lead to waste and the accumulation of decaying material, with a high BOD which could adversely affect the fish by reducing available oxygen.

Many species show a reduced appetite, or even inappetence, as they attain sexual maturity; hence it is not necessary to feed at a high level all the time. The frequency of feeding also varies between species: salmonids, for example, feed several times a day whereas halibut are more appropriately fed twice a week.

Malnutrition in this context would mean the feeding of an inappropriate diet which does not meet the fish's nutritional requirements even though the quantity fed may be correct. This would be uneconomical, as well as affecting the fish's welfare. Any changes in feeding routines should be gradual.

As fish are continuously in water, there would seem to be little chance of suffering from thirst. However, to be able to maintain their fluid balance it is essential that fish should be kept in water of the correct degree of salinity. An inability to maintain the fluid and electrolyte balance is analogous to terrestrial species having no access to drinking water.

Freedom from Thermal or Physical Discomfort

Temperature fluctuations which would not be significant to terrestrial animals in air can seriously affect fish in water. It is necessary to provide water at a constant temperature. Any changes should be minor and gradual, so that the fish can adjust its metabolism slowly. There is a limited temperature range in which fish can thrive. Low temperatures (down to 4–5°C) are not a risk but there will be stress as the temperature rises, either from the temperature itself or from the reduced oxygen content of the warmer water, and disease will become more prevalent.

Fish can also suffer from sunburn and possibly optical damage (they have no eyelids). To avoid ultraviolet radiation in bright sunlight, they need access to deep water or shade.

The absolute chemical composition of the water and changes in that chemistry are vital to all animals which live in water. Most fish can tolerate a range of water conditions but are more likely to thrive if conditions are within the species' preferred range and are constant. To avoid distress, incoming water should be of constant quality and any unavoidable changes should be introduced gradually.

It is important that the water should be free from suspended solids which can abrade the gill epithelium and damage the mucus layer of the skin.

Freedom from Pain, Injury or Disease

Although fish have a local reaction to pain, it is not known whether they have any central, conscious awareness of that pain as the CNS has little or no thalamus and neocortex (which is the pain perception route in higher animals). However, it is correct to assume that there is some pain recognition and fish should be handled accordingly. This is in keeping with practical experience, which shows that fish which are badly handled are stressed and take time to recover from that stress. No surgical procedure should be carried out on fish without appropriate anaesthesia.

Similarly all holding units and handling systems must be designed to minimise the risk of injury to the fish. This is particularly important during handling as the external mucous layer of the skin, which is important to fluid balance and disease control, is very fragile and damage to it would certainly cause welfare problems.

Freedom from disease is not only in the interest of the fish but also of the farmer. The spread of disease from fish to fish can occur very rapidly, particularly after stress or at elevated water temperatures. Fish cannot evade infection when they are in holding facilities. It is important that those who are carrying out day-to-day management procedures are able to recognise signs of disease very early and know how to initiate full diagnosis and treatment procedures as rapidly as possible. It is also important that the risks of disease be kept down by other good management procedures, e.g. only bringing in fish with a known SPF (Specific Pathogen Free) status.

Freedom from Fear and Distress

Facilities must be designed to minimise the risk of predation by birds or aquatic animals. Their presence will alarm fish, and may cause self-inflicted damage as they panic to evade the predator.

Fish are capable of hearing sub-water sounds and it is good practice to minimise adventitious noise levels.

Freedom to Express Normal Patterns of Behaviour

Normal behaviour patterns — swimming, feeding, shoaling etc. — are usually possible. The one behaviour pattern which could be adversely affected would be courtship rituals. However, in many situations fish are harvested before they achieve sexual maturity. In fact as growth tends to slow down or even stop at that time it is only brood fish which will be kept to sexual maturity. They are not kept in intensive conditions and the only adverse effect would be an inability to swim to spawning grounds.

Freedom from Stress or Suffering when Transported

This can involve the removal of fish from one tank or pond to another on the same farm or, at the other extreme, it can involve transport by air for thousands of miles. In either case suitable precautions are required. For a short distance a net or mobile tank is adequate. As the duration of movement increases, so does the need for more sophistication.

There must be adequate oxygen in the water of the container. This can be by saturation, or by continuous gasing of the water through air stones. Sedation of the fish with a suitable chemical, e.g. tricaine methane sulphonate (MS222), might be advantageous. Reduction of water temperature will quieten the fish to some extent, reduce the metabolic rate, the oxygen demand and also reduce the waste product released into the water. All these procedures should be considered as they will reduce the stress and hence improve the welfare of the fish involved.

Freedom from Stress or Suffering when Slaughtered

If the fish are to be transported immediately prior to slaughter, then the techniques suggested in the previous paragraph must be considered. However, the fish cannot be chemically sedated if they are for human consumption.

Slaughter should be rapid with as little prior disturbance as possible. Techniques include narcosis with carbon dioxide, electrical stunning and physical stunning. Of these the latter is the most commonly used and is probably the most rapid and satisfactory where it can be employed. Electrical stunning is probably preferred in rainbow trout.

Physical stunning involves a firm blow with a small, heavy club on the top of the head immediately anterior to a line connecting the rear edges of the operculae and posterior to the eyes. If the fish is a pet fish and has to be killed in the surgery or in front of owners, physical stunning, dislocation of the neck, or severing the spinal cord, whilst being the most rapid, are not aesthetically acceptable. Narcosis by reduced temperature or carbon dioxide solution followed by an injection with pentobarbitone may be the most satisfactory.

Summary

Although less well understood than other livestock, fish are conscious, sentient animals. Good, responsible management and husbandry will ensure that farmed fish are kept in acceptable conditions with due allowance for their welfare. It should be remembered that different species can have widely different environmental requirements.

In some countries codes of practice for aquaculture are being developed. These should be studied and, where appropriate, used by all those involved in fish culture.

References

Report of the Technical Committee of Enquiry into the Welfare of Animals Kept under Intensive Livestock Husbandry Systems. HMSO, London. (1965) Cmnd 2836.
Report on Priorities in Animal Welfare Research and Development. (1988) Farm Animal Welfare Council, London.
Seamer, J. (1992) Transport of Live Animals for Slaughter. *Veterinary Record* **130** (2), 38.

11

Legislation Affecting Farmed Fish

KEITH TREVES BROWN and ALASTAIR GRAY

The Aims of Legislation

Legislation concerned with fish does not differ from that concerning other vertebrates in its broad aims, which are:

- Animal welfare, including prevention of cruelty;
- Prevention of the spread of infectious or contagious diseases;
- Prevention of the supply of unwholesome foods of animal origin;
- Control of the distribution and use of veterinary medicinal products.

These aims are not mutually exclusive. For example, controls on biological medicinal products ensure that the products do not spread disease; withdrawal periods applied to non-biological medicinal products prevent the distribution of foods which contain excessive residues; and requirements for medicines to be safe for the target species are an aspect of welfare.

Regardless of the original intent, legislation is sometimes applied so as to protect national economic interests and the aims become 'non-tariff barriers to trade'. The prevention of such developments is one of the principal purposes of the European Communities (EC), and they have enacted a considerably body of legislation in this area. Conversely, in the USA during the 1970s all attempts at control of disease through federal restriction on fish movement was opposed. This led to each state producing its own legislation with, in some cases, obvious political and economic aims.

Because this book is concerned with fish medicine world-wide, and because the EC is the only supranational legislating body, this chapter will survey mainly EC enactments. Almost the only individual country to have its own legislation covering fish is Norway, and the situation there is summarised in Chapter 12. Legislation in other countries is mentioned in the appropriate species chapters. The general headings in this chapter will be of use to fish veterinarians when determining which aspects of national legislation may be relevant to aquaculture.

Welfare

This is an aspect of legislation which is almost universally neglected where fish are concerned. There is no EC legislation on the welfare of farmed fish; but there is an enactment covering the welfare of experimental animals, and because it defines animals as vertebrates it does include finfish.

Directive 86/609/EEC **on the approximation of laws, regulations and administrative provisions of the Member States regarding the protection of animals used for experimental and other scientific purposes** puts first among its aims the elimination of disparities between member state laws which may affect the functioning of the Common Market. Only secondarily does it aim to minimise the number of animals used (including the avoidance of unnecessary duplication of experiments) and ensure the welfare of such animals as are used. Authorisation of experiments by member state governments is made mandatory and there are provisions covering the choice of species, their welfare and the need for anaesthesia. Article 9 is of particular interest to veterinarians as it covers the action to be taken at the end of an experiment and specifically recommends that a veterinarian should advise on whether the animals should be kept alive, and if so under what conditions.

Prevention of the Spread of Disease

Directive 91/67/EEC **concerning the animal health conditions governing the placing on the market of**

aquaculture animals and products is an extensive hygiene measure intended to control a wide range of diseases. It provides general health specifications for aquaculture animals and products (e.g. eggs) which may be marketed for culture or for human consumption.

The directive includes lists of diseases of farmed finfish, molluscs and crustacea which are subject to governmental control or eradication ('notifiable diseases'). These lists form an annex to the directive, which means that they may be changed without serious procedural difficulties. Initially the diseases of finfish in the annex were:

A disease for which an EC survey was already in progress with a view to Community-wide eradication:
    Infectious haematopoietic necrosis.
Additional disease(s) for which Community-wide movement controls are specified in the directive:
    Viral haemorrhagic septicaemia
    Infectious salmon anaemia will probably be placed in this annex.
Diseases for which member states are entitled to exact local zoo-sanitary measures subject to Community approval:
    Infectious pancreatic necrosis
    Spring viraemia of carp
    Bacterial kidney disease
    Furunculosis in Atlantic salmon
    Enteric redmouth disease
    Gyrodactylosis
    Myxobolosis (whirling disease).

Approved zones and approved farms in non-approved zones, are designated, meaning that they are free from these listed diseases, and procedures for designating them are established. Systems of health certification are laid down for the movement of consignments into and between approved premises and for importation from outside the EC ('third countries'). There are also provisions allowing for member state eradication schemes.

This is an extensive and important measure effective from 1st January 1993. Veterinarians advising fish farmers in the EC should familiarise themselves with it and with any legislation enacted by their own member states in compliance with the directive.

A very similar system operates in Canada under the Federal Fish Health Protection Regulations. Farms may be 'certified' after inspection and microbiological examination of sample fish by registered fish health officials. In both the EC and Canadian systems the certification is for freedom from specified diseases; it offers no guarantee of general hygiene.

***Council Decision 90/495/EEC* To set up an epidemiological inquiry to determine the incidence of infectious haematopoietic necrosis (IHN) in the Community with a view to eradication** is probably the only multinational scheme aimed at the eradication of a specific fish disease. It provides for surveys in each of the member states which will be financed 50% by the Community. An eradication campaign will follow if the findings suggest it is feasible.

Prevention of the Supply of Unwholesome Food

Fish, like other foods of animal origin, may become unwholesome due to:

- Post-mortem deterioration in unsatisfactory storage conditions, especially temperature;
- Post-mortem contamination;
- Being given foods contaminated with toxic materials, e.g. aflatoxin, heavy metals;
- Slaughter while containing medicinal residues.

There are a number of EC enactments which aim to prevent the supply of unwholesome foods of animal origin, either by defining wholesomeness in terms of limits for contaminants, or by controlling feedstuffs and medication.

***Directive 70/524/EEC* concerning additives in feedstuffs** established a registration procedure at the EC level. The word 'additive' means a substance which is not itself a feedstuff (although it may be nutritional, e.g. synthetic vitamins) and which is to be added *routinely* to the feed of normal healthy animals. The definition includes colours, preservatives and antioxidants, gelling agents, minerals etc. It also includes medicinal products which are fed prophylactically, notably coccidiostats for poultry, and it includes growth promoters. Additives which have been approved in the EC procedure are placed in one of two annexes to the directive, with specifications of the species and ages of animals for which they are approved, the limits for the levels of incorporation in feeds and, where appropriate, the withdrawal periods to be applied. Additives are usually placed in Annex II initially, and member states then have the option of licensing or refusing to license their use. Within five years the additive must be transferred to Annex I or withdrawn from the market. Once it is in Annex I, member states must grant market authorisation if application is made.

This directive is of great importance in the mammalian and avian fields. It has had limited impact on fish farming so far, although it seems probable that growth promoters for fish will be developed in due course. Annex I does, however, contain entries for two important colouring agents in salmon and trout: canthaxanthin ($C_{40}H_{52}O_2$ — EC no. E161g) and astaxanthin ($C_{40}H_{52}O_4$ — EC no. E161j). In both cases, the maximum content is 100 mg/kg of complete feedstuffs. The mixture of canthaxanthin with astaxanthin is admitted provided that the total concentration of the mixture does not exceed 100 ppm in the complete feedstuff. Use is permitted from the age of 6 months onwards for either agent.

***Regulation 2377/90/EEC* laying down a Community procedure for the establishment of maximum residue limits (MRLs) of veterinary medicinal products in foodstuffs of animal origin** establishes four annexes, viz.:

Annex I   Substances for which MRLs have been established (by the procedure laid down in the regulation).
Annex II   Substances for which it is agreed that no MRL is necessary.
Annex III   Substances with provisional MRLs.
Annex IV   Substances for which an MRL cannot be established because '. . . residues . . . at whatever limit, . . . constitute a hazard to the health of the consumer.'

Annex III contains the very large number of substances already in use in veterinary medicine for which no MRLs had been established at EC level when the regulation came into force. (Products containing them should nevertheless have had withdrawal periods assigned to them in compliance with Directive 81/851/EEC.) The regulation provides that provisional MRLs shall apply for only a limited time during which a definitive MRL should be agreed and the substance transferred to one of the other annexes.

It is notable that among the first substances to be assigned to Annex II is a fish medicine, hydrogen peroxide.

Both this regulation and Directive 70/524/EEC

mentioned above are intended to prevent the marketing of foods of animal origin containing hazardous residues of veterinary medicinal products; but the approaches to this end form an interesting contrast. The directive applies only to orally administered additives, and specifies incorporation rates and withdrawal periods in the annexes. Regulation 2377/90 establishes MRLs, which will be applicable irrespective of the formulation, dose regimen and the route by which the substance is administered. It remains the responsibility of a member state regulatory authority to assign a withdrawal period to each product containing the substance to ensure that the MRL will be met.

***Directive 74/63/EEC* on the fixing of maximum permitted levels for undesirable substances and products in feedstuffs** has an obvious application in preventing unwholesome food of animal origin reaching the market since many undesirable substances, such as heavy metals, in addition to being toxic to animals may in smaller quantities be cumulative. The directive provides for the creation of an annex which is a list of undesirable substances and their permitted levels.

***Directive 90/167/EEC* laying down the conditions governing the preparation, placing on the market and use of medicated feedstuffs in the Community** has considerable bearing on fish medication since the commonest method of administration is in feed. The directive protects human health by preventing misuse of medicated feeds. It contains provisions covering the premises in which medicated feeds may be compounded, and their labelling and packaging. Supply is restricted to veterinary prescription and only in quantities suitable to treat specific disease outbreaks.

At the time of writing a Code of Hygienic Practice for the Products of Aquaculture is being drafted by the Codex Alimentarius Commission. This international body, sponsored jointly by the World Health Organisation (WHO) and the Food and Agriculture Organisation (FAO) of the United Nations, is responsible for setting standards of wholesomeness of human foodstuffs. The Code as currently drafted offers little positive advice on hygienic production, but it should form an important checklist of issues to be borne in mind in all aspects of aquaculture from the choice of site for a farm to hygienic methods of slaughter and processing of produce.

Control of Medicines

The EC framework legislation covering veterinary medicinal products is mainly concerned with 'market authorisation' — the licensing of products before they may be launched on the market. Before market authorisation is granted, the applicant must furnish evidence of the safety, quality and efficacy of the product. Safety in this context includes:

- Safety for the target species.
- Safety for the operator using or administering the product.
- Safety for the consumer of products of the treated animal.
- Safety for the environment.

The criteria of safety, quality and efficacy applied in the licensing of veterinary medicinal products, and the procedures for applying for market authorisations, are of little concern to the practising veterinarian. However, a market authorisation will give detailed specifications for the labelling and use of the product and these are of concern to a veterinarian prescribing it.

Safety to the target species. Most legislative systems make provision for post-marketing surveillance or 'pharmaco-vigilance'. Pre-launch testing rarely shows up all the problems which can arise with a medicinal product and so the recording, examination and analysis of suspected adverse reactions (SARs), which include lack of efficacy, makes an essential contribution to ensuring safety, quality and efficacy. Complete and accurate reporting of SARs by practising veterinarians is fundamental to the process.

Safety to the operator. This is normally addressed by a requirement for appropriate warnings and recommendations as to protective clothing or equipment to be used when administering the product. Here veterinarians have an important role to perform in drawing farmers' attention to the warnings and precautions attaching to any medicinal products they prescribe. This is of particular importance for fish farmers because formulations for fish feed medication usually contain a higher concentration of active ingredient than is the case for mammals and birds.

Safety to the consumer. This means all those aspects of medicinal residues already discussed under Prevention of the Supply of Unwholesome Food. Before a market authorisation is granted, a withdrawal period has to be assigned to the product and included on the product literature and labels. Where fish are concerned the withdrawal time for any given formulation will vary not only with species but also with water temperature. Under some legislative systems a fixed time is assigned. A concept which is becoming more widely adopted, however, is that of 'degree-days'. This means the sum of average daily water temperatures. For example, a withdrawal period of 120 degree-days means:

24 days at a steady water temperature of						5°C
15	" " "	"	"	"	"	8°C
12	" " "	"	"	"	"	10°C
10	" " "	"	"	"	"	12°C
8	" " "	"	"	"	"	15°C

with appropriate adjustments where the water temperature is variable. It is a responsibility of the prescribing veterinarian to ensure that a fish farmer understands the withdrawal period which must be applied before the stock is harvested.

In Norway, any drug usage in fish must be reported to the authorities, who will then assay samples *before the fish are harvested* to ensure freedom from residues.

Safety to the environment. Of particular importance in fish medication is safety to the environment because chemicals used as baths for farmed fish cannot afterwards be recovered from the water, and medicated feeds are rarely eaten in their entirety. In consequence any drug usage will result in a measure of water pollution, and water-flow will spread the pollution, possibly to highly susceptible ecological communities or human water supplies. The veterinarian has a responsibility to prescribe only sufficient drug and to advise on its correct storage and the safe disposal of unused drug or medicated feed.

***Directive 81/851/EEC* on the approximation of the laws of the member states relating to veterinary medicinal products** requires each member state to institute a regulated market authorisation system based on the demonstration of safety, quality and efficacy. It also instituted the EC Committee on

Veterinary Medicinal Products (CVMP) and a multi-state authorisation system through that body. The system has been little used overall; and it has not been used at all for fish products — not least because of the diversity of fish species farmed in different member states.

Directive 81/852/EEC **on the approximation of the laws of the member states relating to analytical, pharmaco-toxicological and clinical standards and protocols in respect of the testing of veterinary medicinal products** lays down the standards of safety, quality and efficacy to be applied in the assessment of products.

These two directives are the basic regulators of the veterinary pharmaceutical industry in the EC. Although they may pass unnoticed by the average practising veterinarian, they are in fact the assurance of the safety, quality and efficacy of the products used. In both directives the phrase, 'veterinary medicinal products' is defined excluding immunological products and excluding feed additives as defined in Directive 70/524 (see page 174).

Directive 90/677/EEC **extending the scope of Directive 81/851/EEC on the approximation of the laws of the member states relating to veterinary medicinal products and laying down additional provisions for immunological veterinary medicinal products** is a relatively brief enactment extending the controls (and hence the assurances to the practising veterinarian) to immunological products. For such products, safety requirements include the demonstration of freedom from extraneous pathogens, viral, bacterial or mycoplasmal. Live vaccines, of which there are few for fish, must be shown to be adequately attenuated and hence both safe for the inoculated animal and without any tendency to revert to virulence on transmission to other individuals. Efficacy must always be shown and this involves more detail than normal for immersion vaccines for fish: safe dilution rates, efficacious exposure times, and satisfactory renewal or replenishment rates must all be demonstrated.

Legislation, and particularly EC legislation, is never static and complete. The House of Lords (the upper house of the UK Parliament) has commented that the above directives and others not mentioned here have their present form due to a lack of mutual trust between the regulatory authorities of the member states. At the time of writing discussions are well under way towards the only ultimate answer to this problem: the creation of an EC regulatory agency.

References in the Official Journal of the European Communities

Legislation

Journal references

Directive 86/609/EEC: No. L358 of 18.12.86 pp.1–28.
Directive 91/67/EEC: No. L46 of 19.2.91 pp.1–13.
Decision 90/495/EEC: No. L276 of 6.10.90.
Directive 70/524/EEC: No. L270 of 14.12.70 pp.1–11.
Directive 84/587/EEC: No. L319 of 8.12.84 pp.13–23.
Regulation 2377/90/EEC: No. L224 of 18.8.90 pp.1–4.
Directive 74/63/EEC: No. L38 of 11.2.74 pp.31–33.
Directive 90/167/EEC: No. L92 of 7.4.90 pp.42–46.
Directive 81/851/EEC: No. L317 of 6.11.81 pp.1–15.
Directive 81/852/EEC: No. L317 of 6.11.81 pp.16–28.
Directive 90/677/EEC: No. L373 of 31.12.90 pp.26–28.

Further Reading

Bernoth, E.-M. (1990) Marketing authorisation of fish drugs — Current status and future intentions. *Journal of Veterinary Medicine B* **37**, 401–406.

12

The Veterinary Approach to Salmon Farming in Norway

ROLF NORDMO

Norway is well known for its fjords, mountains and rivers. Most of the rivers are famous as excellent salmon rivers and as such are visited by fly-fishers from all over the world. Such an environment is also favourable for the intensive cultivation of salmon and the development of Norwegian salmon farming since the early 1970s has been spectacular. In 1979 the production of Atlantic salmon *Salmo salar* was 4142 tons, whereas in 1991 it reached 150,000 tons. During this period both veterinarians and fish farmers have had to learn from experience.

Farming Systems

The combination of rivers and fjords has strongly influenced the structure of fish farming in Norway, with smolt farms located near rivers or lakes and with sea farms in the fjords.

Farming of Smolts

Smolts can be bred either on land-based farms or using net-pens in lakes and rivers. Land-based farms are more common and are described in this chapter.

Egg collection and hatching

Eggs are collected either from cultivated fish or from fish which are caught wild in the local fjords or rivers each autumn. In both cases the fish are kept in net-pens or in land-based basins until they become ripe for stripping. The stripping period is typically from October to November. Stripped eggs and milt are allowed to fertilise *in vitro*.

Fertilised eggs are sold on to smolt farms, where they are placed in hatcheries. Some smolt farms

have their own stock of breeding animals, but most farmers buy fertilised eggs for hatching. The hatching period varies according to the water temperature, but is most commonly in January. Salmon eggs hatch at 450–500 degree-days in Norway. After hatching, the fry live on their yolk-sac for 2–3 weeks; after this, they become free-swimming and start feeding.

Growth period

Growth periods vary considerably from farm to farm. Some farms use heated water and artificial light regimens to increase growth rate; others produce their smolts at low water temperatures. These variations in farming conditions typically result in 1 year smolts (S1s) or 2 year smolts (S2s). Some 'supersmolts', which smoltify after approximately 6 months, have been produced.

Smoltification

Smoltification of Atlantic salmon in Norway takes place in April to May; the fish are then moved from the freshwater smolt farms to the marine farms, either within one company or to a different one. S1s have an average weight of approximately 40 g when sold and S2s weigh approximately 200 g.

Marine Farms

Most marine farms in Norway are in the fjords or among the islands along the coast. The production is dominated by sea-cage systems. The net-pens are of different kinds but the principle is the same (Fig. 12.1). All types of sea-cage farming are based on a natural exchange of water through the

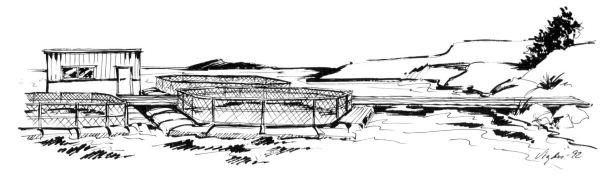

FIG. 12.1 A typical salmon farm with sea cages.

pens; the quality of sites is therefore highly variable, according to local conditions such as tide and streams.

The dimensions of a marine farm are usually expressed in terms of volume; the typical size is either 12,000 or 20,000 m^3, according to Norwegian law.

Growth period

After their release into sea water, the fish are fed over the next 18–24 months on commercial salmon diets. After 2 years in sea water the salmon weigh 3–5 kg.

Slaughter takes place throughout the year, the busiest period being from October to December. This means that most farmers keep two generations of salmon in sea water at the same time.

Location

Some of the farms are anchored close to the land and can be served from a landing. Others are located in the middle of the fjord or open sea and can only be served by boat. During the first 10–15 years of farming in Norway most farmers had their farm in the same place year after year, with the two generations of fish at the same site. Following the introduction of serious infectious diseases, most farmers now co-operate so that each location is used for one year-class at a time. In addition, each location is left fallow for a year after the production period to improve the microbiological condition of the site (Fig. 12.2).

Instead of using different parts of the fjords for their farms, the farmers in one region now typically use the same part of the fjord for the same generation of fish. In this way large regions of the fjord systems can be rested for long periods.

Land-based farms for adult fish have been proposed to control water conditions more efficiently and avoid a major spread of infectious disease. The ever-increasing concern about the potential for pollution by fish farms has also motivated the development of land-based farms, but they are not yet common in Norway.

General Husbandry

Smolt Farms

As fish farming deals with aquatic organisms, the major concern in husbandry is water quality. It will never be possible to offer fish in farms the same conditions as in nature (i.e. 100% saturation of water with oxygen and very low stocking densities). Hence, in fish farming there is a compromise between the needs of commercial farming and the needs of the animal.

Poor husbandry typically leads to gill disease, fin rot, skin erosion, shortening of the gill cover and reduced growth. One of the major tasks for the veterinarian is to make the farmer aware of obvious husbandry errors and advise him of improvements for the system. A knowledge of water chemistry and limnology, as well as of day-to-day farm management, is essential.

As smolt farms in Norway are located near rivers or lakes, the water supply tends to be of surface water from the nearest surface resource. In most of Norway surface water is acidic; a very low total alkalinity reduces the buffering capacity

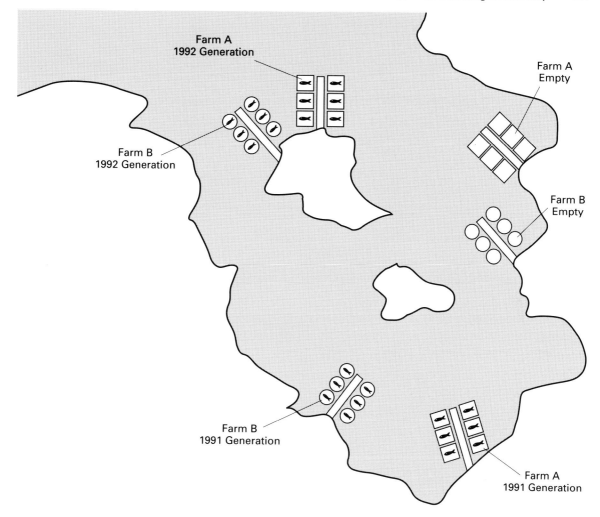

Fig. 12.2 Coordinated alternate use of different localities.

of the water. Some farms use ground-water, either as their only resource or mixed with surface water.

Smolt farms located near the coast can stabilise the pH of the fresh water with small amounts of sea water. Such mixtures have sometimes caused severe outbreaks of both vibriosis and furunculosis and the practice is therefore *not* recommended. In those regions where the water quality *demands* such stabilisation, procedures for sterilising the sea water are of major importance. These include ultraviolet irradiation, ozonisation or heat.

Poor water quality seldom causes severe mortality on fish farms in Norway except for the effects of acidification and labile aluminium. Acidification has caused severe losses in the southern part of the country.

Supersaturation

Poor water quality often has a multifactorial aetiology. In some cases, however, sudden deaths may be caused by a single factor, such as supersaturation of gases. If water is heated to increase the growth rate of the fish, it is essential that the water is then aerated to eliminate supersaturated gases. Faulty pumps (which allow air in through leaky gaskets) may also cause supersaturation.

Ammonia/ammonium

Farms which recirculate water should be aware of the high risk of ammonia poisoning. The LC_{50} (4 days) for ammonia is temperature-dependent;

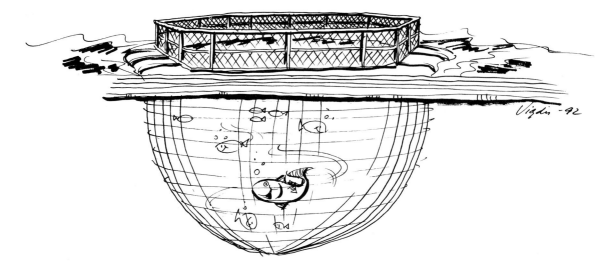

FIG. 12.3 Low stocking density and optimal rearing conditions are the most important actions to prevent diseases.

values between 0.03 and 0.15 mg/l have been recorded. Sub-lethal effects of ammonium have been observed at concentrations as low as 0.005 mg/l.

Labile aluminium

Acid rain, a problem seen in parts of Norway, can mobilise aluminium from the ground and force the aluminium towards toxic forms. The most toxic forms are found when the water pH is around 5.0–5.5. Toxic effects are often observed in the snow-melting period in regions where the buffering properties of the water are low. Calcium, sodium chloride and humus provide protection against the toxic effects of aluminium.

Other parameters

Humus is seldom a problem in fish farming in Norway, and may even have a protective effect against some metals. Small particulate matter can cause gill damage, which may be seen where mining occurs near the water source.

Stocking density and water demands

Optimal stocking density varies according to the size of the fish. Common densities are shown in Fig. 12.4.

As water is seldom the limiting factor in Norwegian fish farming, most farms are run with

COMMON STOCKING DENSITIES FOR SALMON	
Average weight	**kg fish/m³ water**
Less than 2 g	4–6
2–5 g	6–10
5–10 g	10–15
20–30 g	15–20
Smolts	20–30

FIG. 12.4 Common stocking densities for salmon.

a 100% flow-through system. Water demands vary with temperature and with the size of the fish (Fig. 12.5).

Marine Farms

Marine farms may be in a fjord or in open waters off the coast. Fjords with poor water exchange are not suitable for fish farming. Farms located away from the coast (off-shore) have the best water quality conditions, although local tidal streams influence the suitability of the site. In the early days of intensive fish farming, most of the farms were in the fjord systems but recently the trend has been to move to off-shore sites. Finding the best place for farming involves a compromise between the needs for good water quality and for protection against stormy weather.

Salinity

Salinity in the fjords can vary widely according to rain and snow-melting. A fall in salinity due to

FRESHWATER DEMANDS OF SALMON ACCORDING TO FISH SIZE AND TEMPERATURE (in litres/minute/kg fish)									
Temp (°C)	Average weight of fish (g)								
	1	2	4	6	10	20	100	1000	4000
2	0.2	0.2	0.2	0.1	0.1	0.1	0.1	0.1	0.1
4	0.3	0.3	0.2	0.2	0.2	0.2	0.1	0.1	0.1
6	0.4	0.4	0.3	0.3	0.2	0.2	0.2	0.1	0.1
8	0.6	0.5	0.4	0.4	0.3	0.3	0.2	0.1	0.1
10	0.8	0.7	0.6	0.5	0.5	0.4	0.3	0.2	0.2
12	1.0	0.8	0.7	0.7	0.6	0.5	0.4	0.2	0.2
14	1.2	1.0	0.9	0.8	0.8	0.7	0.5	0.3	0.2
16	1.5	1.3	1.1	1.0	0.9	0.8	0.6	0.4	0.3
18	1.8	1.6	1.4	1.2	1.1	0.9	0.7	0.5	0.4

FIG. 12.5 Based on an oxygen saturation of 95% in the inlet water. Oxygen content in the outlet water is a minimum of 5 mg O_2/l.

sudden snow-melting is often followed by a fall in temperature. The combination has caused severe losses in some farms. The temperature and salinity changes are normally limited to the surface layers of the fjords.

Algae

Algal blooms have created problems in Norway's fish farms in the past. Mortalities occur when the algae cause a lack of oxygen and/or toxin accumulation in the water.

Other parameters

The stocking density and size of the fish in each pen also contribute to the water quality. The biomass in sea farms should not exceed 15 kg/m^3. Daily removal of dead fish is also extremely important for both water quality and disease control.

Legislation

The major legislation affecting aquaculture in Norway is *Act No. 2 of 6 December 1968*, concerning control measures against diseases in freshwater fish, which applies until it is repealed or replaced by regulations given in *Diseases in Aquatic Organisms* (Provisional Act of 22 June 1990), the objectives of which are the prevention, control or eradication of diseases in aquatic organisms. This Act applies to such diseases as are specified by the King at any time and only in the Norwegian economical zone. As regards seawater species, the Act applies only to aquatic organisms in captivity.

The owner or other person responsible for aquatic organisms must notify the veterinary officer if there is any reason to believe that such organisms are suffering from, or have died of, the diseases to which the Act applies. It is prohibited to offer for sale, to sell, give away, purchase, receive or release live aquatic organisms if there is any suspicion that they are suffering from or infected by any of those diseases.

The Minister may issue regulations concerning the importation (including the complete prohibition of such importation) of live aquatic organisms or used packaging material, used fishing gear and other items which may be contaminated by infectious agents. The regulations may determine that the importer shall be liable to cover expenses connected with importation and subsequent control procedures and the Ministry may order that aquatic organisms, products or articles which are imported in contravention of regulations issued pursuant to the Act shall be returned or destroyed at the importer's expense without compensation from public funds, even if the item belongs to someone who has not contravened or been an accessory to contravening the regulations.

It is prohibited to establish new installations for hatching eggs or for rearing aquatic organisms, or to expand existing installations, without the prior approval of the Ministry.

The veterinary officer, or anyone the Ministry so empowers, shall have access to localities or installations where such diseases to which the Act applies may occur, and may carry out such

CONTROL MEASURES AGAINST DISEASES IN AQUATIC ORGANISMS APPLIED TO LISTED DISEASES	
Group A	**Group B**
Viral haemorrhagic septicaemia (VHS) Infectious haematopoietic necrosis (IHN) Herpes viroses Other rhabdoviroses Crayfish plague Bonamiosis in bivalves Gill disease (Iridovirosis) in bivalves Martelliosis in bivalves	Bacterial kidney disease (BKD) Whirling disease (Myxosomiasis) Furunculosis *(Aeromonas salmonicida* subsp. *salmonicida)* Gaffkaemia Infection with human-pathogenic *Edwardsiella* spp. Infectious *Gyrodactylus salaris* Infectious *Anguillicola* spp. Infectious pancreatic necrosis (IPN) Infectious salmon anaemia (ISA) Mycosis with *Ichthyophonus hoferi*
Group C	
Burned spot disease Cold-water vibriosis *(Vibrio salmonicida)* Mycobacteriosis Kidney fungus (*Exophiala* spp.) Infection with *Thelohania contejani* Septicaemias with other *Aeromonas* spp. Swim-bladder fungus Ulcerative dermatic necrosis (UDN) Systemic infection with other *Vibrio* spp.	Erythrocytic inclusion body syndrome (EIBS) Hexamitosis Nocardiosis Pancreas disease Proliferative kidney disease (PKD) Septicaemias with other *Pseudomonas* spp. Ulcer disease (atypical *Aeromonas salmonicida*) Vibriosis *(Vibrio anguillarum)* Yersiniosis (ERM)

FIG. 12.6 Control measures against diseases in aquatic organisms applied to listed diseases.

investigations as are deemed necessary. Anyone who wilfully or through gross negligence violates or fails to comply with any regulations, orders or provisions given in the Act, or who attempts to do so or is an accessory thereto, will be fined, or imprisoned for up to 3 months, provided that more rigorous punishment is not applicable.

Control measures against diseases in aquatic organisms apply to listed diseases categorised in three groups (A, B and C) as shown below. *Group A* diseases must be reported immediately to the nearest veterinary officer. Diseases in *Groups B and C* are reported immediately or monthly, according to the previous occurrence of the disease in that region. Based on reports from local veterinarians, the authorities give their instructions to prevent spread of the disease. In general, Groups A and B lead to strict restrictions in the trade and movement of the affected fish. Group C diseases do not normally lead to any restrictions but exceptions may be made for diseases not yet diagnosed in Norway. The disease groups are shown in Fig. 12.6.

The most common of these are described below in the Major Diseases section. The only Group A disease diagnosed in Norway is crayfish plague, which occurs in two river systems in the south of the country; all catching of crayfish from these river systems is forbidden. Several Group B diseases have been diagnosed: BKD, whirling disease, furunculosis, infectious *Gyrodactylus salaris*, ISA and IPN.

A number of regulations and circulars published by the Norwegian government are listed in Appendix I at the end of this book. Some control the use and storage of fish medicines as well as the monitoring of fish health status. Measures have been adopted to ensure that fish are only slaughtered when they have exceeded the recommended withdrawal time for any medication which they may have been given. There is also an Animal Welfare Act which applies to fish.

Legislation affecting fish farming in Norway is administered by the Ministry of Fisheries (Act No. 68 of 14 June 1985, relating to the breeding of fish and shellfish), the Ministry of Environment (Pollution Control Act of 13 March 1981, No. 6), the Ministry of Agriculture (Provisional Act concerning Control Measures against Diseases in Aquatic Organisms, 22 June 1990, No. 44) and the Coast Directorate (Act No. 51 of 8 June 1984 relating to harbours and fairways).

In order to operate a salmon sea-farm in Norway, licences must be obtained. Due to over-production, no new licences are being issued at present but old licences may be transferred to new owners. Applications to establish fish farms are sent to the Regional Fishery Officer (*Fiskerisjefen*), who administers and co-ordinates the application with relevant ministries and directorates.

Major Diseases

Viral Diseases

Infectious salmon anaemia (ISA)

This disease was first notified from a smolt farm in 1984, where it was diagnosed on parr ready for smoltification the following spring. The fish were kept in fresh water but had been exposed to large amounts of sea water. Today (Dec 1992) 78 fish farms in Norway have 'restricted' status due to ISA.

It is believed that the disease is caused by a virus; thus no effective therapy is available. Stress and bad husbandry conditions can provoke out-breaks. To prevent spread both within and between farms, diseased fish should be slaughtered as soon as possible.

Infectious pancreatic necrosis (IPN)

IPN was diagnosed for the first time in Norway in 1975. In 1987 the causative virus (IPNV) was found in 401 of 697 farms tested. IPNV has also been isolated from wild salmon but the spread in wild salmon is expected to be far more limited than in farmed fish. Serotypes isolated are Ab, Sp and N1.

IPN combined with other pancreatic disorders is an increasing problem in Norwegian fish farming. It mainly manifests on smolts following their release into sea water. Because it is known that the virus will be transferred both horizontally and vertically, all parent fish in the national breeding system are tested for IPNV. Eggs from positive parents are destroyed before hatching.

Bacterial Diseases

Bacterial kidney disease

BKD was first diagnosed in Norway in 1980. It is not known whether the disease was introduced with farmed fish or from wild salmon. Outbreaks have been sporadic and this may indicate that the bacterium is present in the wild salmon population and that the disease manifests due to intensive cultivation.

There are no vaccines available. Diseased fish are treated with erythromycin, sulphonamides or oxytetracycline. Injection of erythromycin into parent fish before spawning has been used but such treatment will not eradicate the disease and eggs from infected fish should be destroyed.

Furunculosis

Furunculosis is widespread in Norway. After some sporadic outbreaks in the Numedalslagen river from 1966 to 1977, the disease was introduced to fish farms in 1985 when infected smolts were imported. Since then it has developed to become one of the major causes of stock loss.

The disease is prevented by use of good husbandry practices combined with vaccination. Effective treatment is provided by antimicrobials, though during the past few years an ever-increasing resistance problem has reduced the efficacy of the commonly used drugs.

Vibriosis and yersiniosis

Vibriosis, cold-water vibriosis and yersiniosis are effectively prevented in Norway by the use of vaccines. When outbreaks occur, the diseases are treated with antibacterial agents.

Parasites

Whirling disease

Whirling disease is not regarded as a major problem in Norwegian salmon; it is mainly recognised as a disease affecting rainbow trout raised in earth ponds. However, salmon are thoroughly checked for the presence of whirling disease since all salmon intended for export to the US must be certified as originating from a farm which is free from the disease.

Infectious Gyrodactylus salaris

It is believed that *Gyrodactylus salaris* was imported in 1970. Since then the parasite has

THERAPEUTIC AGENTS IN NORWEGIAN SALMON FARMING

Anthelmintics

Drug	Indication	Dosage active substance	Withdrawal time	Remarks
Praziquantel	Intestinal tape-worm infection	5 mg/kg/day 1–2 days	14 days	Mixed with feed
Albendazole	Intestinal tape-worm infection	5 mg/kg on days 1 and 4	30 days	Mixed with feed. Not registered for fish. Withdrawal under evaluation
Fenbendazole	Intestinal tape-worm infection	5 mg/kg on days 1 and 4	30 days	Mixed with feed. Not registered for fish. Withdrawal under evaluation

Organophosphates

Drug	Indication	Dosage of drug per m^3 of water	Withdrawal time	Remarks
Dichlorvos	Sea lice	<5°C: 3–4 ml 5–10°C: 2–3 ml 10–15°C: 1–2 ml >15°C: 1 ml	14 days	Very toxic Carcinogenic
Metriphonate (trichlorphon)	Sea lice	<6°C: 300 g 6–10°C: 100 g 10–14°C: 50 g 14–18°C: 15 g	21 days	The toxicity of the solution will increase with time Teratogenic

Anaesthetics

Drug	Indication	Dosage of drug per 10 litres of water	Withdrawal time	Remarks
Benzocaine 20% solution in an organic solvent e.g. ethanol, propylene glycol	Stripping, weighing, vaccination, sorting etc.	2.5 ml Upkeep: 1.5–5 ml	21 days	Concentrate: 200 g benzocaine per litre organic solvent (Gives 20% solution) Added in small quantities to container holding fish The water must be oxygenated
Chlorbutanol 30% solution in ethanol	Stripping, weighing, vaccination, sorting etc.	10 ml	21 days	Concentrate: 300 g chlorbutanol per litre ethanol (Gives 30% solution) Added in small quantities to container holding fish The water must be oxygenated
Tricaine methanesulphonate	Stripping, weighing, vaccination, sorting etc.	0.5–0.8 g	21 days	Gives an acidic solution. May be dissolved in buffer or sea water before use The water must be oxygenated.

Medical disinfectants

Group	Drug	Indication	Dosage of drug per 10 litres of water	Remarks
Iodophor	Various compounds	Disinfection of eggs	100 ml in 10 minutes	For the disinfection of newly fertilised eggs use 90 g NaCl Not to be used under or after hatching
Organic chloro-compounds	Chloramine T 1% and other compounds	Gill diseases and fin rot on fry and smolts	Acid water: 2.5 ml in 1 hour Neutral water/ alkaline water: 10 ml in 1 hour	Concentrate is made from 10 g Chloramine T dissolved in 1 litre of water just prior to use (Gives 1% solution)
Quaternary ammonium compounds	Benzalkonium chloride 10%	Gill diseases and fin rot on fry and smolts	Neutral water: 0.075 ml in 1 hour Hard water: 0.2 ml in 1 hour	

FIG. 12.7   *continued*

THERAPEUTIC AGENTS IN NORWEGIAN SALMON FARMING

Medical disinfectants

Group	Drug	Indication	Dosage of drug per 10 litres of water	Remarks
Aldehydes	Formaldehyde 37%	Ectoparasites on fry and smolts *Costia* in sea water	Therapeutic: 2.5 ml in 30 minutes Prophylactic: 1.7 ml in 30 minutes	Prophylactic treatment is repeated every 14 days Solutions with precipitates must not be used
	Formaldehyde 29.5%	Ectoparasites on fry and smolts *Costia* in sea water	Therapeutic: 3.1 ml in 30 minutes Prophylactic: 2.1 ml in 30 minutes	Allergenic. Possible carcinogenic effect. No documented effect against *Chilodonella*
Antiseptic dye	Malachite green oxalate 1%	External fungi on eggs, fry and smolts Ectoparasites on fry and smolts	67 ml in 20 seconds or 2 ml in 1 hour	Concentrate made from 10 g malachite green powder in 1 litre of water (Gives 1% solution) Teratogenic. May cause abnormalities on fry Not to be used on adult fish due to minimum withdrawal time of 1 year
Salt	Sodium chloride	Ectoparasites on fry and smolts	100–150 g in 10–20 minutes	Possible effect against *Chilodonella* and *Gyrodactylus salaris*

Antibiotics and chemotherapeutics

Drug	Indication	Dosage	Withdrawal time	Remarks
Oxolinic acid	General bacterial infections	Fresh water: 100 mg/kg divided over 5-8 days Sea water: 200-350 mg/kg divided over 5-8 days	>12°C: 40 days 8–12°C: 40–60 days <8°C: >60 days	Other regimes with both higher and lower dose are in use. Medicated feed pellets and Aqualets* are being registered Withdrawal time under evaluation
Flumequine	General bacterial infections External and general bacterial infections in fry and smolts	Fresh water: 100 mg/kg divided over 5-8 days Sea water: 125–200 mg/kg divided over 5–8 days 5 g soluble powder 10% (= 0.5 g flumequine) per 10 litres water in 3 hours	>12°C: 40 days 8–12°C: 40–60 days <8°C: >60 days	Dosage and withdrawal time under evaluation Medicated Aqualets under registration Water needs oxygenation
Oxytetracycline hydrochloride	General bacterial infections	800–1000 mg/kg divided over 8-10 days	>12°C: 60 days 8–12°C: 60–180 days <8°C: >180 days	Not to be used on adult fish intended for slaughter
	Infections on parent fish	As pure compound (i.e. 0.75-1 kg pellets per 100 kg fish a day, 7-10 days)	>12°C: 60 days 8–12°C: 60–180 days <8°C: >180 days	Not registered for fish
	Bacterial gill infections, fin rot and experimental general treatment of fry and smolts	10 mg oxytetracycline hydrochloride per kg. i.p. 2 g oxytetracycline hydrochloride (eqv. 10 g soluble powder 20% per 10 litres of water) in 2 hours	>12°C: 60 days 8–12°C: 60–180 days <8°C: >180 days	Water needs to be oxygenated. Not registered for fish
Furazolidone	General bacterial infections Hexamitosis	750 mg/kg divided over 10 days	>12°C: 40 days 8–12°C: 40–90 days <8°C: >90 days	Possible carcinogenic effect. Should not be used if alternatives are available

FIG. 12.7 *continued*

THERAPEUTIC AGENTS IN NORWEGIAN SALMON FARMING				
Antibiotics and chemotherapeutics				
Drug	**Indication**	**Dosage**	**Withdrawal time**	**Remarks**
Erythromycin	To prevent vertical transfer of BKD	20 mg/kg i.p.	>9°C: 40 days <9°C: >80 days	Used on parent fish Not registered for fish
Tribrissen Vet. powder	General bacterial infections	75–100 mg powder/kg daily (eqv. 5 mg trimethoprim, 25 mg sulphadiazine/kg daily) for 5–7 days	>12°C: 40 days 8–12°C: 40–90 days <8°C: >90 days	Allergic reactions are reported due to inhalation of dust
Dihydrostreptomycin sulphate. Several products registered for veterinary use	Bacterial gill infections and fin rot in fry and smolts	0.2 g dihydrostreptomycin (or 0.8 ml procainebenzyl/ penicillin/ dihydrostreptomycin) per 10 litres of water in 2 hours Repeat 1–2 times with 2 days interval		Water must be oxygenated. Pure preparations or combinations with procaine benzyl penicillin

* 'Aqualets' (A. L. Labs, Oslo) is a novel delivery system which gives medication to fish inside a double core extruded bran and capsule rather than providing the medication in the feed or coated outside the feed pellets.

FIG. 12.7 Therapeutic agents used in Norwegian salmon farming. Source: Tonje Høy and Tor Einar Horsberg, *Fiskehelse* pp. 354–356 (1990).

spread to several rivers and fish farms. The major concern is related to the ability of the parasite to almost eradicate wild salmon populations. In farmed fish the disease is controlled by preventing contact with wild fish, combined with the use of formalin.

Tapeworm

Infections by *Eubothrium crassium* are effectively controlled using praziquantel *per os*.

Sea lice

Infestation by *Lepeophtheirus salmonis* is increasingly prevalent. The traditional treatment has been by use of dichlorvos or metriphonate. Several farmers have recently reported reduced efficacy of these chemicals, which may be due to a resistance developing against organophosphates. Treatment with hydrogen peroxide (which is preferable from an environmental point of view) is showing encouraging results.

Clinical Diagnosis

The approach to clinical diagnosis has to be a combination of clinical, macro- and microscopic findings with demonstration of the pathogens. Disease problems in fish are often multifactorial.

Records are very important on fish farms. The fish farmer should always be able to provide the veterinarian with detailed notes on the following:

- Delivery date for fish in each pen.
- Genetic origin for all fish.
- Vaccination history.
- Number of fish and average weight in each pen.
- Stocking density.
- Amount and type of feed given.
- Dates, type, and duration of medications.
- Pattern of mortality (mortality curves and death rates).

The normal diagnostic procedures used by the veterinarian on the fish farm are described in Chapter 5. The approach to diagnosing diseases in Norway varies from region to region: some veterinarians do most of the diagnostic work themselves, whereas others collect diseased fish and have the whole fish sent on ice to a diagnostic laboratory. Most need to co-operate with a diagnostic laboratory in order to demonstrate pathogens. The material selected should always be from individuals showing obvious signs of illness. The first-time diagnosis of notifiable diseases by a veterinarian always has to be verified by one of the official diagnostic laboratories of the Central Veterinary Laboratory.

Therapy

The Norwegian Act of 20 June 1964 No. 5, which states that only veterinarians can treat diseased animals and prescribe medicines, applies to the treatment of farmed fish at all stages of the life-cycle. It also covers the use of medicinal disinfectants and prophylactic treatment for fungi and ectoparasites. All medicines for farmed fish are distributed via pharmacies. The Health Directorate has given some feed mills permission to distribute certain types of medicated feed, but only if it has been prescribed by a veterinarian. By law, all importation and distribution of medicines is administered by the Norwegian Medicinal Depot (NMD). This monopolistic situation makes the sales figures very reliable.

All prescriptions of medicines for farmed fish must be presented on an authorised prescription form. The veterinarian is obliged to send copies of all issued prescriptions to the Fish Directorate, Division of Quality Control, once a week. Pharmacies and feed mills are also obliged to use the same authorised form when receiving prescriptions via telephone, and to send copies of any prescriptions to the same directorate monthly. Through this system the authorities are able to exercise extremely reliable control over the use of drugs in aquaculture.

Before a fish farmer may slaughter salmon intended for human consumption, he must obtain permission from the Fish Directorate. Such permission is only given if the withdrawal period for the last used drug has been exceeded. Through the authorised prescription system, the Fish Directorate can easily check the time and drug usage before they give permission to slaughter the fish.

Due to a lack of registered drugs for use in aquaculture in Norway, it was common to prescribe the 100% active pharmacological preparation of different drugs. This medicine was then combined with the feed by the fish farmer himself. As the availability of licensed medicated feed and pre-mixes has now increased, the prescription of pure substances is forbidden by the Health Directorate (Directive IK — 3/92 dated 31 January 92). In addition to this Directive, the Society of Veterinarians dealing with Fish Diseases (AVF) has agreed to use documented medicines only, according to their agreed code of practice.

Figure 12.7 shows the therapeutants most commonly used in Norwegian salmon farming.

Prevention of Disease

The use of medicines is necessary in the farming of animals but it must not detract from the importance of disease prevention through good husbandry. The prevention of disease has been and always will be one of the major tasks for Norwegian authorities, fish farmers and veterinarians. It is widely accepted that the prevention of diseases, rather than their treatment, gives great benefits both economically and environmentally.

Prevention may be specific or non-specific. Non-specific measures are those that improve the general constitution of the individual, either by enhancement of genetic resistance to diseases or by improvement of husbandry conditions. Specific prevention is mainly by vaccination.

Husbandry Conditions

Non-specific prevention of disease has been an object of great concern over the last few years. High stocking densities, inadequate feeding and failure to remove dead fish daily have optimised the growing conditions of micro-organisms and parasites. In addition, fish which are thus stressed become more susceptible to disease.

In Norway, it is recommended that the stocking density of Atlantic salmon should not exceed 15 kg/m^3. Since dead fish shed bacteria into the water and become a source of infective material for other fish, it is essential that dead fish are removed daily. New methods of removing dead fish, using net bags under the pens, have reduced the stress to the fish and also made the job practicable for the farmer. With these new methods there are no objections to removing dead fish daily.

Immunostimulants and Optimised Feed Compositions

Fish feed also contributes to well-being and resistance against disease. In addition to optimising the feed composition with regard to the traditional nutrients, a lot of new compositions with varying iron and fatty acid content have been developed. Non-specific immunostimulants, such as glucan, have also shown good impact on the general resistance to disease and it is expected that new products will be developed in the coming years. Research work in the field can tell us more about the needs of the fish and it should be borne in mind that fish populations on an optimal diet are less susceptible to disease than those given sub-optimal diets.

Genetic Resistance

Several investigations in Norway have shown that there is a genetic factor in resistance against several common diseases. The major problem in such studies is to measure the quality of the factors. One crucial question is whether those families of fish that are resistant to one disease will show resistance to other diseases, and whether the resistance is negatively correlated with other desirable properties.

Specific Prevention by Vaccination

One of the most successful preventive measures against diseases has been specific prevention by vaccination. The limitations of vaccination compared to non-specific methods is the limited number of diseases where effective vaccines have been developed. In Norway, vaccination of fish started in 1977 and the total volume of vaccines used had reached 75,000 l in 1991.

Vaccination can be by injection, immersion, bath or spray, or via the oral route. The efficacy of vaccination is influenced by the quality of the vaccine, the ability of the fish to develop immunity, and the conditions under which the fish are vaccinated. It produces very good protection against some diseases.

Vaccination should be avoided during smoltification and other stressful periods as the immune response will be reduced. It is obvious that the fish will be stressed during vaccination but this stress should be limited as much as possible. Diseased or medicated fish should *not* be vaccinated. Care should also be taken in farms with latent infections. Severe outbreaks of both furunculosis and vibriosis have been demonstrated in conjunction with vaccination.

It has been recommended that salmon are not vaccinated at water temperatures lower than 8°C. Recent investigations in Norway have demonstrated that vaccination against cold-water vibriosis is effective at lower temperatures (down to 4°C). Other investigations have shown that the secondary response, as demonstrated at revaccination, is less dependent on temperature. It is therefore supposed that revaccination may be carried out at lower temperatures than the primary immunisation. However, these results have not been documented in field trials.

Almost all smolts sold in Norway are vaccinated against vibriosis, cold-water vibriosis and furunculosis. This is because the buyer of the smolt will demand documentation on vaccination. The questions of which strategy to choose are discussed every year and several procedures are followed. It is not possible to set up one regimen as the only applicable one, as several regimens may give the same results. The important thing is to use a method that is recommended and documented as effective.

Most farmers have their smolts vaccinated during autumn against vibriosis and cold-water vibriosis. The size of the fish at this time makes the immersion method most suitable. The fish are then revaccinated by injection against vibriosis and cold-water vibriosis during the spring. In addition, the fish are vaccinated against furunculosis. The spring vaccination takes place in February, March and April and in good time before smoltification. The vaccines used are mainly combination. In choosing the right time for vaccination there is a need for compromise between the need for protection for as long as possible (encouraging late vaccination) and the need to start before smoltification occurs (encouraging early vaccination).

Following these regimens it is expected that the fish will have an acceptable protection against vibriosis, cold-water vibriosis and furunculosis during the first year in sea water. To improve protection against furunculosis during the second summer season, a booster is recommended. Such vaccination has been carried out using the injection method, but the size of the fish makes the application rather difficult and this has led to the development of oral vaccines. Such vaccines are not yet approved by the authorities but may be used as part of field trials. For fish staying in sea water for two winter seasons it would also be of use to boost protection against cold-water vibriosis.

Vaccination against yersiniosis is recommended only in those areas where the disease is recognised as a problem. Major outbreaks have been demonstrated in smolts shortly after introduction to sea water. Outbreaks have also been demonstrated in smolt farms. In such farms vaccination by immersion during the first year of life is recommended.

Side effects

As with all other handling of fish, vaccination can lead to undesired side effects. These could be due to properties of the vaccine or to the vaccination procedure. To minimise them, vaccination should be carried out under the following rules:

- Do not vaccinate fish during smoltification.
- Do not vaccinate diseased fish.
- Starve the fish for 48 hours before vaccination.
- Work as aseptically as possible.
- Be sure not to over-anaesthetise the fish.
- When using the injection method, be sure to apply the vaccine correctly.

To test a population, vaccinate a small number of fish and have them observed for a week before the rest of the population is vaccinated.

References

Gjedrem, T., Salte, R. and Gjøem, H. M. (1991) Genetic variation in susceptibility of Atlantic salmon to furunculosis. *Aquaculture* **97**, 1–6.
Gjedrem, T. (1986) *Fiskeoppdrett med framtid*, pp. 65–67. Landbruksforlaget, Oslo.
Poppe, T. T. (1990) *Fiskehelse*, pp.336–356. John Grieg Forlag, Bergen.

13

The Veterinary Approach to Salmon Farming in Scotland

TONY WALL

Scottish salmon farming has grown very quickly during the last 20 years but unfortunately the problems have kept pace with this increase in production. Fish farmers often have their stocks insured against loss from disease but this cover is only valid if good husbandry practices are followed, especially appropriate stocking densities and regular disease monitoring. Poor husbandry and management are often responsible for triggering off the relatively few diseases which have become common in the industry.

The best farms are managed by stockmen who appreciate the importance of sound farming practices and patient observation. For the visiting veterinarian, the difficulty might be in identifying the husbandry conditions that have initiated an outbreak of disease. Diagnosis and treatment are often quite straightforward but the underlying management problems need to be corrected as well. Thus it is important for the veterinarian to have a broad understanding of salmon farming systems and general fish husbandry.

Farming Systems

Fresh Water

Atlantic salmon eggs are stripped from farmed broodstock in fresh water, usually in November, and are incubated in the dark in specialised housing. There are two main methods of incubation. In the most satisfactory the eggs are spread out on trays, one or two eggs deep, with water flowing over them. This method is time-consuming as dead (white) eggs must be removed individually. In the second method the eggs are stored in jars, many layers deep, with water flowing up from the bottom of the jar. Removal of dead eggs from these jars is not possible and so the spread of fungus is controlled by the use of Malachite green, a chemical of questionable safety for the operator.

The time of the eggs hatching into alevins is dependent on the temperature of the circulating water. For Atlantic salmon this is 390–400 degree-days. To increase the rate of early hatching some units may heat the water up to 10–12°C. This higher temperature is often extended to include first feeding of the alevins, and can be combined with a recirculation facility to reduce heating costs. Raising water temperatures can increase the spread of fungal infection (*Saprolegnia* spp.) in the eggs and parasitic disease later on in the fish. The recirculation of the warmer water will be more likely to infect disease-free stock with water-borne pathogens from other sources in the hatchery. Any impairment in the water quality will be highlighted at these higher temperatures and special care must be taken to monitor oxygen, ammonia and suspended solids.

Early hatching and first feeding will increase the number of smolts ready for the sea in the following spring (15 months hence). These 1 year (S1) smolts, though smaller on sea entry than fish ready for the sea in 2 years time (S2 smolts), are less prone to fungal and parasitic conditions in fresh water and will make valuable space available for the following year's fish.

Most freshwater hatcheries rear their fish to smolt stage in circular tanks with a constant water flow. This capital intensive system maintains a more controlled environment than the alternative system using freshwater cages. These freshwater cages will produce low-cost smolts which adapt rapidly to similar seawater cages. Control of fungal and parasitic disease is more difficult in such cages, especially as wild fish can act as disease vectors.

Collection and removal of dead fish will be undertaken less frequently than in tanks.

Feeding systems in fresh water are usually automatic with a 'top-up' by hand twice a day. This combines small frequent feeds, necessary for the young fish, with careful observation at hand-feeding time.

In the spring, the presence of two generations of fish (smolts ready for the sea and the following year's newly hatched first feeders) may cause problems. These generations need to be kept quite separate. However increasing water temperatures, shortage of water and a large biomass of fish eating increasing amounts of food can cause serious depletion of oxygen levels, so that artificial aeration or oxygenation may be necessary at this critical time.

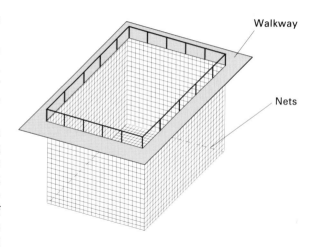

Sea Water

In Scotland smolts are transferred to the sea from late April to early June. When they are physiologically prepared for the change to the hyperosmotic environment of the sea water, they become longer and thinner and lose their parr markings, becoming silvery.

The following points must be considered when choosing a seawater cage site:

(a) Full salinity is desirable (33–35 parts per thousand) for maximum growth. Fresh water from nearby rivers may inhibit fish growth, increase the risk of parasites and cause temperature fluctuations.

(b) The site should be as deep as possible (at least 3 times the net depth at low water) to ensure an adequate dispersal of fish faeces and to guard against the extremes of temperature found in shallow waters.

(c) The site should be sheltered from the prevailing winds and within easy access of the shore.

(d) To avoid fish damage by abrasion against the nets, the maximum current should be 0.6 m/sec.

Most salmon are grown in pens or cages, in groups of 8–20, at the sea-site. The cages are usually steel 12 or 15 m square with nets suspended below the walkways up to 12 m deep. The nets are weighted to ensure the sides are vertical, giving maximum volume. This is rarely achieved and often the nets are folded and distorted into a cone

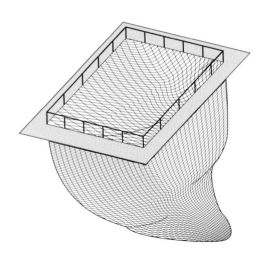

FIG. 13.1 (a) Ideal but rarely achieved net shape. (b) Distorted net shape commonly seen, especially with high currents, and heavily fouled nets.

shape by tidal flow and local currents (Fig. 13.1). This factor is important when calculating stocking densities, as the volume available to the fish will be much reduced, especially with heavily fouled nets. Predator nets hung from the outside of the walkways and over the top of the water from the handrails will reduce seal and bird attacks respectively.

Pumping sea water ashore to land-based tanks is an alternative to floating pen groups, although it is not a common system. It is probably less viable

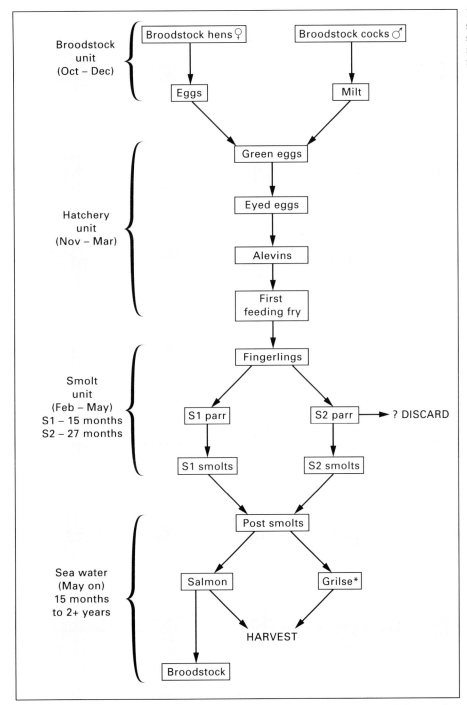

FIG. 13.2 Diagram to represent life-cycle of farmed salmon. * Grilse are sexually mature salmon after 12–15 months in the sea.

due to the high cost of pumping and the capital cost of the unit but it does have the advantage that the fish can be more closely observed and controlled.

Most salmon will be harvested after 15 months (grilse) or else after 2 years in the sea, according to the desired harvesting programme. The fish farmer generally receives the best price for fish weighing 3–5 kg. Meanwhile the broodstock, selected from S1 stocks for fast growth, disease-free status and slow sexual maturation (to reduce the grilse ratio), will be transferred from the sea

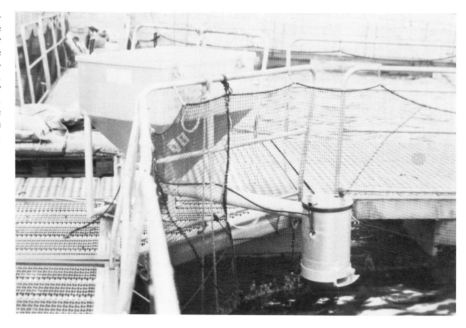

FIG. 13.3 A modern automatic feeding system. The pellets are propelled over the cage area but they are not necessarily evenly distributed over the surface. Consequently the bigger fish get most of the food. This system should only be an accessory — the main feeding being done by hand.

water to a freshwater broodstock unit to await stripping in late autumn. These brookstock will have spent at least two years in the sea (Fig. 13.2).

General Husbandry

Atlantic salmon require a high level of environmental and disease control for successful farming and this will be reflected in the quality of the husbandry.

Feeding

Most salmon feed is manufactured dry pellets, though some sea farms on Shetland feed freshly prepared wet diets. It is important in the freshwater period to offer feed little and often. Automatic feeders are designed for this purpose but hand-feeding is still essential twice a day which allows careful observation of the stocks and a check that excess food is not accumulating on the bottom.

In the sea, hand-feeding 2 or 3 times a day is the most efficient method of delivering the feed to all the fish at the same time and reducing competition for food. This is just not possible on some large seawater units and so farmers will rely to some extent on automatic feeders (Fig. 13.3). This can increase the chance of bimodality of fish size because of uneven distribution of food, with

the result that a feeding hierarchy is established and the smaller fish are underfed. The farmer then has to grade the fish for size, which is stressful and may initiate a disease outbreak.

Feeding to a strict ration and not to appetite is important in the sea, to reduce the chance of pancreas disease and avoid wasting expensive feed. Reduced feeding levels or even withholding food may be necessary during very high summer temperatures to reduce the biological oxygen demand (BOD) caused by the high levels of food and faeces. Starvation can also be useful to reduce the BOD before a stressful procedure such as grading, sea-lice treatment or even before the introduction of a medicated feed at the start of a disease outbreak.

Water

Special care must be taken in the hatchery and smolt unit to measure temperature, dissolved oxygen and pH daily. In Scotland pH can fall dramatically due to snow melts and spates (high river levels from increased rainfall). Oxygen demand will be at its highest in the freshwater smolt unit in the spring, prior to smolt transfer to the sea, due to high biomass and rising temperatures. At this time spates introducing increased suspended sediment can adversely affect respiration of eggs and young fish. Where the waters flow over peat land, the organic matter they collect can exert an oxygen demand and further increase respiratory distress.

In the sea, with less extreme temperatures and with the flushing effects of tides and currents, water quality will usually deteriorate only if husbandry is poor — for example, heavily fouled nets causing poor water exchange, high oxygen requirements from the organic material on the nets, high stocking levels and overfeeding. Treating nets with an anti-fouling product is expensive but may be worthwhile, especially in post-smolts during their first summer in the sea, to avoid net changing and the consequential crowding of fish.

Stocking Levels

These are central to good husbandry and will be determined to some extent by water quality, maximum water temperatures and feeding rates. The presence of endemic disease may necessitate a lower stocking density. In the smolt unit, densities should not be higher than 20 kg/m^3. Paradoxically at significantly lower levels (less than 10 kg/m^3) there is an increase in territorial behaviour which is suppressed at the higher stocking densities. This territorial behaviour can lead to fighting and fin nipping often associated with dorsal fin damage.

Stocking densities in the sea should never be more than 15 kg/m^3 — indeed this is often a condition of any insurance cover. This may need to be reduced further on a site with endemic furunculosis, high seawater temperatures and a rapid build up of a sea-lice burden. Due to increased competition for food, size variation will be greater in these more highly stocked cages which leads to stressful grading procedures.

Grading

Fish are graded to ensure even growth and to avoid aggression. In fresh water this can be achieved with little stress and trauma. It may be necessary to grade every 3 months in the smolt unit to ensure that each tank contains fish of a uniform size. When competition from larger siblings is reduced, middle-sized fish will have the best chance of achieving S1 status rather than

lingering to become S2 smolts. The smaller grade can then be discarded to allow more room for the bigger, faster growing fish.

Handling and grading fish in the sea is more stressful. For this procedure net volume is usually reduced and the fish are crowded in a part of the net to facilitate handling, which also increases the danger of external abrasion. Net changing, grilse grading, sea-lice treatments or moving fish, are all potentially hazardous and can trigger off an outbreak of bacterial or pancreas disease.

Mortality Removal

Removal of dead and moribund fish and investigation of the cause of death is vital to any disease monitoring. Dead fish are a source of infection and should be removed at least weekly or preferably daily during disease outbreaks.

Removal of dead fish from the sea cages is fraught with difficulties and as yet no satisfactory method has been devised. Collection by divers is often the best but it is expensive and unlikely to be used often enough on most farms. 'Socks' sewn into the bottom of the net will collect some of the dead fish but small smolts may not roll into them (Fig. 13.4). If large numbers are involved, the sock may be too small. A modified system using a cone that fits into the mortality sock has now been developed, but most of the same disadvantages are still present. Lifting the nets to remove dead fish is very labour intensive and can stress the fish.

An increase in the mortality level is often the

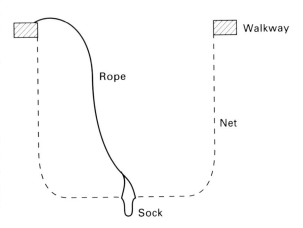

FIG. 13.4 Cage showing mortality sock for collection of dead fish. The sock is brought to the surface by the rope in the cage.

first indication of a potential problem. Collection of dead fish needs to be more frequent during disease outbreaks and periods of high risk. All dead fish should be disposed of carefully to ensure they are not a danger to other fish stocks.

Site Rotation

Special attention must be paid to the rotation of sites and fallowing periods. Mixing year classes in the same pen group or siting groups in close proximity will lead to disease overlaps. In the sea-site, newly arrived smolts will have a reduced chance of survival if disease or lice are endemic in the older fish. The fallowing of whole sea lochs for up to 6 months is desirable and will often involve the co-operation of a number of fish farms.

Methods of Slaughter

In Scotland most fish are initially stunned with a blow on the head or narcotised with carbon dioxide in water. This preliminary action will vary depending on the requirements of the purchaser but should be both humane and hygienic. To satisfy the needs of the smoked fish industry, the majority of salmon are now exsanguinated by severing a gill arch after loss of consciousness. The incorrect disposal of this waste blood may lead to a recycling of disease.

Record Keeping

Record keeping is an essential part of the management of fish stocks. It should provide information regarding feeding, fish numbers and weights, mortalities, disease outbreaks and medication. Movements of fish on to the farm and their origin need to be noted. Water quality parameters (e.g. oxygen, pH, temperature and ammonia) should be noted regularly.

Stock Origin

Good husbandry will take into account the quality and disease status of any fish brought on to the farm. These fish should be the result of mating from an adequate number of broodstock to avoid inbreeding (a minimum of 40 males and 40 female fish). A strain of fish producing a low level of grilse (the term for salmon when they become sexually mature after 12–15 months in the sea) will be desirable as sexual maturity causes a decrease in the quality of the flesh. Salmon are always harvested before they reach sexual maturity to avoid the deleterious effects of the developing secondary sexual characteristics on the taste and appearance of the fish (e.g. dark skin, increase in muscle water, decrease in muscle protein). The production of sterile triploid female salmon (instead of the usual diploid condition) will overcome the maturation drawbacks but a number of other problems have arisen with these fish. Stress testing smolts for freedom from furunculosis (see diagnosis) and examination for parasites before seawater entry will give some confidence to the buyer. Certificates to show that stock are free from infectious pancreatic necrosis (IPN) and bacterial kidney disease (BKD) are usually required by hatchery and sea-site managers.

Notifiable Diseases

There are eight diseases in the UK which are notifiable under the Diseases of Fish Act 1937. Of these, only IPN, BKD and furunculosis are commonly seen in Atlantic salmon in Scotland. Whirling disease is mainly a condition of small rainbow trout in earth ponds and is not perceived as a threat to the Atlantic salmon industry. Movement orders are placed on farms known to be infected with IPN, BKD and whirling disease. This applies to furunculosis only if a clinical outbreak is discovered. In the case of ERM, no movement restrictions are imposed.

A movement order will be enforced for 30 days, restricting the movement of live fish, eggs or feed. It can be renewed for another 30 days if necessary in order to establish a diagnosis of the disease concerned. If the notifiable disease is confirmed, a designated area order (DAO) is placed on the farm or site. The DAO reinforces the restrictions on the movement of live fish and eggs from the site and these will only be lifted after a number of negative tests have been carried out or after a period of fallowing.

Major Diseases

The major diseases to which salmon are susceptible vary according to whether the stock is in fresh

FIG. 13.5 Aquatic diseases.

AQUATIC DISEASES		
Fresh water	**Fresh and sea water**	**Sea water**
Costia infection	Furunculosis	Lice infestations
Trichodina infection	IPN	Pancreas disease
White spot disease		Fading smolt syndrome
Fin rot	Myxobacterial skin infections	Vibriosis
Saprolegnia infection	BKD	Algal blooms
Bacterial gill disease	ERM	Tapeworms
Gas-bubble disease		
Sphaerospora infection		

or sea water (Fig. 13.5). The most common diseases seen in the freshwater period are due to ectoparasites, fin rot and saprolegnia fungus. Eggs are particularly susceptible to changes in water quality, especially temperatures over 13°C, high suspended solids and low pH. Vertical transmission of IPN and BKD organisms can occur with no effect on the egg.

Viral

Infectious pancreatic necrosis

The IPN virus can cause mortalities of up to 25% in yolk sac fry and first feeders, depending on the strain of virus present. Confirmation of the disease will lead to a restriction of movement order (made by the government on the farm to prevent the spread of disease) which can have serious consequences for a smolt unit hoping to sell fish.

Clinically affected fish may show spiral swimming, darkened skin, exophthalmos, haemorrhages in the caecal mass and mucous in the stomach and gut, but usually no signs are observed.

The use of recirculation systems in the hatchery can spread the disease to disease-free stock.

Smolts entering the sea can succumb in large numbers to this disease, but other causes (inadequate smoltification, transport and handling damage) must also be considered. The virus can often be isolated from healthy stock — especially its less pathogenic strains; indeed it appears to be ubiquitous in the sea. There is some evidence to suggest that IPN virus may lead to immunologically compromised fish which are susceptible to outbreaks of pancreas disease. The virus can be transmitted vertically via the sperm or egg or horizontally through the water.

Bacterial

Bacterial gill disease

BGD is associated with poor freshwater quality, especially the presence of uneaten rotting food, organic suspended solids and low oxygen levels. An irritation of the gill lamellae with an excess of mucous secretion leads to a secondary bacterial invasion of the gills — often of the *Chondrococcus* species

Fish with bacterial gill disease show respiratory distress, making exaggerated movements of the gill covers. Mucous and secondary fungal infections may be seen protruding from underneath the gill covers. Examination of the gills reveals them to be swollen and grey. Heavy losses can occur.

Bacterial kidney disease

BKD has been recorded on over 20 farms in Scotland. It is caused by the gram-positive bacteria *Renibacterium salmoninarum* and is transmitted through the eggs via water. It is a chronic disease causing a small persistent number of mortalities in the sea, although losses can be higher in freshwater parr.

The clinical signs are darkening of the skin, lethargy, exophthalmos, anorexia and ascites. White focal lesions are seen in the kidney at temperatures over 10°C. Below 10°C a diphtheritic membrane can be seen over the kidney and other abdominal organs.

Vibriosis

Infection caused by the ubiquitous gram-negative bacteria *Vibrio anguillarum* is usually secondary, initiated by surface damage, descaling or ulceration. The bacteria can often be cultured from open ulcers caused by predator damage, net descaling and rough handling, but it is rarely the primary cause of death. The feeding of contaminated trash-fish diets may cause an outbreak of vibriosis. The main clinical signs are lethargy, skin darkening, shallow bleeding ulcers and anaemia.

Furunculosis

The Gram-negative bacteria *Aeromonas salmonicida* is endemic on the majority of salmon farms in the sea. It is also present in the freshwater systems and in a large number of wild stock, but it generally poses a less serious problem in freshwater. This bacteraemic and haemmorrhagic condition can range from peracute infections to a chronic form. Fish may also be carriers.

Susceptibility to furunculosis is increased by high stocking densities, poor water quality and high temperatures. Concurrent diseases, especially lice infestation and external damage, will increase spread and mortality. In fresh water abraded fins can be a route of entry for the bacteria.

The clinical and post-mortem signs will vary depending on whether the condition is acute or chronic. Lethargic but well grown fish are often seen in the corners of cages (cf. in pancreas disease these lethargic fish are usually thin and wasted). Some skin swellings may be seen along the dorsum and flank and there may be a change in behaviour, with aberrant swimming patterns and a lack of shoaling. Appetite is often reduced, but not always. As this disease is most often seen at higher water temperatures, the metabolic rate and hence the appetite may be very good for the unaffected fish in the cage or tank and they appear to be feeding well.

Fish removed for post-mortem examination may show no gross pathological change in the per acute cases. In the acute stage only a few petechial haemorrhages may be seen in the pancreatic fat or on the musculature of the flank. In longer standing chronic infections, large haemorrhages are seen especially on the swim-bladder and other internal organs. The swim-bladder is often the organ to show the most consistent features of thickening and haemorrhage in the subacute to chronic form. In chronic cases, boils or furuncles appear as necrotic areas of muscle which may burst through the skin, releasing a thick bloodstained material. The posterior gut mucosa is often inflamed, and bloodstained faeces can be expressed from the anus.

It may be unrealistic to expect sea-sites to remain free from this condition but good farming practices can reduce more serious consequences. Freshwater systems should be able to eradicate the disease given a disease-free water source, as all the smolts will be removed to the sea at the same time in the spring. This will enable the next year class to be farmed entirely separately so that cross-infection can be avoided.

Myxobacterial skin infections

These are common in both freshwater and saltwater situations. Opportunistic invasion by these bacteria is seen when pre-existing lesions due to rough handling, over-crowding, fin damage, eroded snouts and predator damage are present. *Caligus* sea lice can cause sufficient skin damage to allow a secondary infection to occur. Large, shallow, uncovered tanks may lead to ultraviolet light damage around the dorsal fin. This typical saddleback lesion is usually associated with myxobacteria. Fish often appear grey and slightly fluffy from an excess of mucous (best seen when fish are still in the water).

Enteric redmouth

ERM has been seen in salmon although it is primarily a disease of trout. It causes haemorrhages and skin hyperaemia around the head and mouth. No severe mortalities have been recorded in sea water.

Fungal

Saprolegnia

Saprolegnia often infect eggs, alevins, parr and smolts in fresh water. Raised white lesions like cotton-wool are seen initially on the head and dorsum, later spreading over the body of the fish. Fin damage, trauma following handling or poor water conditions associated with overfeeding and overstocking may lead to infection from the motile

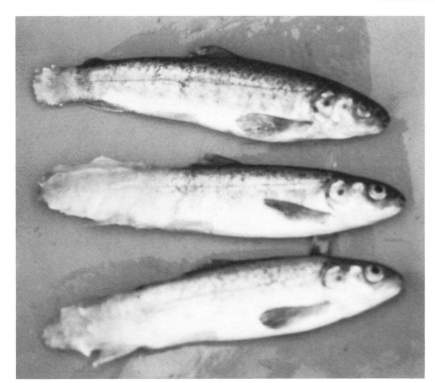

FIG. 13.6 Salmon parr showing complete erosion of the tail fin with secondary overgrowth of *Saprolegnia* fungus. As in all fin erosions, poor water quality and insanitary conditions are often initiating factors — although sexual precocity in the male can be responsible.

spores present in the water. Precocious male parr are particularly susceptible to *Saprolegnia* (Fig. 13.6). Eggs infected with *Saprolegnia* will be grey and fluffy and should be removed to avoid spread.

Sphaerospora *infection*

Salmon fry and fingerlings on a limited number of watercourses (especially fish of a Norwegian origin) become infected by spores released from wild fish, usually in the spring — consequently most of the mortalities occur in the early summer with rising water temperatures. Swollen grey kidneys are often seen in affected fish along with abdominal distension and gill pallor. As the spores are transmitted from wild stock, the eradication of the disease is not practicable. However, good stress-free husbandry will ensure that losses are minimal.

Parasitic

Costia (Icthyobodo necatrix)

Ichthyobodo necatrix is a common organism parasitising the gills and skin and causing gill

damage, skin irritation and scale loss. It is often seen at higher temperatures and the first signs can be a sudden increase in mortalities. Higher losses are more likely to occur in first feeders and fry where epizootic gill infestations can develop rapidly. These parasites are often found over body surfaces in older parr and smolts, causing insidious losses and sub-optimal performance. These older fish are sometimes seen 'flashing' (turning sideways and exposing the silvery flank). *Costia* can also be transferred to the sea and any parasitised fish must be treated, ideally 2 weeks before transfer to minimise stress.

Trichodina

These ciliated protozoal ectoparasites can cause severe damage in both fresh and sea water. The organism parasitises the gills and skin, causing irritation and scale loss, and can result in high mortalities. It will occur in the same environmental conditions as *Costia*, from which it can be differentiated only by microscopic examination.

Fɪɢ. 13.7 (a) Ventral posterior aspect of salmon
showing infestation of
marine lice *Lepeophthierus
salmonis*. Large numbers
of lice are common in this
area but will rarely cause
ulceration. (b) Areas of skin
and muscle erosion on a 700
g post-smolt in the sea caused
by infestation of the salmon
louse *Lepeophthierus salmonis*. The large ulcerated
area will kill this fish due
to failure to osmoregulate.
Arguably the most impor-
tant condition affecting
salmon in the sea, it has
profound welfare implica-
tions due to the extensive
superficial damage to the
fish and the chronic nature
of the condition.

(a)

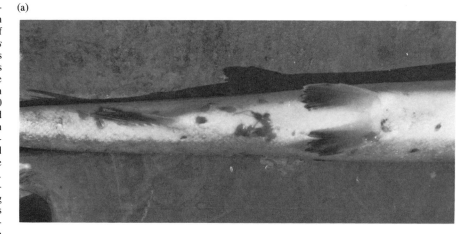

(b)

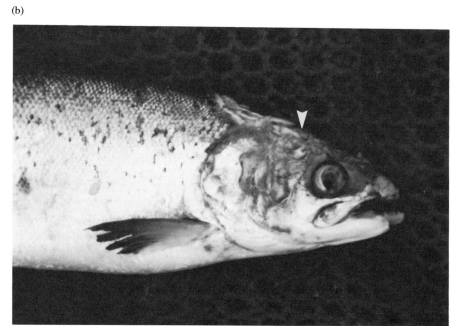

White spot

A disease caused by the ciliated protozoa
Ichthyophthirius multifiliis is sometimes seen in
fresh water on young salmon, causing the typical
raised white spot up to 1 mm in diameter. Skin
damage may be severe, with rupture of the skin.
Heavily infested fish are a dirty-grey colour.
Osmoregulatory failure can lead to death.

Most ectoparasites will be seen in conditions of
low water flushing, which generally induces poor
water quality parameters.

Lice infestation

This is arguably the most important clinical
condition seen in salmon in sea water. The
stressful nature of this parasite on the fish can
initiate other disease conditions.

Lice infestation caused by the salmon louse
Lepeophtheirus salmonis will remove mucous and
skin, especially along the dorsum, gill covers and
anal fin where most of the motile adult and pre-
adult lice are seen. The thinner scale-free skin at
the back of the head may become ulcerated (Figs

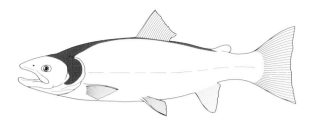

FIG. 13.8 Adult lice distribution over surface of salmon. Darker shaded areas are those most heavily parasitised. Although a large number of adult lice are seen anterior to the anal fin, they rarely cause ulceration similar to that seen on the head.

13.7 a, b, 13.8). Infections from other water-borne pathogens and osmoregulatory failure will reduce the chances of survival for severely damaged fish. Less severely affected fish will show a grey 'collar' over the head and gill covers. The smaller immature stages of the louse are found on the ventral abdomen and flanks; they are non-motile and vary in size from a tiny pinhead to 3 mm. These juvenile stages do not cause the same damage as the older lice. *Lepeophtheirus salmonis* spend most of their life-cycle on the salmon with only a brief free-swimming nauplius stage.

Caligus elongatus is the other species which affects Scottish salmon in the sea. These lice can move from wild salmon and other species to farmed salmon at any stage of the life-cycle and can quickly increase to a severe infestation, which makes the control of *Caligus* species more difficult. The effects of *Caligus* infestation are less severe than *Lepeophtheirus*, the latter producing the large areas of skin ulceration. However, large amounts of mucous production, myxobacterial infections and intense irritation are common.

Adult *Caligus* lice are about half the size of the adult *Lepeophtheirus* and to the naked eye may be confused with the pre-adult *Lepeophtheirus*. By their irritation, both types of lice cause the fish to jump constantly and eat less, predisposing them to other diseases such as furunculosis and pancreas disease (Fig. 13.9a). Moribund fish with chronic wasting diseases or blind fish can be expected to have high lice burdens.

Tapeworms

These parasites are an increasing problem on some sea sites in Scotland. The adult tapeworm *Eubothrium* spp. is found in the anterior intestine and pyloric caecae of salmon at all stages of their growth. The intermediate host is a copepod which can occur in fresh or sea water. Thus the parasite can be transferred from fresh water or the cycle may be completed in the sea. There is no clear evidence of a decrease in growth in those fish affected, nor can these worms infect man, but it may be necessary to treat the fish because of their unsightly appearance at gutting.

Miscellaneous

Gas-bubble disease

This is seen in freshwater systems using bore-hole water or heated recirculating systems. Super-saturated nitrogen or oxygen will cause gas emboli affecting eyes, gills, skin and brain, mainly in alevins. Sometimes tiny bubbles can be seen around the eyes of these fish. Emboli behind the eye will produce exophthalmos. If this condition is present, a silver sheen of gas bubbles will form on the skin of a hand placed in the supersaturated water.

Fin rot

Endemic in most smolt units, this disease is easily seen on the dorsal fin when observing fish in a tank. The fin may have just an excess covering of grey mucous but in more severe cases the whole fin is eroded, leaving a reddened ulcerated stripe. This type of angry open lesion can be associated with *Aeromonas salmonicida* infection (furunculosis) and culture from this type of lesion may yield the organism. Fin rot can also affect the other fins, especially the pectoral and tail fins. In these cases broken fin rays are common and the whole fin has a ragged appearance. Secondary myxobacterial and fungal infections can develop on the previously damaged fin. Secondary fungal overlay (so-called peduncle disease) is typically seen on the tail, especially in precocious male parr.

The causes of fin rot are varied. Stocking densities below 10 kg/m^3 can cause an increase in aggression and fin nipping. Overstocking, which tends to decrease water quality, can lead to fin damage. Roughened tanks and excessive handling may abrade the pectoral and tail fins. The problems are also exacerbated in freshwater tanks by conditions of high light intensity where tanks cast dark

FIG. 13.9 (a) Lateral view of head of salmon affected with pancreas disease. Note large numbers of lice over the gill covers which will be difficult to control even with organophosphorus treatment. This fish has an anterior subcapsular cataract often seen in salmon with pancreas disease. This type of cataract can be seen in salmon where there is a failure to osmoregulate. (b) Salmon smolt removed from sea cages alive in December. This fish had pancreas disease and was one of the hundreds in the cage corners near the surface. Note the advanced emaciation. The ragged fins and areas of descaling are the result of net abrasion due to the fish's weakened state.

(a)

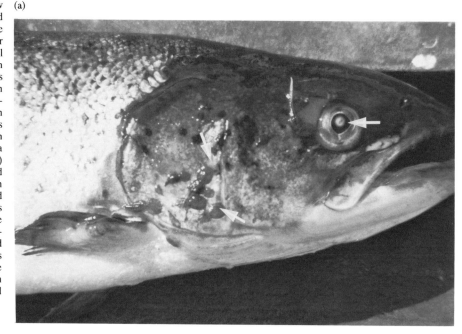

(b)

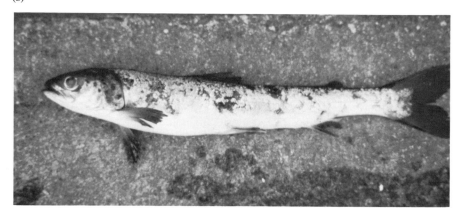

shadows on the fish instead of even, subdued lighting.

Eye damage

Eye damage and loss of globe is commonly caused in fingerlings by cannibalism from other fish. It is seen in early summer as the temperature rises and the fish are getting hungrier. It will be necessary to reduce light intensity and increase the amount of food.

Pancreas disease

Degeneration of the exocrine pancreas tissue causes a wasting condition of farmed salmon. This

disease has been experimentally transmitted in the laboratory but so far no infective agent has been identified. The occurrence of the disease spreading along a group of cages would suggest that cage-to-cage transmission is possible. It is often related to changes in management and stress, e.g. increase in pellet size of feed after a period of starvation, or grading and handling the fish.

It can affect any age of fish in the sea. The pattern of disease is quite variable — in some cases all the fish in a cage can refuse feed at the same time and this may be accompanied by a sudden increase in mortality. More usually there are increasing numbers of thin, anorexic fish found in the corners of the cages (Fig. 13.9b). These lethargic fish will often attempt to feed but will spit out the pellet. There are often large numbers of lice on these fish which can be quite resistant to the usual treatment, acting as a source of re-infection for the other fish. At this stage, long yellow faecal casts may be seen floating in the water or attached to the anus of some affected fish.

Mortality rates are quite variable and many of these thin, lethargic fish recover if graded off from their hungrier neighbours and fed frequently on small sized pellets. Gross post-mortem changes are few. A slight concavity at the ventral aspect of the flank may indicate a lack of food in the gut. In the chronic form there is an absence of any abdominal fat. Histopathology of the pancreatic tissue is essential for confirmation of the diagnosis.

Fading smolt syndrome

This condition has become increasingly important over the last few years. Smolts that have been in the sea for 2–3 months suddenly stop eating, become emaciated and die. It is more common in bigger, fat smolts and some evidence would suggest that it might be initiated by cold water in the hatchery prior to sea transfer. These fish, although having the morphological appearance of smolts, may not be physiologically prepared for the sea. This theory is supported by the fact that these fish will recover if they are transferred back to fresh water. The condition has encouraged some hatchery managers to grow smolts which are lean and fit at transfer time.

The syndrome is different from 'pin-heads', which are fish that have never adapted or fed in sea water and will die during the first weeks of transfer.

Algal blooms

Catastrophic fish kills can be caused by the sudden increases in algae which can occur in freshwater cage systems and are often attributed to overfeeding, with an increased level of nitrogen and phosphorus in the water. In sea water, high salinities and long periods of sunshine can cause an increase in algal numbers. The algae can kill fish by the mechanical effect on the gills, by the release of toxins in the water or by exerting

biological oxygen demands as conditions cease to be suitable and large numbers of the algae die off.

Handling, net changing and sea-lice treatments

These routines frequently precipitate mortalities in the sea. All the procedures involve crowding the fish with the risk of trapping them in folds of the net. The sudden effect of shallowing a net which may usually be over 10 m deep can be very stressful to the fish — especially on a bright sunny day. Widespread panic and burrowing may lead to suffocation, the skin becoming so damaged and with such massive scale loss that osmoregulatory failure may result. Even small abrasions will be routes of entry for bacteria such as *Aeromonas* and *Vibrio* spp. Sea-lice treatments using the organophosphorus dichlorvos may predispose to this sudden panic reaction, often resulting in large fish kills.

Clinical Diagnosis

The order in which diagnostic tests should be performed is shown in Fig. 13.10. The initial

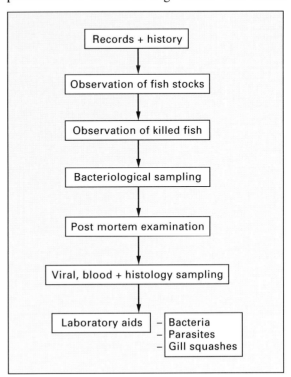

FIG. 13.10 Flow chart showing sequence of events leading to diagnosis.

RECORDS AND HISTORY	
Numbers and Weight of Fish	Are the fish growing quickly or slowly? (This will affect the stocking densitites)
	How often and when were they last weighed?
Stocking Densitites	
Mortality Numbers	Increasing or decreasing?
	What is the frequency of dead removal?
Sick and moribund fish	Have these been seen?
	For how long?
Behaviour	Are the fish behaving normally, (e.g. swimming, shoaling, stacking in the water column, not crowding in corners?)
Water	Check the following parameters over the last month
	Temperatures
	Oxygen levels
	pH
	Salinities
Weather Conditions	Have there been any of the following?
	Spates (will affect suspended solids and pH)
	Snow (melt will affect pH)
	Storms (can cause net distortion and fish damage)
Handling	Grading?
	Use of fish pumps?
	Net changing?
Feeding	Date of manufacture of feed?
	Type of feed. (High energy diets can cause fatty livers)
	Pellet size?
	When was the pellet size changed? (Sudden increase in pellet size may initiate an outbreak of pancreas disease)
	Frequency of feeding:
	manual?
	automatic?
	Food conversion rate? (Will be depressed with chronic parasitism or stress)
Diseases	History?
	Bacterial sensitivities? (Change in sensitivity may denote a new focus of infection rather than a renewed outbreak of an existing one)
	Concurrent diseases and treatments?
Stock Origin	From which hatchery or broodstock?
	Was the disease status checked before purchase?
Fish Type	Triploids are slower growing and more susceptible to cataracts and sea-lice treatments.
	Some Norwegian strains are more susceptible to pancreas disease or *Sphaerospora* infection.
Site	When was the site last fallowed?
	For how long?
	What is the proximity of other farms and what is their disease status? (Some bacteria can survive for over 30 days in sea-water — especially in dead fish — and may travel many miles by tides and currents in that time.)
Wild Fish	Is there contact with farmed stock?
	What is the disease status of the wild stock? (Herring and mackerel can carry large numbers of *Caligus* lice. Wild salmon are often carriers of furunculosis)
Divers	Do the divers at mortality collection report any unusual behaviour, e.g. lethargy, abnormal swimming, crowding on the bottom?

FIG. 13.11 Records and history.

impression of the farm, and the stockman's history and opinion of the problems are very important. Keep your hands in your pockets and start by asking lots of questions! (Fig. 13.11.)

Observation of Fish Stocks

Examination of freshwater hatchery and smolt unit fish is usually easy (Fig. 13.12). Alevin examination can be achieved by sucking them into a glass tube. Fish in cages can be more difficult to see, especially on stormy days and with cloudy water; polaroid glasses may be helpful. Fish will take time to return to normal behaviour after they have been disturbed, so be patient.

Examination of Killed Fish (Diseased and Healthy) (Fig. 13.13)

An overdose of benzocaine or tricaine methane-sulphonate (MS222) anaesthetic is the most

OBSERVATION OF FISH STOCKS	
Are fish well grown or thin?	Are they of mixed sizes?
	Consider metabolic problems such as pancreas disease, chronic parasitism and faulty feeding
Discoloured or abnormally shaped yolk sacs	Consider faulty first feeding, poor substrate for the alevins, overcrowding or water quality
Shoaling and stacking in the water column	Fish should be well distributed in the water volume
	Stress such as handling and predator attacks will cause loss of normal shoaling pattern
	Furunculosis may often be suspected early in a clinical outbreak of aberrant swimming patterns
	Consider the lighting/shading — can lead to fish crowding and only partial use of water volume
	Are the fish crowding round the water inlet? Consider lack of oxygen
	Are the fish crowding round the automatic feeders? May be too hungry
	Are fish being swept towards the central outflow? Consider weakened fish or too fast water-flows. Fish should be able to maintain their position in the tank
Surface/skin changes	Abrasion, ulceration, ragged fins, fin rot?
	Lice damage?
	Predator damage?
	Evidence of fungal infections in freshwater systems?
	Circular pox lesions?
Blind fish	Dark, moribund non-feeding fish which swim slowly on the surface and in corners
	Do not confuse with pancreas disease: fish can show similar behaviour but are not blind
Flashing	Spend time observing freshwater stocks to determine this
Feeding	Are all the fish feeding? Vigorously?
	Are any spitting out food?
	Is distribution adequate to ensure all fish get well fed?
	Is the food fresh and stored properly?
	Overfeeding can lead to environmental water problems and fatty livers
	Sexually maturing fish become less inclined to feed

FIG. 13.12 Observation of fish stocks.

humane method of killing small groups of fish without damaging any organs. However, it may depress some ectoparasite activity (e.g. *Costia* and *Trichodina*) making diagnosis more difficult, in which case stunning by a blow on the head will be more satisfactory.

Bacteriological Sampling

Take bacteriological samples before detailed post-mortem examination, to avoid contamination.

Sampling for suspected bacterial conditions will be mainly from the kidney, skin lesions (including abscesses and ulcerative dorsal fin lesions), heart blood and rectal mucosa. The kidney is the organ that will most consistently yield any suspected pathogens.

The samples should be taken from moribund, newly killed fish (Fig. 13.16). If only dead fish are available, the suspected pathogens may still be grown but will probably be heavily contaminated.

Post-mortem Examination

- Has the fish been *feeding*? Is there food in the stomach? Faeces in the rectum? Yellow mucosal castes of dead cells in the hind-gut are indicative of not feeding.
- Note any *peritoneal fluid*. This may be excessive in amount (e.g. in BKD) or it may be blood-stained (e.g. in furunculosis).
- Is *abdominal and pancreatic fat* present? This may help to establish if the condition is chronic or acute.
- Note any petechial or larger *haemorrhages* — often seen on liver, flank, pancreatic fat and swim-bladder. Reddening of the mucosa of the terminal rectum is common in bacterial diseases. The *colour of the liver* can be misleading. Light-coloured livers are not uncommon in healthy farmed fish. The *colour of the flesh* will depend on whether the pigment, astaxanthin, is incorporated into the diet.
- *Heart examination* may reveal enlargement or even rupture — possibly associated with pancreas disease or septicaemia.
- *Swim-bladder* The size of this organ is quite variable although it may be grossly enlarged causing abdominal distension and swimming abnormalities. More usual diseases of the swim-bladder are a thickening of the wall and haemorrhages, often due to chronic bacterial infection.

EXAMINATION OF DEAD FISH	
Shape	Is there any spinal deformity?
	Jaw deformity? (Common in triploids)
	Thin body and big head (pinhead)? (May not be feeding but note that triploid fish are longer and leaner than their diploid counterparts)
	Abdominal distension/ascites — consider BKD, PKD, exophiala
Fins	Look for evidence of fin rot, abrasion, rough handling and erythematous, ulcerated dorsal fins
	Missing or damaged pectoral fins can be associated with water-flow and quality as well as tank shape
Gills	Should be a deep pink/red colour. Note any gross overlay of fungus or mucous — may indicate a water problem
	Haemorrhages on the gills may be caused by a septicaemia or rough handling prior to death
	Small discrete nodules on the gills may be the glochidia, of freshwater mussels
	Incomplete gill covers are related to overstocking at the alevin stage
Skin	Note any ulceration or scale loss. Fish dying from any cause will frequently lose scales, leading to skin ulceration, from rolling around on the net or tank bottom. (Fig. 13.14). Histological examination of the margins of these lesions will reveal no inflammatory response
	Skin swellings — boils/furuncles
	— haematomas often seen associated with damage
	Skin darkening — can be a generalised reaction to stress, disease or blindness
	Note fungal infections or saddleback disease
	Assess lice burden on seawater salmon. Three or four adult *Lepeophtheirus* on a 50g smolt is cause for concern, whereas a 2 kg salmon may have 5 times that burden without undue consequences
	Nose damage can result from handling and lice treatments
	Predator damage — seal bites will cause large deep V-shaped lesions, usually on the lower flanks (Fig. 13.15)
	Damage from diving birds may be a penetrating stab wound or a bilateral area of scale loss where the fish has been squeezed by the beak
Eyes	Corneal oedema and ulceration may occur after rough handling. The proximity of the spherical fish lens to the cornea can result in secondary cataract following corneal abrasion
	The lens of the fish will normally go cloudy due to post-mortem change after a few hours at ambient temperature
	This change is much slower in fish stored on ice
	Some wrasse species, present in cages to reduce lice burdens, may cause eye damage to the salmon
	Note any exophthalmos possibly caused by a septicaemia, IPN or gas-bubble disease. Iris haemorrhage at the irido-corneal margin may be caused by rough handling before death or erythrocyte fragility. Phthisis bulbi may be the consequence of a bacterial endophthalmitis or penetrating corneal injury
Bacteriological sampling	Take bacteriological samples before detailed post-mortem examination, to avoid contamination
	Sampling for suspected bacterial conditions will be mainly from the kidney, skin lesions (including abscesses and ulcerative dorsal fin lesions), heart blood and rectal mucosa. The kidney is the organ that will most consistently yield any suspected pathogens
	The samples should be taken from moribund, newly killed fish (Fig. 13.16). If only dead fish are available, the suspected pathogens may still be grown but will probably be heavily contaminated

Fig. 13.13 Examination of dead fish.

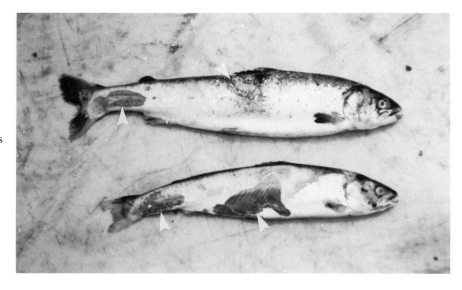

Fig. 13.14 Dead post-smolts recovered from the bottom of the cages. In these cases the scale and skin loss (arrows) due to abrasion on the net bottom is an agonal change and no inflammatory process is involved. *Vibrio* organisms are ubiquitous in the marine environment and may sometimes be isolated from these areas.

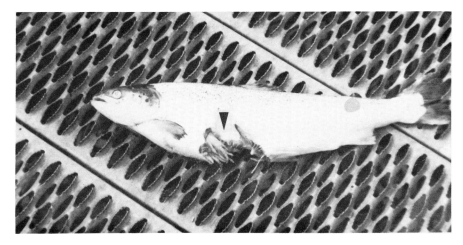

FIG. 13.15 Seal bite (arrow) in a 1 kg grower. As well as the damage inflicted by the bite, these predators can cause considerable stress and trigger off other disease conditions.

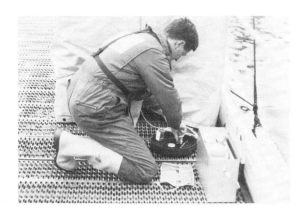

FIG. 13.16 It is necessary to take samples for histology and bacteriology on the sea cage site in newly-killed fish. The task is easy in good weather!

- *Kidney* should be dark coloured and concave. Small paired whitish spots on the surface of the kidney are normal; they are the Corpuscles of Stannius. Note any grey, swollen convex kidneys (possibly due to PKD or BKD), discrete greyish swollen lesions (possibly BKD, exophiala), diphtheritic membrances over the kidney and other organs (possibly BKD) and haemorrhages (septicaemias).
- Note any *tapeworms* in the abdominal cavity or gut.
- Enlargement of the *spleen* can occur in furunculosis and BKD. The colour is cherry red with furunculosis and dark red with BKD.

Other Sampling

Virus isolation. Usually involves kidney samples or ovarian fluid (from broodstock) placed in clean, dry universal containers without preservative. Samples should be kept on ice to arrive at the laboratory within 24 hours.

Blood sampling. This can be undertaken in anaesthetised fish or immediately after stunning. Blood can be withdrawn into a syringe from the heart or the caudal vein between the anus and tail. The use of vacuum blood collection methods will often collapse the blood vessel in a small fish.

Blood smears. These can be obtained by cutting off the tail in a very small fish, previously anaesthetised or killed. These procedures must be carried out humanely.

Histology samples. Take routinely in the majority of cases. These should only come from moribund or healthy fish which have been killed within the previous 30 minutes — not dead ones.

Preserved samples should be less than 5 mm in any direction. The easiest obtainable preservative will be 10% buffered formal saline. If none is available, use 9 parts of full salinity sea water and one part formaldehyde 40%.

Samples routinely taken will be gill, kidney, liver, muscle, heart, spleen. Other organs will be preserved and examined as necessary. In very small fish, open the abdomen and preserve the whole fish. Kidney samples can be collected in small fish by cutting a 'steak' — including muscle and skin.

Basic Laboratory Aids for the Veterinary Practitioner

It is advisable to plate out from the target organ directly onto a tryptone soy agar plate (TSA). Agar paddles in bottles which can be incorporated with sugars for selective fermentation are an aid to the diagnosis of suspected bacteria (Fig. 13.17).

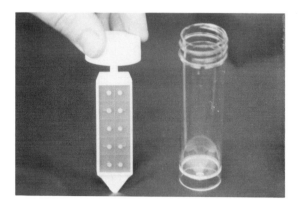

FIG. 13.17 These agar paddles with sugars for selective fermentation can be useful in identifying bacteria, especially *Aeromonas salmonicida*. They can also be used as transport media as they are easier than agar plates to keep uncontaminated. (Permission granted by Bionor.)

Swabs in charcoal transport media should be avoided — they seem to decrease the viability of some organisms when they are subsequently plated out. An ordinary swab without transport media will give better results if plated out on the same day before it dries out.

Incubate any plates at 20–22°C. If an incubator designed for growing mammalian bacteria is used, the temperature may not become low enough during the summer. In this case grow the bacteria on a bench top in a warm room.

The most commonly grown bacteria will be *Aeromonas salmonicida*, which usually produces a brown pigment in the agar. Occasionally strains can be encountered that do not produce the brown pigment. Some strains can take up to five days to produce colonies. The latex agglutination test is an easy useful indication of the presence of *A. salmonicida* (Fig. 13.18).

Sensitivity discs are available including the commonly used antibacterials — oxytetracycline, oxolinic acid, potentiated sulphonamide and amoxycillin.

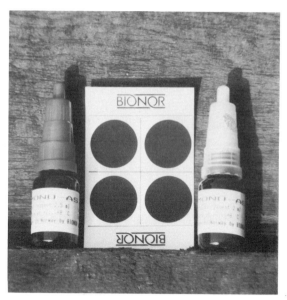

FIG. 13.18 Latex agglutination test for *Aeromonas salmonicida*. (Permission granted by Bionor.)

The intensive nature of salmon aquaculture leaves little room for second chances if the laboratory results are less than perfect. If possible, the above methods should be performed in parallel with those at a more specialist laboratory for confirmation of the results.

Parasite checks. Checks must be done regularly in fresh water, especially during periods of elevated water temperatures, at the first signs of flashing or an increase in mortalities. It will be necessary to check alevins and fry every week during the summer. Samples should be taken from sick fish, and some healthy controls should also be sacrificed for sampling.

A superficial scraping from a freshly killed fish along the dorsum and over the gills will be sufficient to detect any parasites present. Leaving the prepared slide of mucus and a drop of water to warm up for a minute or so will improve the motility of some of the parasites and make detection easier.

To make lice counts on seawater salmon, pick off the lice with forceps, or scrape them off a killed fish with a wooden spatula. They can be preserved in 10% buffered formal saline for later investigation. With the use of a hand-lens, they can be split into age groups and sexes to evaluate the optimum time for treatment.

Gill squashes. Useful in diagnosing some gill disease, especially bacterial gill disease and parasites. It can be helpful in estimating the amount of mucus, bacteria and gill debris but it is not a useful method for detailed examination of gill structure. A small piece of gill without the arch is placed on a slide with a drop of water. The structures are teased out and a cover-slip is placed over the specimen.

Stress Testing

To ensure that smolts are free from furunculosis on leaving the hatchery, a stress test can be carried out which will reveal the carrier state if present. Isolate and inject a number of smolts with a steroid (usually prednisolone) and then gradually increase the water temperature to 18–20°C over 10 days. The fish are killed at the end of 2 weeks from the start of the trial and sampled bacteriologically for evidence of furunculosis.

In practice, mortalities due to *A. salmonicida* will be seen before the end of the trial if the disease is present. As only a proportion of the population is used in this trial, it can do no more than act as a guide to the presence of furunculosis. However, it can also give valuable information regarding the presence of other diseases which may appear following the administration of the immunosupressive drug.

Therapy

The veterinarian responsible for prescribing medications for fish needs to be aware of the legislation governing their use. Practically speaking, the use of such medication is restricted to those compounds for which the regional water purification board will grant a licence — the so-called Water Discharge Consents. It will matter little that the veterinarian may wish to prescribe a specific drug or chemical: if there is no water discharge consent for that compound, then it cannot be used. It is the responsibility of the farmer to ensure that any drug used has a water discharge consent but contact between the veterinarian and the purification board can help to resolve any conflicts of interest.

The licensed products that are available for use in salmon are few — four antibacterials and one pesticide. These compounds have withdrawal periods relating to time and water temperature (e.g. 400 degree-days can be either 40 days at 10°C or 100 days at 4°C). The use of unlicensed products or licensed products used outside the data sheet recommendations will automatically carry a 500-degree day withdrawal period.

Although every effort must be made to ensure the use of accurate and effective treatments that have been tried and tested, the rapid emergence of new diseases may sometimes necessitate the use of unlicensed new drugs. Insurance or professional indemnity must be carefully considered by the practitioner in charge of health care and prescribing. It is also important for the practitioner to check up-to-date information about drug side-effects and environmental and human safety, which are rapidly becoming limiting factors in prescribing.

Drugs can be administered to fish by water-bath treatment, in-feed or by injection.

Bath Treatment

This method usually involves the use of chemicals that can be potentially harmful. Fish should be starved for at least 12 hours to lower the metabolic rate and reduce oxygen consumption. The decrease in faeces in the water will reduce the biological oxygen demand from this organic matter and also decrease ammonia levels. The artificial increase of oxygen levels is usually necessary as many of the chemicals are reducing agents, i.e. they cause a decrease in the available oxygen. It is important to monitor oxygen levels during a bath treatment.

Ideally, a small number of fish should be treated initially to assess the effects. Observation at all times is essential and the procedure must be abandoned if fish appear unduly stressed. Unfortunately, the more the fish are in need of treatment, the greater will be the danger from that treatment.

In the bath method, the water is turned off for the treatment period. In the related **flush** treatment the water is left running so that the medication gradually becomes more dilute. In practice, bath and flush treatments are often combined — 20 minutes of bath treatment and then a slow flushing out after starting the water source again.

Protective clothing should be worn by staff and water discharge consents may be needed for the therapeutic agent.

Formaldehyde solution (34–38% w/w solution)

Used in fresh water for ectoparasite infestations, and possibly for sea-lice treatments (but the volume needed is often impractical).

Dose. 150–250 ppm for 1 hour. Use the lower level in soft water.

Formaldehyde is a reducing agent and will remove oxygen from the water, especially at high temperatures. Avoid splashes to the face. Any white precipitate of *para*-formaldehyde is toxic to fish and must be filtered off.

Malachite green (zinc free)

Used in fresh water as an anti-fungal agent for eggs and for fish, and in the treatment of *Ichthyophthirius* infections (white spot). Has some effect against *Costia*.

Dose. 1–2 ppm for 30–60 minutes.

This is a respiratory poison and repeated treatment can be cumulative causing fish losses. The safety of the compound to humans is in doubt and the operator should wear protective clothing.

Formaldehyde/malachite green solution (Leteux-Meyer mixture)

Used in fresh water especially against *Ichthyophthirius* (white spot) infections and for parasitic infections associated with secondary *Saprolegnia* fungus.

Dose. 1 ppm malachite green and 150 ppm formaldehyde for up to 1 hour.

Chloramine T

Used in fresh water mainly against bacterial gill disease. It has some activity against ectoparasites and fungus. As a disinfectant it is useful in the control of fin rot.

Dose. 2.5 ppm up to 20 ppm for 30–60 minutes. Use at a lower rate in soft water with low pH. Do not mix with formalin.

Benzalkonium chloride

This surfactant is used for removing mucus and debris from the gills and skin of fish (bacterial gill disease and superficial myxobacterial skin infections). It is especially useful for removing debris attached to the gills after a spate.

Dose. 1–4 ppm for 1 hour. Use lower level in soft water.

This is toxic and quite stressful to the fish. The treatment may need to be abandoned if the fish show undue signs of distress. Oxygen levels will show a moderate reduction.

Sodium chloride

Safe and effective for treating fungus and ectoparasites in fresh water. This treatment is mainly used on very small alevins showing early signs of costiasis.

Dose. 1–2% for 30 minutes or 0.1–0.2 ppm permanently. Use the lower dosages for salmon fry.

The main problem with sodium chloride is the huge amount needed for medicating even a small smolt unit.

Dichlorvos (Aquagard: Ciba Geigy)

Organophosphorus compound for treating sea-lice (*Lepeophtheirus* and *Caligus*).

Dose. 1 ppm active dichlorvos (or 2 ppm of the 50% Aquagard) for up to 1 hour.

This product is dangerous to fish and humans: training on the effective and safe use of this chemical is essential. Follow codes of practice for pesticides and advise regional river purification board. Be prepared to abandon treatment if the fish show undue stress (e.g. gasping, rolling, burrowing). Provide additional oxygen. Withdrawal period: 4 days.

In-feed Medications

The four licensed antibacterials are incorporated into the feed for administration to fish. They are used to treat bacterial infections in both fresh water and sea water.

The drug is surface-coated on the food pellets with the addition of fish oil or gelatin, and the process is usually carried out in the feed mill. In urgent situations the farmer may mix the drug with the food pellets at the farm. Licensed products should be used if available.

All dosages below are of the *pure* drug, and are based on the weight of fish (kg).

Amoxycillin

Used mainly for furunculosis infections which are resistant to other antibiotics.

Dose. 40–80 mg/kg for 10 days. The higher dosage rate is more effective and is recommended.

This palatable drug is the newest antibacterial for fish. In some ways it is also the most disappointing and often produces only temporary relief from a furunculosis outbreak. This is possibly related to its rapid excretion by the fish — there is no long period of protection and the fish are more susceptible to reinfection. The short withdrawal period (50 degree-days) is useful if medication is necessary before slaughter. Up to 20% of the drug is lost in the surface coating of the pellets at the feed mill.

Co-trimazine (potentiated sulphonamide or trimethoprim/sulphadiazine)

Dose. 30 mg/kg fish for 7–10 days. Withdrawal period: 400 degree-days. Fairly unpalatable. The fish will become increasingly reluctant to eat the medicated feed as treatment progresses — especially at lower water temperatures with a reduced feeding rate. Do not overdose. Avoid any concurrent treatments, especially dichlorvos — this combination of drugs can be dangerous.

Oxolinic acid

Widely used for furunculosis but the causal organism now shows increasing evidence of resistance.

Dose. 10 mg/kg for 10 days. This rate appears satisfactory in fresh water but a dosage rate of 30 mg/kg is necessary in sea water. (Note that this is not in the data sheet.) Withdrawal period: 500 degree-days. The long-term safety of these older-style quinolones is currently being reviewed.

Oxytetracycline

Widely used; however the common pathogens are now showing signs of increasing resistance.

Dose. 75 mg/kg of fish for 5–10 days.

Other antibacterials

Unlicensed antibacterials occasionally used as in-feed medication include:
Furazolidone — unpalatable. 75 mg/kg.
Erythromycin — sometimes used in the control of BKD with equivocal results, only suppressing the disease. In-feed dosage is 100 mg/kg daily for 7–10 days.

Fenbendazole

This can be used as an in-feed treatment for the adult tapeworm *Eubothrium* spp. The dose is 6–8 mg/kg repeated in 48 hours if necessary. A transient inappetance can occur after the second dose.

Injection

Antibiotics may also be administered by injection, especially oxytetracycline (25 mg/kg intraperitoneally) and co-trimazine (125 mg/kg intraperitoneally). The sites of injection are usually intramuscular or intraperitoneal (Fig. 13.19).

As these are unlicensed preparations in salmon, their use should be restricted to broodstock which will not be used in human consumption. Long-acting tetracyclines have been used on broodstock which will be killed after stripping the eggs and milt and this can be a valuable treatment in the control of furunculosis, as these fish will be eating very little prior to their sexual maturation. Individual injection may be the only method of administering the antibiotics. 20 mg/kg of long-acting tetracycline injected intraperitoneally should be effective and safe. Care should be taken that the fish are not overdosed, as 50 mg/kg can cause liver damage and death.

Fig. 13.19 Injection sites for fish.

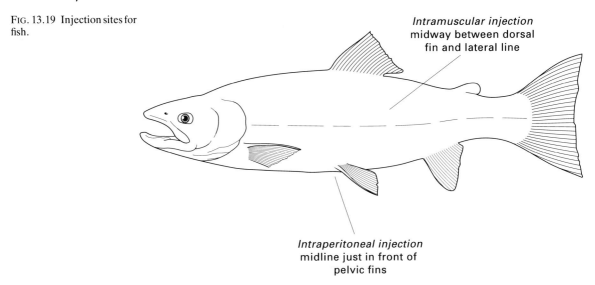

Intramuscular injection midway between dorsal fin and lateral line

Intraperitoneal injection midline just in front of pelvic fins

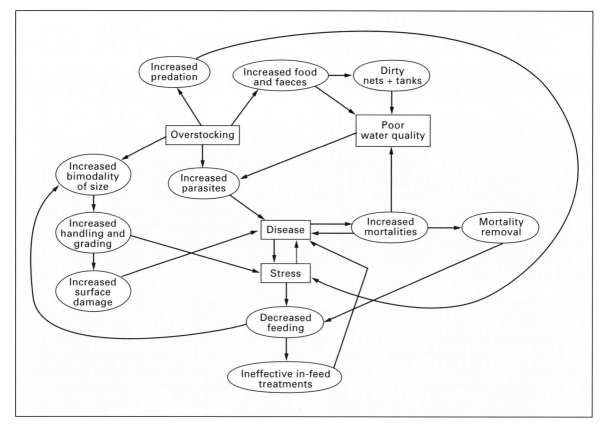

FIG. 13.20 Relationships between stocking rates, water quality and disease. If increasing water temperatures and the presence of endemic diseases are taken into account the problems will be magnified.

Prevention of Disease

The prevention of disease is the veterinarian's most important job. Patient, careful observation of fish stocks is essential. Initially every effort must be made to ensure stocking densities and water quality are correct. If either of these factors are wrong, a cascade of events may occur precipitating a disaster (Fig. 13.20).

Water quality

Oxygen levels, pH and flow rates and, if necessary, suspended solids and ammonia must be monitored. Ammonia levels can become critical if water-flow is reduced or if the water is recirculated. Check for any accumulation of rotting feed — this indication of overfeeding will reduce water quality. Clean nets will increase the water-flow and reduce the biological oxygen demand caused by the organic matter.

Stocking rates

Fish grow quickly in the summer months during high temperatures and cages can soon become overstocked. Only grow the number of fish in a cage which will achieve the terminal stocking density without thinning. Minimise handling and allow smolts plenty of room during that first 6 months in the sea.

Fresh water tanks should be well shaded with no shadows to ensure utilisation of all the available water volume.

Only with low stocking densities can the effect of endemic diseases such as lice infestation and furunculosis be kept to a minimum.

Handling/grading

Any handling, however careful, will lead to some stress and superficial damage. This is more likely to happen in an overcrowded system with faulty feeding methods.

If possible, avoid grilse grading at high summer temperatures — but if it is unavoidable the prophylactic use of antibiotics should be considered.

The use of wrasse may reduce the frequency of lice treatments and the consequent damage from handling.

Feeding

Over-reliance on automatic feeding systems, especially in the sea, can result in large differences in the size of the fish. Hand feeding is preferred

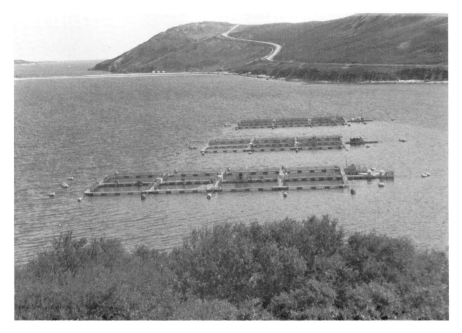

FIG. 13.21 Three cage groups on the Scottish mainland each containing eight cages 15 m square. Each group is separated by about 100 m. Groups of cages in such close proximity must be treated as one unit containing only one year class, with adequate fallow periods.

and allows good observation of the stock while preventing overfeeding. Avoid a sudden increase in pellet size in seawater smolts as it can precipitate an outbreak of pancreas disease.

When first feeding the alevins the timing and amount must be accurate to reduce yolk-sac disease and ensure good water quality.

Mortality removal

In cages this must be carried out at least once a week — and daily during a disease outbreak. This removes a source of infection to other fish, while examination of the dead fish often gives the first warning of imminent trouble. Freshwater tanks are designed to make removal of dead fish easier so that it can be done daily. Moribund fish should also be examined and removed.

Separation of year classes and fallowing

Both these practices (Fig. 13.21) reduce the chance of the cross-over of infection from one year to the next. Experience shows that even a break of 4 months — from the final harvest in January to smolt arrival in May — can decrease bacterial and lice infection and markedly increase the chances of smolt survival.

Clean nets and tanks

This will help to maintain good water quality and remove pathogens that may be present. Nets and tanks should be disinfected before re-use. Hand nets should be soaked in a disinfectant before being used on different groups of fish.

Hygiene and disease

Staff and visitors should be aware of the dangers of spreading disease. Suitable boots and overalls should be supplied for each unit (Fig. 13.22).

Workers handling mortalities should not feed fish later on the same day.

Dead fish must never be dumped in the sea. It is both anti-social and self-defeating.

Waste blood and other slaughtering by-products must be disposed of safely: either chemically sterilised before returning to the sea or on shore at an approved site.

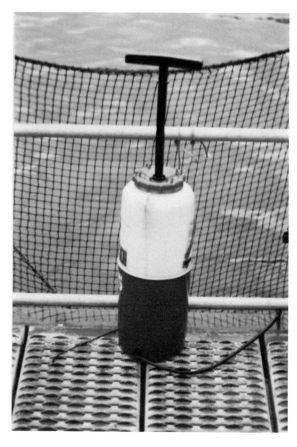

FIG. 13.22 A simple method of disinfecting boots and oilskins. These procedures may have limitations but they will heighten the awareness of the importance of hygiene to farm staff and visitors.

Control of vermin and disposal of spoilt food is important.

The exclusion of wild fish from farmed salmon stock is necessary to reduce the risk of transfer of disease. A high percentage of wild fish carry pathogens, e.g. furunculosis and BKD, which can be potentially serious for farmed stocks.

Precautions must be taken to reduce the introduction of disease to the hatchery from infected eggs. As well as testing the brookstock for diseases carried in the egg, it is common practice to disinfect the surface of the egg to remove any possible pathogens.

Prophylactic antibiotics

These can sometimes be justified in the routine treatment of smolts prior to transfer to a seawater site with endemic furunculosis. This strategy will depend on water temperatures and the previous disease history of the farm. For this reason it is essential to keep good records of sensitivity patterns for the strains of bacteria present.

Vaccines

These are available against vibriosis, enteric red mouth and furunculosis. At the moment only the *Vibrio* and ERM vaccines are effective, but these diseases are not usually a major threat to salmon stocks. The current furunculosis vaccine gives only a low level of protection and the majority of salmon stocks in Scotland are not vaccinated. A higher level of protection seems to be obtained using the intraperitoneal route of administration rather than the immersion method. The development of an effective furunculosis vaccine would be very welcome.

Sea-lice control

Effective monitoring of sea-lice numbers and their treatment will greatly reduce the stress and spread of other diseases. Sea-lice infestation must be one of the most important factors in initiating other disease conditions in the sea.

In any salmon farming system there will be pathogens present which can cause overt disease given the right conditions. The overuse of chemicals and drugs can bring its own problems and usually medications are no more than an aid to good farming. It is self-evident that fish farmed under good environmental conditions will stay healthy.

Salmon farming in Scotland has been a rapidly expanding industry over the last 20 years and has brought many benefits and employment to the remote areas. However, problems have unfolded with the growth of the industry and it will be important to tackle not only improved husbandry and therapy but also the environmental and welfare issues which are emerging.

Appendix
Guidelines on the Welfare of Farmed Fish: A Personal View by Tony Wall

Welfare is measurable and is necessarily a moral consideration. The welfare of an animal concerns its state as it attempts to cope with its environment (Fig. 13.23). If it fails to cope, then there is a welfare problem. Coping can be defined as the normal regulation of body-state and emergency responses.

The fact that one measurement may be normal (e.g. growth) does not necessarily mean that welfare is good. Nor does there have to be physical damage to indicate that welfare is poor.

Animal welfare can be considered in terms of the five freedoms defined by Brambell (1965) with the additional two proposed by Seamer (1992). Although fish are aquatic and differ considerably from other species normally dealt with in veterinary practice, the seven freedoms can still be used as a framework for the consideration of fish welfare.

Freedom from Thirst, Hunger and Malnutrition

• Transfer of fish from fresh to salt water entails changes in osmoregulation. Every effort must be made to ensure that the minimum number of parr are transferred with the smolts — they will not be able to adapt to concentrated sea water and will die off over the summer. $S\frac{1}{2}$s and $S1\frac{1}{2}$s can pose a problem as large losses can be expected.

Rainbow trout transferred to sea water must be of sufficient size to adapt to the new environment with the minimum of losses.

INDICATIONS OF POOR WELFARE		
Reduced	**Increased**	
Life expectancy	Body damage	Adrenal activity
Growth	Disease	Behavioural anomalies
Reproduction	Immuno-suppresion	Self-narcotisation

Fig. 13.23 Indications of poor welfare.

Feed must be of good quality to ensure adequate growth and minimal disease. Poor quality feed will result in increased levels of food being given with increased production of faeces and the risk of reduced water quality.

The area of feeding highlights the difference between the requirements of ectotherms and homeotherms. There are occasions in the life of some fish when feeding reduces or ceases and most fish are adapted to go without food for long periods.

There are circumstances when it may be appropriate to reduce or withhold food from fish e.g. when administering antibiotics, before handling procedures and in response to disease.

Freedom from Thermal or Physical Discomfort

- Aquatic poikilotherms are more dependent on their environment than homeothermic terrestrial animals. The quality of the water is all important and to a large extent this depends on the standard of husbandry (net changing; tank cleaning; correct feeding, absence of uneaten food; and stocking levels).
- *Temperature*: ensure that there are no sudden changes. High temperatures cause stress and reduced oxygen levels.
- *Oxygen levels* should be near saturation.
- *Ammonia levels* and suspended solids should be low.
- *pH fluctuations* should be avoided if possible.
- *Salinity fluctuations* should be avoided for Atlantic salmon.
- *High stocking levels* cause poor water quality, skin abrasion, fin damage, increased competition for food and a higher level of disease.
- *Shading* of shallow tanks and cages reduces ultraviolet light damage and lessens fear and apprehension in the fish.
- *Tidal flows* over 0.6 m/sec cannot be tolerated by caged salmon and should be avoided.
- Sudden vibration of tanks or noisy engines can initiate panic in newly transferred smolts, with accompanying trauma.

Freedom from Pain, Injury and Disease

- *The amount of pain* that fish perceive is not known but in the absence of further research they must be given the benefit of the doubt.

- *Anaesthesia* will be necessary for all surgical procedures.
- *Injury can be caused* to the delicate external mucous layer of the fish by prolonged crowding and rough handling, especially at grading.
- *Fin clipping* (usually for identification) may cause pain as well as injury and is not recommended.
- *Injury can be reduced* by the proper design of holding units and handling systems.
- *The effects of disease* will be reduced by daily observation of stocks by experienced personnel capable of recognising signs of ill-health and initiating appropriate action. The facilities must allow adequate observation of the stocks.
- *Disease-free stock* should be used for farming whenever possible.
- *Disinfection* of equipment and personnel decreases the risk of disease transfer.
- *Dead and dying fish* should be removed, killed and disposed of hygienically.
- *Fallowing sea-sites* and the *separation of year-classes* reduce disease transfer.
- *Chemical or bath treatments* often involve stress. Crowding should not be excessive and the fish should be observed constantly. Oxygen levels should be monitored and additional oxygen should be available.
- There is an over-riding responsibility to treat diseased fish, or as a last resort to slaughter them. The use of unlicensed compounds can highlight the conflict between welfare of the fish and the responsibility of the river boards for discharge controls.

Freedom from Fear and Distress

- *Predation*, especially by birds and seals, will cause fear and distress as well as injury to the fish. Access by predators must be denied.
- *Grading* by any method is stressful and should be kept to a minimum. However, it must be recognised that lack of grading will lead to a disparity in sizes, with cannibalism and dominance by the larger fish, and sub-optimal performance by the smaller ones. The use of passive graders, where the fish are not handled, is beneficial in some circumstances.
- *Shading* shallow tanks will reduce fear and will mimic the lighting conditions found in the natural habitat.

- *Stress* can be minimised by gradual changes in husbandry (especially food quality and quantity) and in water quality.

Freedom to Express Normal Patterns of Behaviour

- *Tanks and cages* must be big enough to allow swimming and shoaling.
- *Maturing fish* will not be able to express normal courtship rituals in a farmed situation. These fish should be removed and killed.

Freedom from Stress and Suffering when Transported

- *Careful handling* of the fish and adequate oxygenation of the water are essential.
- *Starvation* of the fish for 24 hours prior to transfer will reduce biological oxygen demand and maintain good water quality.
- The use of *sedation* to reduce stress may be appropriate during handling before transportation.
- *Sudden changes* in temperature and pH should be avoided.

Freedom from Stress or Suffering when Slaughtered

Slaughter

Appropriate equipmentand adequate training of personnel in slaughter techniques are essential.

The slaughter method used should:

— render the fish insensible instantaneously and as efficiently as possible;
— prevent the fish recovering from the above.

Even the recommended methods have practical limitations and it is important that research is directed at slaughter methods in food producing fish.

- *Methods used for salmon include*:
  stunning, with or without bleeding;
  carbon dioxide narcosis, with or without bleeding;
  bleeding alone.
- *Stunning*: Using a club, deliver a single hard blow or series of short sharp blows midline just behind the eyes. This may be followed by cutting all four gill arches on both sides to ensure rapid bleeding. This method is effective in producing sufficient instantaneous brain damage.
- *Carbon dioxide narcosis*: The fish are placed in a bath of sea water previously saturated with carbon dioxide. This saturation can only be determined in practice by measuring the fall in pH. Narcosis is attained after 1–2 minutes.
  If these fish are returned to sea water, they will recover. For this reason bleeding after carbon dioxide narcosis is essential, cutting all four gill arches on both sides.
- *Bleeding alone*: Some or all gill arches are cut without prior stunning or narcosis. The fish are bled out in the water. There is an increase in activity and muscular spasms for up to 4 minutes.
- *Methods used for trout include*:
  electric shock;
  placing fish in an ice slurry;
  killing fish in air (anoxia);
  carbon dioxide narcosis (as for salmon).
- *Electric shock* using a pulse of direct electric current. There is instantaneous immobilisation of the fish. This method can cause fracture of the spine and haemorrhages in the flesh of electrocuted fish. Care must be taken to ensure operator safety.
- *Ice slurry*. The fish are placed in ice and water at about 2°C. They become torpid and eventually death is by anoxia.
- *Killing in air (anoxia)*.

Specific Issues

- *Moribund fish*. Some disease conditions (especially pancreas disease and lice infestation) often have a high morbidity rate, leaving large numbers of moribund anorexic fish on the water surface. These fish should be removed and humanely destroyed. An overdose of anaesthetic or manual stunning are appropriate methods of destruction.
- *Surplus fish* (usually smolts and parr) should be destroyed in a humane manner. Anaesthetic overdose is the method of choice.
- *Sampling live fish*, e.g. for parasites or blood collection, should be carried out under anaesthetia.

When fish are to be killed prior to sampling, *anaesthetic overdose* is the method of choice. However, this procedure may reduce ectoparasite motility.

Stunning and destruction of the brain (*pithing*) is an alternative to anaesthetic overdose. (Telangiectasis in the gills can occur after stunning but if this artefact is expected it can also be ignored.)

Decapitation or *cervical dislocation* without brain destruction may not cause immediate insensibility as fish are tolerant of prolonged hypoxia.

Diagnostic and other investigative procedures:

There are certain specific procedures where the welfare of individual fish is compromised in order to maintain the health and welfare of the stock as a whole. e.g. 'Stress testing' for the detection of specific pathogens and salinity tolerance testing.

- *Stress-testing* (mainly for furunculosis). This procedure involves injecting a sample of the population with corticosteroids under anaesthesia and increasing the water temperature to 18–20°C over 10 days. The carrier state will thus become manifest as clinical disease.

  These fish often become grossly infected with fungus and parasites. Tail and fin erosion can be severe. However, by eliminating the carrier state, specific pathogen-free fish will be farmed. This will reduce disease and improve welfare in the long term.

  It is recommended that stress-testing is encouraged. The fish should be treated vigorously for any parasitic or fungal disease and good water quality should be maintained. Alternative methods of identifying the carrier status of common fish diseases should be investigated.

- *Challenge in salt water.* A small sample of smolts can be challenged in sodium chloride solution (usually 33–40 ppt) to determine if they are ready for the sea. This method is used to estimate the optimum transfer time of the bulk of the smolts to the sea. The test fish should be observed carefully and removed from the salt water at the first signs of their inability to cope with their new environment.

- *Broodstock.* Stripping broodstock for milt and eggs should be carried out under anaesthesia.

Anaesthesia and Tranquillisation

- *Applications*:
  Handling broodstock.
  Grading, sorting and weighing fish.
  Sampling fish.
  Vaccinating and injecting fish.

- *Products available*:
  Benzocaine (ethyl *p*-amino benzoate) $C_9H_{11}NO_2$).
  —Insoluble in water. First dissolve in ethanol, methanol or acetone.
  —Stock solution (100 g benzocaine in 1 litre of solvent as above) should be stored in dark glass at room temperature.
  —Neutral in solution.
  Tricaine methane sulphonate, (ethyl *m*-amino benzoate) $C_{10}H_{15}NO_5S$).
  —The only compound licensed for fish.
  —Soluble in water.
  —Causes acidic solution which must be buffered to avoid physiological stress to fish.

- *Buffering*
  In fresh water, buffering of tricaine methane sulphonate is required. Sea water has a very high buffering potential, so additional buffering is not required. Phosphate-buffered saline (0.1 M) may be used as a buffer for tricaine methane sulphonate in fresh water.

- *Method*
  —Fish should be starved for up to 12 hours prior to anaesthesia to prevent regurgitation.
  —Anaesthetic agent should be added to an aerated container and a few test fish should be placed in solution.
  —Anaesthesia has occurred when fish lose all righting reflexes and reflex activity (although gill covers should continue to open and close). Good anaesthesia will occur in 60–120 seconds.
  —Aerated recovery tanks must always be available at the same time. Good recovery will take 60–120 seconds.
  —Fish which have recovered should be observed for a few hours before the majority are anaesthetised.
  —Water temperature, size of fish and genetic origin all play a role in anaesthesia. For this reason fish should be monitored constantly during anaesthesia and recovery.

- *Dosages*
  Tricaine methane sulphonate and benzocaine:
  (a) 1:12,000 solution for surgical anaesthesia. 1:20,000–1:30,000 for tranquillisation.
      or
  (b) Add either anaesthetic agent, a small amount at a time, and observe the loss of reflexes of the fish.

References

Brambell, F. W. R. (chairman) (1965). *Report of the Technical Committee to Enquire into the Welfare of Animals Kept Under Intensive Livestock Husbandry Systems.* Cmnd 2836. HMSO, London.

Broom, D. M. (1988). The Scientific Assessment of Animal Welfare. *Applied Animal Behaviour Science* **20**, 5–19.

Broom, D. M. (1991). Animal Welfare: Concepts and Measurement. *Journal of Animal Science* **69**, 4167–4175.

Brown, L. A. (1988) Anaesthesia in fish. In: *Tropical Fish Medicine: Veterinary Clinics of North America: Small Animal Practice.* **18**(2), March pp. 317–330.

Cawley, G. — See Chapter 10 (Welfare) in this book.

Farm Animal Welfare Council. *Pain and Stress in Fish.* Report of a seminar held at Stirling University, 11th May 1990.

Kestin, S. C., Wotten, S. B., Gregory, N. G. (1991). Effect of slaughter by removal from water on visual evoked activity in the brain and reflex movement of rainbow trout (*Onchorhynchus mykiss*). *Veterinary Record* **128**, 443–446.

National Farmers Union of Scotland (Fish Farming Section). *Codes of Recommendation for the Husbandry and Welfare of Farmed Fish.*

Scottish Salmon Growers Association: *Guidelines for the Humane Slaughter of Farmed Atlantic Salmon.*

Scottish Society of the Prevention of Cruelty to Animals: Fish Farming in Scotland in 1990. Preliminary Study by Dr J. Remfry.

Seamer, J. (1992). Transport of live animals for slaughter. *Veterinary Record* **130** (2), 38.

World Society for the Protection of Animals (Scientific Advisory Panel). *Pain Assessment and Euthanasia in Ectotherms.*

14

The Veterinary Approach to Trout

ANDY HOLLIMAN

From their natural location in the western half of North America (almost all populations are found west of the Continental Divide), the rainbow trout (*Oncorhynchus mykiss*) and its anadromous form, the steelhead, have been transported all over the world. It is in demand both as a sport fish, in self-sustaining freshwater populations, and for commercial culture. In the United States and some European countries trout culture has the longest history of any form of fish culture. More recently it has expanded into Australasia, Japan, South America, Canada and South Africa. Of all the salmonids, none is as amenable as the rainbow trout to captivity or so tolerant of different temperatures, salinities and relatively low oxygen levels. These characteristics, together with its fast growth rate, make it the preferred species for freshwater farming of table fish.

The origin of large-scale trout farming goes back to the Danish earth ponds of the 1930s. By the end of the 1960s, raceway farms, pioneered in the USA, spread first to Brittany and then to Italy. These two types of farms are responsible for 98% of European portion-size production. Nonetheless, other rearing systems, notably tank and cage systems, the latter in both fresh and salt water, are of importance in many parts of the world.

Trout is marketed in a limited number of forms. Fresh trout is the main product, either gutted or ungutted, and a recent development is the production of filleted trout. It is also sold frozen, mainly in portions, or smoked. Hot smoking is mainly restricted to freshwater trout; cold smoking is suitable for trout raised in sea water.

Italy, Denmark and France are the major European producers of portion-sized trout (200–250 g), each producing about 30,000 tonnes per annum; they are followed by Spain, the United Kingdom and Germany, each producing about 16,000 tonnes. In Scandinavia, particularly Finland (20,000 tonnes), there is a significant production of large trout (1–2+ kg), principally sea-grown, competing in a market dominated by salmon. In the United States the leading producer of portion-sized trout is Idaho (over 20,000 tonnes).

Farming Systems

The farming cycle of the rainbow trout can be conveniently sub-divided into three stages: incubation, fry rearing and on-growing.

Incubation

This stage relies on a supply of high quality water, ideally from a spring or borehole at constant temperature. Incubation may be carried out in hatchery trays or baskets held in series in plastic or fibreglass troughs resting 3 cm above the bottom, and supplied with water from a feeder channel. A litre of eggs requires an inflow of 3–5 litres/minute; a tray of 10,000 eggs requires 5,000 litres/day. An alternative system is the jar or vertical incubator, usually of fibre glass or plastic and holding from 5–100 litres of eggs.

Fry Rearing

After hatching the fry are transferred to rectangular or circular fry tanks, usually of fibreglass or plastic, with an inflow pipe, a central outflow and an overflow pipe. The standard size of a rectangular tank is 2 m × 2 m × 50–60 cm deep.

At about 1 month old the fry can be stocked at 25 kg/m^3 with a water through-flow of 1 litre/minute/1–1.3 kg, this reducing to 1 litre/minute/2.5 kg as the fry reach 10 g size. After reaching 500 fish/kg they can be held in any form of tank or raceway but should not be placed in earth ponds until 16 weeks post-fertilisation, as a precaution against whirling disease.

On-growing

The three major enclosures for land-based farms are ponds, raceways or tanks.

Earth ponds

This traditional system (Fig. 14.1) was developed in Denmark and comprises a single or double series of earth ponds, excavated on a level site and relying on gravity feed. The ponds are supplied from a watercourse via an inlet channel. Each pond discharges to an effluent channel and finally to the river further downstream. The ponds are usually unlined but if the substrate is porous the bottom can be covered with a layer of clay. Sometimes they are lined with polyethylene sheeting.

A typical pond size is 30 m × 10 m × 1 m deep at the intake, sloping to 1.5–2 m at the outflow. Flow rates are quite slow at 1–1.5 litres/second, resulting in 3–6 water changes per day. Average stocking density is 2 kg/m^3.

Advantage

- Very cost-effective where land is fairly flat, inexpensive and easily excavated.

Disadvantages

- Requires a level site.
- Requires regular cleaning to avoid build-up of food/faeces.
- Fish not easily observed.
- Husbandry procedures such as chemical treatments, grading and harvesting are not very easy.

Raceways

This is the original North American system. Raceways (Fig. 14.2) come in a variety of designs and sizes and consist of a series of parallel channels, often sub-divided by screened sluices. Typically they may be 30 m long × 2.5 m wide × 0.7 m deep and constructed of concrete or brick. They rely on high flow rates of clean water.

Advantages

- Economy of land use.
- High stocking density.
- Ease of grading, harvesting and treatment.

Disadvantages

- Require high flow rates.
- Hygiene problems lower down the system.
- Fish waste energy swimming.
- Damage to fish caused by concrete walls.

Tanks

Usually circular and constructed of concrete, corrugated metal or fibreglass, often in prefabricated sections; tanks are typically 4 m in diameter and 0.75 m deep. The concrete base slopes from the circumference to a central drain. They can be dug into the ground or kept above ground, and are usually covered with netting to deter birds. Water enters through a peripheral inlet at about 4 litres/second and flows in a circular fashion before leaving at a central outlet comprising a stand-pipe surrounded by a screen.

Advantages

- Easily erected and maintained.
- Inflow and outflow arranged to be self-cleaning using vortex effect.
- Each tank individually controlled via valves.
- More uniform distribution of fish.
- Can be covered if necessary.
- Ability to use single structure for virtually whole growth cycle if necessary.

Disadvantages

- Cost.
- Chemical treatments less easy to apply.
- Not well suited to automatic handling.

Cage systems

In recent years cage systems have become popular in some parts of the world. Whether in

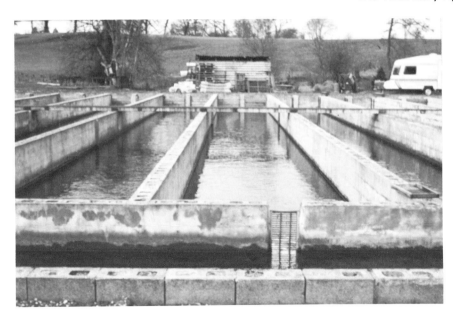

FIG. 14.1 A Danish earth-pond system.

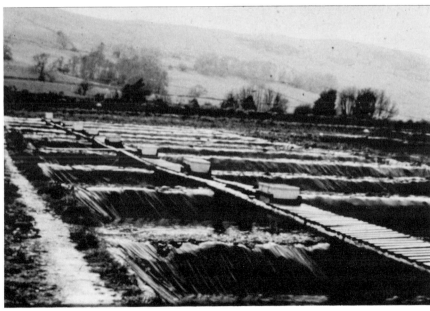

FIG. 14.2 Raceway system for trout production.

fresh water or sea water, the basic construction is the same, although more sophisticated designs have started to appear for sea water use.

Simple cages consist of cube-shaped nets suspended from a square or rectangular floating collar which may also serve as a walkway, facilitating fish observation and handling. Nets or wires may be used above the cages to discourage birds. Cages may be fastened together to form large rafts of up to 30 units. Trout can be transferred to cages with a mesh size of 5 mm^2 at about 4–5 g (smaller mesh leads to fouling problems) and can be grown to 25 g in the same cage at densities no greater than 2–3 kg/m^3. At 25 g, they can be held at 15–20 kg/m^3 if the mesh size is 12 mm^2.

Advantages

- Cost-effective if adequate water circulation and depth.

Disadvantages

- Need adequate water exchange.
- Need adequate depth.

- Low mechanical failure.
- Stable environment.
- Cages may be joined for increased stability.

- Need sheltered site.
- May need boat access.
- Difficult to service in bad weather.
- Medication difficult.
- Fouling of mesh.
- Artificial aeration may be difficult.

General Husbandry

Trout require a plentiful supply of good quality water. Compared with other farmed species, they have higher oxygen requirements and are more sensitive to ammonia, carbon dioxide and suspended solids.

Any farm plan must take into account the available water supply and the target production figure. Figures for available water should be based on lowest known flow rates over as many years as possible. An excess in mid-winter may be a drought situation in summer. Areas upstream of any proposed farm site must be examined for evidence of heavily fertilised farmland, other intensive farming systems, factories, mine workings, etc., all of which could catastrophically reduce water quality at any time.

As a rough estimate, a production figure of 10 tonnes per annum requires at least 4.5 million litres of water per day (50 litres/second), this figure being temperature-dependent. The tapping of a high quality underground water supply, for example borehole water, should be considered essential as a hatchery supply.

Abiotic Factors

The most important input to a farm in terms of water quality is oxygen. Extreme pH, ammonia and suspended solids constitute some of the more potentially damaging factors in the water supply.

Oxygen

It is recommended that the minimum dissolved oxygen concentration for trout is 5.5 mg/l, or 7 mg/l for eggs. Low levels cause high mortality (Fig. 14.3); reduced oxygen concentrations over a long period can cause disease. In general, the smallest fish on a farm require the best oxygenated water and the greatest water supply: their oxygen requirements are greater than larger fish per unit weight, as a consequence of the surface area/volume ratio.

100×10 g fish at $10°C$ need approximately 300 mg O_2 per hour.

10×100 g fish at $10°C$ need approximately 200 mg O_2 per hour.

1×1 kg fish at $10°C$ needs approximately 160 mg O_2 per hour.

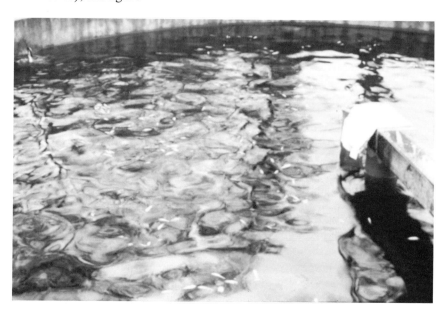

FIG. 14.3 Surface of a circular tank, showing a fish kill caused by reduced dissolved oxygen in the water supply.

CONCENTRATIONS OF AMMONIA WHICH CONTAIN AN UN-IONISED AMMONIA CONCENTRATION OF 0.025 mg/l						
	pH value					
Temperature (°C)	6.5	7.0	7.5	8.0*	8.5*	9.0*
5	63.3	20.0	6.3	2.0	0.66	0.23
10	42.4	13.4	4.3	1.4	0.45	0.16
15	28.9	9.2	2.9	0.94	0.31	0.12
20	20.0	6.3	2.0	0.66	0.22	0.088
25	13.9	4.4	1.4	0.46	0.16	0.069
30	9.8	3.1	1.0	0.34	0.12	0.056

* Concentrations of ammonia derived for pH values above 8.0 may be too stringent if the concentration of free carbon dioxide in the water is very low.

FIG. 14.4   Concentrations of ammonia which contain an un-ionised ammonia concentration of 0.025 mg/l.

Temperature

Temperature will have a major controlling influence on rates of embryonic development, growth, oxygen consumption, efficiency of food conversion etc. Trout have rather lower preferred temperatures than other freshwater species. The optimum water temperature for incubation of eggs is 13°C, and for growth of trout it is around 16°C.

pH and ammonia

Trout prefer water in the pH range 7–7.5, but tend to survive in water of low pH better than non-salmonids. On the acidic side of pH 5.5, the pH of the water can, in itself, be harmful to fish. In waters draining acidic bogs or afforested catchments or as a result of acid rain, the water may be extremely acidic and may also contain dissolved aluminium in toxic concentrations.

The recommended maximum concentration of un-ionised ammonia in water for trout is 0.025 mg/l (Fig. 14.4).

Suspended solids

Solids in suspension may be inorganic or organic in origin. Concentrations of inert suspended solids up to 25 mg/l seem to have no harmful effects, provided that the solids remain in suspension.

The Farming Cycle

Broodstock

These are usually held in raceways or large ponds using high quality water, at much lower stocking densities and lower feeding rates than required for production fish. However, they are fed well prior to spawning and are usually stripped manually at 3 years old. Stripping is much easier under anaesthesia. Anaesthetic must be rinsed off afterwards because the smallest residue affects sperm motility. It is important to avoid breaking the eggs or allowing any blood contamination as this may block the micropyle and reduce fertilisation success. The technique is to strip the male first, followed immediately by the female, into a plastic container with no trace of detergent or disinfectant. The optimum ratio is 1 ml of milt to 8,000 eggs (10,000 eggs 5 mm in diameter occupy 1 litre). Milt and eggs are gently stirred with clean, dry hands, taking care to avoid direct sunlight or any temperature shocks at this stage. After fertilisation the eggs are water-hardened for 10 minutes before transfer to incubator trays or bottles.

Hatchery

The newly fertilised or 'green' eggs remain sensitive to temperature shocks and physical movement for 15–18 days, when the eyes become visible as two black dots. From the 'eyed' stage until hatching the eggs are relatively tough and can withstand sorting, handling and transport. Unfertilised or damaged eggs can be killed by 'shocking' the eyed eggs, which involves pouring them to another container held 40–50 cm below. Healthy eggs remain undamaged and are returned to trays or jars to continue development.

The incubation period of eggs from different females at the same temperature can vary by as much as 5–6 days. In general the incubation period is approximately 300 degree-days. Poor hatchability occurs at temperatures much above 18°C or below 4°C. The newly-hatched yolk sac fry will continue to absorb yolk for 2–6 weeks, depending on temperature, before reaching the swim-up stage and actively feeding.

Commencement of feeding is a critical period. Some managers offer feed whilst the fry are still in hatchery troughs but others wait until transfer to fry tanks. Fry must be fed well using the smallest crumbs, and all excess removed. Once accustomed to feeding, food is offered little and often for 20 hours per day via automatic feeders. Such a system is essential for good fry production. Body weight will double every week or so and the diet is adjusted accordingly. An increase in diet size is to be avoided if it proves too big for some of the fish.

Fry tanks

At 500 fish/kg the fry can be moved to tanks or raceways but, as previously mentioned, must not be stocked into earth ponds until about 16 weeks post-fertilisation (7–8 cm). Management changes required during this period involve alterations in feed rates and pellet size and possibly adjustments to water-flow rate and depth. In any trout population a hierarchical structure is established, resulting in differential growth rates and a big variation in individual size. Tail and fin nipping is a likely consequence. This can be much reduced with regular grading (starving fish for 12 hours beforehand) but the procedure will stress fish unduly if carried out too frequently and will result in reduced growth rates. A suitable regime is to grade once in the fry tanks, once on transfer to larger tanks and two or three times whilst growing.

Floating cages

At 4–5 g, trout can be transferred to floating cages in fresh water. Automatic feeding saves on both time and labour; the amount and frequency of feeding is controlled by the size and number of fish, the required growth rate and water temperature. Additional hand feeding should be offered to ensure that the farmer is observing his fish for at least a part of each day.

Rainbow trout are generally too small at the end of their first summer feeding to tolerate full strength sea water (32–34 ppt salinity) but may tolerate a 50:50 dilution (14–19 ppt salinity). By the end of the autumn, they can probably tolerate full strength sea water if they have reached 100 g, albeit with an increased risk of stress-induced bacterial disease. There are two distinct phases during the acclimatisation of rainbow trout to sea water: an adjustive phase characterised by increased plasma osmotic concentration and a regulative phase during which control is established over osmotic concentration by active ion secretion through the gills.

In Scandinavia, where sea cages are very popular for large trout production, the sea is too cold for growth in late winter and early spring, and it can freeze. Consequently, fish are transferred in April at 700–800 g when 2+ years old and are harvested in November/December at 3+ kg. The average salinity at these sites is 19 ppt.

Fish Farm Effluent

The production of wastes by farm fish and the discharge of pollutants are not insignificant. It has been estimated that the production of 1 tonne of fish involves the same discharge of waste (ammonia, nitrates, nitrites, suspended solids and BOD) as 1 day's discharge of treated sewage from a town of over 300,000 people.

The quality of fish farm effluent is influenced by the nature of the water supply (spring, borehole, river); the effects of the fish on the water; and the treatment process employed. The extent and ability of a river to dilute and transport fish farm effluent depends on the river's characteristics, the magnitude of the effluent discharge and whether wastes are in suspension or in solution.

Increased suspended solids and BOD through a farm can be controlled by settlement and this is often the only form of effluent treatment on a farm. With freshwater cages, problems arise mainly when intensive production is centred on small bodies of water. Little flushing action takes place within a cage unit and solids may sediment. The increased levels of phosphorus and nitrogen will stimulate algal growth and possibly an algal bloom which may pose a toxic threat. Over 10 kg of phosphorus per tonne of fish per annum is produced as a waste product. Phosphorus is the main element linked with the eutrophication of natural waters and concentrations >25 ppm have been linked with algal blooms. As a general rule, lakes suitable for freshwater culture should have a total turnover time of less than 1 year.

The main effort to reduce pollution in recent years has been directed towards improving fish feeds. The use of high-energy extruded pellets has significantly reduced feed requirements; in addition, the phosphorus content of feeds has been reduced by a third and the production of suspended solids reduced by over a half.

Legislation

International exchange of cultured fish species is increasing rapidly, facilitating the dissemination of serious infectious diseases. Effective programmes of prevention and control are necessary to prevent the spread of fish disease agents within and between countries. The extent to which individual countries institute and enforce such controls is quite variable and indeed some countries impose no control measures at all.

United States of America

Fish health certification is the responsibility of the Fish and Wildlife Service. All salmonids entering the country must be checked for whirling disease and viral haemorrhagic septicaemia. There are no uniform guidelines or regulations governing fish disease control: each state has developed its own.

Canada

All provinces are united under the Fish Health Protection Regulations, which are enforced by Fish Health Officials. The regulations apply to all facilities from which live and dead cultured fish, eggs of cultured and wild fish, and products of dead cultured fish of all species belonging to family Salmonidae, will be shipped into Canada or from one province to another.

United Kingdom

The Diseases of Fish Act 1983 absolutely prohibits the importation of live salmonids. Salmonid eggs may only be imported under licence, and the importation of ungutted salmonids is prohibited.

A number of diseases affecting rainbow trout are deemed to be notifiable (infectious haematopoietic necrosis, infectious pancreatic necrosis, viral haemorrhagic septicaemia, whirling disease and bacterial kidney disease) and the Ministry of Agriculture, Fisheries and Food has powers to prohibit the movement of fish from farms where a notifiable disease has been suspected or confirmed.

Scandinavia

Health control programmes have been in place in most of the Nordic countries for a number of years.

In Denmark, no importation of live freshwater fish and their products can take place without special permission from the Veterinary Department of the Ministry of Agriculture. Denmark has a voluntary eradication scheme for the control of viral haemorrhagic septicaemia.

In Sweden all importers of live fish must be licensed and be able to show disease-free status for at least 3 years. Finland prohibits the importation of all live fish and fish eggs. Norway launched a national fish health programme for salmonids in 1991, in an attempt to reduce disease losses, and membership of the programme is mandatory for certain categories of fish farms.

European Community (EC)

From 1 January 1993, any current legislation within the member states of the EC will become redundant as Community-wide legislation is adopted. Directive 91/67/EEC defines the animal health conditions governing the placing on the market of aquaculture animals and products. The geographical area of the EC is to be divided into continental and coastal zones, each of which is strictly defined. Zones may have either approved or non-approved status. Member states will be able to restrict introductions of susceptible species to those originating from sources of at least equivalent or better health status.

Australia

Australia is remarkably free of many of the serious infectious diseases which limit rainbow trout production in other countries. At present there is no policy common to all the states for the control of disease outbreaks, notification requirements or compensation for farm owners, and the extent of veterinary involvement is variable from state to state. The importation of fish, fish eggs and fish products is covered by the Commonwealth Veterinary Quarantine Inspection Service, and requires Ministerial approval. To date, none have been imported.

Major Diseases

Viral Diseases

The most important viral diseases of trout are infectious pancreatic necrosis (IPN), viral haemorrhagic septicaemia (VHS) and infectious haematopoietic necrosis (IHN). Diagnosis is based on typical symptoms and pathology, and viral isolation in tissue culture.

Infectious pancreatic necrosis (IPN)

The spread of this virus has been associated with international traffic in eyed ova. It is absent from Australia and New Zealand.

It is principally a disease of fry and fingerlings; mortality can be high from 2–12 weeks of age but is unusual in older fish and falls to zero in adults. Signs include swollen abdomen, exophthalmos, dark pigmentation and spiral swimming. Clinical disease can be induced in growing fish by stressful procedures such as transport and grading. Disease outbreaks may be associated with poor water quality allied to high stocking density. The virus can be recovered from apparently healthy fish and it appears that survivors of outbreaks become disease-free carriers for life. Horizontal and vertical transmission occur.

Diagnosis is based upon age of fish and symptoms, virus isolation in tissue culture, and histopathological examination.

Viral haemorrhagic septicaemia (VHS)

The virus is widely disseminated in Europe and is probably endemic in wild fish species near infected sites. Until recently VHS virus was thought to occur only in Europe but was first isolated in North America from Chinook salmon (*Oncorhynchus tshawytscha*) and Coho salmon (*Oncorhynchus kisutch*) in 1988 and again in 1989. The virus was morphologically and serologically indistinguishable from typical European strains. In 1990 it was also isolated from Pacific cod. Its occurrence from four unrelated locations near the marine environment in Washington suggests that the virus is enzootic in portions of the Pacific Ocean.

The brown trout (*Salmo trutta*) is highly resistant to disease and is likely to be the natural host. In rainbow trout the earliest fry stages and broodstock appear to be resistant. The most susceptible stage is from fingerling up to 200–300 g size. Rapid, high mortalities can occur in the acute stages.

Acute, chronic and nervous forms of the disease are recognised, each merging into the other. Signs include anorexia, erratic swimming, swollen abdomen in the more chronic stages and defects of balance in the nervous form. Disease outbreaks have been linked with many stress factors including water quality, transport, stocking density etc. VHS is typically a disease of poor environmental conditions. Infection in rainbow trout in sea cages has been observed in France, Denmark and Norway.

Lateral transmission appears to be the main route of spread, via the introduction of diseased stock or water from an infected site. There is no conclusive evidence of vertical transmission.

Infectious haematopoietic necrosis (IHN)

This is widespread in the salmon producing areas of North America. It has been recorded in Japan for many years but was not detected in Europe until 1987 in association with heavy mortalities of rainbow trout yolk-sac fry and fingerlings in Italy and France. Cases have also been reported in Belgium and Germany.

IHN typically affects early feeders and growers, usually at low water temperatures (10°C), often in the spring as temperatures are rising; outbreaks are rarely seen above 15°C. Mortality can be high in young fish at 10°C. Typical signs include exophthalmos, pale gills, swollen abdomen and trailing faeces. Infection can occur both through the water and from parent carriers to fry. Surviving fish may become lifelong carriers and shed virus in their sexual fluids.

Bacterial Diseases

Enteric redmouth (ERM)

All salmonids world-wide are potentially susceptible to the organism *Yersinia ruckeri*. It is present in the guts of carrier fish, in low numbers in the aquatic environment, and it can survive for up to two months in pond mud. The disease presents as a haemorrhagic septicaemia, often stress-associated, which in the acute form resembles other bacterial septicaemias. Affected fish may show reddening of the mouth, and the cutaneous petechiation may be intense. In the chronic disease, fish may darken and show bilateral exophthalmos. Internally, there is evidence of splenomegaly and diffuse haemorrhages through the viscera and musculature, into the gut and onto the swimbladder wall.

Cold-water disease (Peduncle disease)

The bacteria, *Myxobacterium*, *Flavobacterium* and *Chondrococcus* have been associated with a variety of disease conditions. Members of these various genera are all pigment producers. Their precise reservoir is unclear but they are presumed to occur naturally in the aquatic environment.

The organism in cold-water disease is *Cytophaga psychrophila (Flexibacter psychrophilus)*. Many of the early reports of this condition came from the USA's Pacific north-west, in hatchery-reared salmonids. More recently the condition has been described in New Zealand and some European countries, including France. It is a serious infection, typically occurring at temperatures below 10°C and primarily affecting juvenile fish. In the acute form fish may darken and die without any surface lesions. More commonly, surface lesions are seen in the peduncle area but may also occur on other areas of the trunk and head. There may be yellowish margins to eroded fins, and underlying tissues can be extensively eroded. The caudal fin may be lost. The disease can progress to septicaemia. Long thin bacteria are present within the lesions, and moist, yellow spreading colonies appear on *Cytophaga* agar within 3 days at 20°C.

Fry mortality syndrome ('fry anaemia syndrome')

Cytophaga psychrophila (or a closely related bacterium) is the causative agent and Lorenzen *et al.* (1991) have proposed the name Bacterial Fry Anaemia (BFA) for this condition. It occurs in many European countries and the United States, though it has only been reported in the last decade.

Fry are typically affected at 5–7 weeks post-feeding at temperatures of 8–14°C, and mortalities peak after two weeks. Outbreaks may last one month, with mortalities up to 70%. Signs include lethargy, anorexia, exophthalmos and corkscrew swimming; gills are pale and internally there is pallor of liver, splenomegaly and an empty gut. Histopathologically there is focal necrosis of the liver, kidney and heart. Long, slender rod-shaped bacteria can be seen in most organs and in smears of spleen, kidney and blood. The disease responds well to antibiotic therapy.

Columnaris disease

All species of freshwater fish world-wide are susceptible to *Chondrococcus columnaris* — fish are a natural reservoir of this bacterium. It is principally a disease of warm-water fish but is well recognised in rainbow trout held at temperatures greater than 14°C, and is associated with stressors such as crowding, handling, external injury etc. The optimum temperature for an outbreak is thought to be 20–30°C. Gills are affected first, exhibiting yellowish necrotic areas progressing from the tips to the base of the filaments. Body lesions appear at the base of the dorsal fin or occasionally the pelvic fins and extend to the body surface as necrotic areas, sometimes with the characteristic appearance of a saddle. The condition may become systemic and invade the kidney. Long, thin bacteria are present in the lesions: they have a tendency to form columns when seen in wet preparations of diseased tissue, and they form dry yellowish colonies on *Cytophaga* agar after 3 days incubation at 20°C.

Bacterial gill disease (BGD)

Several genera, including *Flexibacter*, *Flavobacterium* and *Cytophaga*, have been implicated

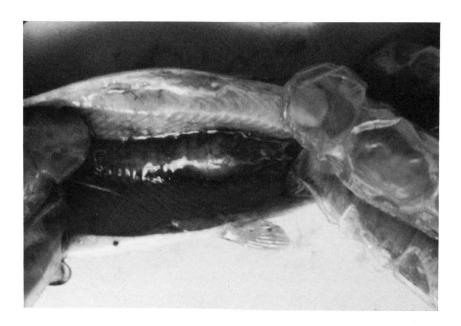

FIG. 14.5 Bacterial kidney disease in a rainbow trout.

in this condition, which is thought to be a secondary infection following gill alteration due to water quality aberration. Rapid extensive colonisation of the gill lamellae by filamentous bacteria occurs, initially at the tips, resulting in lamellar hyperplasia. Mortality levels, due to asphyxia, can often be high. Gills are examined for the presence of clubbing of gill lamellae and masses of long, thin bacteria, especially at the tips of lamellae.

Bacterial kidney disease (BKD)

The causative organism is *Renibacterium salmoninarum*. Most salmonid species in North America, Europe and Japan are susceptible and it has been observed in wild and farmed fish in both freshwater and marine environments. Acute disease is very unusual, and typically this is a chronic systemic infection, seldom manifesting in fish less than 6 months old. Mortality may be significant but is rarely rapid. Signs include anorexia, swollen abdomen, exophthalmos, cloudy cornea and skin ulceration. In rainbow trout skin and eye lesions may be more common than 'typical' kidney lesions. Focal white lesions may be found in kidney, spleen and heart (Fig. 14.5).

Increase in water temperature in the spring seems to serve as an important trigger to infection, and freshwater cage sites typically show clinical disease at this time. Both horizontal and vertical transmission have been shown to occur. High stocking density markedly increases the rate of horizontal spread and poor environmental conditions increase the severity of the clinical episode.

Renibacterium salmoninarum has very fastidious growth requirements and is a very slow growing bacterium. It fails to grow on tryptone soya agar (TSA) at 20°C, even after two weeks incubation. Optimum growth temperature is 15–18°C and up to six weeks incubation may be required. KDM2 medium or SKDM medium are both widely used.

Streptococcosis

Various (unclassified) streptococci are implicated in this disease, which occurs in both freshwater and seawater fish in South Africa, Australia, USA, Japan and Italy. It is of major importance in South Africa and Japan.

The disease is a haemorrhagic septicaemia, usually stress mediated, typically seen at 18–25°C, and signs include exophthalmos, darkening, splenomegaly and haemorrhagic enteritis. Diagnosis is by isolation from a variety of organs on TSA at 25–35°C for 24–48 hours.

Furunculosis

This is mainly a freshwater problem. Rainbow trout are less susceptible than Atlantic salmon and

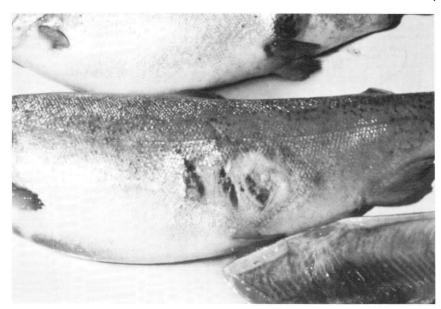

FIG. 14.6 Furuncles on the skin of a rainbow trout.

brown trout. The disease occurs in Europe, America, Asia and South Africa and the organism is *Aeromonas salmonicida* ssp. *salmonicida*, which has long been regarded as an obligate fish pathogen and will persist in carrier fish on an infected farm. Wild fish may serve as the source of infection for a farm, and physical damage, adverse environmental conditions and high stocking density will all increase transmission and infection rate. Clinical disease may occur in sea water when carrier fish are transferred to a marine site and are subjected to abnormal stress factors.

The peracute form of furunculosis usually affects fingerlings: the fish darken and die rapidly, and bacterial foci may be seen in heart, kidney and gill tissue. The acute disease may affect fish at any age. Clinical signs include anorexia, darkening for 2–3 days, and acute haemorrhagic septicaemia. Internally there will be splenomegaly, pale liver and soft kidneys, with haemorrhagic lesions.

In the chronic form, seen in older fish, there is septicaemia with or without furuncles (red, raised, fluid-filled lesions on the flanks — Fig. 14.6) which may ulcerate. Such changes have been reported in association with acute disease in Norway. There may be haemorrhages at the fin bases. Internally there is evidence of intestinal inflammation and haemorrhage in various organs.

A. salmonicida is very difficult to culture from carrier fish. From clinically affected stock, primary isolation should be made from kidney on TSA or brain heart infusion agar (BHIA) at 20–25°C for 24–48 hours. The majority of strains produce a brown diffusing pigment on these media.

Other diseases caused by *A. salmonicida*. Two other subspecies of this bacterium exist, namely ssp. *achromogenes* and ssp. *masoucida*. The former is often termed 'atypical' *A. salmonicida* and causes ulcerative diseases in salmonids and other species in both freshwater and marine environments. The latter has been isolated from salmonid fish in Japan.

A series of disease outbreaks involving heavy losses in fingerling brown trout and sea-trout have been described associated with the achromogenic strain. Signs of disease differed markedly from those of furunculosis. Shallow skin ulcers on the flanks were typical and there was an absence of internal gross pathology.

Motile aeromonad septicaemia

This problem is common world-wide and all freshwater fish species are susceptible. Motile aeromonads are a ubiquitous component of the aquatic environment and also a normal inhabitant of the gut of fish. However, it should be emphasised that the role of motile aeromonads as fish pathogens has not been clearly defined, and they show wide variation in virulence amongst different isolates. The most virulent motile aeromonads belong to *Aeromonas hydrophila* and not *A. sobria*.

Disease occurs most frequently in warm waters with a high organic load, in association with stressors such as handling, parasitism and low oxygen. Signs are of a haemorrhagic septicaemia and include haemorrhages on the flanks and vent and over internal surfaces. Kidney liquefaction is often a feature. In sub-acute and chronic cases, shallow necrotic erosions and ulcers are evident externally. There is necrosis of haematopoietic tissue of kidney and spleen and focal necrosis in heart, liver, pancreas and muscle.

Primary isolation for diagnosis should be made from kidney on TSA incubated at 20–25°C for 24–48 hours. The significance of isolating this organism must be considered with regard to its widespread occurrence in the environment.

Pseudomonad septicaemia

The *Pseudomonas* spp., particularly *P. fluorescens*, are common world-wide, mainly in fresh water, and all species of fish are susceptible. *P. fluorescens* is very common in fresh water with a high organic load. The disease is stress-mediated, manifesting as a haemorrhagic septicaemia. The signs and diagnosis are as for motile *Aeromonas* septicaemia.

Vibriosis

Vibrio anguillarum occurs world-wide, principally in marine environments, and is a major cause of infection in farmed fish and is typically a disease of salmonids in seawater cages. It is usually stress mediated, with haemorrhagic septicaemia. Rainbow trout appear to be more susceptible to infection than Atlantic salmon. The disease is usually seen at temperatures greater than 11°C, and may occur in fresh water when fish are fed marine offal. Clinical signs are virtually indistinguishable from those of other septicaemias and include lethargy, anorexia, congested fin bases and deep necrotic ulcerated skin lesions in more chronic cases. Diagnosis is by isolation of the organism from kidney on TSA with 1% NaCl at 20–25°C for 24–48 hours.

Fungal Diseases

There are very few significant mycotic diseases of rainbow trout.

Saprolegnia *infection*

Saprolegnia infection of dead trout eggs and its subsequent spread to adjacent live eggs can be a serious problem, necessitating the frequent use of malachite green. Systemic infection of yolk-sac fry can also occur and involves all organs. Infection is common in spawning salmonids and precociously mature salmonids, and this effect is thought to be related to sex hormones. Susceptibility to infection can be greatly increased as a result of integument damage (e.g. handling), trauma or primary infections causing skin lesions (e.g. bacterial/parasitic infection).

Signs of the disease include focal grey–white skin patches. The lesions are often circular, extend out radially, and may become brown due to entrapped silt. They are randomly distributed over the body.

Pathology includes superficial dermal necrosis and oedema with epidermal sloughing, resulting in fluid imbalance and circulatory shock. Involvement of muscle layers is rare. Inflammatory responses are weak or absent.

Because of the prolific growth of saprophytic fungi once a fish is dead, isolates must be made from living or freshly-killed fish. Identification is based on the presence of characteristic filaments and sporangia in wet smears; culture is on conventional media.

Ichthyophonus *infection*

The taxonomic classification of this organism as a fungus is now widely accepted. It is an internal obligate pathogen. Infection of rainbow trout occurs via the oral route when fed trash fish, and the effects can be catastrophic. Penetration of the gut mucosa results in invasion of other organs producing a systemic granulomatosis, particularly in liver and heart where it appears as raised white nodules. Each granuloma has a well developed capsule and a significant component of epithelioid cells and macrophages. Trash fish should be steam sterilised or avoided altogether as the only sensible means of control. A marine cage system is open to any locally endemic disease, including *Ichthyophonus*.

Parasitic Diseases

Important parasites in rainbow trout are classified in Fig. 14.7, where they are grouped in accordance with their main areas of attack (skin and gills, gut, skeletal system, viscera and musculature). They are considered here in detail in the same order:

Ichthyobodo (Costia) necatrix

Common world-wide, this is primarily a freshwater parasite but now firmly established as a serious parasite in the marine environment. Many fish species are affected and it is of major importance in fry. The parasite is found on skin and gills causing epithelial hyperplasia and excess mucus production, appearing as a bluish-white film on the body surface. Symptoms include respiratory distress, anorexia, flashing and occasionally sudden death.

Ichthyophthirius multifiliis

This is perhaps the most ubiquitous parasite of freshwater fish and is common world-wide. In the last ten years it has extended north and is now well established in cold water as far as northern Finland. Many fish species are affected.

The disease is known as 'Ich' or 'white spot'. Organisms within the epidermis set up an acute to sub-acute dermatitis with hyperplasia, often producing characteristic white spots — a response typically seen in persistent heavy infections. In primary infestation a high degree of compatibility is maintained between host and parasite. The disease is particularly common at temperatures higher than 17°C and is often associated with adverse water quality. All ages of fish are susceptible but the smaller the fish, the more severe the pathological effects.

Trichodinids

This group of peritrichous ciliates includes *Trichodina, Trichodinella* and *Tripartiella*. They are common world-wide and affect many fish

RAINBOW TROUT: IMPORTANT PARASITES	
Body area	**Parasite**

Skin and gills	Protozoa:
	    Ichthyobodo (Costia) *necatrix*
	    Ichthyophthirius multifiliis
	    Trichodinids *(Trichodina, Trichodinella, Tripartiella)*
	    Chilodonella
	    Paramoeba
	Metazoa:
	    Gyrodactylus
	    Dactylogyrus
	    Argulus
	    Lernaea

Gut	Protozoa: *Hexamita (Octomitus)*
Skeletal system	Protozoa: *Myxosoma cerebralis*

Viscera and musculature	Protozoa:
	    PK'X'
	    Ceratomyxa shasta
	Metazoa:
	    Diplostomum spathaceum
	    Diphyllobothrium

FIG. 14.7 Important parasites of the rainbow trout.

species, in both fresh water and salt water. Freshwater forms are more common on the skin and marine forms on the gills. It is typically a disease of fry and growers resulting in mild sub-acute dermatitis and hyperplasia. Signs include respiratory distress, flashing and jumping. Serious losses in sea cages have occasionally been reported, and the disease is often associated with poor water quality and high stocking density.

Chilodonella

Many fish species world-wide are affected by this parasite. Its effects are similar to those of the trichodinids but gill lamellar hyperplasia is more generalised. It can be a particular problem at 5–10°C.

Paramoeba

These protozoa are found on salmonids farmed in sea water in Tasmania and North America. When temperatures are in the range 12–20°C and salinities approach 35%, all or most of the fish in seawater cages can become infected over several weeks, resulting in up to 50% mortality. The pathology is of a mucoid branchitis and symptoms include anorexia and respiratory distress. Freshwater baths elicit a dramatic recovery.

Gyrodactylus spp.

These are primarily skin parasites, occasionally found on gills, and are common world-wide, affecting many fish species. They can reproduce rapidly if conditions are favourable and the disease often reflects poor husbandry conditions. They are found regularly in association with protozoa. Signs include ragged fins, excess mucus and scale damage. Sporadic outbreaks may occur with a low mortality.

Dactylogyrus spp.

These gill parasites are also common world-wide, and affect many species of fish. The flukes are capable of inducing focal gill hyperplasia and occasionally emaciation when present in high numbers.

Argulus spp.

This branchiuran crustacean is sometimes called the 'fish louse'. Again, it is common world-wide and it affects many freshwater fish species. It is a parasite of the skin and fins and is mainly found in warm, still waters. It is an ocasional parasite of rainbow trout. The life-cycle includes a free-swimming larva which attaches to fish; the adult is able to leave the host and swim freely. When present in large numbers the parasites cause severe local inflammation and epithelial damage and obvious discomfort. They are thought to play a role in the transmission of a number of other diseases.

Lernaea spp.

This copepod crustacean is sometimes called the 'anchor worm' and it affects many host species, world-wide. Focal haemorrhage, ulceration at point of attachment and secondary bacterial infection are not uncommon. The anchor may penetrate vital organs in fish less than 20 mm long. It has been reported that 'heavy' infections of *L. cyprinacea* may cause the death of yearling rainbow trout, although infestation on stocked rainbow trout in a Utah reservoir in the USA did not affect the survival of the stocked fish — probably because the fish were too large for the parasite to penetrate vital organs when first parasitised.

Hexamita (Octomitus)

This protozoan is found in Europe and North America and particularly affects salmonids. It is parasitic in the gall bladder and intestine and has been associated with exophthalmos, distended abdomen, ill thrift and occasional high mortality. It can be found closely apposed to the brush border but with no discernible pathological change in the underlying epithelium.

Myxosoma cerebralis

This major protozoan parasite is a member of the Myxosporea and is of serious economic importance in Europe and America: it is the causative agent of whirling disease. First detected in Europe in 1903, it apparently entered the USA in either live or frozen trout in the early 1950s.

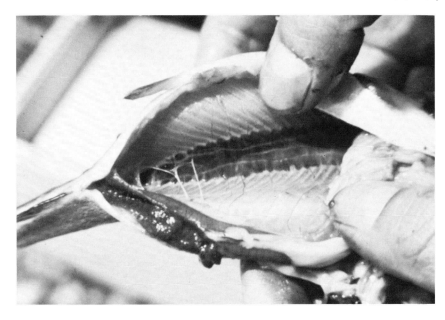

Fig. 14.8 Proliferative kidney disease.

Once within the fish, spores are formed in the cartilage of the head and vertebrae, producing spinal deformities, lysis and typical whirling if the auditory capsules are involved. There may also be altered pigmentation of the posterior half of the body. As cartilage is replaced by bone in growing trout, they become refractory to disease.

The tubifici oligochaete intermediate hosts live in the mud bottoms of earth ponds. To control the problem, therefore, it is now customary to raise trout in troughs, tanks or concrete channels before putting them out into earth ponds at a time when the cartilage has ossified (approximately 8 weeks post-feeding or 6 cm long; if contamination is heavy then 12 weeks or 10 cm long).

Proliferative kidney disease (PKD)

PKD is present in most areas of the world where trout are farmed. Most cases have been diagnosed in rainbow trout but other species of wild and farmed fish have been affected. It is probably the most economically damaging disease affecting UK trout production, causing losses estimated at £1 million in 1986.

PKD is caused by a myxosporean parasite, termed PK'X', and the kidney is its main target organ (see Fig. 14.8). Signs include exophthalmos, abdominal distension with ascites, melanosis and anaemia. Internally the kidneys are grossly enlarged

and mottled; there is pallor of gills and liver, splenic enlargement and occasional petechiation. Histological changes are most marked in the kidney. There is evidence of destruction of renal excretory structures within areas of chronic diffuse inflammation, haematopoietic hyperplasia and occlusion of blood vessels. The heavy host reaction and apparent failure to complete spore development in rainbow trout lends support to the idea that PKX is a myxosporean parasite of some other fish living in the water with juvenile salmonids.

All three kidney functions are impaired — waste excretion, maintenance of fluid balance and blood cell production. Death results from renal failure or anaemia. Mortality can range from 0–90% but may be as low as 2–5% in good quality water conditions and if the water temperature does not remain high for any length of time. However, infected fish are prone to various forms of stress and often succumb to secondary diseases. Recovered fish show almost complete healing.

All fish are susceptible in their first summer in infected water and in the UK fingerling rainbow trout become infected between May and October. On an infected site 100% of trout will carry PKX cells. Clinical disease is seen between 12–18°C and is more rapid and more severe at the higher temperature. In France the disease appears at temperatures lower than 15°C. During the winter, the infectious stage appears to be absent or below the threshold levels necessary to induce infection.

Ceratomyxa shasta

Restricted to the west coast of North America, this parasite mainly affects Chinook salmon (*Oncorhynchus tshawytscha*) and Coho salmon (*O. kisutch*), but also rainbow trout. There may be granulomatous lesions in almost any soft tissue, particularly the intestine, and occasionally body wall musculature. Signs include distended abdomen, exophthalmos and anorexia. Mortality may be high.

Diplostomum spathaceum *(the 'eye fluke')*

The strigeoid metacercariae of this digenetic fluke are found in the retina, vitreous and lens of the eye. The first intermediate hosts are *Lymnaea* spp. of snail and the final host is a piscivorous bird (primarily *Larus* spp.). The fluke attacks species of freshwater fish in Europe and North America, and rainbow trout are particularly susceptible.

Invading cercariae may produce a line of inflammation along the flanks of infected fish, resulting in irritation and flashing. Widespread migration of high numbers of larvae may be lethal. Larval flukes may be found in many tissues but will only

mature in the lens, where several hundred may be found. Generalised cortical liquefaction may occur as the flukes migrate to the anterior cortex of the lens. Signs include cataract, blindness, darkening of affected fish and reduced growth rate (Fig. 14.9). Fish are often found swimming at the sides of ponds.

The failure of cercarial transmission between snail and fish at temperatures below 10°C has been reported, and it has been shown that migration of the diplostomules to the lens rather than penetration of the fish that is inhibited at water temperatures below 10°C. Consequently, infection is a summer phenomenon in temperate climates. The optimum temperature for the establishment of infection in fish is 17.5°C.

Diphyllobothrium *spp.*

There are two species of interest: *Diphyllobothrium dendriticum* and *D. ditremum*. The first intermediate host is usually a copepod crustacean and the final hosts for these two species are piscivorous birds. The pathogenic stage of these cestodes is the plerocercoid.

Diphyllobothrium spp. have been associated with disease in several species of freshwater fish in both Northern Europe and North America. Mortalities in rainbow trout and other salmonids

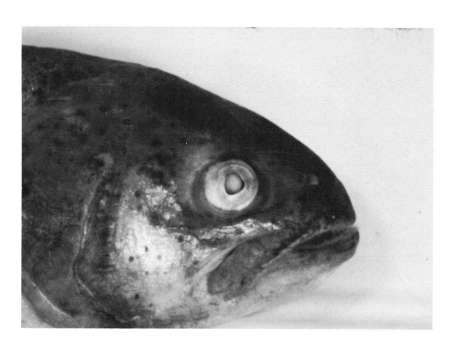

FIG. 14.9 Eye fluke.

in three lakes in Washington, USA, have been described. Mixed infections of *D. dendriticum* and *D. ditremum* have been observed in cultured rainbow trout in Scotland without significant pathological effect. An epidemic in brown trout (*Salmo trutta*) and rainbow trout in a reservoir in Western England caused by plerocercoids of *Diphyllobothrium* spp. has been described. Heavy losses of both species occurred and mortality appeared to be related to the number of plerocercoids present.

The disease is a feature of cage-reared fry and fingerlings in lakes and reservoirs. Some freshwater lakes are unusable for cage culture for this reason. The plerocercoids are found free in the abdomen or in cysts amongst the pyloric caecae, liver, gonads and muscle. The plerocercoids of *D. dendriticum* invoke a significant inflammatory response and a significant humoral response in rainbow trout.

Large numbers may be tolerated without significant effect, although they may act as stressors. However, large numbers in small fish are likely to be associated with some pathology, e.g. visceral adhesions and occasional mortalities. Up to 500 worms may be present in any one fish. No control is possible because of the feeding of trout on natural zooplankton copepods.

Nutritional Diseases

Vitamins

Trout have an absolute requirement for all known water-soluble vitamins (except *p*-aminobenzoic acid) and for vitamins A, E and K among the fat-soluble vitamins (Fig. 14.10). Intensive trout production demands vitamin supplementation of the diet, the stability of which is one of the main factors affecting the diet's shelf life. Several vitamins are susceptible to breakdown during production and storage, e.g. C, B_1, B_2, B_6, E.

Water-soluble vitamins. In general these are present at very low levels in fish diets and are highly vulnerable to leaching in the water before consumption. Fish stores are depleted rapidly, necessitating constant supply to prevent deficiency symptoms. However, the clinical frequency of deficiencies of single water-soluble vitamins is low.

The general features of such deficiencies include poor growth and darkening of the body.

Pyridoxine (B_6) is important in trout because of their high protein requirement; and a deficiency in pantothenic acid affects cells with a high energy expenditure and undergoing mitosis. Fish are unable to synthesise vitamin C from glucuronic acid. The vitamin is necessary for tissue formation and repair (e.g. wound healing), for calcification of bone and for increased disease resistance.

Fat-soluble vitamins. Vitamin A is essential for the normal structure and function of the eye and gill and for the general maintenance of differentiated epithelia. Vitamin D_3 (cholecalciferol) is at least three times as effective as vitamin D_2 (ergocalciferol) in satisfying the requirements of trout for vitamin D. Vitamin K is involved in cellular metabolism.

Vitamin E activity is present in several tocopherols; the most biologically active form is α-tocopherol. One function is as a lipid-soluble anti-oxidant, protecting phospholipid-containing biological membranes. It also protects against the toxic effect of free radicals. High mortalities have been reported in rainbow trout fry 6–10 weeks post-feeding, with evidence of muscle degeneration and necrosis. The lesions were similar to those previously described in salmonids and other species with vitamin E/selenium deficiencies. It was concluded that vitamin E supplementation at 400 IU/kg prevented mortalities and myopathy in rainbow trout fry and that currently recommended minimum requirements for vitamin E may be insufficient under some practical conditions.

Fatty acids

Rainbow trout require a dietary supply of linolenic acid (C_{18}). Trout are able to elongate the carbon chain and further desaturate this fatty acid to the highly unsaturated 20- and 22-carbon fatty acids. Deficiency diseases can be prevented by the addition of 1% linolenic acid (12.3ω3) to purified diets. Deficiency signs include poor growth rate, caudal fin erosion and shock syndrome.

Lipoid liver degeneration (LLD)

This disease is associated with the feeding of rancid diets low in vitamin E (typically diets

VITAMIN DEFICIENCY			
Vitamin	Requirements (mg/kg diet)	Deficiency signs	Notes/risks
Water-soluble Thiamine (B$_1$)	10	Anaemia Aberrant swimming Convulsions Eye pathology	High levels of thiaminase in many fresh fish (e.g. clupeids) Losses during storage
Riboflavin (B$_2$)	5–15	Anorexia Reduced growth Cataract and corneal changes	Leaching into water Losses during storage
Pyridoxine (B$_6$)	5–15	Erratic and spiral swimming, epileptiform seizures	
Pantothenic acid	40	Anorexia Low growth rate Ocular changes and gill disease Gills become clogged and exudate-covered, the lamellae fuse and show epithelial hyperplasia especially at the distal end of filaments	Leaching into water
Niacin	150	A type of photosensitisation or sunburn following ultraviolet exposure	
Biotin	1.0	High mortality Short clubbed gill lamellae Blue slime disease	Deficiencies are very rare
Cyanocobalamin (B$_{12}$)	0.02	Anaemia	
Folic acid	5	Severe anaemia	
Vitamin C (ascorbic acid)	100	Spinal lordosis and scoliosis Opercular and lamellar deformation Increased susceptibility to fracture Failure of wound healing Haemorrhages around eyes	Leaching into water Losses during production (up to 40%) and storage (up to 90%) More stable forms of ascorbic acid are now being added to fish diets
Fat-soluble Vitamin A	Young trout 2500–5000	Anaemia Twisted gill opercula Exophthalmos Corneal and retinal pathology	
Vitamin D	1600–2400	Poor growth Increased liver lipid Tetany of white skeletal muscle	
Vitamin E	30 IU/kg diet of vitamin E acetate in the presence of adequate selenium	Anaemia Ascites Mortality	
Vitamin K	5–10	Anaemia Visceral haemorrhage	

FIG. 14.10 Vitamin deficiency signs and risks in trout.

containing high levels of unsaturated, readily oxidisable fats) and has been described as a significant problem in rainbow trout on Norwegian fish farms. It has been shown that the addition of α-tocopherol and vitamin C to rancid diets prevents the development of LLD and microcytic anaemia.

The main feature is the accumulation of ceroid in hepatocytes, causing a homogenous yellow-orange discoloration of the liver. Death results from the cumulative effects of liver dysfunction and anaemia due to increased red blood cell fragility. Mild cases may show a complete recovery. Significant pseudobranch pathology has been noted in association with LLD in rainbow trout.

Pansteatitis

This describes a generalised inflammatory infiltration of adipose tissues. It is associated with the feeding of certain types of fish oil or unsaturated fatty acids of fish origin in a diet poor in vitamin E, and may be a reflection of disordered fat metabolism. The main presenting signs are swimming aberrations, discoloration and high mortality after minimal stress. The swim-bladder is often swollen and full of viscous fluid. Histopathological lesions are found in the brain, heart, spleen, kidney, skin, skeletal muscle and invariably in the pancreas and swim-bladder.

Nutritional eye diseases

Vitamins B_1, B_2 and A, the amino acid methionine and zinc have all been associated with eye pathology. Vitamin premixes added to feeds generally contain ample B_1, B_2 and A, and so deficiencies are rare today, but amino acid or mineral deficiencies are still possible as some feed manufacturers may be forced to change to inadequately tested ingredients.

The eye pathology related to vitamin A deficiency is unique in being the only nutritional eye pathology of salmonids that involves exophthalmos and the retina as well as the cornea. No true cataract is formed. B_1 deficiency is associated with clouding of the cornea, leading to total blindness, whilst B_2 deficiency results in cataract formation originating in the post-subcapsular lens cortex with some involvement of the cornea, which becomes progressively thin and cloudy.

The cataract associated with zinc deficiency is the only cataract shown to have a developmental pattern which varies with the age of the fish. Methionine deficiency is also associated with cataract formation, resembling that seen in vitamin B_2 deficiency. However, there is no corneal involvement.

Aflatoxicosis

Aspergillis flavus is a blue-green mould capable of growing on oil-seeds and producing toxic metabolites which act as potent carcinogens in trout. Aflatoxin at 0.01 parts per billion produces neoplastic change (malignant hepatocellular carcinoma) in rainbow trout over a relatively short period. The tumour can involve biliary and vascular tissue and occasionally metastasises to spleen, kidney and gills. Acute exposure to aflatoxin may produce a generalised haemorrhagic syndrome or acute liver necrosis.

Feed compounders are aware of the need for great care in the selection and storage of oil-seeds. The condition is now rarely seen except in developing countries where the storage of seeds in humid, tropical conditions is still a serious problem.

Clinical Diagnosis

A thorough diagnostic investigation of any disease outbreak will require the full range of veterinary skills, i.e. epidemiology, clinical examination, post-mortem and laboratory examination.

No single sign is specific for any one condition and not all signs are present in every case of disease. However, a good clinical history and clinical examination provide a vital first impression before laboratory results are complete.

Epidemiological Considerations

Factors to be taken into account include water quality (temperature, oxygen, pH, flow rates and salinity changes) and management practices such as stocking density, feeding rates, changes in feeding practices and recent on-farm usage of chemicals. Good record-keeping is essential. Mortality rates are of particular interest, and mortality patterns can be revealing:

Sudden high mortality — toxic insult or sudden water quality deterioration.
Mortality rising steadily to peak followed by steady fall — typical of bacterial or viral infection.
Chronic losses over an extended period — typical of a parasite problem.

FIG.   14.11 Post-mortem findings.

POST-MORTEM FINDINGS		
Organ	**Post-mortem finding**	**Probable cause**
Kidney	Focal or diffuse swelling	BKD, PKD, nephrocalcinosis
Liver	Haemorrhage/congestion	Bacterial/viral septicaemia
Spleen	Congestion and enlargement	ERM, furunculosis, 'fry mortality syndrome'
Heart	Inflammation	Streptococcosis
	Focal nodules	BKD
Gut	Contents mucoid and bloodstained	Bacterial septicaemia
	Contents mucoid, thick or thin:	IPN
	Nodules on wall	Larval parasites
	White membrane around gut or other organs	BKD, streptococcosis
Muscle	Cysts or granulomata	Parasite infection
	Focal nodules	Tumour
	Haemorrhage	Bacterial/viral septicaemia

Clinical Diagnosis

Behavioural changes

- Increased activity at surface/gulping.
- Crowding at inlets/outlets.
- Listlessness on surface or at edges.
- Flashing or scraping.
- Abnormal swimming — whirling or spiralling.
- Inappetence.

Gross pathology

- *Cataract* — eye fluke, nutritional deficiency.
- *Exophthalmos* — BKD, nephrocalcinosis, gas-bubble disease.
- *Fin and tail erosion* — external protozoa, *Flexibacter/Cytophaga* infection.
- *Swollen abodmen* — BKD, PKD, neoplasia, bacterial/viral septicaemia.
- *Skin ulceration/haemorrhage* — bacterial/viral septicaemia, BKD.
- *'Cotton-wool' growth on skin* — *Saprolegnia*.
- *Trailing faecal casts* — bacterial/viral infection.

Post-mortem Examination

See Fig 14.11 for a summary of post-mortem findings.

Therapy

Fish diseases are caused by a wide range of infectious organisms. Viral diseases are not susceptible to control by chemotherapy. The control of fish parasites, particularly ectoparasites, by chemotherapy is feasible but the range of available treatments is limited and there are environmental problems associated with their use. Systemic parasite infections, e.g. *Myxosporidia* and *Microsporidia*, are much more refractory to treatment and effective chemotherapeutants are lacking.

There is increasing recognition of the need to regulate the use of chemotherapeutants in aquaculture. A more responsible approach has been encouraged in recent years and this has seen a surge of interest in areas such as drug kinetics, tissue residue levels, environmental impact etc.

Despite the wide range of drugs now available in human and veterinary medicine, the range of medicines licensed for aquaculture use is very limited. Current legislation for the licensing of new products is complicated, expensive and slow and the next decade is unlikely to see many new licensed products.

Therapy of Viral Diseases

No effective chemotherapeutants are available for use in aquaculture and control must rely on other management techniques, as already described. The effect of ultraviolet (uv) irradiation on fish pathogenic viruses has been studied and infectious haematopoietic virus has been shown to be particularly sensitive to UV but the susceptibility of infectious pancreatic necrosis virus was found to be low.

Therapy of Bacterial Diseases

Tetracyclines

Oxytetracycline is the most widely used but resistance is widely encountered, and residues may persist for several weeks under medicated fish cages. Recommended withdrawal times vary from 350–500 degree-days. There is a bio-availability of 5.6% at oral doses of 75 mg/kg.

Potentiated sulphonamides

These have been widely used in many countries in the last 15 years, and resistant strains of bacteria have begun to emerge in recent years. Recommended withdrawal times vary from 350–400 degree-days.

Quinolones

First-generation quinolones are active against Gram-negative organisms; second-generation quinolones show extended antibacterial activity. Bacterial resistance develops quite rapidly to first-generation quinolones (e.g. nalidixic acid, flumequine and oxolinic acid). Only low frequency chromosomal mutational resistance to the newer quinolones has been recognised and is not thought to be a significant clinical problem. Plasmid-mediated resistance does not occur.

Recommended withdrawal time is 500 degree-days, and under medicated cages oxolinic acid residues disappear within one week of the end of therapy. The bio-availability of oxolinic acid is 13.6% at an oral dose of 75 mg/kg. A dose of 10–30 mg/kg fish is generally recommended.

Nitrofurans

Drugs such as furazolidone and nifurpirinol have been widely used for many years, but use is now discouraged as a result of the link between nitrofurans and oncogenic and mutagenic compounds. Nitrofurans also show anti-protozoal activity and are used successfully to control *Hexamita* infections.

Erythromycin

This is considered the drug of choice for the control and treatment of bacterial kidney disease (see 'Preventive Measures'). Optimum dosages and durations and types of treatment for the maximum clearance of the pathogen from the host and the maximum reduction of mortality still need to be determined. There is evidence that *Renibacterium salmoninarum* can gain resistance to erythromycin.

Benzalkonium chloride

This has strong antibacterial properties and is used widely for the control or suppression of bacterial gill disease. Therapeutic levels approach toxic levels, particularly in soft water, and fish may die from the treatment.

Chloramine-T

This is an effective chemical for the control of Bacterial Gill Disease (BGD), and toxic levels are well above treatment levels. It is also an effective protozoacide and fungicide.

When stressors such as concomitant parasite infestations or low oxygen levels are present a second and possibly a third treatment may be necessary.

Therapy of Fungal Diseases

Most fungal infections of rainbow trout are external and are thought to be secondary or opportunistic invaders. Fungal infections of hatchery-reared fish have been adequately controlled for many years with formalin or malachite green. However, because of concern over the toxicity of these two fungicides, potential alternatives are being sought. In the USA, formalin is the only registered aquatic fungicide; malachite green is not approved for use and is unlikely to be registered because of its potential teratogenicity.

The use of formalin and salt is described below in 'Therapy of Parasitic Diseases'.

Malachite green

This organic dye is a very effective fungicide at extremely low concentrations and has been widely used for over 50 years. No effective alternative has yet been found. It is estimated that over 1,000 kg p.a. are used in the United Kingdom.

Malachite green is available as the oxalate or hydrochloride salt and should be zinc-free for aquaculture use. However, there is great potential for variation in the origin and quality of the dye. This may explain the wide diversity in concentration and exposure times suggested by different workers over the years. It may be used either as a bath or flush treatment, taking care to ensure even distribution and adequate aeration. Recommended dosages, using 50% malachite green, include:

Bath (1 hour):   Fry and fingerlings: 4 ppm
                 Adults: 2 ppm
Flush: Eggs: 4 ppm for 1 hour using a
                 continuous drip.
                 Earth pond: 10 ppm added
                 gradually over 2 hours.

However, Alderman (1985) suggests that an achieved 1.0–2.0 ppm active ingredient exposure in a flush treatment should be adequate for all normal situations in rainbow trout culture.

Therapy of Parasitic Diseases

With very few exceptions, the limited range of chemicals available has been in use for many years.

Malachite green

Malachite green is also an effective anti-protozoal agent and it acts synergistically with formalin. Use at 0.1 ppm. Two or three doses may be added over a period of 7–10 days.

Formalin

Formalin (a solution of 40% formaldehyde) is used extensively for external parasite infections, especially protozoa. It should be stored in dark containers, and discarded if any white precipitate (*para*-formaldehyde) is present. Formalin itself is an irritant and may induce significant gill damage: aerate during treatment and reduce dose levels at high water temperatures.

It acts synergistically with malachite green. For treatment of *Ichthyophthirius*, at least one re-treatment after three days is required to ensure eradication of the parasite.

Recommended dosages:

Hard water: 250 ppm for 1 hour
Soft water: 160 ppm for 1 hour
Elevated water temperatures: 125–150 ppm for 1 hour
As a long-term treatment for ponds: 15–25 ppm.

Organophosphates

Two applications, one week apart, are usually sufficient to treat monogenetic trematodes and crustaceans. Note that resistant strains of parasites may develop. Organophosphates are not licensed for use with food fish and there is concern regarding the safety of handlers, fish and the environment.

Metronidazole and related compounds

These are used to treat intestinal infections with the flagellate *Hexamita* but are not licensed for this use. They are added to food at 0.25–1% for three days or dissolved in water at 5 ppm of active ingredient.

Salt

Sodium chloride is used as a 3% bath for removal of external parasites and fungi. Treatment time should not exceed 30 minutes and should be terminated at the first signs of stress.

Chloramine-T

This chemical is active against protozoa and monogenetic trematodes. (See 'Therapy of Bacterial Diseases' above.)

Prevention of Disease

With problems of antibiotic resistance, legal constraints on the use of chemotherapeutants and their cost, the old adage 'prevention is better than cure' was never more valid than today.

Reduction of Stress

If a fish cannot avoid or overcome stress, its stress response will be both prolonged and exaggerated and its state of health will be impaired. Stressors include management procedures such as

ANTIMICROBIALS USED IN TREATMENT OF TROUT DISEASES		
Antimicrobials	**Dose (in food for 10 days unless stated)**	**Disease**
Benzalkonium chloride	1–2 mg/l of water for 1 hr	Bacterial gill disease
Chloramine-T	8.5 mg/l of water for 1 hr	Bacterial gill disease
Chlortetracycline	50–75 mg/kg fish	Bacterial septicaemia
Erythromycin	25–100 mg/kg fish	BKD, streptococcal infection
Flumequine	6–12 mg/kg fish	Bacterial septicaemia
Furazolidone	25–75 mg/kg fish for 10–20 days	Bacterial septicaemia
Nifurpirinol	10–50 mg/kg fish	Bacterial septicaemia
Oxolinic acid	5–10 mg/kg fish	Bacterial septicaemia
Oxytetracycline	50–75 mg/kg fish	Bacterial septicaemia, streptococcal infection
Potentiated sulphonamide	30–60 mg/kg fish	Bacterial septicaemia
Sulphonamides	200 mg/kg fish	Bacterial septicaemia
* Dose given as active component per kilogram of fish		

FIG. 14.12 Antimicrobials used in treatment of trout disease.

netting, grading, handling, vaccination, chemotherapy, transport and sudden temperature shock. They also include environmental factors such as overcrowding, poor water quality, social interaction between fish and exposure to new holding facilities. Many of these procedures are unavoidable but sensible precautions would include the following:

- Reduce time taken to net, grade and transport.
- Carry out potentially stressful procedures in colder months (but not necessarily vaccination).
- If repeated stresses are unavoidable, allow sufficient recovery period between them.
- Withdraw food 2–3 days prior to a stressful procedure, to reduce oxygen requirement.
- Use mild anaesthesia to promote survival during severe stress.
- Use dilute salt solutions (approx. 5 g/l NaCl) during severe stress to reduce stress response.
- Avoid exposure to water-borne pollutants. A facility to shut off water-flow temporarily and to aerate the water is useful.

Recommended Management Practices

Management practices conducive to fish health include the following:

- Buy stock from disease-free sources, and disinfect ova.
- Use quarantine procedures.
- Keep accurate farm records (e.g. flow rates, temperature, pH, ammonia, feed levels and stocking densities).
- Store feed properly and use before expiry date.
- In the hatchery, check regularly for parasites and also for damaged tails (sensitive indicators of stocking density and water quality).
- Pick out dead eggs and discard bad batches.
- At first feeding, the timing, feed size, rate and distribution are critical to avoid starvation.
- Earth ponds should be dried and disinfected at least once a year.

Disinfectants

Iodophors are good for farm use, diluted to 250 ppm available iodine as a general disinfectant and 100 ppm for disinfecting ova. However, organic matter and soil will reduce or completely neutralise the effects and they are not recommended for ponds. Transport tanks should be disinfected after use, and nets and graders washed and disinfected before use in different ponds and tanks. For egg disinfection, the pH of the iodophor is adjusted and buffered to 6–7.5 with sodium bicarbonate (proprietary preparations are available). Eggs are immersed for 10 minutes with occasional agitation and then rinsed thoroughly in clean running water. Use 1 volume eggs to 10 volumes disinfectant. This is effective against the major fish viruses but will not penetrate the egg membrane, thus allowing IPN to survive.

Vaccination

Vaccines have become accepted as a major tool in fish disease control, following their introduction into the USA in 1976. In the last few years they have been licensed and are in widespread commercial use in most European, Scandinavian and many other countries world-wide. This is inevitable in view of the widespread misuse of antibiotics and the increased concern about the environmental impact of chemical usage. In the UK, about 80% of trout farms use vaccines directly, or indirectly as a result of purchasing vaccinated stock.

Vaccines against vibriosis, enteric redmouth and furunculosis are currently available, whilst vaccines against columnaris disease and *Aeromonas hydrophila* septicaemia may soon be available. In terms of efficacy, the vaccines against ERM and vibriosis are highly effective but there is still some concern over the effectiveness of furunculosis vaccines as the protection afforded is by no means high. Many technical problems have been encountered with viral vaccines but hope lies with the fast developing technology of genetic engineering. Because of the pressure on anti-parasite treatments, work on anti-parasite vaccines is continuing apace and the long term looks optimistic. The development of a commercial vaccine against *Ichthyophthirius* infection is a distinct possibility, but much work remains to be done before a vaccine against *Ichthyobodo necatrix* is developed.

Reasons for vaccine breakdown have been cited as poor husbandry/excess stress; fish sick or in poor condition (especially gill damage plus immersion vaccines); fish too small (optimum size 4.5 g+); insufficient time allowed for immunity to develop (protective immunity takes 14–21 days to develop at 10°C); or short-cuts in procedure.

Chemo-prophylaxis

Whilst in general the administration of chemo-therapeutants, especially antibiotics, to a group of healthy fish is not recommended, there are specific instances where the procedure may be of value. The following regimes have been suggested.

Proliferative kidney disease (PKD)

If malachite green therapy is commenced at the first visible signs of kidney enlargement, three doses of 100 ppm-minutes duration will prevent any further development of disease in that year. However, tissue residues may persist, and a withdrawal period of 600 degree-days is suggested. This treatment regime is unsuitable in warmer parts of France due to high water temperatures and pH factors. Treatment must be continued weekly for up to 6 months, making control more difficult.

Bacterial kidney disease (BKD)

This is among the most difficult of bacterial fish diseases to control. The pathology and epizootiology remain poorly understood. Avoidance is the best control, remembering that both vertical and horizontal transmission are possible. Broodstock should be tested free of infection, using coelomic fluid in the female and injected with 20 mg pure erythromycin/kg prior to spawning, resulting in significant intra-ovum antibiotic levels. After spawning, the eggs are surface disinfected with iodophor, and the fry may be treated with erythromycin shortly after first feeding.

More research is needed to optimise adult injection regimens for the accumulation and retention of the antibiotic in the eggs. Controlled studies in hatcheries are also necessary to assess the value of the procedure for preventing vertical transmission. To avoid horizontal transmission, different age groups should be kept well segregated on a farm, and the farm disinfected during any fallow period.

Further Reading

Textbooks

Roberts, R. J. and Shepherd, C. J. (1986) *Handbook of Trout and Salmon Diseases*. (2nd edn) Fishing News Books, Blackwell Scientific Publications Ltd, Oxford.
Stevenson, J. P. (1987) *Trout Farming Manual*. (2nd edn) Fishing News Books, Blackwell Scientific Publications Ltd, Oxford.
Sedgwick, S. D. (1990) *Trout Farming Handbook*. (5th edn) Fishing News Books, Blackwell Scientific Publications Ltd, Oxford.
Solbe, J. (1988) *Water Quality for Salmon and Trout*. The Atlantic Salmon Trust, Pitlochry, Perthshire.

Publications and Journals

Fish Farmer
Fish Farming International
Trout News (Directorate of Fisheries Research, MAFF, England)
Journal of Fish Diseases
Bulletin of the European Association of Fish Pathologists
Diseases of Aquatic Organisms
Journal of Aquatic Animal Health
The Progressive Fish Culturist
Journal of the Fisheries Research Board of Canada
Journal of Fish Biology

References

Alderman, D. J. (1985) Malachite green: a review. *Journal of Fish Diseases* **8**, 289–298.

Lorenzen, E., Dalsgaard, I., From, J., Hansen, E. M., Hørlyck, V., Korsholm, H., Mellergaard, S. and Olesen, N. J. (1991) Preliminary investigation of Fry Mortality Syndrome in rainbow trout. *Bulletin of the European Association of Fish Pathologists* **11(2)**, 77–78.

Pickering, A. D. (1989) Fish husbandry and stress. *Trout News* **8**, 12–14.

15

The Veterinary Approach to Channel Catfish

MIKE JOHNSON

Farming channel catfish (*Ictalurus punctatus*) is a relatively young industry, but much of the groundwork that led to the industry's popularity and rapid growth was developed before the 1960s. Channel catfish were cultured as early as 1910 by the Kansas State Fish Hatchery and the first reported spawning in captivity was in 1892. Much of the pioneering work for use of the species in small-scale aquaculture was conducted at Auburn University in the 1950s by Dr Homer Swingle and his students. Prior to Swingle's work, most of the channel catfish fry produced were raised in federal and state hatcheries to stock public reservoirs or sport-fishing ponds.

The initial growth in farm-raised channel catfish occurred in Arkansas during the early to mid 1960s. The state's production reached an early peak of approximately 7 million kg of fish from 4047 ha of ponds in 1966. The subsequent decrease in production was attributed to the lack of a supporting infrastructure (feed mills, marketing, processing, etc.) to develop and promote further growth.

In Mississippi, only channel catfish fingerlings were raised commercially before 1965. The state's commercial production of farm-raised channel catfish began that year with a single pond of 16 ha. The growth of the industry has been rapid, increasing 2400% since 1975. During 1991 over 186,000 metric tons of food-size catfish were sold compared to about 2,600 metric tons in 1975.

Channel catfish are raised in over 68,000 ha of ponds located in at least 17 American states. Mississippi is by far the largest producer, with over 41,278 ha of catfish ponds, and many factors make it an ideal state for the purpose. There are large tracts of flat land well suited for pond construction and soils rich in clay, with abundant high quality water supplies from aquifers close to the surface. The climate provides a catfish growing season of more than 200 days, and the larger farms can afford the initial large capital investment of approximately $10,000 per ha. There are also five major feed mills, many hatcheries, and numerous processing plants — all important components of a successful growing agriculture industry.

Farming Systems

At present the pond culture of fish and shrimp is the most popular aquaculture system in the world, and more than 95% of the channel catfish in the United States are produced in ponds. Ponds offer an inexpensive natural ecosystem that degrades fish waste products and supplies oxygen by diffusion and photosynthesis. However, for pond culture to be successful and competitive, the growing season must be long and the land inexpensive. Pond culture requires large tracts of flat land (Fig. 15.1) with soils high in clay content to hold water. Additionally, the water source must be of high quality and of adequate and dependable supply.

Pond Types

There are two types of pond used in channel catfish production: watershed ponds and levee ponds. Levee ponds are by far the most common; they are similar to irrigated rice fields but are rectangular in shape and the four embankments are much higher. The ponds are relatively shallow, with level bottoms, and the water source is usually a shallow aquifer (ground-water). Most watershed ponds are irregular in shape and usually have one main levee in the dam; they may be relatively

FIG. 15.1 Aerial view of channel catfish ponds in the Mississippi Delta.

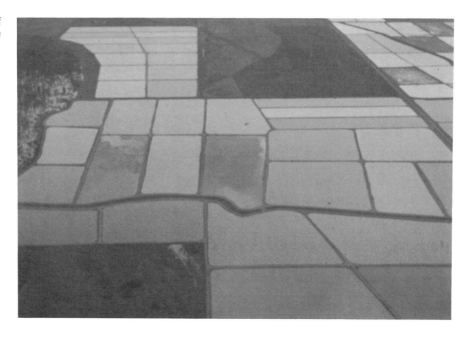

shallow on one side and 3–4 m deep near the drain. The water source is usually entirely from run-off, although pumped water from streams, reservoirs, or aquifers is sometimes used.

Site Selection

Large tracts of flat land allow ponds to be built adjacent to each other, which makes construction and management more economical. Soil composition should be at least 20% clay. Sandy soils or areas with limestone streaks and gravel beds may cause excessive seepage of water and should be avoided. Constantly adding water to leaky ponds not only adds to the production costs but may also affect the incidence of certain diseases that are strongly temperature-dependent (see Enteric Septicaemia). Land previously used for crops should be tested for pesticide levels, especially in the low areas of the fields where water collects. Watershed ponds should be built to avoid run-off from lands used for agriculture. Some herbicides may not directly affect the fish but are highly toxic to phytoplankton, thus creating an oxygen depletion.

Pond sites should be away from rivers and streams that may overflow the levees. Flooding of ponds will allow fish to escape, contaminate ponds with trash fish, and possibly introduce pollutants

and disease organisms. Pond site selection should allow for proper drainage and all ponds should be capable of being drained completely without the effluent entering another pond.

Pond Size

Most levee ponds are about 7 ha of water built on about 8 ha of land. Most producers build units of four 7 ha ponds on 32 ha of land, and water is supplied to all four ponds in one unit by one central well. However, there are many variations in pond size depending on topography, production goals, type of farm (fingerling or food fish), construction costs, property lines and personal preference. Fingerling ponds and broodstock ponds range from 0.8 to 4 ha; food fish ponds average 5 to 10 ha.

There are advantages and disadvantages to using large ponds for catfish production. Large ponds (greater than 4 ha) are proportionally less expensive to build because less land is devoted to levee construction. Oxygenation of the water is greater in large ponds, because waves increase surface area for gas transfer, but wave-induced erosion of levees is more severe. Water quality problems, such as low dissolved oxygen concentrations and high levels of ammonia or nitrite, are easier to manage in small ponds. Diseases are more manageable in small ponds because it is easier to detect the initial stages of an epizootic, treatments are easier to administer, and disease outbreaks are more likely to be contained. Harvesting fish from small ponds is more efficient and manageable because smaller numbers are involved.

The average pond depth is 0.9–1.2 m and the optimum depth is 1.2 m. Deeper, sheltered ponds are more prone to thermal stratification in summer and thus are more likely to suffer from oxygen depletion. Wind is usually sufficient to prevent stratification in shallow ponds and oxygen from the air is more likely to be mixed throughout the water column. Shallow ponds are also easier to harvest.

Water Source

The quality and quantity of the water source dictates the profitability of a channel catfish operation and determine the size, type and management of a farm. Ground-water is the best source for a levee pond operation: it is usually free from pollutants and wild fish. The absence of wild fish greatly decreases the chance for fish pathogens to enter ponds through the water source. Ground-water is usually devoid of oxygen, but is quickly oxygenated once it is pumped into a pond.

Intensive culture of channel catfish requires large amounts of high quality water. Wells supplying 7,500–11,000 litres/minute are required for four 7 ha ponds.

Some optimal and tolerated ranges of water quality parameters for channel catfish are listed in Fig. 15.2. These values are only guidelines, since variables such as fish health, age and size need to be considered. Additionally, interaction of these variables needs to be considered on a daily basis before recommending optimal levels.

General Husbandry

Species Selection

There are at least 50 species of the family Ictaluridae in North and Central America. Channel catfish is the most commercially important Ictalurid species in the United States because it possesses several traits that make it a good species for culture. It does not reproduce readily in a culture pond environment, yet reproduction can be controlled because it is very easy to spawn. Sufficient numbers of fry are produced yearly for restocking and the fry readily accept artificially prepared feeds at 3 days of age. Channel catfish are a hardy fish; they tolerate crowding and adapt well to various culture environments. Finally the most important attribute of the farm-raised channel catfish is its mild flavour, light texture and lack of fishy odour.

Channel catfish account for almost all the farm-raised catfish in the United States but blue catfish (*Ictalurus furcatus*) is a potentially valuable commercial species. Some strains of blue catfish grow at about the same rate or faster than channel catfish to the size desired by commercial processors (0.5–0.7 kg), after which blue catfish grow faster. The dressing-out percentage of blue catfish is higher at 60–62% compared with 58–62% for channel catfish. Blue catfish are more resistant to

WATER QUALITY PARAMETERS FOR CHANNEL CATFISH		
Variable	**Optimal level**	**Tolerated level**
Salinity	0.5–3 ppt	0.01–8 ppt
Temperature 24–14°C	0–40°C	
Dissolved oxygen	5–15 ppm	2 ppm–300% saturation
Total alkalinity	20–400 ppm as $CaCO_3$	<1 to >400 ppm as $CaCO_3$
Total hardness	20–400 ppm as $CaCO_3$	<1 to >400 ppm as $CaCO_3$
Carbon dioxide	0 ppm	Depends on dissolved oxygen concentration
pH	6–9	5–10
Un-ionised ammonia	0	<0.2 ppm as N
Nitrite	0	Depends on chloride concentration

Fig. 15.2 Water quality parameters for channel catfish. Note: Prolonged exposure to non-optimal conditions may be tolerated but can result in reduced growth, impaired reproductive performance, or increased susceptibility to disease. *Source*: Tucker and Robinson (1991).

Edwardsiella ictaluri infections and channel catfish virus, but are more susceptible to the parasites *Ichthyopthirius* and the bacterium *Cytophaga columnaris*. Blue catfish are easier to harvest but do not grade well and have sharp spines making them more difficult to handle. They require a year longer to reach sexual maturity and are more difficult to breed because of the large size of broodfish (5–13 kg).

Other species of catfish have been cultured commercially, but each species has one or more characteristic that limits its economic importance. Flathead catfish (*Pylodictus oliveris*) are very important as predator species in reservoirs, lakes, and rivers but are extremely cannibalistic, making them unprofitable for aquaculture. White catfish (*Ictalurus catus*) is the most hardy of all but grows slower and has a poorer dressing-out percentage than channel catfish. Bullheads (*Ictalurus nebolosus*) and other species are more tolerant of poor water quality than most other ictalurids, but grow slowly and have a low dressing-out percentage.

Broodstock Management

The ultimate goal of any animal production facility is improved production efficiency and higher yields. One way to accomplish this is through the use of proper breeding programmes. The livestock and poultry industries are testimonials to the success of good, sound breeding programmes. However, the relatively young channel catfish farming industry has yet to take significant advantage of the improved biological potential that selective breeding programmes can provide.

At present, many managers unintentionally select broodstock with undesirable traits. Selection is often based simply on certain phenotypic traits, such as size. The source of these broodstock are food fish ponds that have been through several production cycles. Fish of various year classes and sizes may be in the same pond. In selecting broodstock by size from these ponds, the manager may inadvertently be selecting for slow-growing fish that are adept at escaping the seine.

Producers should try to develop a sound breeding programme based on some minimal guidelines in selecting broodstock for reliable spawning:

- Select broodstock of at least 3 years of age and weighing 1.5 kg. Channel catfish of 4–6 years

of age weighing between 1.8 and 3.6 kg are excellent spawners. Older, heavier fish are more difficult to handle and produce fewer eggs in proportion to body-weight.
- Select domestic broodstock. Wild fish are less likely to be reliable spawners.
- Avoid selecting fish with a history of exposure to channel catfish virus and *Edwardsiella ictaluri* epizootics.
- Select only fish of a known age.
- Select males and females from different ponds and preferably from different farms. This helps avoid inbreeding.
- Keep accurate records of spawning success, fry survival, and growth rates of fingerlings and food fish. If possible, try to keep records on disease outbreaks in groups of fingerlings.

Brood fish should be sexed annually so that the proper ratio of males and females can be stocked in each pond. Males and females are identified by their secondary sex characteristics; it is simpler if the fish are mature and if they are examined during or just prior to the breeding season. Males have a thickened, broad, muscular head with thickened lips, and are more darkly pigmented on the lower jaws and abdomen. The urogenital pore of the male forms a fleshy papilla and serves for both sperm and urine release. The female has a more slender head and a robust, well-rounded, white abdomen. The genital opening of the female is separate from the urinary pore but both lie in a groove or slit covered by folds of skin. A small probe can be used to sex smaller fish by determining whether the genital and urinary pores are separate or common.

Female channel catfish spawn once a year; males can spawn two or three times. Most large-scale fingerling producers stock broodstock ponds with male to female ratios of 2:3 or 1:2. Optimal spawning success can be obtained by following the guidelines below:

- Move the broodstock each year into ponds that have been drained and refilled.
- Place broodstock in ponds with very little perimeter traffic.
- Sex and move broodstock in the late winter or early spring when water temperatures are cool to minimise handling stress.

- Broodstock should be on a good plane of nutrition all year.
- Stocking rates of broodstock should be less than 2,000 kg/ha to optimise spawning success.

Channel catfish spawn when the water temperature remain consistently above 21°C. Sudden drops below 21°C or increases above 30°C may cause the fish to abandon their nests. Spawning only occurs in sheltered areas or special 'spawning containers' such as milk cans, ammunition cans, or small kegs or drums. Spawning containers are not placed into the broodstock ponds until water temperatures have stabilised. This minimises the chances of obtaining early spawns, which often contain many infertile eggs. Two or three containers are used per four pairs of broodstock since not all fish will spawn at once. Containers are checked every other day for the presence of spawn. Approximately 6,000 eggs/kg of female are produced. The male remains in the container to protect and oxygenate the fertilised eggs. Spawns are removed from the container as soon as they are found and are transported to a hatchery.

Egg and Fry Production

Commercial hatcheries in Mississippi generally operate for approximately 10 weeks beginning in late April or early May. Optimal temperatures for hatching eggs and rearing fry are 25–28°C. Lower temperatures delay the hatching time and lead to fungal invasion of the egg masses. Temperatures greater than 28°C may promote congenital defects in the embryo, increase the incidence of invasion of the eggs by bacteria, or increase the incidence of channel catfish virus epizootics in the fry.

Water supply is an important consideration in designing a hatchery. Although either surface or ground-water sources are used, ground-water is preferred: its quality and temperature are constant, the water is free of turbidity, and it is less likely to be contaminated with pesticides. The water source should be of sufficient hardness (greater than 5 ppm calcium as $CaCO_3$) to promote hatching success and fry survival and vigour.

Egg masses are usually dipped in a 10% betadine solution before being placed in the egg-hatching trough in baskets, typically constructed of galvanised or rubber-coated hardware cloth. Slowly rotating paddles or bubbles from airstones create a current that circulates fresh oxygenated water through the egg mass. Channel catfish eggs hatch after 6–8 days, depending on the temperature. Colour indicates the stage of development: during normal development, eggs change from yellow to pink to red-brown. Newly hatched fry (called sac fry) fall through the egg basket to the bottom of the trough. Three to four days later the fry will have absorbed their yolk and begin swimming (swim-up fry). Swim-up fry must be fed at intervals of 2–4 hours, usually on a commercial catfish or trout fry starter ration containing 50% protein. They are fed for about seven days after swim-up and then transferred into nursery ponds. Egg-hatching troughs and fry troughs should be cleaned and sterilised before receiving new egg masses or fry.

Nursery ponds are usually stocked at approximately 150,000–250,000 fry/ha. The receiving pond must be rid of all resident fish and insects that can prey on the fry. Nursery ponds should be fertilised to increase phytoplankton growth, which prevents growth of aquatic weeds and promotes the growth of zooplankton as a natural food source for the fry. The fry are fed 2–3 times daily the first few weeks. Feed is distributed around the shoreline and they begin to accept supplemental feeds once the natural food supply becomes limiting, though several weeks may pass before the fry are seen feeding on the supplemental feed. At this stage they are classified as fingerlings (Fig. 15.3). Survival rates of 80% from fry to fingerling are considered good.

Fingerling Production

Food fish are harvested and fingerlings restocked year round. After fingerlings reach 12–20 cm, they are harvested and stocked at lower densities in food fish grow-out ponds. Stocking rates are usually 10,000–25,000 fish/ha but can vary from 5,000 to over 35,000 fish/ha. Higher stocking rates require a higher level of management skills, sufficient aeration equipment, adequate water supply, and quick disease recognition and treatment.

Food Fish Production

Two production strategies are used in raising channel catfish to food size: single crop and

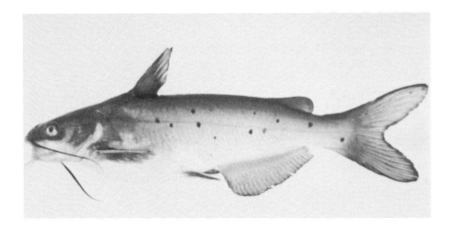

continuous production. The single crop scheme consists of growing a single cohort of fingerlings and then seining all the fish in the pond. The pond is either drained or not, depending on the production schedule. A new cohort of fingerlings is then restocked for grow-out. In the continuous production strategy, large fish are selectively harvested with a grading seine and then the pond is restocked with small fingerlings to replace those removed. However, this method has its inherent problems. After a few years in production the farmer may be unable to make an accurate estimate of the number of fish of a certain size, the stocking density, or standing crop of fish in that pond. Good records are essential and computer programmes are available. However, accurate estimates of harvest size and numbers are difficult and time-consuming. Diseases are also easily transferred from different groups of fish in ponds managed under the continuous production strategy and water quality is poor due to the high feeding rates.

Despite its disadvantages, the continuous production system remains the most commonly used strategy. Large standing crops of fish are always present, feeding rates are high, and production per unit pond area is, in theory, greater. At a given time more ponds will contain fish in a continuous production system than in a single harvest system. Therefore, when fish are unmarketable due to off-flavour, a producer using a continuous production strategy may have more ponds full of marketable fish than a producer using a single crop strategy.

Transport of Channel Catfish

Transporting live fish is an integral part of the channel catfish industry. Fish may be moved at any life stage, and proper handling and transporting is very important to the success of a producer. Mishandling or stressing the fish during transit may result in dead fish upon arrival or stress-related infectious diseases shortly following delivery.

The goal when transporting is to move as many fish, or weight of fish, in as little water as possible, since it is unprofitable to move water. However, the fish must not be crowded to the point that water quality deteriorates and stresses the fish. The weight of fish that can be safely transported depends on many factors: size and type of tank, types of aeration, duration of the transport, water temperatures, and fish size. Listed below are some principles of transporting fish. (Additional detailed information can be found in the References.)

- Use insulated tanks for transporting fish on long trips, particularly in hot weather. Large tanks should have internal baffles to minimise turbulence within the tank.
- Three types of aeration systems are used to maintain adequate dissolved oxygen concentrations in hauling tanks: surface agitators, diffused air and diffused oxygen. The choice of aeration depends on the hauling system and needs of the transport.
- Hauling tanks should be filled with clear well water. Well water is free from phytoplankton and other organisms that can consume oxygen.
- The water in the hauling tank should be within

3°C of the source water in which the fish are held before hauling.

- Water temperatures can be decreased by adding ice. Approximately 1 kg of ice per 10 litres of water will reduce the water temperature by 6°C.
- Maintain at least 5 ppm dissolved oxygen in the hauling tanks at all times.
- Always acclimatise fish to a change in water temperature. This involves changing the temperature of the hauling water by less than 1°C/2 minutes until the water temperatures are equal.
- Use sodium thiosulphate at the rate of 7.4 ppm for each ppm of any chlorine in the ice.
- Use a defoaming agent at the rate of 7.4 g/100 litres of water. Excessive foam decreases oxygen transfer at the water surface.
- Add sodium chloride to the hauling water at the rate of 0.2 kg/100 litres (0.2%) to reduce osmoregulatory distress.
- Withhold feed for 1–2 days prior to transporting because fish with empty stomachs consume less oxygen.

Nutrition

Channel catfish have a relatively simple gastrointestinal tract and the contribution of microbial-synthesised nutrients to the total dietary nutritional requirement is minimal. Most nutrients must be provided in the diet.

Types of feeds utilised

Currently the ability of feed manufacturers to adjust nutrient levels in feeds for various life stages of channel catfish is limited. Logistics make the manufacture, storage and distribution of several different feeds impractical. For example, some large channel catfish farms may feed 180–220 t of catfish feed a day during the peak growing season. Even if various nutrient levels of feed were available, producers are not equipped to store large quantities of different lots of feeds. However, as the industry evolves, improved feeding strategies using adjusted nutrient levels for various life stages, different seasons, and for various environmental factors may prove efficacious and profitable.

Feedstuffs from animal and plant origin are combined to meet the nutritional requirements of channel catfish. Those of animal origin are usually of better protein quality than those of plant origin. Soybean meal is the primary plant feedstuff because of the quality of its essential amino acid profile; others are cotton-seed meal (glanded and glandless) and peanut meal. Corn, wheat middlings, rice, rice bran and milo are used as inexpensive sources of energy and to improve pellet quality. The primary animal feedstuffs are menhaden fish meal, meat-and-bone meal and blood meal. Menhaden fish meal is an excellent source of amino acids and improves palatability. Meat-and-bone meal is highly palatable and is usually a good source of inexpensive protein, calcium and phosphorus. Blood meal is high in lysine and is sometimes added to meat-and-bone meal to improve protein quality.

Feeding strategies

Channel catfish fry absorb their yolk-sac 3–5 days after hatching. They then begin actively swimming in search of food. Fry are fed a meal-type feed containing 45–50% protein (primarily from fish meal). Many producers use trout or salmon starter feed. The fry are fed to satiation and frequently (8–10 times daily). Some producers feed fry every hour. Excess feed is removed daily from the troughs to prevent the deterioration of water quality parameters.

Fry are usually stocked from the hatchery into ponds at 8–10 days after swim-up. Feeding fry in large nursery ponds is frustrating since the fry may not be seen for weeks; however, they should be fed and the feed should be spread over a wide area of the pond. Whether the feed is being consumed in appropriate amounts or serving as a nutrient for the production of natural food organisms is debatable.

Fry start feeding obviously when they reach 2–5 cm in length, after which they are considered fingerlings. Fingerlings are usually fed a 35–36% protein feed in small-sized crumbles or small floating fingerling pellets. Most producers prefer using a feed that floats because feeding the fish is usually the only time the producer can see the fish. Assessing feeding activity is thus the only reliable way to monitor health of channel catfish.

Larger fingerlings are usually fed by mechanical

blowers that blow the feed out over the pond. Typically the feeds are 32% crude protein and the fingerlings are fed at 3% body-weight. Feeding rates are adjusted weekly at a 2:1 feed conversion. Feeding twice a day optimises growth but may be impractical on large commercial catfish farms. Feeding rates may be as high as 200 kg of feed/ha/day but because of water quality problems many producers limit feeding rates to 100–125 kg/ha/day.

Brood fish must be fed throughout the year to optimise spawning success. They are usually fed a 32% protein feed at 1–2% body-weight daily. Some producers supplement the feeding of brood-stock with forage fish, such as fathead minnows (*Pimephales promelas*), stocked in late winter or early spring at 2,000–4,000 fish/ha. Where per-mitted, tilapia (*Oreochromis* spp.) also make excellent forage for food fish: approximately twenty pairs of adults are stocked per hectare in late spring or summer and rapid reproduction, supplying sufficient numbers of forage for brood-stock. At colder temperatures tilapia are easily caught by broodstock and below 10°C tilapia are unable to survive. Thus, tilapia will not become established in the pond.

Feeding activity of channel catfish is directly related to water temperature. Consumption is greatly reduced below 10°C and, a common practice of many producers is to stop offering feed in the winter, due to both poor feeding activity and muddy levees which makes delivering feeds to the ponds impossible. During the winter channel catfish may go 40–60 days with no supplemental feed. However, it has been shown that they can lose up to 9% of body-weight during the winter if not fed. Winter feeding also benefits the overall health of the fish going into the spring.

Because of the decreased metabolism in cold water, feeding rates and the protein percentage of the feeds are decreased. Fish are usually fed a 25% protein feed, given in the afternoon when water temperatures are highest. Producers who feed their fish during the winter may limit feeding to every other day, every third day, or once a week.

Major Diseases and Clinical Diagnosis

On an annual basis, 8–10% of pond-raised channel catfish are lost due to disease. Annual losses to infectious diseases are estimated to cost the industry up to 20 million dollars annually. These values do not take into account losses due to morbidity, poor feed conversion, and decreased growth. Fingerling-sized fish account for over 90% of the total number of disease losses; however, food-size catfish account for over 55% of fish lost by weight.

Many fish pathogens are found normally in channel catfish production ponds but it is not until the fish are stressed that disease outbreaks occur. Stress is caused by poor water quality, poor nutrition, excessive handling and many other factors.

Serious disease losses can occur due to bacterial, fungal, viral or parasite infections. However, bacterial infections account for over 50% of all the disease losses in the channel catfish industry.

Viral Diseases

There are only two known viral diseases of channel catfish: channel catfish virus and catfish reovirus. The pathogenicity of catfish reovirus is low and it does not cause high mortalities. Very little is known about the pathogenesis or epizootiology of this disease, and catfish reovirus has not been reported outside California.

Channel catfish virus disease (CCVD)

CCVD is caused by a highly virulent herpes virus that can result in up to 100% mortality in channel catfish fry and young fingerlings. CCVD occurs during the summer when water temper-atures are above 24°C. Acute epizootics are often associated with stressors, such as handling or poor water quality.

Gross clinical signs are characterised by a distended abdomen, exophthalmia, and petechial haemorrhages on the body and base of the fins. The abdominal cavity is filled with a clear to yellowish fluid, the liver is usually pale and the spleen enlarged and congested. However, all or none of these clinical signs may be present. Secondary bacterial infections are common. Histologically the kidney, spleen, and liver are oedematous and necrotic. Hepatocytes develop intracytoplasmic inclusion bodies.

Channel catfish virus is host specific and other

species of catfish seem to be refractory to natural infections. Different strains of channel catfish show differential susceptibility.

Isolation of the virus from the liver, spleen or kidney is performed using a channel catfish ovary cell line; brown bullhead cells can also be used. The characteristic cytopathic effect of syncytial formation occurs within 12–24 hours if cells are incubated at 25°C.

In theory, CCVD can be managed by lowering the water temperature, but catfish farmers have little control over hatchery and pond water temperatures. At present, management of the disease relies upon hatchery sanitation and quarantine and disposal of infected fry.

Bacterial Diseases

Enteric septicaemia of catfish (ESC)

Edwardsiella ictaluri is an obligate bacterial fish pathogen, which accounts for over 45% of fish lost in the industry. Fingerlings and yearling fish are most commonly affected, and mortality rates in a population can run as high as 80%. Large losses are associated with heavy stocking, poor water quality, recent copper treatments and concurrent infection with *Trichophyra*. The disease is seasonal, occurring in spring and autumn when the water temperatures are between 22 and 28°C. Concurrent columnaris infections occur in a significant number of ESC infections.

ESC occurs in acute or chronic forms. Acute ESC is characterised by a typical bacterial septicaemia with necrosis and inflammation of multiple organs. Chronic ESC (Fig. 15.4) is characterised by the classical 'hole in the head' or a bump on top of the head at the cranial foramen. Necrosis and inflammation of the internal organs may not be as evident in chronic ESC.

Gross lesions of channel catfish with ESC include petechial and ecchymotic haemorrhages around the mouth, fins, opercular flaps and ventral surface. Slightly raised to depressed punctate red or tan to white nodules may also be evident, covering the dorsal and lateral trunk. Infected catfish often have exophthalmia and ascites. An ulcer or white soft swelling may be present on the dorsum of the head. Slight depigmentation with

underlying haemorrhage may be evident over the cranial foramen.

Gross lesions of the internal organs are evident in the liver, anterior and posterior kidney, and spleen. These tissues may appear congested, mottled, swollen and necrotic with multiple haemorrhages. Lesions are characterised by necrosis and inflammation of the various organs. Principal lesions are usually evident in the intestine, olfactory sacs, liver, skin and brain. Meningioencephalitis may be evident involving the olfactory bulb, olfactory tracts and brain. Nephritis, ocular lesions and myositis may also be observed.

The pathogenesis of *E. ictaluri* is not known. It is a Gram-negative, cytochrome oxidase-negative bacterium that is weakly motile. Motility is lost above 30°C. It is fairly host specific for channel catfish but has been isolated from other catfish species. The bacterium can survive in water for 8 days and mud for 4 months but it is not known if it can reproduce in water or mud. Histological findings suggest the intestinal mucosa and olfactory mucosa may be the sites of entry.

E. ictaluri can be isolated readily from the kidney, liver and brain by using brain/heart infusion or blood agar. Small white bacterial colonies (2 mm in diameter) develop following incubation for 48 hours at 28°C. Diagnosis is based on physical and biochemical characteristics, indirect fluorescent antibody techniques, or ELISA.

Columnaris disease

Flexibacter columnaris (now known as *Chondrococcus columnaris*) accounts for approximately 30–35% of the bacterial disease outbreaks seen annually in cultured channel catfish in Mississippi. *C. columnaris* is a long, slender, pigmented, Gram-negative rod that is strictly aerobic. It is ubiquitous and normally found in the pond environment. Infections often follow stress due to poor water quality, handling, concurrent bacterial infections, proliferative gill disease or winter kill, and can be internal or external. External infections usually precede internal infections of columnaris.

Epizootics of columnaris occur most often in spring and autumn in Mississippi and other southeastern states when water temperatures are between 10 and 24°C. However, disease outbreaks can occur throughout the year and concurrent

FIG. 15.4 (a) Chronic cutaneous lesions of fish infected
with *Edwardsiella ictaluri*.
(b) Granulomatous lesion
on the top of the head which
gives the name 'hole-in-
the-head' disease.

(a)

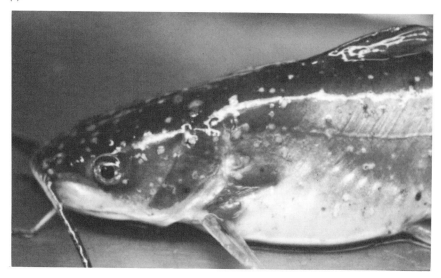

(b)

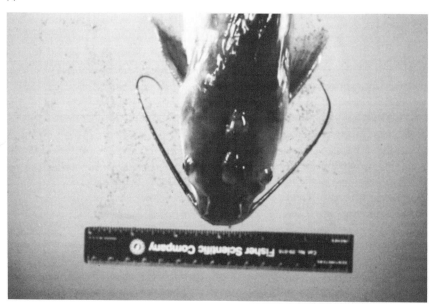

infections of columnaris and *E. ictaluri* are not
uncommon. Columnaris usually affects fingerlings;
larger fish can also be affected but the disease
tends to be less severe in older fish.

Lesions are commonly seen on the gills but may
also be evident on the head, body and fins, or
in the mouth. Gross lesions on the gills are
characterised by yellow-brown necrotic tissue at
the distal end of the gill filament. Lesions extend
to the gill arch as the disease progresses and may
appear as focal infarcts or encompass the entire
gill arch. Gross lesions on the skin begin with pale,
discoloured grey-white plaques which can progress
to large necrotic ulcers with extensive loss of the
surrounding tissue and musculature. Frequently,
the pale discoloration begins at the base of the

dorsal fin, covering as much as 20–25% of the fish, giving the characteristic shape of a saddle — hence the frequently used name 'saddleback'. Histologically, lesions are characterised by sloughing of the gill epithelium or the gill filaments, congestion, multifocal haemorrhages and vast necrosis of the gills and dermis.

A rapid presumptive diagnosis can be made when sufficient numbers of the bacteria are present from a skin or gill scraping. *C. columnaris* bacteria move by flexing or gliding and form 'haystacks' or column-like masses (hence the specific epithet, columnaris). Gross lesions in the mouth occur as yellow-brown patches that may only focally invade the skin. Systemic infections involving columnaris can only be detected by isolating the bacteria on appropriate media. Isolation can be made on a low nutrient agar such as Ordal's or Cytophaga agar incubated between 25 and 29°C. Colonies are flat and spreading, with rhizoidal edges and a clear, characteristic yellow colour.

Motile aeromonad septicaemia

The highest incidence of *Aeromonas* infections occurs in spring and autumn, but disease outbreaks can occur throughout the year. As with columnaris, predisposing stress is usually associated with disease outbreaks of *Aeromonas*. Environmental factors associated with *Aeromonas* epizootics include high nitrite levels, high temperatures, low dissolved oxygen, high ammonia and excessive handling and crowding. Both *Aeromonas sobria* and *A. hydrophila* may be isolated from affected fish and cannot be differentiated on clinical signs.

Species of *Aeromonas* are short, Gram-negative, fermentative rods, which are motile by a single flagellum. They are ubiquitous in most natural waters and more prevalent in waters with high organic loads. They can be isolated routinely from water, mud and the digestive tract of channel catfish. There is controversy about the classification of motile aeromonads due to the existence of phenotypically, genotypically and antigenically diverse members. *Aeromonas liquefaciens* and *A. punctata* are now grouped into the species *A. hydrophila*, which differs from *A. sobria* by hydrolysing esculin and fermenting both salicin and arabinose.

There may be several clinical forms of this disease: skin lesions with internal infections, skin lesions only, and acute mortalities with no lesions. Gross clinical signs of aeromonad infections are characterised by multifocal petechial and ecchymotic haemorrhages over the body. Dermal ulceration with haemorrhage and inflammation may be evident. Erosion of the underlying musculature may be extensive. Exophthalmia, ascites and frayed fins are common characteristics. Petechial haemorrhages and congestion may be observed. The liver and kidney may be pale, swollen and friable. Histologically, there is extreme tissue destruction and necrosis.

There is evidence of a carrier state in channel catfish and that the virulent aeromonads are carried in the intestinal tract and shed when fish are stressed. Experimentally, the route of infection has been demonstrated to be via the digestive tract or uninjured skin under crowded conditions at high temperatures.

Isolation of *Aeromonas* from liver or posterior kidney can be made on TSA, blood agar, or any general-purpose bacterial culture medium. Incubation temperatures are best at 25–29°C for 24–48 hours. Biochemical characteristics are used to confirm the diagnosis. Interpretation of *Aeromonas* isolates from fish can be confusing if the sample is not fresh. *Aeromonas* will overgrow *E. ictaluri* in culture, especially when isolated from dead fish.

Parasites

Protozoan parasites account for almost all of the parasitic disease losses seen in channel catfish culture. Although some of those protozoans are obligate parasites, most are facultative and only pose health problems to fish under stressful conditions.

Ordinarily most protozoan parasites cause no significant damage when present in small numbers. However, in large numbers they may decrease oxygen transfer at the gill surface. Some may feed on the epithelial cells and mucus and a few (e.g. *Ichthyophthirius multifiliis*) actually attach to or burrow under the epithelial cells, severely damaging the gills.

Bacterial disease outbreaks often are diagnosed with concurrent infestations of large numbers of protozoan parasites. The bacterial disease probably weakens the fish, making it more susceptible to infestation by the protozoans, but sometimes the parasite may be the primary agent in causing fish mortality.

In most cases, treatment of parasitic infestations is warranted only if there are large numbers of parasites. Treating fish for parasitic infestations that are concurrently infected with a bacterial or viral pathogen can stress fish and increase mortality. Therefore, a thorough diagnosis is imperative before treating for external parasites. The exception to this rule is *Icthyophthirius multifiliis*, which must be treated *immediately* if found on catfish.

Ichthyophthirius multifiliis *(Ich)*

'Ich' is the most pathogenic external parasite of cultured channel catfish. It is a ciliated protozoan and adults have a large C-shaped macronucleus. Infections of this organism are often grossly visible as small, raised white spots on the skin and gills. Depending on the temperature and health of the fish, mortalities maybe as high as 100%.

Ich has a biphasic life-cycle and is susceptible to treatment during only two life stages within this cycle (free-living stages). The free-swimming infective tomite burrows under the epidermis of the skin or gills. Within days the parasite develops a mouth and is called a trophozoite; it feeds on the body fluids and epidermal cells. The mature trophozoite leaves the fish and swims until contacting substrate suitable for cyst formation. Cell division begins as early as one hour after encystment. Up to 2,000 theronts are formed within the cyst. When cell divisions are complete, the cyst ruptures and the theronts, then called tomites, actively search for a fish host. Tomites have 48 hours to find a host or they will die. The life-cycle can be completed in less than four days if ambient water temperatures are between 21 and 27°C. Treatments are only effective in the two free-swimming stages and not when the parasite is on the fish or encysted.

Epizootics occur most often in the spring when water temperatures are between 21 and 26°C. However, epizootics have occurred in the winter when water temperatures were as low as 5°C. The infective stages of Ich supposedly do not survive above 28°C but epizootics of this disease are seen in the summer, though rarely.

Trichodina

Trichodina is the most common parasite of channel catfish and is often considered an ectocommensal causing minimal damage. Many different trichodinid species can infect a fish at the same time and members of the genus are easily recognised by their denticular ring. There is a seasonal incidence of heavy infestations in the spring and fall, and large numbers most often occur in debilitated fish. In such numbers the parasite may cause mortalities.

The pathogenesis of *Trichodina* is unknown, but heavy infestations of the gills can cause increased mucus production. This, along with large numbers of parasites residing on the gill surface, probably reduces oxygen transfer at the gill surface, thus further debilitating the fish. Treatment of *Trichodina* with copper sulphate, potassium permanganate or formalin is usually effective.

Ichthyobodo (Costia) necatrix

Ichthyobodo is a small flagellated protozoan, about the size of a red blood cell, and looks like a tear drop when attached to the gill or skin of the fish. It can be present throughout the year but is most common during colder weather. It is an obligate parasite and is often found on the gills or skin of apparently healthy fish; it seems to cause problems only when it occurs in large numbers. Stress is a major predisposing factor for the occurrence of epizootics. Large numbers of *Icthyobodo* have often been seen with PGD infected fish. Increased mucus production on the skin of fish infected with *Ichthyobodo* give the fish a characteristic white–grey to bluish coloration.

Evidence suggests that this parasite penetrates and feeds upon the live cells of the host. Histologically, there is hyperplasia and necrosis of the gill epithelial cells. Oedema or spongiosis may be evident in the epidermis of skin infestations. Diagnosis is best made from gill or skin scrapings while the protozoan is still alive. Treatment with copper sulphate, formalin or potassium permanganate is usually effective.

Trichophyra

Trichophyra is a suctorian protozoan with a broad, round body covered with tentacles. A few of these parasites are commonly found on the gills of channel catfish with no apparent ill effects. However, in moderate numbers *Trichophyra* may cause severe swelling and ulceration of the gill tissue, and the resulting blood loss may cause anaemia. Large losses of channel catfish have been observed with concurrent infections of *Trichophyra* and ESC. Diagnosis is made by microscopic examination of gill scrapings. Copper sulphate is the only effective treatment.

Proliferative gill disease (PGD) or 'hamburger gill disease'

PGD can occur throughout the year but is most prevalent in spring and autumn when water temperatures are between 16 and 21°C. The disease occurs most often in new ponds or ponds that have been drained, dried and refilled, but its prevalence in older established ponds is increasing. PGD can be transmitted to channel catfish from pond water and mud from ponds where catfish have been diagnosed with the disease. Its incidence can be quite high and it appears to be increasing.

Subclinical infections are difficult to diagnose unless tissues are examined histologically.

The disease is characterised by marked inflammation of the gills with various degrees of necrosis, chondroplasia and chondrolysis of the gill cartilage. The name 'hamburger gill disease' describes the way in which the swollen, friable gills bleed easily when touched (Fig. 15.5). The clinical signs are associated with a myxozoan parasite reported to resemble *Sphaerospora* species.

More recently a triactinomyxid myxozoan (*Aurantiactinomyxon* sp.) has been identified in water from ponds of PGD-infected channel catfish. This same myxozoan was present in the intestinal epithelium of an oligochaete worm found in pond mud samples. The worm, *Dero digitala*, normally lives in the pond mud and may be present in numbers as high as 300–1,000/m². The worms are 0.3–0.6 cm long, and channel catfish exposed to worms harvested from a pond undergoing a PGD outbreak develop gill lesions and parasites in the gills characteristic of PGD. Fry exposed to squash suspension of the worms also develop PGD.

The gills appear to be the initial route of infection. The organisms spread to other organs including kidney, liver, heart, brain, spleen and intestines. The most common gross clinical sign is

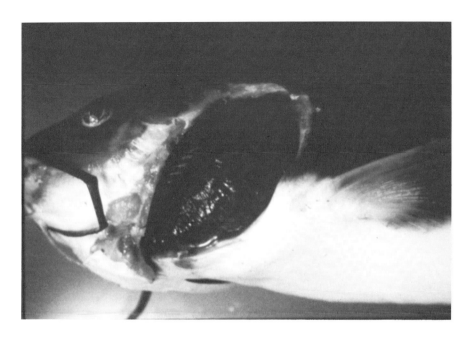

FIG. 15.5 Proliferative gill disease or so-called 'hamburger-gill disease'.

the swollen, friable gills. Gill lesions reduce respiratory efficiency and fish may be at the surface gasping for air, even when dissolved oxygen concentrations are high. The fish may be weak and observed resting in large numbers at the water bank. Mortalities may be very acute and occur within 2 days of exposure. Histologically there is a moderate to severe branchial hyperplasia and branchitis. Chondroplasia and extensive haemorrhage may also be prevalent in the gills. PGD parasites may or may not be abundant.

A presumptive diagnosis can be made by microscopic examination of gill filaments demonstrating filament cartilage hyperplasia, chondroplasia and chondalysis. However, PGD can only be confirmed by identification of the causative parasite after histological examination. There is no treatment but good water quality and high dissolved oxygen levels must be maintained to keep mortalities to a minimum. Treatment with chemicals commonly used for external protozoan parasites may cause a significant increase in mortality.

Diseases of Uncertain Aetiology

Red spot or red fillet syndrome

This syndrome is usually seen as red spots in the fillet of dressed whole fish or fillets (Fig. 15.6).

Other forms include small petechial haemorrhages in the fillet, multifocal large red spots throughout the fillet, uniformly pink fillets, purple and red spotted fillets with a rotten odour, fillets with red streaks, and whole fish with a red fillet on one side and a fillet of normal colour on the other. No matter what the form, affected fish are viewed as unwholesome by the channel catfish processor and often rejected. Rejection rates through the processing plant on a daily basis have been reported from 2–10%.

Lesions of a similar nature have been described grossly and histologically following an acute oxygen depletion due to, for example, a phytoplankton die-off in the pond. These lesions of haemorrhage and necrosis of the musculature were similar to what is observed in many of the fillets presented by some processing plants.

Many of the case histories of red spot are associated with higher than normal mortalities in nets used to hold fish overnight in ponds after seining. Similar lesions in channel catfish muscle have been observed in fish affected with PGD. Again the fish were suffering from a functional tissue hypoxia due to the marked swelling of the gills. Research into this problem is continuing, but red spot appears to be primarily a function of low environmental dissolved oxygen, increased exercise, blood acidosis and warm water temperatures.

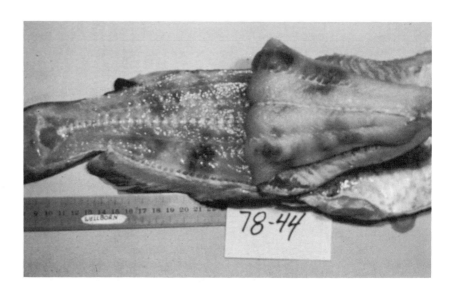

FIG. 15.6 Fillet of channel catfish affected by 'Red Spot' due to severe handling stress.

Winter kill ('winter fungus', 'winter mortality')

Heavy losses of channel catfish can be attributed to this syndrome. Often farmers do not submit fish for diagnosis due to winter kill since there is no known cure. Mortalities are chronic and highly variable. Fish affected are usually of harvestable size, although fingerlings are affected as well.

The causes of winter kill are unknown; however, the underlying factor appears to be stress. Previous disease outbreaks, bouts of low dissolved oxygen and exposure to high nitrite levels during the summer and early autumn seem to predispose fish to winter kill in the late autumn or winter when water temperatures are below 16°C. Fish may appear to have recovered from previous disease outbreaks, but subsequently develop winter kill. Poor water quality may also stress the fish and predispose them to winter kill, probably by decreasing the fish's ability to adapt to cooler or cold water temperatures. Recent reports suggest that *Saprolegnia* sp. is the causative agent of winter kill in fish immunocompromised by rapid drops in water temperatures (Fig. 15.7).

Gross characteristics of affected fish include dry depigmented areas of skin, endophthalmia, and areas of external mycosis on the skin and gills. All or none of these clinical signs may be evident. Occasionally, bacteria can be isolated from the posterior kidney and liver, and a variety of external parasites may be present.

There is no effective treatment. Potassium permanganate to remove external fungal infections is usually ineffective at cold temperatures; it may temporarily remove the fungus, but at cold water temperatures the immune system of channel catfish is suppressed, healing is slow, and fungal infections often recur or bacterial infections develop. Effective fish disease treatments during warmer months and proper water quality management may reduce subsequent losses to winter kill. Fish should be fed throughout the winter to ensure optimum nutritional status.

Anaemia ('no-blood' or 'white-lip' disease)

The clinical signs of a severe idiopathic anaemia are variable but packed cell volumes are often below 10% (sometimes as low as 1%): clinical signs include pale gills and internal organs, mottled skin, ascites, a pale ventrum, fluid in the stomach, and pink to straw-coloured blood. Mortalities may be either acute or chronic depending on ambient dissolved oxygen concentrations. In Mississippi, anaemias are usually detected in late summer to late autumn; in Alabama and Georgia the disease is predominantly seen in the late spring and summer. It is not known whether these differences in occurrence reflect dissimilar aetiologies between locations.

No pathogenic agents have been consistently associated with this condition. In Alabama the disease has been linked to the diet: when healthy fish were given a suspect feed, they developed an anaemia within 7 days with haematocrits of 1–9%. Anaemia may also develop when fish are given feed contaminated with micro-organisms that

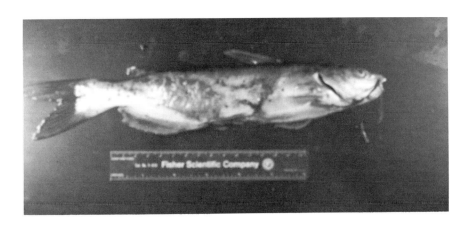

FIG. 15.7 Channel catfish with fungus infection on lateral skin associated with 'winter-kill' syndrome.

convert folic acid to pteroic acid. (Pteroic acid is a folic acid antagonist; hence, red cell maturation ceases.) Severe idiopathic anaemias in channel catfish may be associated with vitamin B_{12} and folic acid malabsorption. A mild, but variable, anaemia develops when channel catfish are exposed to high concentrations of nitrite. Mild anaemias are also associated with infections of *E. ictaluri*.

Severe idiopathic anaemias in Mississippi are sporadic, occurring on only one or two ponds on a farm. Since all the fish are fed the same diet on a farm, it is doubtful if the anaemia is feed related. Usually the affected fish are 0.5 kg or larger; smaller fish seem unaffected and continue to feed. However, variable anaemias affecting all sizes in a pond do occur. The producer rarely knows that there is a problem until dissolved oxygen concentrations drop to marginal levels. Many cases of anaemia are first noticed by the channel catfish processors because of pallor of the fillet. Processors prefer not to buy anaemic fish because of their marked white colour and they claim shelf-life is reduced. If such fillets are purchased, they are usually marketed as frozen, value-added products.

The best a channel catfish producer can do when faced with a pond of anaemic fish is to keep the water well aerated. In Alabama and Georgia they recommend changing feed, and not using feed that has been stored for long periods of time. If the anaemia is feed-related, the problem may quickly resolve simply by using a new batch of feed. Similarly, anaemias occurring during systemic bacterial or viral infections will resolve after the infectious disease is controlled. Nevertheless, it is often not possible to identify the underlying cause of the anaemia. In such instances, the only recourse is to attempt to maintain optimum environmental conditions until the problem resolves. In particular, dissolved oxygen concentrations should be maintained as near saturation as possible by providing adequate supplemental aeration.

Non-infectious Diseases

Water quality can directly affect the health of the fish. In particular, levels of dissolved oxygen, ammonia and nitrites may be responsible for certain non-infectious diseases.

Hypoxia

Dissolved oxygen values which fall below 4 mg per litre should be considered as a factor in fish health. At such levels there may be adverse effects on weight gain, feed consumption, feed conversion, reproductive performance and disease resistance. Low levels of dissolved oxygen below 1 mg/l are lethal if exposure lasts more than a few hours (Fig. 15.8). In channel catfish ponds, there may be wide fluctuations from more than 15 mg/l in the afternoon to below 3 mg/l by dawn. These daily changes are common and are a result of the dense algal populations found in commercial ponds.

Concentrations of dissolved oxygen at dawn are

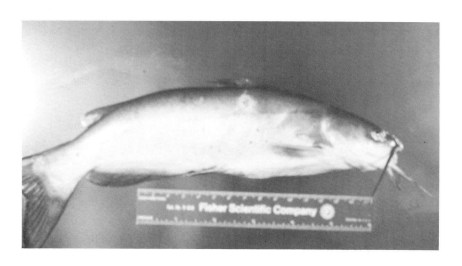

FIG. 15.8 White depigmented areas with red patches on channel catfish skin due to low levels of dissolved oxygen in the water. The lesions develop several days after the critical stress.

usually highest in spring and decline as the growing season progresses. In spring, the lower feeding rates, fish standing crop and water temperatures (oxygen solubility is greater at cooler temperatures) account for the higher oxygen concentrations; during the summer the dissolved oxygen levels are at their lowest at dawn due to the higher water temperature, higher feeding rates and higher fish standing crop. All these factors combine to make the period from mid-July to September the most critical time for oxygen depletion. Monitoring dissolved oxygen levels several times daily and throughout the night is routine practice in all ponds, and mechanical aeration with pump-sprayers, large paddlewheels, and diffused air systems is common during the summer and early autumn in heavily stocked culture ponds.

Ammonia

Channel catfish excrete ammonia as the principal nitrogenous waste product following protein catabolism. High levels of un-ionised ammonia in the environment lead to ammonia toxicity, the actual mechanism of which is unknown. High ammonia levels decrease growth rates, reduce feeding activity, increase water uptake and serum corticosteroid levels, increase dissolved oxygen requirements, and possibly cause degenerative changes in the gills.

Treatment of high ammonia levels is not feasible in large channel catfish culture ponds. Exchanging water ('flushing') has little effect due to the large size of most commercial culture ponds and the dynamic biological processes in the pond. The best approach is the use of reasonable feeding rates and not to feed over 100–125 kg/ha per day for extended periods.

Methaemoglobinaemia ('brown blood disease')

This problem occurs when channel catfish are exposed to high concentrations of nitrite (NO_2^-) in the culture ponds. Nitrite occurs as an intermediate in the processes of nitrification and denitrification, and concentrations in the pond may vary from 0 to 20 ppm NO_2 or more. Concentrations are highest in the cooler months, due to a decrease of ammonia assimilation by phytoplankton populations and the differential effect low temperatures have upon bacteria involved in nitrification. Nitrite levels have been known to increase from 2 ppm NO_2 to 16 ppm NO_2 in 24 hours.

The nitrite ion is actively transported into the circulatory system by lamellar chloride cells in the gills. Channel catfish concentrate nitrite in the blood so that concentrations found in the plasma are greater than concentrations found in the surrounding water. Once in the blood, nitrite causes the oxidation of the haem iron in haemoglobin. This results in the formation of methaemoglobin, which is not capable of combining with oxygen. This creates a functional anaemia, in which there is a loss in the ability of the haemoglobin in the red blood cell to bind with oxygen rather than an actual loss of red blood cells.

Clinically the blood turns a characteristic dark brown colour, and the gills appear chocolate-brown. As with proliferative gill disease, the fish suffer from hypoxia even when dissolved oxygen concentrations are high. Fish may be listless, lying on the pond bank, or gasping for oxygen.

Methaemoglobin concentrations may vary from 5% to over 90% of total haemoglobin in channel catfish. Slight browning of the blood and gills is evident when methaemoglobin levels range from 25–30%. Exposure to sublethal levels of nitrite have been shown to increase the susceptibility of channel catfish to *Flexibacter (Cytophaga) columnaris* and *Aeromonas* infections.

This is one of the few diseases that is preventable and also easily treated if it occurs. Chloride and nitrite compete for the same uptake sites in the chloride cell; therefore, the rate of nitrite uptake and subsequent methaemoglobin formation is influenced by the ratio of nitrite to chloride in the external water environment. A nitrite : chloride molar ratio of 1:10 will keep haemoglobin levels near normal. Channel catfish farmers are advised to keep the chloride concentration in their ponds above 50 ppm; they should monitor nitrite concentrations, and use sodium chloride as an economical, simple management plan to prevent methaemoglobinaemia.

Therapy

Antibiotic Treatments

The United States Food and Drug Administration has approved only two antibacterials for use in channel catfish: Romet® (sulphadimethoxine–ormetoprim, Hoffman-La Roche, Inc., Nutley, NJ) registered for treating *Edwardsiella ictaluri* infections and Terramycin® (oxytetracycline, Pfizer Inc., New York, NY) registered for treating *Aeromonas hydrophila* infections.

Romet-30 (RO-5) is a 1:5 mixture of ormetoprim and sulphadimethoxine. The premix is incorporated into feed which is fed to deliver a dosage rate of 50 mg of active ingredient/kg of fish per day for 5 days. There is a 3 day withdrawal period following treatment before slaughter.

Terramycin is added to feed and fed to deliver 55–82 mg of active ingredient/kg of fish per day for 10 days. There is a 21-day withdrawal period following treatment before slaughter.

Both Romet and Terramycin have their limitations. Depending upon the formulation, Romet can be unpalatable to channel catfish unless a high level of fish meal is incorporated into the Romet medicated feed. Terramycin is heat labile and destroyed during the extrusion process in manufacturing floating feed; therefore the drug is usually incorporated only into sinking feeds. Practical limitations associated with the use of these two antibacterials make the approval of new efficacious chemotherapeutants to treat *E. ictaluri* infections of considerable importance to the success of catfish producers. The most serious consideration is the rapid development of antibiotic-resistant strains of bacteria isolated from diseased channel catfish.

Chemical Treatments

Copper sulphate

Copper sulphate pentahydrate ($CuSO_4 \cdot 5H_2O$) is registered for use in waters used to produce food fish as a herbicide and algicide. It is also used to control ectoparasites, such as *Ichthyobodo, Trichodina, Ambiphyra, Trichophyra* and *Ichthyophthirius*. It comes in granules or powders and is considered 100% active for the purpose of calculating treatment rates.

The chemistry of copper sulphate in water is complex and it can be highly toxic to channel catfish under certain conditions, particularly in waters of very low alkalinity, hardness, pH, salinity and decreased organic matter. (Larger fish are usually more resistant.) As a general rule copper sulphate should not be used in waters with a total alkalinity of less than 50 ppm as $CaCO_3$. Treatments are determined by dividing the total alkalinity by 100: the answer will be the ppm of copper sulphate pentahydrate that should be used. Where the total alkalinity is greater than 300 ppm, treatment with copper sulphate may not be effective because the copper forms insoluble complexes and rapidly precipitates out of the water column. Following heavy rainfall, total alkalinities should always be checked again prior to a copper sulphate treatment because the additional water from the rainfall may dilute the pond water and thus decrease the total alkalinity.

Copper sulphate is a potent algicide and the algae die-off causes oxygen depletion, which is more severe in warmer waters. Great care should therefore be exercised when treating waters during the summer months: supplemental aeration is essential. In addition, the use of copper sulphate pentahydrate stresses fish and makes them more susceptible to ESC, so that it should not be used during the ESC temperature window (22–28°C).

Potassium permanganate

Potassium permanganate is registered for use in waters used to produce food fish as an oxidising agent and a detoxifying agent. It is also used to treat external columnaris and fungal infections and to control ectoparasites. The chemical is not effective against the parasite *Trichophyra*. Potassium permanganate comes in powder form and is considered 100% active.

Potassium permanganate is toxic to fish and algae, and very expensive. Therefore it is imperative that the chemical be used properly and at the right dose. As it is consumed by organic matter, the higher the organic load in the water the higher concentration of potassium will be needed.

Rates for pond treatments range from 2–12 ppm, depending upon the organic load in the water. The amount needed to treat a pond can be determined by a 15-minute potassium permanganate demand test. Under most circumstances it is best to start with a 2 ppm treatment and add more chemical at intervals until the correct dose is achieved. The goal is to keep a wine-red colour in the water for 10–12 hours. If the colour changes before 10 hours, a second treatment may be required. Judging the correct colour is more of an art than science: if too much chemical is used the fish die; if too little chemical is used the treatment is ineffective. The following day fish should be checked again to determine the effectiveness of the treatment.

Prevention of Disease

Most commercial culture of channel catfish is conducted in large ponds on large farms. The time-consuming tasks associated with everyday activities such as feeding, harvesting and water quality testing leave little time for comprehensive programmes for monitoring fish health. Consequently, when an epizootic is first detected, the disease often has already progressed to the point where therapy will be expensive and may not be as effective as it would have been if initiated earlier. Obviously prevention, rather than treatment, should be the goal in fish health management. Disease incidence may be reduced by providing a good environment, ensuring adequate nutrition, and preventing stresses related to overcrowding or improper handling. To a degree, common diseases can be anticipated on a seasonal cycle (see Fig. 15.9) and preventive measures should be aimed accordingly.

Regrettably, economical and practical considerations limit the extent to which these stressors can be minimised under commercial conditions. The following checklist represents an idealised perspective and the suggestions must often be compromised for practical reasons. The best general advice is to use common sense and prevent situations that will lead to increased incidence or severity of diseases.

Breeding

- Do not use wild fish for broodstock. They may be easily stressed by routine husbandry practices, more susceptible to disease, and less tolerant of poor water quality.
- Avoid strains of channel catfish that are more susceptible to diseases. For example, the Rio

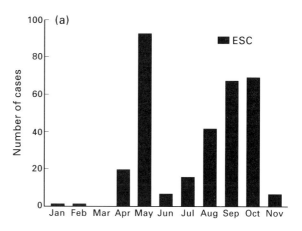

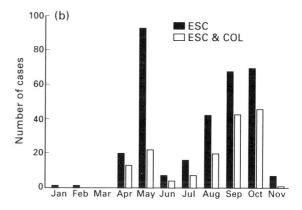

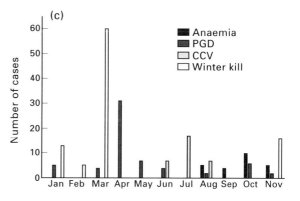

FIG. 15.9 (a) Demonstrating seasonal incidence of ESC at the Stoneville Fish Disease Diagnostic Laboratory, Stoneville, Mississippi in 1991. (b) Demonstrating incidence of total ESC cases in comparison to cases of ESC with concurrent Columnaris infections at the Stoneville Fish Disease Diagnostic Laboratory, Stoneville, Mississippi in 1991. (c) Seasonal incidence of anaemia, PGD, winter kill and CCV (at the Stoneville Fish Disease Diagnostic Laboratory, Stoneville, Mississippi in 1991).

FIG. 15.10 (a) A parasite between the secondary filaments is visible and also the marked intralamellar bridging (clubbing) can be seen. (b) A close-up of the parasite using H+E stains.

(a)

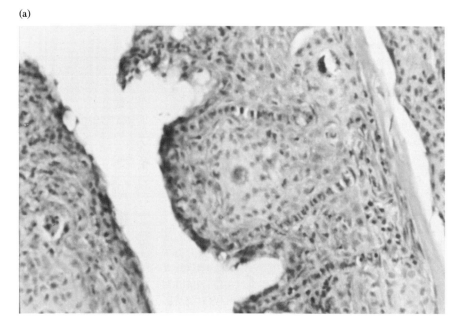

(b)

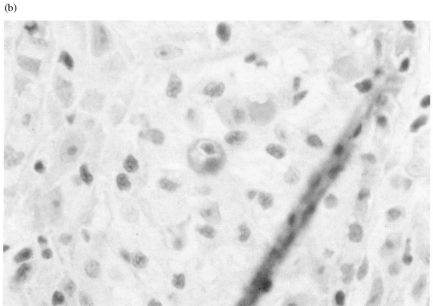

Grande strain is more susceptible to channel catfish virus.

- Prevent inbreeding which may decrease the disease resistance of a fish. Select broodstock from as many different geographical areas and egg masses as possible.
- Keep good records of hatching percentage, fry survival and growth, and fingerling and food fish performance. Cull strains of brood fish which produce progeny that perform poorly and are more susceptible to disease.

Hatchery Management

- Keep the water temperatures between 25 and 28°C.

- Make sure there is adequate dissolved oxygen and water-flow in the hatchery.
- Make sure there is a minimum of 5 ppm calcium hardness for optimum egg hatchability and fry survival.
- Make sure total gas pressure is below 105%.
- Avoid surface waters which may contain diseases or pollutants.
- Sanitise equipment and troughs before introducing the next batch of eggs.
- Avoid overcrowding, which stresses the fry and makes them more susceptible to channel catfish virus.

Fry and Fingerlings

- Avoid overcrowding fish in nursery ponds: overcrowding increases the incidence of channel catfish virus and ESC (stay below 300,000/ha).
- Maintain adequate water quality by maintaining dissolved oxygen concentrations above 5 ppm.
- Observe fish closely when water temperatures are within the ESC window (22–28°C). A rapid diagnosis of ESC with early administration of proper medicated feed will reduce fish losses.
- ESC stresses fish, making them more susceptible to columnaris. A rapid diagnosis of ESC with early administration of medicated feed will therefore also reduce losses to concurrent infections of ESC and columnaris.
- Have fish checked for parasites before ESC season (Fig. 15.10). Losses due to ESC are greater in heavily parasitised fish.
- Vaccinate channel catfish for ESC with proven vaccines that are currently being developed.
- Avoid handling fingerlings when water temperatures are extremely warm. The dissolved oxygen concentrations will be lower in warm water, and also fingerlings are more easily stressed in warm water. Handle in the early morning when water temperatures are coolest.
- Drain ponds and allow them to dry between year classes of fingerlings to decrease the transmission of disease.
- Have fingerlings examined before purchase to determine their state of health. Do not buy fish heavily parasitised or markedly malnourished. Avoid fish infected with PGD and ESC.

Food Fish

- Maintain adequate water quality. Keep dissolved oxygen concentrations above 5 ppm.
- Do not decrease water levels in ponds in winter (a practice carried out to decrease levee erosion caused by winter winds). Water temperatures change more rapidly in shallow ponds and rapid decreases in water temperature stress catfish.
- Use a single harvest strategy. Diseases are more easily transferred using the continuous production strategy. However, other economic considerations may favour continuous production.
- Methaemoglobinaemia is a preventable disease. Keep chloride concentrations well above 50 ppm and measure water quality parameters daily or at least every other day.
- Keep feeding rates below 100–125 kg/ha.
- Routinely examine fish to determine their state of health (e.g. parasitic load etc.).
- Check gills of food fish before stocking fingerlings. If food fish are undergoing a subclinical PGD epizootic, delay stocking pond.
- Under the continuous production strategy seine the pond often to remove marketable fish. Large fish in the pond convert feed less efficiently, cannibalise small fingerlings and can act as reservoirs of disease. Large fish in a pond seem more predisposed to winter kill and anaemia.

Further Reading

Boyd, C. E. (1990) *Water Quality in Ponds for Aquaculture.* Auburn University Agriculture Experiment Station, Auburn, AL.

Burgess, W. E. (1989) *An Atlas of Freshwater and Marine Catfishes*, p. 784. T. F. H. Publications, Neptune City, New Jersey.

Dunham, R. A., Hyde, D., Masser, M., Plumb, J., Smitherman, R. O., Perez, R., Rambaux, A. C. and Rezk, M. (1992) Comparison of Cultural Traits of Channel Catfish, *Ictalurus punctatus*, and Blue Catfish *I. furcatus*. *Research and Review: A Compilation of Abstracts of Research on Channel Catfish.* Catfish Farmers of America.

Lewis, D. H. (1985) Principal diseases of farm raised catfish. Southern Cooperative Series *Bulletin* No. **225**, 17.

MacMillan, J. (1985) Infectious Diseases. In: *Channel Catfish Culture, Development in Aquaculture and Fisheries Science*, Vol. 15 (Editor Tucker, C. S.), pp. 434–441. Elsevier Science Publishers, New York.

Plumb, J. A. (1985) Principal diseases of farm-raised catfish. Southern Cooperative Series *Bulletin*No. **225**, 9.

Rogers, W. A. (1985) Principal diseases of farm-raised catfish. Southern Cooperative Series *Bulletin* No. **225**, 26–27.

Schwedler, T. E., Tucker, C. S. and Beleau, M. N., (1985) Non-infectious diseases. In: *Channel Catfish Culture, Development in Aquaculture and Fisheries Science*, Vol. 15 (Editor Tucker, C. S.), pp. 497–541. Elsevier Science Publishers, New York.

Tucker, S. and Robinson, E. H., (1991) *Channel Catfish Farming Handbook*. Van Nostrand Reinhold, New York.

16

The Veterinary Approach to Marine Prawns

IAN ANDERSON

The term shrimp is more commonly used in the Americas to refer to species in the family Penaeidae, while marine prawn (or prawn) is more common in Asia-Pacific. In this chapter the two words are used to mean the same thing (prawn) and refer to species in the genera *Penaeus* and *Metapenaeus*.

Total world production of prawns from farms was estimated variously to be 509,000 or 564,800 t in 1989, constituting 26% of the total world harvest of prawns. In 1981 farm production accounted for only 2.1% of the total. With all the tropical shrimp fisheries exploited to their maximum sustainable level, any increase in supply to the market place will come from increased farm production. Figure 16.1 shows the production of farmed prawns by country.

The farming of prawns began in South-east Asia where prawns were harvested as an incidental catch from tidal fish ponds. A few farmers enclosed areas of mangrove swamps with earthen walls specifically to grow prawns. Sluice gates were

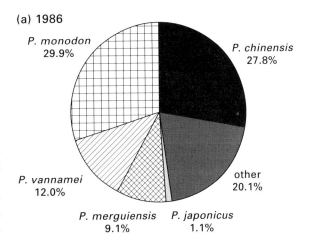

(a) 1986

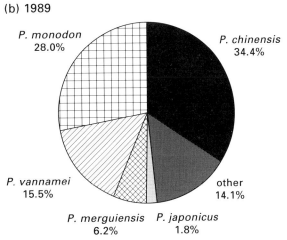

(b) 1989

FIG. 16.2 Total production of farmed prawns and shrimp by species in 1986 and 1989. For a total production of (a) 298, 573 tonnes in 1986. (b) 509, 367 tonnes in 1989.

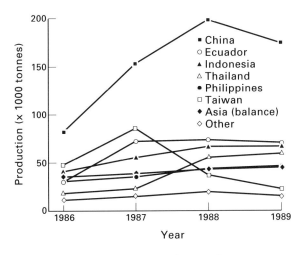

FIG. 16.1 Production of farmed prawns by country.

constructed to allow water to enter at high tides. Small prawns entered the enclosure and grew without any feeding by the farmer. Nets placed over the sluice gate caught marketable prawns as they migrated to the sea on ebb tides at dusk or at night. Modern prawn farming began in the late 1970s and early 1980s when fishermen and hatcheries started to supply large quantities of juvenile prawns or prawn fry to farms. The Japanese were the first to control the breeding and artificial rearing of a prawn species. Artificial rearing methods are now widespread and prawn farms are found in more than 40 countries. These farming systems are normally prawn monocultures.

Prawn farmers use a number of different penaeid prawns. The important ones by total production, distribution and value are:

Black tiger prawn	— *Penaeus monodon*
Chinese white shrimp	— *Penaeus chinensis*
Western white shrimp	— *Penaeus vannamei*
Banana prawn	— *Penaeus merguiensis*
Indian white prawn	— *Penaeus indicus*
Blue shrimp	— *Penaeus stylirostrus*
Kuruma prawn	— *Penaeus japonicus*
Southern white shrimp	— *Penaeus schmitti*

Figure 16.2 illustrates the relative importance of each species in terms of production.

A number of other species have been reared experimentally or at low levels of production. Figure 16.3 lists many of the shrimps and prawns cultured or bred in the world, their natural distribution and the countries where they are farmed. *Penaeus chinensis*, a species more tolerant of colder temperatures, is cultured in northern and southern China and most of China's reported production of prawns is from this single species. *P. vannamei* is the most commonly cultured species in Central and South America, while *P. monodon* is the most common species in Taiwan and the Asia-Pacific. Both species are hardy; they tolerate a range of environments and perform well in ponds and at high density. *P. monodon* is the fastest growing and largest of the common penaeid prawns: average weights of 30–35 g have been achieved in pond culture after 90–100 days from stocking as post-larvae which would weigh as little as 0.019 g. Most

SOME OF THE PRAWNS AND SHRIMP FARMED THROUGHOUT THE WORLD			
Species			
Scientific name*	**Common name**	**Natural distribution**	**Cultured in**
P. monodon	Giant (black) tiger prawn	Indo-West Pacific	Taiwan, SE Asia[†], China, Australia, India, Vietnam
P. chinensis (*P. orientalis*)	Chinese white shrimp or Oriental shrimp	West Pacific	China, Korea
P. vannamei	Western white shrimp	Eastern Pacific	Ecuador, Central and South America
P. merguiensis	Banana prawn	Indo-West Pacific	SE Asia, India, China
P. indicus	Indian white prawn	Indo-West Pacific	SE Asia, India
M. ensis	Greasyback shrimp	Indo-West Pacific	Taiwan
P. stylirostris	Blue shrimp	Eastern Pacific	Central and South America
P. japonicus	Kuruma prawn	Indo-West Pacific	Japan, Korea, Taiwan, Italy
P. aztecus	Northern brown shrimp	Western Atlantic	USA
P. duorarum	Northern pink shrimp	Western Atlantic	USA
P. setiferus	White shrimp	Western Atlantic	USA
P. penicillatus	Red-tailed prawn	Indo-West Pacific	China, Taiwan
P. semisulcatus	Green tiger prawn	Indo-West Pacific and Eastern Mediterranean	Taiwan
P. esculentus	Brown tiger prawn	Indo-West Pacific	Australia
P. schmitti	Southern white shrimp	Western Atlantic	Central and South America
P. californiensis	Yellow-leg shrimp	Eastern Pacific	USA
M. dobsoni	Kadal shrimp	Indo-West Pacific	India
* P = Penaeus, M = Metapenaeus.			
† SE Asia = Indonesia, Philippines, Thailand, Brunei, Singapore and Malaysia.			

Fig. 16.3 Some of the prawns and shrimps farmed throughout the world.

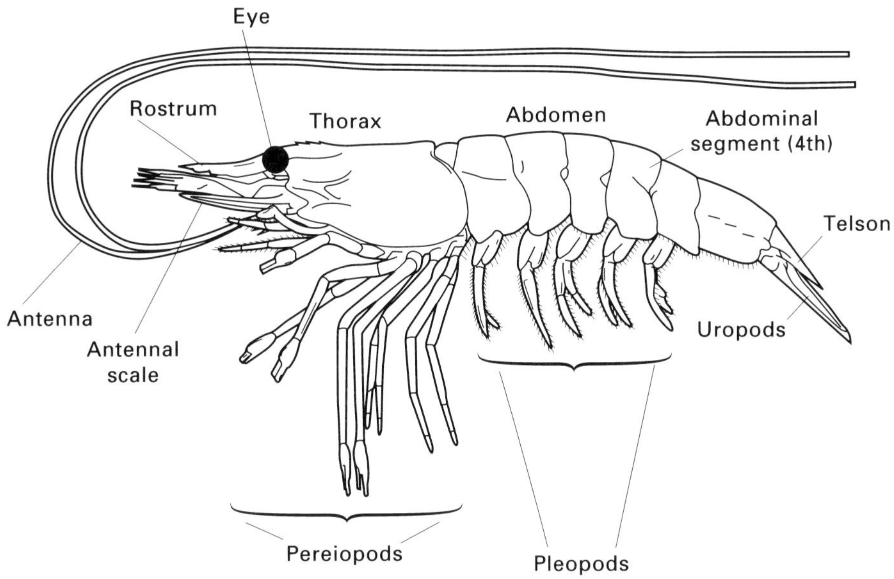

FIG. 16.4 External anatomy of a prawn.

references in this chapter will be to this black tiger prawn.

The various species have different attributes which make them attractive to the farmer. The most common factors are that the fry or brood-stock are available locally and that there is an existing local market for the species. Selection can be for a specific characteristic: some prawn species prefer stable salinities close to full strength sea water, other species tolerate a wide range of salinities; some are bottom or benthic feeders, others swim in the water column. Some are selected because of a valuable export market — for example the Kuruma prawn in Japan can realise US$100/kg at certain times of the year.

General Biology

Penaeid shrimp belong to the order Decapoda (Class Malacostraca), the largest order of crus-taceans. Order Decapoda (ten legs) contains the familiar crayfish, lobsters and crabs. A chitinous exoskeleton or cuticle covers the prawn entirely. Muscles attach to the inner surface of the cuticle. Movement of the appendages and abdomen (tail) is possible because the exoskeleton is divided into separate plates or tubes connected by thin, non-chitinised and flexible cuticle. Muscles and cuticle act together as a lever system.

Externally the prawn can be divided basically into the thorax and abdomen (Fig. 16.4). The thorax (or head) is covered by a single, immobile carapace which protects internal organs and sup-ports muscle origins. The eye stalks and eyes, the sensory antennules and the antennae (all paired) arise rostrally. The walking legs or pereiopods are the thoracic appendages. Gills are formed from sac-like outgrowths of the base of the walking legs and sit in branchial chambers on either side of the thorax. The carapace extends laterally to cover the gills completely. The abdomen has the obvious segmentation of invertebrates. A pair of swimming legs or pleopods arise from each of the six abdominal segments. A tail fan comprising a telson, which bears the anus, and two uropods attaches to the last (6th) abdominal segment. A rapid ventral flexion of the abdomen with the tail fan produces the quick backward dart characteristic of prawns.

The cuticle which is secreted by an epidermal cell layer, consists of chitin and protein in which calcium carbonate and calcium phosphate have been deposited. Pigments are deposited in the cuticle for colour and pigment cells or chromat-ophores are present in the hypodermis. Parts of the digestive tract are lined by chitinous cuticle.

Prawns grow by periodically shedding their cuticle (termed moulting or ecdysis). The epidermis detaches from the inner cuticle layer and begins to secrete a new cuticle, while the old cuticle is moulted. Immediately after moulting the new

Fig. 16.5 Internal anatomy
of a prawn.

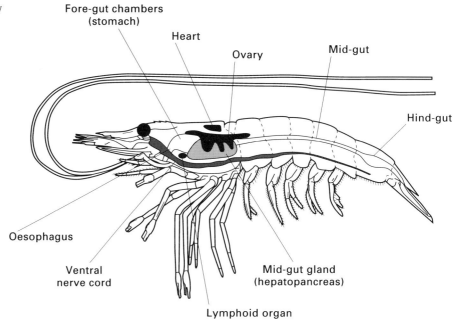

Fore-gut chambers
(stomach)

Heart

Ovary

Mid-gut

Hind-gut

Oesophagus

Ventral
nerve cord

Mid-gut gland
(hepatopancreas)

Lymphoid organ

cuticle is soft and is stretched to accommodate the increased size of the prawn. Note that actual tissue growth within the prawn is continuous between moults.

A simple, single-chambered heart delivers haemolymph (blood) to open haemal sinuses via a simple, open-ended arterial system. There are no return venous vessels. From the tissues and haemal sinuses, the haemolymph passes through the gills prior to returning to a pericardial sinus. Haemolymph enters the heart through pairs of slit-like openings in the heart wall before it is pumped into the arteries again. Haemocyanin (0.17% copper) dissolved in plasma is the respiratory pigment. The blood cells (haemocytes) are involved in clotting, phagocytosis of foreign particles and cellular inflammation. The haematopoietic tissue is found in sheets or nodules throughout the thorax. Paired lymphoid organs are closely associated with the circulatory system, but have an unclear function. Lymphoid organs may act as a 'filtering organ' for blood.

A straight digestive tract consisting of an oesophagus, fore-gut chambers (or stomach), mid-gut and hind-gut opens ventrally on the thorax (Fig. 16.5). The fore-gut and hind-gut are lined by chitin. A large mid-gut gland or hepatopancreas, an anterior caecum and a posterior caecum arise

from the mid-gut. The fore-gut functions as an ingestion, grinding, straining, mixing and filtering complex. Fluid and particles, 1 μm and smaller, enter the mid-gut gland from the fore-gut chambers. The mid-gut gland is responsible for synthesis and secretion of digestive enzymes, the absorption of nutrients, accumulation and metabolism of calcium, copper, lipids and glycogen, and inactivation of potentially toxic metals. The autolysis of the mid-gut gland is rapid at death.

Prawns are diocious, with paired gonads lying in the dorsal part of the thorax or the thorax and abdomen. They usually mate and spawn at sea. The timing of mating in relation to moulting and spawning follows one of two sequences according to the structure of the thelycum. The thelycum is a special seminal receptacle for the storage of spermatozoa located between the 5th pereiopods on the ventral surface of the thorax of the female. In *P. japonicus*, *P. monodon*, *P. chinensis* and other species with the thelycum modified for internal storage of sperm ('closed thelycum'), mating occurs just after the female moults. At this time the male can insert the spermatophore (encapsulated spermatozoa) through the soft cuticle of the thelycum. In the 'open thelycum' penaeids, which include *P. vannamei*, *P. stylirostris* and *P. setiferus*, the spermatophore is attached to the exterior of the thelycum of a hard-cuticle, fully mature female only hours before she spawns. Prawns spawn directly into the sea water, and the eggs are fertilised by the stored spermatozoa at the moment of spawning.

Life-cycle

The development of penaeid prawns is complex. Larvae hatching from the fertilised eggs pass through a series of moults and metamorphic stages before becoming adult-like (juveniles). Juveniles continue to grow and moult as they develop into mature adults.

Each distinct life stage has a different behaviour, environmental requirement and nutritional needs. It is important to understand the early development stages when investigating disease problems in hatcheries. The generalised developmental biology described here most closely follows that of *P. monodon*, though it can be applied to all species. Details of time and nursery habitat (always coastal) can vary.

The eggs gradually sink to the bottom. Hatching of the first stage, the nauplius, occurs about 12 hours later. The larval stages consist of three to six nauplius, three protozoa and two or three mysis substages depending on actual species, each representing a moult. This larval development period varies with temperature and feeding levels but is usually 10–14 days. Mysis III larvae moult to become post-larvae (PL) which have all the appendages and organs seen in adult prawns.

Prawn larvae are naturally planktonic in behaviour. Swimming is possible using antennae in nauplii, antennae and thoracic appendages in protozoa and thoracic appendages in mysis larvae. The normal adult slow swimming using the pleopods (abdominal appendages) is seen in the post-larvae. Nauplii are about 0.3 mm long at hatching and are characterised by being totally planktonic and positively phototaxic; they exist entirely on their own egg yolk. The larvae begin to feed as protozoea. They are filter feeders and consume any particle of the correct size (8–200 μ); in hatcheries, unicellular algae are typically provided as food. They are approximately 1 mm in length, with a narrow elongated thorax and abdomen, and a loose-fitting carapace. Paired eyes, a rostrum and feeding appendages are present for the first

time. The second metamorphic change is seen when the third protozoea stage moults into the first mysis stage. Mysids have five pairs of functioning pereiopods (thoracic appendages). The carapace now covers all the thoracic segments. The mysids swim in a more adult manner and actively seek out phytoplankton and zooplankton to feed on. The final metamorphosis is to the post-larvae stage, where a full complement of functioning appendages are present.

Post-larvae are given a numerical suffix which indicates the time in days since metamorphosis. For example, a PL15 has been a post-larva for 15 days. Post-larvae continue to moult as they grow. They migrate shoreward and settle in nursery areas close to shore or in estuaries, where they grow quickly to juvenile and sub-adults, tolerating the variable physico-chemical environment. Sub-adults migrate back to sea where they finally mature to mate and spawn. Penaeid prawns are rarely older than two years.

Farming Systems

It is hard to generalise about the systems used to breed and rear prawns and shrimp. Actual details vary from country to country and species to species. Basically there are three types of on-growing farms: intensive culture systems in which prawns are raised in high density in tanks and raceways; semi-intensive systems where prawns are stocked at moderate densities in ponds, cages and occasionally tanks and where artificial food is fed; and extensive culture systems utilising large, low-density ponds or enclosures in natural bodies of water in which little or no management is practised or even possible. Prawn hatcheries are intensive or extensive (larger tanks and lower stocking densities) and will supply prawn fry (PL20–35) to the farm for on-growing to market size. Fry or early juveniles caught in the wild may be used for stocking in extensive culture systems and occasionally semi-intensive farms. The majority of prawns are farmed in earth ponds where they are fed on artifical diets and their water is aerated.

Hatcheries

There are three basic types of prawn hatchery found throughout the world: the communal culture method, the Taiwanese style and the western intensive or 'Galveston method'. In the simplest terms these three classifications refer to the density of larvae stocked in the larval rearing tanks and the size of those tanks. Larvae would be stocked at 30–50 per litre in the communal culture method, while the Galveston and Taiwanese methods stocking would be at 100 or more larvae per litre. Larval rearing tanks would be 10–30 t in the Taiwanese style hatchery, while 2 t tanks are more typical in a western intensive hatchery.

Communal culture method or the extensive hatchery

The extensive larval rearing methods were developed by the Japanese for *P. japonicus*. The method uses large rectangular or square tanks of 40–2,000 t made from concrete. The depth is 1.5–2 m. The idea of communal culture is to utilise a natural diatom (phytoplankton) bloom in the rearing water as food for the larvae. The water is fertilised with nitrates and phosphates to maintain the density of the algal bloom. Mature female prawns are added directly to the prepared tank; they spawn and are then removed. As the larvae get older, rotifer (*Brachionus* sp.) or brine shrimp (*Artemia salina*) nauplii (both zooplankton) are added to the tank water. Minced mussel, clam meat or commercial feeds are used once the prawns metamorphose to PLs. There is no water exchange through the rearing period, though the water depth may be increased by adding clean sea water. The advantage of this method is the low labour input (no algal culture) and the one tank is used for spawning, larval rearing and nursery rearing. The disadvantages are the high initial cost of tank construction, less control and the large number of spawners required for one rearing cycle in each tank.

Taiwanese style hatchery

The Taiwanese style hatchery is based on the 10–30 t square or rectangular concrete tanks used for larval rearing. Nauplii from a spawning tank are stocked at 100–150 per litre. The larval rearing tank may be completely dark or well lit, though a dim light is more usual as it encourages larvae to distribute more evenly through the water column. The rearing water may be managed as a clear or enriched ('dirty') water system. In the clear method, water is exchanged regularly and waste is siphoned from the tank bottom. The larvae feed on food added to the rearing water from the live food production section, e.g. algae and brine shrimp nauplii. In the 'dirty' system, water is rarely exchanged and waste accumulates on the tank bottom. It has been proposed that an ecological balance is maintained between the larvae, algae, micro-organisms and collidal organic particles. Algae and other food are added through the rearing period, and the larvae also eat organic particles in the water. Aeration is provided continuously in the tanks so that the food particles and larvae are maintained in an even suspension. In the 'dirty' system, the initial water level is 70% of the total, and is increased as the larvae get older. Water exchange is only required if the pH falls outside the range 7.7–8.3 or if mortalities begin to occur.

Western intensive hatchery

The western intensive system is a clear-water method where larvae are initially stocked at 100 per litre or higher. The hatcheries are quite compact and essentially they comprise a seawater supply system, an air supply system, a drainage system, a maturation section, spawning tanks, algal culture laboratory, algal culture tanks, brine shrimp hatching tanks, larval rearing tanks and a nursery or post-larval rearing tank area. The actual arrange ment of tanks and other facilities should be based on operational procedures which ensure efficient operation (Fig. 16.6). Hygiene considerations should also influence how the hatchery is designed. For example, the transfer of mature broodstock to spawning tanks should not be through larval rearing areas. All surfaces should be chemically resistant so that disinfection is possible. All floors should be sloping and drainable. All the water and aeration system should be accessible, and be able to be dismantled, disinfected and dried. Electricity for pumps and a freshwater supply for washing are advantageous. The importance of electricity to run blowers or compressors for aeration of algal and larval cultures is such that all hatcheries will have stand-by generators available in case of power failure.

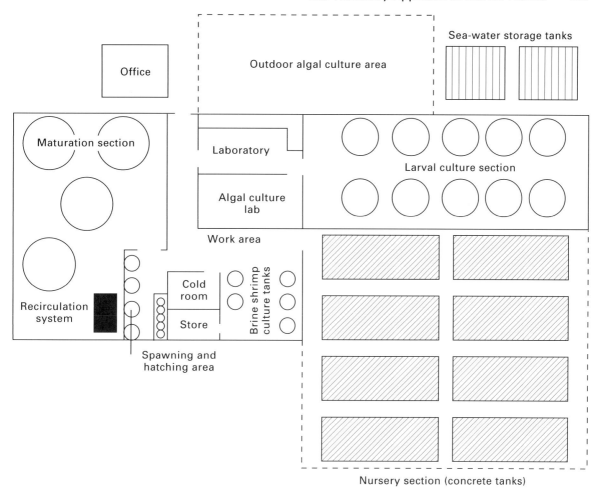

FIG. 16.6 A floor plan of an intensive prawn hatchery.

Sea water supply system. A sea water intake system would include pumps, some form of filtration and storage. The best intake is one that receives water via sub-sand filtration, though the intake pipes can be laid directly on the sea floor if the intake area has a rocky or sandy bottom.

Coarse screen filters are needed over the end of the open intake to prevent fish and marine organisms from entering. The water is then usually pumped to a settling tank prior to further filtration. Settling tanks are elevated to provide gravity fed water to the hatchery. Two settling tanks should be available so that one can be cleaned and disinfected without interfering with the hatchery water supply.

A common form of preliminary filtration is through pressurised sand filters (diatomaceous earth or activated charcoal can also be used) which filter to a nominal 200 μ particle size. Subsequent filtration is recommended for water to be used in spawning and larval rearing tanks, and in live food production. This further filtration is usually with a series of cartridge filters down to 5 μ. Many hatchery manuals recommend further water treatment using ultraviolet light (UV) disinfection and filtration through 1 μ cartridge filters. Water to be used in the starter algae cultures will often be filtered to 0.45 or 0.22 μ (again with cartridge filters) or autoclaved to make it sterile. An alternative to cartridge filtration and UV disinfection is chemical disinfection, by adding calcium hypochlorite to the settling or storage tank water to achieve a concentration of 10 mg/l residual chlorine after 12–24 hours of disinfection. Chlorinated water must be neutralised with sodium thiosulphate to remove any toxic oxidative by-products. The neutralised sea water should be used within 6 hours to avoid excessive increase in bacterial counts. Potassium sulphate may also be used as a chemical disinfectant.

It is important for the hatchery to have sufficient water for its daily use. Pumping capacities and reservoir storage volume should be determined from larval rearing and nursery tank capacities and planned water exchange rates. An even greater capacity is needed if the hatchery is sited in estuarine areas where rain could affect water quality.

Water circulation in the hatchery is closed. The distribution pipes should be drainable or, even better, able to be dismantled and dried. As prawns are very susceptible to metal poisoning, none of the pipes throughout the intake, filtering and tank systems should be of copper, brass, galvanised iron or non-marine grade stainless steel. PVC pipes are common. Water recirculation systems are used in some prawn hatcheries, for example when ambient water temperatures require heating or when oceanic water supplies are limited.

Air supply system. Oil-free blowers (low pressure, high volume) or compressors are used. The air lines are usually PVC pipes. The pipe system should include condensation traps and taps to bleed off water. Air intakes should be away from hatchery areas and have dust filters. Several air blowers should be installed so that the hatchery always has a back-up in case of break-downs.

Drainage system. The drainage system must be big enough in all parts of the hatchery to ensure complete discharge of waste water. The floors and tank outlets must drain to the drainage system properly. Flooding of the hatchery floors should not occur. Drainage systems are usually open and can be used as an aid in larval and post-larval harvesting.

Maturation section. In many instances wild-caught broodstock or spawners are used to supply fertilised eggs for the hatchery. Gravid females with fully mature ovaries are held in spawning tanks and will spawn the first or second night after capture. Blank females (non-gravid) and males are collected, held

in maturation tanks and fed a high quality fresh diet. Ovary maturation and spawning are induced by the removal of an eye or eye-stalk ablation 1–2 weeks before eggs are required.

Maturation sections, as with larval rearing, require oceanic water. Typically a unit will consist of circular tanks 3–6 m in diameter with a black, smooth inner surface. The water depth would be at least 1 m. For *P. monodon* a sandy bottom is recommended, though no substrate is necessary for most species. The section should be well screened to provide a low light intensity and lit to provide a constant photoperiod. A daily water exchange rate of 200–300% is necessary. Ideally, this water would be drawn continuously from the ocean source. In reality, filter and heating costs usually mean that maturation tank water is recirculated. The individual tank can have its own sub-sand filtration or is supplied from a separate recirculation system with a biological filter, settling tank and protein skimmer.

The maturation section also has spawning tanks, feed preparation and storage areas, and a laboratory area where hatched nauplii are counted. Mature mated females are selected from the maturation tanks and placed in spawning tanks. The spawning tanks are fibreglass with an inner food-grade gel coat. They are usually small (150 litres) and may be designed to collect the eggs, which sink to the bottom so that they can be transferred to a hatching container. Otherwise the spawner is removed and the eggs are allowed to hatch in the spawning tank. Mild aeration is supplied. The actual water conditions, temperature and salinity depend on the species of prawn. The phototaxic nature of nauplii is often exploited to concentrate and collect them prior to transfer to larval rearing tanks.

Larval rearing tanks. A range of tank designs are used for larval rearing. Initially 2,000 l to 5 t cylindroconical fibreglass tanks were used, typically with a central standpipe outlet screened with fine mesh (200–500 μ, depending on the age of the larvae); continuous aeration is supplied from the bottom of the cone to mix and suspend larvae and food particles. More common now are long, parabolic 10–20 t fibreglass tanks, which use space efficiently and have excellent characteristics for water circulation (using a central aeration line), cleaning and harvesting. Depending on local ambient air temperatures, submersible water heaters, may be needed to maintain water temperatures overnight and the tanks should be insulated to stop excessive heat loss and high energy costs.

The actual type of tank varies greatly. Concrete or concrete block tanks are not uncommon. Low cost tanks made from plywood, or even bamboo slats, and lined with plastic are used in the Philippines and Thailand. In all instances an even aeration through the tank must be supplied. Subdued lighting is usually recommended and can be achieved by individual tank covers or by enclosing the hatchery. Any tank design needs to consider ease of cleaning, drainage and harvest. In the clear-water intensive hatchery, all food must be provided.

Nursery tanks. Once the larvae metamorphose to post-larvae, PL3–5s are harvested and transferred to nursery tanks. These are larger than the larval rearing tanks; they can be circular, square or rectangular and made from fibreglass or concrete, or lined with plastic. They are designed to provide adequate aeration, to be drainable and to allow easy harvesting. Stocking densities are lower. PL are fed artifical compounded diets or minced fresh foods until they are harvested as PL10–25 or the size required for stocking at the farm.

Live food production section. One of the most labour intensive and expensive activities in a hatchery is the production of food for the larvae to eat. While recent advances have meant artificial micro-particulate foods are available for larvae, hatcheries traditionally rely on a range of unicellular algae and brine shrimp nauplii for food. The mass culture of algae requires large tanks in direct sunlight. These tanks are either inoculated with 500–1,000 l of an axenic algal starter culture of a single species, or filled with unfiltered sea water which is fertilised and the mixed natural algal population is allowed to bloom. The production of algae starter cultures usually follows a sequence comprising inoculation of a pure stock culture into carboys (5 l) and thence into starter culture (500 l or 1,000 l). An air-conditioned algal culture laboratory is present in most hatcheries for the initial transfers and culture. An autoclave or ultrafiltered water is available for culture media

preparation. Pumps can be used to move starter and mass culture media around.

The culture of brine shrimp (*Artemia salina*) involves the hatching of commercially purchased brine shrimp cysts (or eggs). Typically 150–500 l cylindroconical fibreglass tanks are used. The tanks are well aerated and the bottom of the cone is usually transparent. When the aeration is turned off, the hatched nauplii move to the light where they can be drained and harvested into fine mesh sieves.

Farms

Prawn farms can be intensive, semi-intensive or extensive but how farms are classified varies. Generally, intensive culture is in concrete tanks or raceways with stocking densities at 160–200 PL/m^2. Semi-intensive cultures utilise 0.2–5 ha earth or concrete-walled ponds with 20–50 PL stocked per m^2 of pond bottom. In extensive culture 5–20 ha and larger ponds are used with stocking densities at 1–10 PL/m^2.

Intensive farms use ponds, raceways or tanks of 500–5,000 m^2. Pond walls may be earthen, plastic lined or concrete. Often the bottom is left as earth, although sand is used. The Japanese have a circular concrete tank system of 1,000–2,000 t for the intensive culture of *P. japonicus*. This 'Shigueno' type has a sandy substrate on the tank bottom. Due to the high density of culture and high feed inputs, maintenance of the water quality by water exchange and aeration is essential. Intensive prawn farms have the same kind of infrastructure requirements as other intensive fish farm systems.

Semi-intensive farms are the most common system in Asia and the Pacific. The basic farm comprises a pump station(s), primary supply canal or reservoir, grow-out and nursery (optional) ponds, drainage canals, and intake and discharge water control structures in each pond.

The site selected for the semi-intensive farm should have water temperatures of 28°C and greater if tropical species like *P. monodon* and *P. vannemi* are to be cultured. The water salinity should be within the optimum for each species but brackish water (15–25 ppt) is good. Water should come from an unpolluted estuary, river or mangrove creek. The area should have a low evaporation rate and not be influenced by heavy rain or flooding. A freshwater supply is useful for diluting pond water. The soil should be a clay-loam with a pH greater than 5.5. On-site electricity and the other infrastructure requirements of good road access, good communications and local equipment and feed suppliers are other factors to consider. Access to a reliable supply of PLs is essential, and some farms have on-site hatcheries to fulfil this requirement.

The farm layout depends on the topography of the site and location of the water source. Some farms are constructed to allow tidal exchange of water but this limits the ability of the farmer to change water as required. With tidal water exchange, farms do not stock above 20 PL/m^2. More common is a design which depends on pumps to raise the water to an elevated primary supply canal. Water is then gravity fed to the individual ponds. The elevations are such that a drainage canal is built above the high tide mark so that ponds can be drain-harvested at any time. The size of the total pond area, the tidal ranges if the pump inlet is above low water mark and the expected stocking densities influence the pumping capacity and reservoir size required. Pumps are axial or centrifugal and are run by electricity. Diesel-powered pumps and those run from tractor power take-off attachments are also used. Bore-water and beach-well water can supply a farm. Water reticulation from the primary supply canal is varied. Open canals with small PVC pipes supplying individual ponds may be used. Supply canals may be open, concrete culvert-like systems built on pond walls or buried concrete pipes.

Rectangular earth ponds of 0.2–5 ha are common, sometimes with concrete walls. Typical pond depths are 1–1.5 m. Pond walls should slope at 2:1 to 3.5:1, depending on the type of soil used for construction. The inlet and outlet should be at opposite ends and the bottom should slope toward the outlet with a minimum fall of 0.1%. The pond must be able to drain completely. Inlet structures or pipes must be screened to prevent entry of fish (eggs, larvae and adults) and other aquatic animals.

The outlet structure is usually concrete. It can be a monk with wooden boards and screens; it may be a gate built into the pond wall or even a combination utilising concrete walls and PVC drain pipes. The structure should be designed to control the water depth, take water from the pond bottom and allow screens to be attached. It is important that the outlet structure or pipes are large enough to allow rapid drainage for harvesting. Outlet structures in the pond, or more usually in the drainage canal, can be modified to allow harvest nets or cages to be attached and many farms construct a concrete harvest area or catch basin around the outlet structure, which helps to keep the prawns alive at the end of a drain harvest.

Aeration is usual in semi-intensive prawn ponds, particularly overnight and early morning. Dissolved oxygen levels must never drop below 2 mg/l — even a couple of hours at this threshold will slow growth. Paddle wheel aerators of 0.5–3 hp are common and 6 units/ha is usually recommended. The paddle wheel aerators are also important for circulating the pond water. Injection aerators are becoming more common now and in these a propeller at the end of a tube under the pond surface pulls air down into the water, producing fine bubbles which are good for oxygen transfer.

Semi-intensive farming involves feeding artificial diets, although the algal bloom and natural pond productivity are important for good production. Trash fish is used and care is needed to avoid water quality problems. More common are compounded pellet diets which have a high water stability and often include soluble amino acids from prawn head meal or squid meal as attractants. The even spread of the pellets over the pond is important to maximise production. Pellet blowers or modified fertiliser spreaders attached to tractors can be used for feed distribution and it is usual for the layout to allow vehicle or tractor access to all ponds. Wooden walkways in the pond increase the accessible area.

There are some farm systems which have nursery ponds or tanks at the farm. The ponds are small (0.05–0.4 ha) and the PLs are stocked at 60–200/m^2. The prawns are held for up to two months or when they are 1–2 g in size. They are harvested and transferred to the on-growing pond. Covered nursery ponds are used to provide a head start for prawns in sub-tropical regions when stocking in the winter or early spring.

Extensive farms are common in Ecuador, where the ponds are up to 100 ha. A few farms in Southeast Asia and elsewhere have been built to follow this farming system. There is very little water exchange — perhaps 1–5% per day — and the water can be supplied by tidal exchange through sluice gates or with pumps. Normally water levels are 70–100 cm. The prawns feed on natural food present in the pond, though supplementary feeds are used occasionally. Prawn fry for stocking may be supplied from wild-caught prawns or from hatcheries and stocking densities are 1–10 PL/m^2. Again, the principles of good pond design and construction need to be followed. In particular, the pond should be drainable to facilitate an efficient drain harvest.

Traditional extensive farms in Indonesia, China and India have low stocking densities and rely on natural pond production. These farms use tidal water exchange and a partial harvest system, taking prawns of the right size over long periods from the one pond or enclosure. Many of these ponds are being modified and upgraded to semi-intensive pond production methods.

General Husbandry

Each species of prawn has some specific requirements for growth. Similarly, the husbandry is somewhat specific for each species and each type of farming system or country. In the grow-out stage local conditions are an important modifying influence on how the farm is managed. The market for the prawns will influence husbandry of the pond prior to harvest. Details of how each species should be reared will not be given here but some general comments are possible.

Husbandry in the Hatchery

As in all farming, there is a lot of art in the science of prawn hatchery operation but some basic husbandry principles can be stated:

- Use the best broodstock.
- The better the nauplii, the easier it is to get good survival to post-larvae.
- Use clean sea water with bacterial counts less than or equal to 10^3/ml.
- Provide as stable an environment (water quality) in the rearing tank as possible.
- Avoid any sudden changes of pH, salinity or temperature at water exchange or addition of live food.

In the maturation section of the facility, the light intensity and ambient noise levels are kept low. Adult prawns are fed fresh food including mussel, clam, cockle and squid. The ratio of males to females is usually 1:1. The fecundity and viability of spawnings from ablated female broodstock have not been as good as spawnings from wild-caught females. Some farmers prefer post-larvae from wild rather than induced spawnings. Gentle handling and good water is essential for successful spawnings.

A larval rearing cycle in the hatchery begins with a spawning and the preparation of the larval rearing tank. The fertilised eggs or nauplii are washed and disinfected. The nauplii numbers are estimated by sampling and counting, using a microscope. The water in the hatching tank should be within ±0.5°C and ±1 ppt salinity of the water in the larval rearing tank. If it is not, the nauplii need to be acclimatised. The rearing tank has already been cleaned, disinfected, rinsed and dried; before it is used again for larval rearing it is filled with filtered sea water, then drained and refilled. Some hatcheries add EDTA at 10 mg/litre to chelate any toxic metals present in the water. A stock of algae is added and then the nauplii are carefully transferred to the tank.

Feeding of algae, zooplankton and other food follows guidelines established for each species. (Several examples of feeding programmes are given in Fig. 16.7.) The husbandry of the larvae then follows a daily pattern, beginning with water management. Water quality parameters like temperature, pH, salinity, ammonia and perhaps nitrite/nitrate levels are checked. Any sediment in rearing tanks is removed by syphoning. If the hatchery uses a batch water exchange system, new water is then added. The tanks should be checked and the screens over the water outlets cleaned. Water exchange must be done whenever problems are suspected and usually every day after the mysis stage is reached. The actual amount varies from hatchery to hatchery and with the age of the larval culture but a 50% exchange per day is generally adequate in an intensive hatchery. The density of algae and zooplankton is assessed twice a day (the morning measurement is after the water exchange) and appropriate amounts of the food organisms are added. The larvae should be examined several times during the day and night, but always at least once in the morning, and assessed in the sampling

FEEDING SCHEDULES FOR REARING LARVAL PRAWNS				

1. For penaeid prawns

Day	Stage*	Algae (cells/ml)		*Artemia* (nauplii/ml)
		Isochrysis	*Tetraselmis chuii*	
0	N_1–N_3	—	—	—
1	N_3–N_6	75000 (20% yeast)	—	—
2	P_1	100000 (20% yeast)	—	—
3	P_1	100000 (20% yeast)	—	—
4	P_2	100000 (20% yeast)	—	—
5	P_2	75000 (20% yeast)	20000	—
6	P_2	75000 (20% yeast)	20000	—
7	P_3	50000 (20% yeast)	40000	3.0 (frozen)
8	P_3	50000 (20% yeast)	40000	3.0 (frozen)
9	M_1	—	40000	3.0 (frozen)
10	M_2	—	20000	3.0 (frozen) + 3.0 (live)
11	M_3	—	—	8.0 (live)
12	PL_1	—	—	10.0 (live)

2. For penaeid prawns

Day	Stage*	Algae (cells/ml)		*Artemia* (nauplii/ml)
		Isochrysis	*Tetraselmis chuii*	
0	N_1–N_3	—	—	—
1	N_3–N_6	—	—	—
2	N_6–P_1	50000	—	—
3	P_1	80000	20000	—
4	P_1–P_2	80000	20000	—
5	P_2	50000	50000	—
6	P_3	50000	50000	—
7	P_3–M_1	—	80000	—
8	M_1	—	50000	0.2
9	M_2	—	50000	0.2
10	M_3	—	30000	0.5
11	M_3–PL_1	—	30000	1
12	PL_1	—	—	1

3. For *P. merguensis*

Day	Stage*	Algae (cells/ml) *Skeletonema*	*Artemia* (nauplii/ml)	Dry plankton g/m^3
0	N_1–N_3	—	—	—
1	N_4–N_6	2000	—	—
2	P_1	10000	—	—
3	P_1–P_2	10000	—	—
4	P_2–P_3	10000	0.5	—
5	M_1	10000	1	—
6	M_1–M_2	10000	1.5	—
7	M_2–M_3	10000	2	—
8	M_3	10000	2	—
9	PL_1	5000	3	—
10	PL_2	5000	3	—
11	PL_3	5000	3	2
12	PL_4	—	3	2

* N = nauplii; P = protozea; M = mysis; PL = post-larvae.

FIG. 16.7 Feeding schedules for rearing larval prawns.

beaker for appearance, colour and activity. The stage of development of the larvae is determined by microscopic examination and a health check is carried out at the same time, monitoring for ciliates, filamentous bacteria, deformities, bacterial necrosis lesions and any other abnormalities.

Once the larvae have all metamorphosed to post-larvae, they can be harvested and transferred to nursery tanks. Final rearing in the hatchery is at lower stocking densities. Usually more artifical feed is used during the nursery rearing period.

The Husbandry of Prawns in Ponds

There are four important areas to be considered as a pond of prawns is grown for harvest after three to five months: the initial pond preparation, stocking the pond with post-larvae, water management and feeding. The daily routine on a farm is to check the screens on inlets and outlets and clean them, look at the pond water and test it, distribute the food, monitor food consumption, look at the prawns, and exchange the water and feed again as required.

Pond preparation

The pond must be completely sun dried after excess bottom debris has been removed. The pond is then limed, ideally with quicklime to disinfect the bottom. More lime can be added as carbonate of lime or slaked lime if required to raise the pH of the soil and improve pond productivity. The inlet screens must be checked and replaced or repaired if damaged. No fish eggs, larvae or juveniles should enter as the pond is filled with water because they may grow to become predators. Kill any fish present by adding tea-seed cake, or other source of saponin, or rotenone to the partially filled pond. Fill the pond completely and fertilise to get a good diatom algal bloom. The ideal bloom is a green–brown to golden brown colour, with a secchi disk transparency density of 30–40 cm. Inorganic fertiliser with a ratio of nitrogen to phosphorus at 10–20:1 is said to encourage a diatom bloom. Farms may use organic materials, such as chicken manure, suspended in bags as a fertiliser.

Pond stocking

The stocking of PLs is a critical time for the farmer. Good quality prawns should be used. If poor PL survival is suspected, the farmer must decide whether to drain and restock or continue growing the understocked pond. Both decisions will lose the farmer money. A good algal bloom should be established to provide food for the PLs. To minimise acclimatisation stress, farmers should advise the hatchery of the pond water characteristics at least three days before stocking so that the hatchery can adjust its water conditions to within $\pm 3°C$ water temperature, 3–5 ppt salinity and ± 1 pH unit.

Transport from the hatchery and stocking are best done in the early morning to avoid extremes of temperature. The PLs should be acclimatised in a tank beside the pond at a rate of no more than 2.5% of the transport water per minute. Farmers should avoid obtaining PLs from hatcheries which use rearing water temperatures greater than 32°C or antibiotics, or where the PLs are not exposed to light for at least 2–3 days prior to transfer. A group of PLs should be kept in the acclimatisation tank for 2 days to assess initial survivals after transport and stocking; thereafter some PLs can be retained in small cages in the pond for continued survival monitoring until the juvenile prawns can be caught by cast nets at 4–5 weeks.

Water management

The quality of the water is monitored daily, usually at sunrise and again at the end of the day. Temperature, dissolved oxygen (DO), salinity, transparency (secchi disk reading) and pH are measured routinely. Many of these factors are inter-related; for example, if there is a dense algal bloom (secchi disk reading of less than 20 cm) the DO will be low in the morning. A good farmer keeps a record of these parameters and develops an idea of how each pond responds to management and weather changes, so that feeding levels, water exchange rates or fertiliser levels can be adjusted before there is a water quality problem. In general terms the DO should never be below 2 mg/litre, salinity should be around the optimum for the species under culture and the pH should be at

7.5–8.5 in the morning. The bloom density should be maintained at 30–40 cm for at least the first 4 weeks of culture.

Many farmers do not exchange water in the early stages because new water will wash away the PLs' naturally grown foods and also because the strong currents at water exchange can damage the PLs, crushing them against the outlet screens. Initially daily water exchange will be 5–10% of total pond water, depending on the stocking rate and algal bloom. The rate can be increased to 30% per day as the prawns reach market size. A reservoir capacity to exchange 60% per day should be available to avoid problems if the algal bloom grows out of control.

Feeding

With good pond preparation, the natural food present is often sufficient for the PLs for the first 6 weeks. In intensive culture, however, or in nursery ponds or if the pond has not been well prepared, feeding must start immediately. Initial feeding rates are 25% of total prawn biomass but this decreases gradually to 2.5% of total biomass as the prawns reach market size. Manufacturers provide a range of pellet sizes and offer feeding rate tables based on the size of the prawn. The food should be distributed as evenly as possible over the pond.

At first, the feeding rate must be calculated on estimated survival after stocking (80% would be considered normal) and expected growth. From the time the juveniles are caught, feed consumption rates can be monitored using feeding trays in ponds and daily feeding rates are adjusted accordingly. (Overfeeding is expensive and affects water quality.) Fortnightly cast net samples taken at random in the pond should be used to estimate the average weight of the prawns. The total biomass is calculated from the average weight and the estimated survival rate.

Nursery ponds

Nursery ponds are used in some farms to grow PL15–20 to a 1 g juvenile for stocking into a grow-out pond. Nursery pond culture systems have the advantage of increasing the number of harvests from each grow-out pond. The number of juveniles

stocked for grow-out can be estimated accurately at harvest and transfer from the nursery; consequently feeding rates are estimated more accurately. The prawns also have access to natural food twice in the production cycle, which is another saving on feed costs. Because the prawns are larger in grow-out ponds, there are fewer losses to predators. Disadvantages include the cost of extra construction and ponds, and the losses at harvest which count against every farmer having a two-stage rearing system.

Legislation

Prawn farms have caused specific problems in some areas, and it is in these areas where some governments have legislated.

Many prawn farms in South-east Asia were built in the narrow mangrove zone. Except for mangrove forestry, this land was considered unused or unusable and prawn farming became the ideal new industry to utilise it. In many places the mangroves had already gone as the land had been exploited for rice paddies or fish ponds and eventually the importance of the mangrove fringe to protect coastal areas from storm erosion was recognised. It was also appreciated that the mangroves were nursery areas for wild fish and prawns. Some countries now have legislation which limits the amount of mangrove forest that can be used, or which requires a 100–200 m fringe be left.

Rapid development of the prawn farming industry can place a great fishing pressure on wild fry or broodstock of the desirable aquaculture species. This overexploitation and the demands of the local industry have resulted in the introduction of bans on the export of broodstock by some Asian countries.

There are other problems. Too many farms in a small area can lead to severe water pollution. Disease associated with pollution stress has caused big production losses in Taiwan and northern Thailand recently. There is a need to limit the number or size of farms in an area. Water treatment or conditioning may be required before pond water is discharged into natural water bodies.

In the narrow coastal zones of some countries, rice paddies have been developed as prawn ponds. Once the paddies have been contaminated by sea water, long-term soil reconditioning is needed before rice production is possible again. The production of a staple food like rice might be strategically more important than the production of a luxury product for export.

The demand for fish meal for use in pelleted prawn diets has affected some poor coastal communities. Overexploitation of wild fish stocks for fish meal can make it very difficult for local artisans to catch any fish. Their standard of living drops or, worse, they starve. The development of any new industry should take into account the needs of all the community, as well as the economy of the country or the wealth of an individual.

Major Diseases

Most of the serious diseases are described from the hatchery or intensive nursery systems. Fortunately it is at these levels where early diagnosis and therapy are practical. Diseases are seen in juveniles in grow-out systems but are often associated with poor pond fertility, poor pond bottom conditions or poor water quality. Very intensive juvenile culture in tanks or raceways are similar to intensive nursery systems and thus experience similar disease problems.

Disease in Hatcheries

Things happen quickly in larvae and early post-larvae. Disease processes are no exception: all the larvae in a rearing tank can die within 48 hours if appropriate action is not taken as soon as disease is detected. Many commercial hatcheries add antibiotics to culture water routinely because the acuteness of larval disease does not allow time for detection and then successful treatment. Sudden changes in water temperature, salinity and pH, at water changes or addition of food organisms, can cause mortalities as easily as infectious pathogens. Accumulated nitrogenous waste and unutilised nitrates from algal culture media can also cause problems. Disease, poor growth and actual mortalities can be associated with underfeeding. Poor husbandry and water management have an important effect on disease incidence and the success of a larval culture. As a generalisation, disease is common at protozoea III and mysis I substages, and again in early post-larvae (PL1–3). Also, disease is more common in older hatcheries than in new ones.

Early larval mortalities

The spawning of poor quality broodstock can lead to weak nauplii. The survival of these larvae to protozoea I or II can be very low. They do not appear to have the strength to start feeding vigorously. Appendage abnormalities which prevent moulting can also result from a poor quality spawning.

Monodon baculovirus disease (MBV)

Baculoviruses are common in invertebrates. monodon baculovirus most commonly causes disease in PL20–30. Larvae are not affected. The virus infects mid-gut gland tubule cells and mid-gut mucosa. Affected PLs are dark, lethargic, anorexic and often heavily fouled by epicommensal organisms. Diagnosis is on the histological appearance of eosinophilic viral occlusions in the nuclei of mid-gut gland tubule cells. Crowding and poor husbandry in nursery tanks at hatcheries will enhance the severity of the infection. Post-larvae with infections of moderate severity do not transport well and may have high mortalities at initial pond stocking. MBV may be detected in pond-reared juvenile prawns suffering from other diseases.

Baculovirus penaei (BP)

This was the first viral disease of penaeid prawns described. BP causes serious epizootics in larval, post-larval and juvenile *P. aztecus*, *P. duorarum*, *P. vannemei* and others. It is restricted to the USA and the Pacific Coast side of Central and South America. Multiple polyhedral occlusion bodies form in the mid-gut gland tubule cell nuclei. In larvae, BP epizootics are acute with near 100% mortalities in 24–48 hours. Affected prawns stop feeding and growing, and there is epicommensal fouling due to the reduced grooming activity of the sick prawn. In juvenile prawns the disease is more chronic and total mortalities are lower.

Baculoviral mid-gut gland necrosis (BMN)

BMN is another disease caused by a baculovirus but it has been described only from *P. japonicus* and is restricted to Japan, where it is principally a disease of larvae and post-larvae. Mortalities of

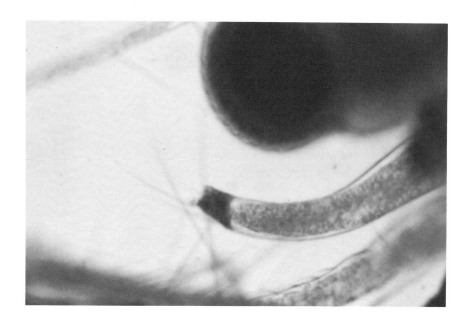

up to 98% by PL20 are reported. Affected prawns have a 'white-turbid' or opaque mid-gut gland. This baculovirus does not produce occlusion bodies, though histologically there is a marked nuclear hypertrophy, and necrosis of mid-gut gland tubule cells. This, with electronmicroscopy, would be diagnostic.

Bacterial necrosis

All ages of larvae are susceptible to this common disease. A progressive erosion of appendages within melanisation (a brown to black pigment) is apparent. Larvae become weak and die. 100% mortality of a larval culture can occur if young larvae are affected but mortalities are low in PLs. The disease appears to be associated with trauma to the cuticle (e.g. heavy aeration), conditions that encourage high number of bacteria in the culture water (e.g. poor hatchery hygiene, high organic loads or contaminated algae) and undefined nutritional and environmental stressors. Bacterial necrosis is more common in older hatcheries. While the aetiology has not been proven, there is a bacterial involvement in the lesions and antibiotics added to the larval culture water do stop mortalities. Diagnosis is on the appearance of the multifocal melanised cuticular lesions on antennae, uropods, pleopods and other append-

ages (Fig. 16.8). Death probably results from a secondary bacterial septicaemia or failure to moult as the old cuticle is held back by necrotic adhesions.

Luminous vibriosis

This is a recently described disease which can cause 100% mortalities in *P. monodon* larval cultures of all ages. At night the movement of affected larvae can be followed because they emit a continuous greenish luminescence. The luminous bacteria *Vibrio harveyi* appears to be responsible. Masses of the bacteria accumulate in the gut and then rapidly multiply and spread to the haemoceole to cause death. Diagnosis is on an increasing mortality rate, luminous larvae and isolation of a luminous *V. harveyi*. Chemical treatment of the disease is limited. Prevention is by good hatchery hygiene and frequent water exchange in larval cultures.

Larval bacterial septicaemia

A systemic bacterial infection is a common terminal event in larvae and PLs following a range of other diseases, poor water quality, wounding etc. Ubiquitous bacteria in the marine environment and bacteria which are part of the prawns'

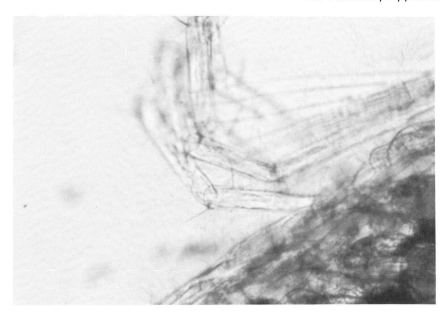

FIG. 16.9 Filamentous bacterial fouling on the pereiopods of a post-larval *P. monodon*.

normal microflora are implicated as the pathogen. These opportunist bacterial pathogens include *Vibrio alginolyticus*, *V. parahaemolyticus*, other *Vibrio* spp., *Aeromonas sp.* and *Pseudomonas* sp. Diagnosis is on detection of large numbers of motile bacteria in the haemolymph of affected larvae. Examination of Gram-stained tissue sections helps detect early infections. Larvae may have a red body colour, will stop eating and are less active. At times the mid-gut gland become opaque white. Severe mortalities do occur. Larval septicaemia prevalence increases with the age of the hatchery.

Filamentous bacterial fouling

Leucothrix mucor, a filamentous bacteria ubiquitous in the marine environment, can foul the surface of larvae and post-larvae. The bacteria does no direct harm; rather, the infestation causes mortalities by impairing respiration, feeding, swimming and moulting. Disease outbreaks are often associated with high organic loads in culture water, low dissolved oxygen levels and the added stress of moulting e.g. protozoea III to mysis I. It is a common secondary infection in PLs with monodon baculovirus disease. Entire larval cultures can die overnight. Early diagnosis is important. Diagnosis is on the identification of filamentous bacteria covering the body surface and gill filaments (Fig. 16.9) in wet preparation examinations.

Larval mycosis

This systemic fungal disease of larvae and post-larvae has been the cause of serious mortalities in hatcheries throughout the world. Protozoeal and mysid stages are most susceptible. A sudden onset of mortalities is seen, often with the entire larval culture dead in 24 hours. Affected larvae contain an extensive, non-septate, highly branched fungal mycelium throughout the body and appendages (Fig. 16.10). It is considered that phycomycete fungi in the genera *Lagenidium*, *Sirolpidium* and *Haliphthoros* are the aetiological agents. It can be very difficult to prevent entry of the small, free-swimming, infective zoospores to the hatchery. Washing the fertilised eggs or nauplii with sterile sea water is an effective preventative method. Larval mycosis can be secondary to bacterial necrosis. The overuse of antibiotics seems to encourage outbreaks in larvae by removing the competitive microflora, allowing the fungus to proliferate.

Protozoan fouling

Another form of epicommensal surface fouling is due to infestation by various sessile peritrichous ciliates (e.g. *Zoothamnium*, *Epistylis* and *Vorticella*)

FIG. 16.10 Fungal hyphae throughout the uropods in a *P. monodon* with larval mycosis.

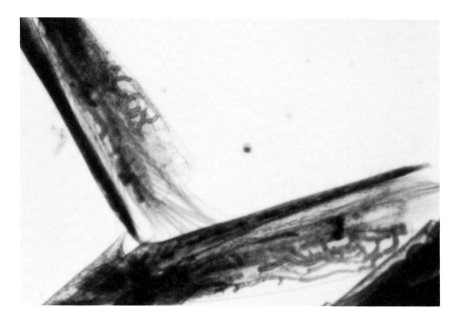

and possibly other types of protozoans (e.g. the suctorians). As in filamentous bacterial fouling, the main effect is the obstruction of gill filament surfaces causing hypoxia and death if the infestation is severe. Clinically affected prawns can be discoloured, are lethargic and may swim to the surface of the tank. High levels of organic waste or high bacterial counts in the culture water result in increased ciliate numbers. High mortalities are only apparent when there are high numbers of ciliates together with low dissolved oxygen levels. Masses of the characteristic protozoa are easily identified on microscope examination of wet mounted larvae or post-larvae.

Disease in Farms

Unless one considers intensive tank or raceway culture, disease in juveniles in a pond or enclosure is usually detected only after a significant number of prawns have died. As a consequence, therapeutic administration of antibiotics or other chemicals is rarely economic. There may be some benefit in saving some of the pond population simply so that the farmer has some money, even though there is no profit. Practically, the farmer can respond to clinical disease by improving husbandry, increasing water exchange and reducing total biomass of prawns in the pond by partial harvesting. The lower stocking densities seen in semi-intensive and extensive systems result in a low prevalence of the disease, but it is seen and can cause devastating loss.

Infectious hypodermal and haematopoietic necrosis (IHHN)

This viral disease is caused by a small RNA-containing picorna-like virus. The most serious disease is described from high density, intensive tank and raceway cultured *P. stylirostris* and *P. monodon*. Its effect on pond-cultured prawns is variable. The signs of the disease are not specific. Infected juveniles show reduced feeding and a behaviour which involves rising to the surface, rolling and then sinking to the bottom. Moribund prawns may have a bluish colour with opaque abdominal muscles. The disease is found in the Americas, but virus-infected prawns have been observed in South-east Asia, Tahiti and Israel. The virus has probably been spread to other countries with the movement of IHHN contaminated hatchery-reared prawns. Diagnosis requires histological demonstration of eosinophilic, Feulgen-negative intranuclear inclusions in tissues of ecto-dermal or mesodermal origin, i.e. not mid-gut gland tubule cells.

Hepatopancreatic parvo-like virus disease (HPV)

The small DNA containing, parvo-like virus most commonly causes disease and mortalities in juvenile prawns. Within 4–8 weeks of onset, accumulated mortalities of 50–100% have been seen in *P. merguiensis* and *P. semisulcatus*. A range of clinical signs are seen, including poor growth rates, anorexia, surface fouling by epicommensals and secondary infections. The severity of the infection is enhanced by the stress of crowding. The virus infects the tubules cells of the mid-gut gland to cause necrosis and atrophy of the gland. Diagnosis is on identification of the prominent basophilic, Feulgen-positive intranuclear inclusion bodies in the tubules cell nuclei. HPV seems to be distributed throughout the Indo-West Pacific.

Shell disease

This is a common, usually non-lethal bacterial disease seen in wild and cultured crustacea, including prawns, all over the world. Grossly the characteristic lesions of brown or black eroded areas are present on the gills, carapace, abdomen and appendages. After each moult the old diseased exuvium is lost. Mortalities may occur when the eroded cuticle extends in the underlaying soft tissue. Death would follow secondary bacterial infections or entrapment in the old exuvium. Damage to the outermost, waxy protective layer of the cuticle permits invasion by ubiquitous bacteria. The bacteria multiply and erode the deeper layers with chitinases. The initial damage is caused by handling or inter-animal trauma, nutritional deficiencies, chemical exposure, pollution, nitrogenous waste products or developmental abnormalities. Shell disease increases in conditions that encourage high numbers of bacteria. In fact, an increase in prevalence of shell disease lesions on the uropods and telson of pond-reared prawns indicates poor pond bottom conditions.

Bacterial septicaemia (vibriosis)

Systemic bacterial infections of juvenile prawns can be seen throughout the world. Bacterial septicaemias have become one of the most common disease problems seen in pond culture but are entirely avoidable. The infection is secondary to severe stress, other diseases, wounds and poor environment. The organisms isolated from moribund prawns are usually *Vibrio* bacteria, which are common in the brackish-water environment. Prawns with septicaemia display non-specific signs which include lethargy, darkening of the body, anorexia, gathering at the pond edge, occasionally reddening of the gills and appendages, and increased cuticular epicommensal fouling. Extensive shell disease lesions may also be present if pond conditions have been poor for some time. In well prepared ponds where farmers provide good water quality and do not over feed, bacterial septicaemias should not be a problem.

Rickettsial infections

Rickettsia-like organisms can cause a systemic infection and disease in prawns. Grossly the prawns are lethargic, collect at the pond edge, have a dark body colour and have secondary bacterial or viral infections. Cumulative mortalities of a pond population may be as high as 90%. In *P. marginatus* and *P. merguiensis*, rickettsial microcolonies are present in the mid-gut gland tubule cells; while in *P. monodon* the rickettsia are more systemic, although principally damaging the lymphoid organ. In practice, control of the disease is very difficult. The source of the infection and the normal host are not known. Treatment of juvenile prawns in ponds does not produce a permanent cure — mortalities begin again as soon as medicated feeds are withdrawn.

Fusarium *(fungus) disease*

This is a mycosis that primarily affects the cuticle and the gills. The fungus, *Fusarium solani*, produces expanding cuticular or subcuticular lesions which are black or brown. Only juveniles and adults appear susceptible to this ubiquitous deutromycete fungus. Up to 10% of prawns can carry the infection in a pond. Mortality rates of 90% have been reported from epizootics in tank and raceway reared *P. californiensis*. The disease has been described from the Americas, Japan, Tahiti and Thailand. Identification of the characteristic canoe-shaped macroconidia (spores) in or on melanised lesions provides a definitive diagnosis of this disease.

Black gill syndrome

Black gills are a clinical sign and not a single disease. It is common to see darkened gills following an accumulation of debris and sediment between the filaments. This is associated with high organic and particulate loads in culture water. There could be some interference of normal respiration as a result. The gills will clean when the prawn is returned to clean water. Darkened gills have also been associated with exposure to toxic chemicals like cadmium, copper and nitrate and to low pH. Black gills are a common clinical sign of IHHN, shell disease, filamentous bacterial, fouling and protozoan fouling. It is important that, at the very least, wet mounted gills be examined microscopically before a diagnosis is made. One specific disease in which black gills are an important clinical sign is *Fusarium* disease.

Haemocytic enteritis (HE)

Haemocytic enteritis describes the histological lesion which characterises this disease. A marked inflammation of the mid-gut with a loss of the epithelial mucosa and proliferation of bacteria in the lumen is seen. Gross signs are non-specific. Affected prawns are lethargic, anorexic, small in size and dark, and their cuticle is often fouled by epicommensal organisms. The disease is common and has been seen in tank, raceway and pond-reared prawns. Experimentally, HE has been shown to be caused by ingestion of a toxic filamentous blue–green algae, but it is probable that several aetiologies will be found for the disease. Anything that damages the mid-gut mucosa to allow the gut bacteria to proliferatate will cause this haemocytic inflammation.

Nutritional diseases

'Black death'. Caused by a vitamin C deficiency it is a well described disease of prawns, characterised by black lesions under the cuticle of the abdomen, carapace, appendages, gills and foregut. Vitamin C deficiency is not seen in prawns with access to natural food, e.g. in ponds with algae.

Blue discoloration. Reported in pond-reared *P. monodon*. Wholesalers do not buy from ponds with a high percentage of blue prawns because they are said to have soft flesh and consumers do not like the colour. The lack of normal colour is due to low tissue levels of the carotenoid astaxanthin, which can be converted by prawns from the β-carotene in plants or algae. Consequently, blue prawns should not be a problem in a well fertilised, productive pond. In tank or raceway systems it may be necessary to add carotenoids to the pelleted diet.

Chronic soft shell syndrome. This syndrome has been described in the Philippines, in pond-reared *P. monodon*. The cuticle of affected prawns remains soft and papery for several weeks after moulting. The disease has been associated with poor pond productivity and an inbalance in dietary calcium and phosphorus. A diet with a Ca:P ratio of 1:1 is the best for prawns.

Muscle necrosis

Muscle necrosis is characterised by white, opaque abdominal muscles. All striated muscle fibres are necrotic. The necrosis follows periods of severe stress because of overcrowding, low dissolved oxygen levels, sudden salinity changes, high temperatures and so on. If the prawns are removed from the adverse environment at initial stages, they can return to normal. Otherwise mortalities will occur.

Clinical Diagnosis

Hatchery

History

A detailed knowledge of husbandry, management and hygiene practices is required before advice can be given on disease prevention. The ages of larvae or post-larvae at the time of mortalities and the pattern of mortalities help define the kind of diseases to consider. Live food production may be a factor: has there been enough food available and has it been contaminated?

Examination of the larvae

Most hatchery technicians will have a good idea of the health of their larvae, even if they do not know the actual cause of the problem. Ask them what they have seen.

Gross examination. Look at the prawns swimming around in a glass beaker. Note degree of swimming activity, colour and evidence of feeding.

Microscopic examination. The most valuable examination of larvae and early post-larvae is a microscopic examination. Most hatcheries will have a compound microscope to count algae and to stage the larvae but it is often dirty and hard to use. The veterinarian's own compound microscope, with at least ×400 magnification, is preferable. Place a drop of water with the larvae on a microscope slide (a wet mount) and cover with cover slip, then examine under the compound microscope. Some workers only use dissecting microscopes, but considerable skill is required to identify gut motility, melanised (brown) appendages and epicommensal fouling at such low magnifications (approximately ×40 maximum). The larvae can be somewhat immobilised by mounting them under a cover slip. Determine the stage of the larvae. Carefully examine the gills, mid-gut, cuticular surface (at edges), antennae and tail fan to check for abnormalities or abnormal function.

Histology. Examination of sectioned larvae and post-larvae is required to confirm viral infections. The fixative of choice is Davidson's although a 10% formalin-based fixative will suffice. Always sample at least 50 larvae for histology. The use of 100 μ mesh nylon filter cloth and small funnels aids the concentration and handling of these very small prawns.

Water quality

Techniques for evaluating sea water quality can be used to check the hatchery supply and larval rearing conditions. Of importance are any changes after addition of new water or food organisms. The number of bacteria in the rearing water and concentrations of ammonia, nitrite and nitrate also need to be checked. Dip slides that incorporate marine agar or TCBS (a media specific for the *Vibrio* group of bacteria) are available. These load a set volume of water and can give an accurate assessment of the number of bacteria in the algal or brine shrimp cultures and the larval rearing water.

Bacteriology

Bacteriology is not common for larvae or rearing water. A mixed bacterial flora is usually grown and interpretation can be difficult. In bacterial septicaemia and luminous vibriosis a single dominant bacteria may be isolated but the method is complicated and requires some special equipment. Collect 10–25 larvae (depending on size) place them on sterile filter paper and wash twice in sterile sea water, then grind the washed larvae in a small tissue grinder or mortar and pestle. Tissue debris is resuspended in sterile sea water, then plated out onto marine agar, seawater trypticase soy agar or TCBS. This isolation of bacteria is important if antibiotic sensitivities are required. Excessive antibiotic use in a hatchery does lead to multiple antibiotic resistances.

Farm

History

Collect the same type of information as for an investigation of fin fish diseases in ponds, tanks or raceways. Consider the source of the prawns, their age, the water quality, mortality pattern, water productivity, feed quality, weather and so on.

Clinical observations

Observe the prawns swimming around and feeding. This cannot be done in ponds. In fact if prawns are visible swimming near the edge of the pond during the day, assume that something is wrong. Dead prawns sink: farmers will only see the dead prawns at the pond edge, while hundreds more will be dead in the middle, out of sight. Use a scoop net to catch lethargic prawns at the pond edge and use a cast net to sample the prawns out in the pond. Collect prawns from the feeding trays or the lift nets which are used to check feed consumption rates. Use a bucket with a portable aerator to keep all the collected prawns alive at the pond. Only use live prawns for post-mortem examinations as there is a rapid autolysis of the mid-gut gland. Even those prawns which have been dead for only a few minutes cannot be used for histology.

Post-mortem examination

Appendage and gill clips. Wet mount and examine microscopically for fouling organisms, bacteria in haemolymph and fungi.

Gross. Examine surface for erosion, melanised areas, soft cuticle and 'firmness' of the body. Cut the abdomen from the thorax, cut the carapace dorsal and ventrally, and divide the entire thorax in half longitudinally. Examine the mid-gut gland, heart, gonads, mid-gut, lymphoid organ and foregut chambers for abnormalities.

Histology. After a detailed history, histology is the most useful aid currently available to diagnose diseases in juvenile prawns. For the veterinarian investigating diseases at the farm it is essential that sick, but live, prawns are dissected and placed in fixative as quickly as possible. Rapid autolysis of the mid-gut gland prevents diagnosis of many of the viral diseases. Injection of fixative into the mid-gut gland and haemoceole first, followed by dissection has been recommended. Another possibility is immediate dissection, bisectioning and, if required, further transections to pieces 1 cm thick, then immersion in cold fixative. A 10% seawater formalin or 10% buffered neutral formalin fixative solution can be used. The best fixative for prawns (and the one to use if at all possible) is Davidson's, followed by storage in 50–70% ethanol. Use 10 times as much Davidson's as tissue for fixation. Fix for 24–72 hours, depending on the size of the prawn. After fixation, transfer to alcohol for storage and transport. The formula for Davidson's fixative, which has the advantage of rapid tissue penetration, is:

> 330 ml 95% ethyl alcohol (ethanol)
> 220 ml formalin (40% formaldehyde)
> 115 ml glacial acetic acid
> 335 ml water.

Store at room temperature.

Bacteriology

Diagnosis of septicaemias may be carried out by bacterial isolation from haemolymph on marine agar, seawater TSA or TCBS agar. Haemolymph can be obtained from the pericardial cavity or median sternal sinus, using a sterile syringe and needle. Surface disinfection of the articulating membranes with 70% ethanol is necessary before sampling.

Other diagnostic tests

Transmission electron microscopy is required for the definitive identification of prawn viruses. Note that cell lines from aquatic crustaceans do not exist. Prawn viruses cannot be grown in the laboratory. Tissue preserved for TEM may be requested by the pathology laboratory to which samples are sent.

The use of a 0.1% malachite green stain aids the identification of baculoviral occlusions in squash preparations of fresh midgut gland. Immunodiagnostics are not generally available or used in diagnostic investigations. Experimental ELISAs have been developed for bacterial and viral pathogens of prawns.

Therapy

The treatment of diseases in prawns follow the principles of chemotherapy in finfish. In hatcheries, the antibiotics or antiprotozoan chemicals are added directly to the culture water in the rearing tank. A prior knowledge of the chemicals' effect on the live food organisms is useful if sudden deterioration in water quality is to be avoided. Teaseed cake and chemicals like formalin can be added directly to tank or pond water on the farms. Therapy in juvenile prawns is usually delivered *per os* with medicated feeds. Prawns may also be exposed to other chemicals such as chelated copper compounds, which are added to control algal blooms. In nearly all cases, chemicals are used in prawns with little or no scientific information on efficiency, safety or withholding times. There are no antibiotics registered or approved by the USEPA or USFDA for use on prawns. Figure 16.11 is a basic guide to the treatment of some common prawn diseases.

The use of antibiotics in hatcheries is ambiguous. Some of the antibiotics used (for example, erythromycin) are not active against the Gram-negative bacteria which cause bacterial necrosis

THERAPY FOR SOME COMMON PRAWN DISEASES		
Disease	**Drug and dose (added to culture water)**	
Bacterial diseases		
In larvae and post-larvae:		
Bacterial necrosis	Furazolidone	10 mg/l
Larval bacterial septicaemia	Nifurpirinol	1 mg/l
	Oxytetracycline	60–250 mg/l
	Nitrofurazone	1 mg/l
	Neomycin	10 mg/l
	Streptomycin	4 mg/l
	Erythromycin	1.5 mg/l
Luminous vibriosis	Sodium Nifurstyrenate	10 mg/l
Filamentous bacterial disease	Cutrin-Plus® (a chelated Cu compound)	0.1–0.5 mg Cu/l
	Oxytetracycline	100 mg/l
	Streptomycin	4 mg/l
	Neomycin	10 mg/l
In juveniles:		
Shell disease	Oxytetracycline	1.5 g/kg feed*
Bacterial septicaemia	Nifurpirinol	100–500 mg/kg feed
Haemocytic enteritis	Nitrofurazone	100–500 mg/kg feed
(antibiotics help reduce the		*when fed at 2–10% of biomass
severity of HE)		to 10–14 days (3–15g OTC/kg prawn)
Fungal diseases		
Larval mycosis	Malachite green (as a daily dose)	6–10 µg/l
	Treflan (trifuralin) – a continuous dose	10–100 µg/l
Fusarium disease	No effective treatment	
Parasite diseases		
Protozoan fouling	Formalin	1.5–2.5 ml/100l
	Chloramine T	5 mg/l

FIG. 16.11 Therapy for some common prawn diseases.

or luminous vibrosis. These antibiotics must alter the microflora in the rearing tank to improve conditions for the larvae in some way. The action is not against the bacteria in or on the prawn larvae. Hatchery workers inhale the fine aerosol created on continuous aeration of the larval rearing tanks. If there are antibiotics in the culture water, the aerosols will contain antibiotics and the bacteria in the upper respiratory tract of the hatchery staff are exposed to low concentrations of antibiotics. This is a good way to develop antibiotic-resistant bacteria.

Therapy of juveniles in ponds should only proceed after consideration of the costs and possible benefits. With such short production cycles, and with the cost of antibiotics and the cost of delaying harvest to ensure no residues remain in the prawn tissues, chemotherapy is not usually economic. More benefit is provided by increasing pond water exchange rates and partial harvesting to decreased pond biomass.

A 'vaccine' for penaeid prawns is available commercially. Invertebrate immunity is simple and non-specific; it does not involve memory or production of immunoglobulins. The 'vaccine' is a mixture of heat and formalin-killed bacteria which are meant to stimulate the non-specific immunity in larvae to increase PL survival. Its use in hatcheries is not common.

Prevention of Disease

As in any kind of aquaculture, the first step to prevention of disease is site selection. Large farms often have a hatchery on site. This may guarantee the farm a PL supply, but there would have had to be a compromise on site selection. A penaeid hatchery needs a stable, oceanic seawater supply. Farms are best supplied by brackish water and are sited on land where the soil permits a low pond construction cost. Management will focus more on the farm section, the money-making end of a combined operation, to the detriment of the hatchery. In these situations, hatchery production can be lower than expected. A stand-alone hatchery and farm would be better.

Hatcheries

In hatcheries, the goal of disease prevention is to minimise stress by providing optimum environment, nutrition and husbandry conditions. Disease epizootics in larval and early post-larval cultures usually involve opportunist pathogens, which proliferate in the intensive culture environment and then infect a stressed and weakened or injured prawn. There is also evidence that the virulence of facultative bacterial pathogens (e.g. *Vibrio harveyi*) increases from cycle to cycle. Successive passages from host to host provide a mechanism where the characteristic of virulence is selected.

In order to limit the spread and adaption or selection of these virulent strains, it is advisable to separate each group of larvae in time (batch culture) and to isolate each group in space. Any vector of contamination (water, workers, equipment, predators and the prawn larvae themselves) must be controlled continuously to prevent vertical and horizontal transmission of pathogens. This theory should form the basis of the approach to hatchery hygiene.

Batch production may be the ideal but it is not easy to synchronise spawning to the point where all the larval rearing tanks in a big hatchery can be stocked with nauplii at the same time. Rearing larval cultures of different ages in adjacent tanks increases the chances of cross-contamination and is not ideal. The aim should be to produce larvae of a similar age in each rearing cycle. If this is not possible, the hatchery should be designed so that the larval cultures of different ages are physically separate. For example, during aeration a fine aerosol from a rearing tank can drift throughout the larval rearing section and contaminate other cultures. Some hatcheries separate large rearing tanks by solid walls and doors; alternatively, fine mesh shade cloth can be hung between the tanks to prevent the cross-contamination.

Movement of people in the hatchery must be controlled, particularly in the larval rearing area. If the same workers are involved in a range of activities, the larval work must be done first.

Footwear is provided for use only in the hatchery. Footbaths or soak mats with disinfectant should be placed between sections and the disinfectant must be changed regularly. Each larval rearing tank has its own set of equipment for sampling and maintenance and this should be washed, disinfected, rinsed and dried daily.

All hatcheries should use break-cycles to help maintain a clean environment and achieve consistent production in the long term. Twice a year, or after three larval rearing cycles, hatcheries should stop operations completely for 3–4 weeks. During the break-cycle all surfaces (walls and ceilings included) and tanks can be thoroughly cleaned, disinfected and dried. Airlines and water pipes should be dismantled or flushed clean, disinfected and dried.

Stocking densities of larvae should be appropriate for the species and the rearing system. Feed for the larvae should be sufficient. (Underfeeding reduces growth and health.) While most hatcheries feed only one species of algae, it is probably better for the health of the larvae to use at least two species, using axenic algal starter cultures. Bacterial contamination of algae culture can be the source of bacterial pathogens for the larvae: aseptic techniques should be used in the algae culture laboratory as long as possible, that is until the outside tank culture, and further bacterial contamination of the larvae should be avoided by using an acid decapsulation of brine shrimp cysts. Reduce nitrate levels in the algal culture media. The algal medium should be similar in temperature, salinity and pH when it is added to larval cultures. Ideally, use algae that form long chains (*Skeletonema* sp.) so that the algae can be harvested and concentrated in a net, then added to the larval tanks as a concentrate.

Broodstock should be treated with 2 ml formalin per 100 litres for 15–20 minutes as they enter the hatchery. Nauplii can be disinfected in a 30-second dip in 20–30 ml/100 l formalin and a 60-second dip in 0.1 mg/l iodophor to prevent MBV infections. This is followed by a rinse in running, filtered sea water for 3–5 minutes. A rinse in filtered sea water or Treflan may be required if there are problems with larval mycosis.

The water used in the larval rearing tanks should be free from sediment. Maintenance of a good quality water supply is probably the single most important factor when selecting a hatchery site. The aim is oceanic water which is not influenced by rivers or pollution. There is increasing evidence to suggest that water treatment to remove as many of the bacteria as possible is not a good idea. The aim in the hatchery should be to supply water with heterotrophic, viable bacterial counts of around 10^3 ml. Bacterial disease problems develop when a single, hatchery-adapted strain of bacteria dominates in the larval culture water. A mixed flora of normal environmental bacteria appears to be suitable. If the hatchery water supply is disinfected by chlorine, the water should be used within 6 hours after neutralisation. Cartridge filters must be removed from their housings each day to be cleaned, disinfected, rinsed and dried. If the cartridges are left in the filter system, they become a source of hatchery-adapted bacteria which colonise and grow on the filter surfaces and then inoculate the larval cultures when the 'clean' water is added.

Skilled observation by experienced hatchery managers and technicians is needed for early detection of poor larval health. Fine tuning of the husbandry and management of larval cultures will be necessary to achieve the 50–80% survival rates to PL stage that all hatcheries expect to produce. The pressures of food production and the maintenance of the physical systems within the hatchery often mean it is not possible for hatcheries to follow ideal husbandry and hygiene practices.

Farms

Good pond construction is as important as good site selection when it comes to the prevention of disease on farms. Ponds must be designed so that they can be drained completely. To prepare any pond properly it must be drained and sun dried; excess organic detritus from the previous production cycle must be removed, and the pond should then be limed to disinfect and fertilise it. There should be sufficient pumping capacity or a large enough water reservoir to exchange water in the ponds as required.

The establishment of a good dense diatom bloom in the pond to be stocked helps to provide a stable environment for the initial part of the rearing cycle. The water used to fill the pond and in subsequent water exchanges must be screened.

Exclude all wild fish, prawns, crabs and molluscs from the pond. Regularly monitor water quality. Provide optimal water quality with good water exchange and proper feeding. Use paddle wheels or other aerators to maintain DO levels during the night at greater than 2 mg/l.

In most pond culture systems the recommended stocking level is not more than 30 PL/m^2. Stock only good quality PLs: they should swim actively; respond to stimuli; have clear muscle (not opaque); swim up-current; be white, grey or dark brown in colour; have straight abdomens, rostrums and antennae; have a clean cuticle; and have a long, skinny body shape.

A Philippino hatchery has reported PL survival rates of 90% and greater in the ponds after stock had passed two stress tests devised by the hatchery:

(1) A random sample of PL are exposed to a 15 ppt drop in salinity. Healthy fry show no mortality over 2 hours and recover in 24 hours to feed.
(2) Expose PL to 10 ml/100 l formalin. No mortalities should be recorded.

Monitor the feed consumption rate using feed trays and monitor growth rates by regular sampling. Alter feeding rates according to the estimated prawn growth and survival rates. Avoid overfeeding and reduce the quantity of feed when insufficient water is available for exchange.

It is important that comprehensive records are kept of water quality measurements, growth rates, survival, feeding rates and harvest weight. Any mortalities or disease should be investigated immediately. Except in the case of rickettsial infections and stocking mortalities due to heavy baculovirus infections, the avoidance of disease on prawn farms is simply a result of good husbandry and management. Well fed prawns in a clean environment and at appropriate stocking densities rarely have disease problems.

Further Reading

Bell, T. A. and Lightner, D. V. (1988) *A Handbook of Normal Penaeid Shrimp Histology*. The World Aquaculture Society, Baton Rouge, Louisiana.

Chamberlain, G. W., Haby, M. G. and Miget, R. J. (1985) *Texas Shrimp Farming Manual*. Texas Agricultural Extension Service, Corpus Christi.

Lim, C. C., Heng, H. H. and Cheong, L. (1987) *Manual on Breeding of Banana Prawn*, 62 pp. Fisheries Handbook No. 3, Primary Production Department, Republic of Singapore.

McVey, J. P. and Moore, J. R. (Eds) (1983) *CRC Handbook of Mariculture, Vol 1. Crustacean Aquaculture*. CRC Press, Boca Raton.

Sindermann, C. J. and Lightner, D. V. (Eds) (1988) *Disease Diagnosis and Control in North American Marine Aquaculture*. 2nd, revised edn. Elsevier, Amsterdam.

Taki, Y., Primavera, J. H. and Llobrera, J. A. (Eds). (1985) *Proceedings of the First International Conference on the Culture of Penaeid Prawns/Shrimp*. Aquaculture Department, Southeast Asian Fisheries Development Centre (SEAFDEC), Iloilo, Philippines.

17

The Veterinary Approach to Carp

RUDOLF HOFFMAN

The common carp (*Cyprinus carpio*) was first cultivated in the old Chinese Empire four or five thousand years ago. It was not until about the 11th century that carp farming became established in Europe, where it followed the spread of Christianity; monks, in particular, farmed the fish and their ponds also served as drinking-water reservoirs for farm animals. Over the next few centuries the main centres for carp farming became Silesia, Bohemia, Poland, Bavaria and parts of France. The industry declined from the late 18th century but was revived in the 1880s.

Today carp are still farmed in ponds in the Far East, though to a lesser extent than other fish. Carp culture is much more important in central and eastern Europe (parts of France, central and southern Germany, Poland, Hungary, Russia, Ukraine, Romania and Croatia) and the Near East (especially Israel and Egypt) and also in North America.

Farming Systems

The cultivation of carp, in contrast to most other species of fish, is relatively extensive. Carp need a large volume of water in proportion to fish biomass; the ponds are quite shallow and therefore need large surface areas.

Carp are often combined with other species, especially tench (*Tinca tinca*), though the choice usually depends on the demands of regional markets. Tench and species such as sheatfish (*Silurus glanis*) are cultivated for human consumption, typically in warmer regions such as Hungary. Other species in these polyculture systems are produced for stocking natural water systems and include tench, pike (*Esox lucius*) and pike-perch (*Lucioperca lucioperca*). The pike also control small feral fish such as minnows, which might otherwise compete with carp for the available food resources in the last year of production. Cyprinid plant-eaters are often introduced to control excessive plant growth in eutrophic ponds, especially east Asian species such as grass carp (*Ctenopharyngodon idella*), silver carp (*Hypophthalmichthys molitrix*) and bighead (*Aristichthys nobilis*). There might also be species of bait fish and ornamentals such as koi and goldfish, and recently carp farmers have become interested in some species of sturgeon for their polyculture systems.

The mixing of so many different species risks the introduction of disease. Imported ornamental and other fish, for example, are potential transmitters of new diseases from their own region. A very important factor is that parasites introduced into new areas are able to find new hosts, and very often cause high losses.

An additional possibility is to combine carp farming with the production of waterfowl. These systems range from the extensive, exploiting wild or semi-farmed geese and ducks, to intensive cage culture of the birds on gratings over the water body. The waterfowl benefit the ecosystem of the pond by fertilising it with their faeces; however, they remove food, especially plants, snails or other molluscs and also small fish, and they transmit diseases, especially via parasites which have fish as intermediate hosts.

Most of the carp's food is produced in the pond, with supplementary artificial feeding according to season and stocking rates. Most of the feed (especially the protein element) is in the form of zooplankton or benthic animals such as rotifers, copepods, tubificids and chironomids, and the production rates of these animal nutrients depend on the natural productivity of the soil, the influence of the weather (especially sunshine) and the use of fertilisers to enhance the primary production of food from plankton. Additives, especially for energy, are commonly in the form of cereals for

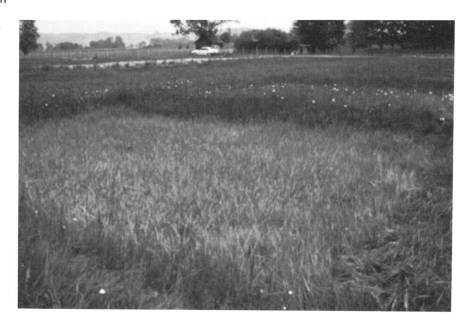

carbohydrates. Commercial feeds to optimise productivity are given mainly in spring and autumn.

In most cases the carp are bred under natural conditions. The spawning ponds (Fig. 17.1) are small at 50–300 m^2 and not deeper than 30–50 cm. They contain plants and are filled with warm water (18–20°C) a few days before the presumed date of spawning. One female and two males are then introduced. Hypophyseal injections are also used in carp production to achieve spawning maturity. One female weighing 5 kg can produce up to one million eggs, which stick to the plants.

The stages in the life-cycle of the carp are given in Fig. 17.2, which shows that carp are transferred to other ponds as they grow (Fig. 17.3). The bigger the fish, the larger and deeper the pond. The time-scale shown in Fig. 17.2 is for the moderate climates of central Europe. In warmer southern areas, the production cycle can be shortened by up to 2 years and is even shorter in subtropical and tropical countries, where very often the preferred size of marketable carp is smaller anyway.

Generally, carp farms are open systems which cannot be isolated from outside influences; including flying birds, which play a role as predators and as transmitters of pathogenic agents. The water body itself is extensive in area and is influenced by its environment: the pH of the water and the fertility of the pond depend on the type of underground soil and also on the catchment area. In contrast to former times, when carp ponds had to be fertilised regularly, the intensification of agriculture has induced in many regions an over-fertilisation of ponds by leaching and run-off from surrounding fields, with a consequent overgrowth of algae.

General Husbandry

For the veterinary approach to carp, farming conditions cause some difficulties. In larger ponds it is not possible to see the fish or to catch samples during the production period in summer. Therefore, even relatively high losses may not be detected before the harvest in autumn when the pond is fished. Furthermore, there are major practical problems in giving oral medication or bath treatments (see Therapy) and therefore it is important to take advantage of all the management stages at which carp are manipulated or transferred to other ponds, using them for intensive health care.

It is especially important in spring to assess the fish for their condition after a long winter before they are distributed over the ponds, and again in the autumn to ensure that the fish are healthy enough to survive the winter — a period without feeding which can be withstood only by fish in

FIG. 17.2 Development of carp.

DEVELOPMENT OF CARP	
Type of pond	**Development stage**
Spawning pond 50–300 m³ 30–50 cm deep 1 female spawner 2 males	*Incubation time:* 4–5 days (4 days at 20°C, or 5 days at 18°C) *Post-hatching:* 3–5 days: start of swimming and exogenous nutrition 7–9 days: end of yolk-sac period *Loss rate:* up to 50%
Fry pond 100,000-400,000/ha	*Period:* 4–6 weeks *Feeding:* plankton (starting with rotifers; later large plankton and water-flies) *Weight:* 1 g at end of period *Length:* 2–3 cm *Loss rate:* 30%
Fingerling pond 20,000/ha	*Period:* 7 weeks, up to end of first winter *Feeding:* plankton and additionally commercial food (especially in autumn) *Average weight:* 250 g at beginning of winter
Production pond (2nd year) 2,000-6,000/ha	*Transfer* at 1 year old to larger ponds in spring *Additional feeding* in spring and autumn *Average weight:* 500 g at end of year
Production pond (3rd year) 400-850/ha	*Additional feeding* in spring and autumn *Harvested* at end of summer *Final weight:* 1250-1500 g

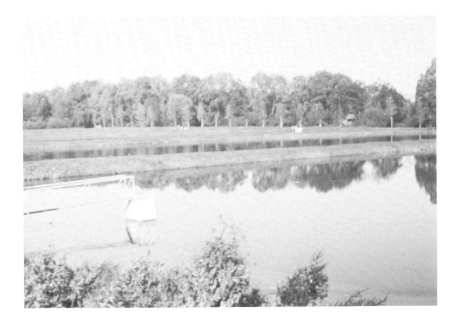

FIG. 17.3 Carp production pond.

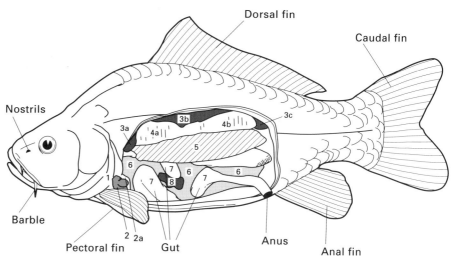

FIG. 17.4 Schematic picture of carp anatomy, (1) gills, (2) heart with atrium, ventricle and bulbous artery, (2a) diaphragm, (3a) head, kidney (3b) middle kidney, (3c) caudal kidney, (4a) cranial swim-bladder, (4b) caudal swim-bladder, (5) ovary, (6) liver, (7) gut, (8) spleen.

good condition. Any undetected diseases may spread towards the end of winter, when the fasting fish have used all of their reserves and are unable to resist infections. At this time water temperature is generally low, but the immune system of carp is able to work efficiently only at temperatures over about 15°C. It is not surprising that many heavy outbreaks of disease occur in the early spring (spring viraemia, coccidiosis) when the carp is relatively unprotected.

Legislation

There is very little legislation specifically for carp, but carp farming is often restricted by natural and environmental protection laws. These may cover the use of therapeutic treatments if there is any danger of a water system outside the farm being affected. Legislation on fish health protection does cover spring viraemia of carp (SVC) which, for example, must be reported to the veterinary administration in Germany. Unfortunately, in most countries only the classical farm fish species are covered by legislation. Polycultural carp farming often includes ornamental species and even koi which belong to the same species as *Cyprinus carpio*, can pass borders without control in some countries if declared as ornamental fish. Therefore the effective prevention of distribution of infectious diseases and parasites does not seem to be possible in most European and Asian countries at present by governmental methods.

Major Diseases

A schematic diagram of the anatomy of a carp is shown in Fig. 17.4.

Viral Infections

Spring viraemia of carp (SVC)

Under field conditions, the outbreak of disease is regularly observed during the spring, even if the virus itself is present throughout the year. The incubation time is between 7 and 60 days, depending on temperature; under field conditions, 14–28 days are reported. Certain factors influence this seasonability. At the end of the winter, the hibernating carp has used most of its reserves and energy. Fish are especially handicapped if there was a strong frosty winter or a mild one with relatively high temperatures but no feeding. As the water temperature rises in spring, energy requirements also increase but often natural food production has not yet taken place. Under these conditions, the carp is more susceptible since active immune reactions start only at higher water temperature from about 14°C upwards.

Outbreaks of SVC depend on the general condition of the fish, the water temperature (the lower the temperature, the more heavy may be the outbreak) and especially on secondary bacterial complications. All transitions from clinically inapparent to total loss may be seen.

The pure viral infection is characterised clinically by dark body coloration, exophthalmos and a distended abdomen. Sometimes petechiae can be observed in the skin. Internal lesions are regularly seen as haemorrhages on serous layers of organs and in muscles. Histologically, necrosis in the haemopoietic tissue, liver and spleen and partial lymphocytic encephalitis are detectable. In the field, further development of the disease is influenced by secondary bacterial infections, which cause the most commonly described lesions such as bloody fibrinous ascites and purulent peritonitis. These secondary bacteria are members of the water flora, especially aeromonads and pseudomonads. More than 50 different strains have been described, but the most common is *A. hydrophila*.

Causal therapy is not possible and the use of antibiotics may control only bacterial complications. Therefore, prophylaxis is important. During the last decade, SVC infection has become a minor problem as a result of a good hygiene programme in most areas. It begins with the regular disinfection of ponds (liming, drying, freezing) and the assessment of individual fish when carp are prepared for the winter ponds, with the removal of all fish which are ill or in a bad condition. In spring, feeding should start as early as possible if no natural food is available. It is also important to control ectoparasites, especially blood-sucking ones, since it has been proven that the SVC virus is transmitted by carp lice and leaches.

Carp epithelioma

This disease was already recognized in mediaeval carp culture and described in Gessner's fish book in 1563. It was mentioned later as carp pox, *Epithelioma papillosum* or *Papillosum cyprinii*. Even at the beginning of this century an infectious genesis was discussed. The viral aetiology was proven only a few years ago in Japan, where a *Herpesvirus* was shown to be the causative agent.

Carp epithelioma can induce marked effects on carp, especially growth retardation, but the most common occurrence is only a superficial skin infection with little effect on fish health. A change in the viral virulence or in the susceptibility of carp must be considered, since high losses were reported in the 1920s. In addition to *Cyprinus carpio*, some

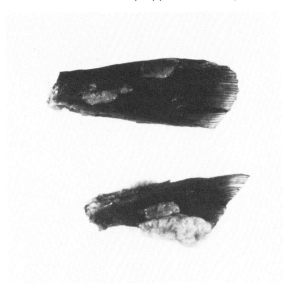

Fig. 17.5 Carp epithelioma, tumours on flukes.

other related cyprinids seem to be affected by the same agent.

The lesions are whitish to opaque, sometimes also pigmented, and consist of irregularly shaped warts up to several centimetres in diameter and a few millimetres thick. (Fig. 17.5). Histologically only the epidermis is involved showing a hyperplasia of epithelial cells, often with intercellular connections. Mitotic figures are common, especially in the superficial parts. Some hyperplastic epithelia can contain intranuclear inclusions of Cowdry type A bodies. Between epithelia, normal mucous cells may be dispersed.

Tumour formation may originate multicentrically on all parts of the body, but metastasis to other organs has never been reported. The hyperplasia may persist over months. Spontaneous regression can take place.

Bacterial Diseases

Carp erythrodermatitis (CE)

Although generally only a local infection, with septicaemia as the exception, CE may induce heavy economic loss. *Aeromonas salmonicida nova* has been determined as the causative agent but some strains of *A. hydrophila* can induce an identical condition.

CE is directly correlated with primary skin

Fig. 17.6 Carp erythrodermatitis; deep ulcer caused
by *A. hydrophila*.

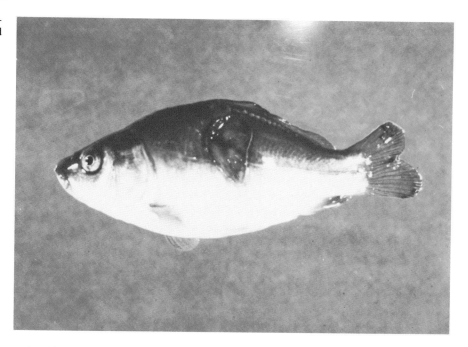

lesions casued by ectoparasites (especially leeches
and lice) which injure the skin, or with small
wounds caused by bad management, usually at
sorting. An intact skin gives an impermeable
barrier: bacteria can infect only debrided areas of
skin. Reduced body condition after a long winter
or after SVC infection can favour the outbreak of
CE. Clinical signs include centrally necrotic areas
on the body surface surrounded by a haemorrhagic
halo. Later there are deep ulcers with a diameter
of up to about 4 cm including skin subcutis and
underlying muscles (Fig. 17.6). The carp's general
behaviour is often normal but these open surface
areas may induce an ionic imbalance due to loss
through the unprotected surface areas. There is
often spontaneous healing but deep, constricted
scars develop and there may be curvature of
the vertebrae and body axis as a consequence.
Affected carp are not marketable for human
consumption and must be removed from the pond.

Other *Aeromonas* and *Pseudomonas* may provoke problems in carp which are emaciated or in
bad condition.

Fungal Diseases

Branchiomycosis

This disease is also described as gill rot. It
is caused by the phycomycete *Branchiomyces*
sanguinis in carp and tench, and also in other
cyprinids, sheatfish and whitefish. Related species
such as *B. demigrans* occur in many freshwater
fish.

Branchiomyces sanguinis is a branching fungus
between 9 and 15 μ in width and the hyphae
grow mainly in the preformed channels of gill
vessels. It can occur in fish of all age classes but
particularly affects younger carp in their first or
second year. Most outbreaks are observed during
summer at water temperatures higher than 20°C,
though some cases have been documented at 14–
16°C. Mortality is relatively high (10–50%).

The exact mode of transmission is still unknown.
Outbreaks are very often associated with bad
environmental conditions, such as overcrowding,
eutrophy of the water with high ammonium (NH_4)
and ammonia (NH_3) depending on pH and temperature, as well as mass development of phytoplankton. It is likely that the infection must be
preceded by initial gill epithelium lesions which
open an entry for the fungal spores.

Affected fish show forced respiratory activity
and the gill lamellae are dark red or whitish.
Microscopically and histologically, the growth of
hyphae inside the gill arteries, veins and lacunae
can be seen, followed by a total thrombosis of the
vessels. As a consequence partial or complete
necrosis of primary lamellae occurs, causing a

reduction in the respiratory capacity. With the lower oxygen content of warm water, very often drastically reduced further by overnight oxygen consumption, affected fish die of suffocation.

Diagnosis can be made easily by squash preparation and histology.

Saprolegniasis

Carp are susceptible to skin mycosis by Saprolegniaceae but severe problems are rare. However, especially during the autumnal fishing and preparation for winter, all carp with even small affected skin lesions should be removed. In most cases these infections are secondary complications of mechanically or chemically induced injuries, so that prevention measures by good management are important.

Parasitic Diseases

Trypanoplasma (Cryptobia) infections

In the carp farm, *Trypanoplasma tincae* is very important for tench, whereas *T. borelli* is relatively harmless for its host, the carp. Both parasites belonging to the flagellates, live in the blood and need intermediate hosts (leeches) of the genera *Piscicola* and *Hemiclepsis*. They are characterised by two flagella, one at each end.

Clinical signs in affected tench include lethargy and emaciation. Anaemia and pale gills occur regularly but atypical movements are relatively rare. Diagnosis can be by proof of the parasite in blood smears.

An oral treatment with methylene blue (60 mg/kg body-weight/day over 4 weeks) or with metronidazol (50 mg/kg body-weight/day) was reported. However, prophylaxis is more important. It consists of regular disinfection of ponds to eradicate the intermediate hosts, the leeches.

Coccidiosis

Coccidiosis in carp may be caused by two different members of Eimeridae, *Eimeria carpelli* and *E. subepithelialis*. Both are very important, especially in young carp.

The disease often occurs during early spring before the carp start to feed. Fish have naturally lost condition during the winter and young carp which weigh less than 25 g are especially susceptible to disease. A mild infection is usually tolerated by older carp.

Clinically, no typical signs can be seen. Emaciation is common and losses often increase rapidly. Fry of only one week old can be affected. Pathological signs are different in each species of the parasite. The typical picture in *E. carpelli* infection is a severe enteritis with red, hyperaemic gut mucosa (enteritis coccidiosis). The parasite multiplies in the lamina mucosa, which is destroyed in large areas. In the case of *E. subepithelialis*, small whitish nodules develop in the lamina submucosa (nodular coccidiosis). They have a diameter of 1–3 mm and contain the oocytes. Clinical signs are less dramatic than in the enteritis type.

Myxosporean infections

For most cyprinids, myxosporean infections of skin, gill or internal organs are common and mostly harmless. Only three are of great importance: *Sphaerospora renicola*, *Myxobolus encephalicus* and *M. cyprini*. The life-cycle is unknown for most species, but recent results indicate that an invertebrate (oligochaete) intermediate host is obligatory, at least for Myxobolidae.

Sphaerospora renicola — myxosporean swim-bladder inflammation. When *Sphaerospora renicola* was first described, it was widely distributed but mostly regarded to be less pathogenic. Later on blood parasites (Csaba-cells) were shown to be a developmental stage of *S. renicola*. More recently, swim-bladder inflammation of carp fry has been shown to be caused by a myxosporidian-like organism which has since been proven to be also a developmental stage. In conclusion, there are three different developmental stages of the same parasite *S. renicola* but the exact mechanisms of transformation between these three phases still have to be confirmed, as well as the question of the probable intermediate host. *Sphaerospora* spores themselves have not been shown to be infective for carp.

Classical *S. renicola* can be found in kidney tubules of carp of all age classes in most European countries and Israel. They are roundish sporogenic pseudoplasmodia, up to 20 μ in size, containing light-breaking granules. In these pseudoplasmodia, sporogenic cells differentiate into mature spores (6–8 μ long, 6.4–8.3 μ wide). Tubule lumina are filled and widened by pseudoplasmodia. Pathological lesions of excretory and haematopoietic kidney occur only in heavy infections. Blood stages, which probably precede the kidney phase, start with a uninucleated primary cell containing a secondary cell which divides to produce 6–8 small secondary cells. These secondary cells start the cycle again after disintegration of the primary cell.

Swim-bladder stages are found only in very young carp and only for a few weeks between June and early August. Their development starts with an uninucleated primary cell and one secondary cell in the swim-bladder endothelia. A rapid multiplication takes place, including the formation of up to 40 secondary cells (containing two tertiary cells) which are probably the linkage to the renal form.

Swim-bladder inflammation is widely distributed and occurs in up to 80% of carp farms. A similar distribution can be seen at the renal sphaerosporosis.

Clinical problems usually develop only from the swim-bladder stages. The infestation of parasites in the swim-bladder wall induces a proliferative inflammation characterised macroscopically by thickening and dimming of the wall of the posterior chamber and histologically by polypoid proliferation of the inner epithelium, oedema, haemorrhages and heavy lymphocytic infiltration. The parasitic stages can be detected only in July and August, whereas the inflammation becomes chronic and persists over some months. This can also explain the former misinterpretation of swim-bladder inflammation as a bacterial or viral problem. Clinically affected carp fry show irregular movement and locomotive disturbances. In survivors, the caudal chamber of the swim-bladder is shrunken. Losses may be up to 50%.

Myxobolus cyprini

M. cyprini is a widely distributed parasite of carp and other cyprinids in Europe, exhibiting a broad variety in its spores. Typical are unequal polar capsules in the slightly oval spore (7.6–9.7 × 10–13.5 μ). The first stages observed are plasmodia inside skeletal muscle fibres. After muscle disintegration, mature spores are distributed through the body.

The problems found in recent years are probably associated with the intensity of fish production. However, no real information exists either on the original distribution area or on introduction of this disease by fish exchanges. Locally, up to 90% of fry and two-summer stocks are affected.

Clinical signs may include swelling of the abdomen due to ascites, exophthalmus and probably an anaemia. Pathologically, releasing of spores from destroyed muscle fibres cause a severe haematogenous and lymphogenous dissemination to all organs. Spores may occlude blood capillaries, inducing local necrosis and haemorrhages. Spores in the liver, spleen or kidney are regularly eliminated by macrophages.

Myxobolus encephalicus

This parasite infects blood vessels (especially capillaries) of the brain and meninges of small carp. Plasmodia adhere to endothelia and are reactively overgrown by the endothelia. The development from plasmodia to mature spores (6.6–12 × 6.3–10.4 μ) takes place under the protection of the endothelia.

M. encephalicus is widespread over Europe, locally with a prevalence of up to 40% of carp farms. Only *Cyprinus carpio* seems to be affected and only fry show problems, which may be serious between weeks 3 and 5. Affected fish show abnormal swimming behaviour, whirling or circling, in a vertical position with head down. Histologically, widening of affected capillaries by proliferating developmental stages and blood congestion are seen, associated with oedema and partial diapedesis of red blood cells, but with no thrombus formation. Losses may reach 100%, probably by emaciation from cessation of feeding. In affected areas, prophylaxis is by strong disinfection of spawning and brood ponds to remove intermediate hosts.

Further pathogenic myxosporeans of lower importance are *Choromyxum cyprini* in the gall bladder of carp and grass carp, and *Thelohanellus nikolskii* (*dogieli*) affecting the skin of carp, which was brought into Europe from East Asia with imported fish. The total number of Myxosporea found in carp is estimated to be about 65, but most are non-pathogenic.

Ciliates

Chilodonella cyprini

Chilodonellosis is similar to *Costia* infection, inducing skin infections. *C. cyprini* is distributed world-wide; it is a holotrichal ciliate with a roundish, heart-like form caused by the slightly retracted lower end. It is 33–70 μ long and 21–40 μ wide. Cilia are arranged in a bundle around the stoma.

Ichthyophthirius multifiliis *(white spot disease)*

This world-wide freshwater ciliate also affects carp. Descriptions of the parasite can be found in Chapter 6.

The intensity of infection in carp ponds depends on population density. Weakened fish are more affected than those in good condition and fry are more susceptible than older fish. Hatching larvae can be endangered if spawners are affected.

The typical lesions are white spots identical to those in other species. In infected carp ponds the disease is progressive, often inducing losses of up to 50% and reduced growth. Acute losses are more typical for fry and fingerlings. The pathology is identical to those in other fish.

Monogenea

Monogenean platyhelminths may be a problem in ponds with insufficient management. The problems they cause are similar to those caused in other fish.

Trematodes

Sanguinicolosis

The adult of the trematode parasite *Sanguinicola inermis* lives in blood vessels and its triangular eggs are distributed by the bloodstream. Miracidia bore actively through gill vessels and leave the fish in search of the intermediate host, a snail. The intensity of the infection depends on the snail density of the pond. The eggs are produced from May to November, with a peak in July. There may be distinct differences between different regions in Europe in the occurrence of this parasite.

Eggs in gill vessels may induce heavy thrombosis leading to gill necrosis and death by respiratory insufficiency. Young fish are particularly affected but older individuals show no clinical effects. The adult parasite in blood vessels apparently does not harm the host. Eggs arriving in organs other than gills (heart, kidney) are encapsulated by the host and undergo degeneration.

Eye diplostomatosis

The second trematode which is important for carp is *Diplostomum sphathaceum*.

The fish is its second intermediate host in a three-host life-cycle, being invaded by the cercariae after they have left the first host, a water snail. The adult parasite lives in fish-eating birds (mews).

The cercariae often leave snails in large masses after an increase in water temperature. Carp fry can be killed if invaded by large masses. Older ones survive but become blind since metacercariae reach for the eye lens. Even if the blind fish is not handicapped in its feeding and development, it is easily caught by predators.

Grass carp are the most susceptible in polyculture. The main method of control is reduction of snail populations in affected regions.

Cestodes

Although large numbers of tapeworms may be found in fish, only three species have great importance in carp. Two of them, *Caryophyllaeus fimbriceps* and *Khawia sinensis*, belong to the Cestoidea: they have undivided bodies and a two-host life-cycle using oligochaetes as intermediate hosts. *Bothriocephalus acheilognathi* (or *gowkongensis*) is a member of Eucestodes, characterised by a scolex and proglottides; its intermediate hosts are copepods.

The original tapeworm of carp is *C. fimbriceps*, which is relatively harmless. *K. sinensis* was introduced to all parts of Europe with the importation of East Asian plant-eaters and caused heavy epidemics. *B. acheilognathi* was also introduced into Europe from the Far East in the 1960s and 1970s: in the first years there were heavy losses, especially in one-summer and two-summer stocks, but during recent years a host–parasite equilibrium seems to have been established and no more drastic losses have been reported.

All three species are influenced by temperature and season in their development, depending on regional climatic conditions. A small burden is tolerated by carp, especially older fish: they are not weakened but they do become parasite reservoirs. Heavier infestations induce emaciation, reduced growth and a swollen abdomen. Locally the gut wall is irritated by the suckers followed by obstipation (*Khawia*) or enteritis (*Bothriocephalus*). Furthermore, toxic products of tapeworms may induce a degenerative process in all parachymatous organs. Mortality can reach 80–100% in young carp.

Nematodes

Nematodes are no problem for carp in most regions except in Russia, where the adult females of *Philometroides lusii* (a member of Dracunculidae which lives in blood vessels and other organs) reside at the end of their life-cycle under the fish's scales. Scaleless carp are not affected.

Leeches

The most important leeches in carp culture are *Piscicola geometra* (Fig. 17.7) and *Hemiclepsis*

marginata, widely distributed hirudineans inhabiting ponds, lakes and rivers. *P. geometra* is also found in brackish waters. The leeches can live on the fish for longer than 4 weeks, sucking the blood with their proboscis and then laying their eggs in cocoons, which are very resistant.

Leeches can be easily transported on fish, and also on the plants or other pond material to which egg cocoons may be attached, so that they become widely distributed. Eutrophic and neglected ponds may harbour high numbers of leeches.

Single leeches are usually harmless except in the case of fry: one leech can kill up to ten fish larvae. Higher numbers on an adult fish can induce anaemia. However, the main danger is in the transmission of parasites (*Trypanoplasma*), bacteria (erythrodermatitis) or viruses (SVC). This transmission is favoured by the injection of contaminated anticoagulants by the leech before blood-sucking.

Crustaceans

Ergasilus sieboldii

This copepod crustacean is a parasite of many freshwater and partially marine fish. In carp culture, slow-moving fish such as tench are more affected than faster ones, such as carp. *Ergasilus*

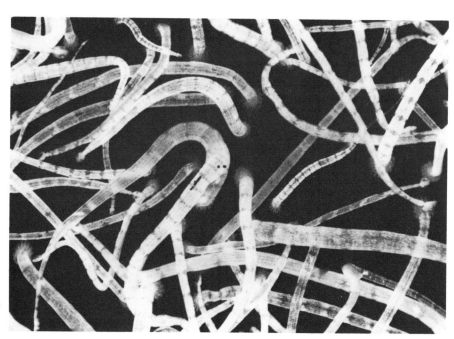

FIG. 17.7 Masses of *Piscicola geometra* removed from carp surface.

may produce two or three generations a year and the females parasitise the fish during warmer seasons. It is a gill parasite, finding its nourishment from the branchial epithelium. The destruction of the gill surface often causes secondary bacterial or mycotic infections and death.

Lernaea *spp.*

Some species of this copepod, especially *L. elegans*, affect fish in carp culture, and lernaeosis is widely distributed in Siberia, Central Asia, Europe, Israel and parts of North America.

The first parasitic phase, by copepodites on the gills, is relatively harmless but mature females become permanent parasites, anchoring themselves under the fish's skin where they cause deep wounds, loss of blood and ions and often secondary bacterial ulceration, frequently inducing mass mortality.

Argulides

The most important Branchiura are Argulides (carp-lice), which are distributed world-wide but are only temporarily on their hosts during blood-sucking. About 50 species of the genus *Argulus* are particularly important. The parasites have a sting connected to a poison gland. This poison has anticoagulating and paralysing qualities which are dangerous only for fry — a few parasites may kill small fish but are relatively harmless to older ones, though high infestations can cause anaemia. The main problem is the transmission of bacteria or viruses which can be on the surface of the sting.

Disorders due to inadequate gaseous exchange

The levels of dissolved gases in the water influence fish health. In carp ponds these levels depend on the degree of trophication, the biomass of algae and macrophytes, the temperature of the water, and light. The processes of assimilation, (increasing oxygen and removing carbon dioxide) during daylight and the reverse effects of dissimilation during darkness can influence fish health very rapidly in the summer.

Oversaturation of the water with oxygen in the afternoon for many days is associated with high blood concentrations of the gas. A sharp decrease in the water's oxygen after sunset can induce *gas-bubble disease* in the fish, since the gas tension in the blood is then higher than in the surrounding water. Death is caused by gas bubbles excreted in the blood vessels inducing embolism in gills and internal organs.

During the night, especially in the early morning before sunrise, oxygen concentrations fall short of the minimal need of about 3.5–4 mg/l and carp may die from suffocation.

High concentrations of carbon dioxide can induce movement disorders in carp (at about 200 mg/l at 15°C). The gas also controls pH levels especially in soft unbuffered water. In the late afternoon pH can increase over the critical value of 10 as carbon dioxide concentrations decrease.

To prevent the negative effects of gas levels, pond water needs to be stabilised: it should be buffered by regular liming in sensitive areas. Plant growth must be controlled, either mechanically, or by chemical means (such as liming) or by including plant-eating fish in a polyculture system.

Ammonia intoxication

The nitrogen cycle and the ionisation of ammonia are described in detail in Chapter 4. Suffice to say here that the higher the pH and temperature of the water, the higher the ammonia toxicity to the fish. High ammonia concentrations become critical at pH > 8.0–8.5. Besides directly damaging the surface of the fish, such concentrations hinder excretion by the gills and an additional auto-intoxication develops. Not all toxicological details have yet been explained, especially concerning whether gill necrosis (as a condition without fungi or other infectious agents) is induced directly by ammonia intoxication. Prevention is possible by stabilisation of pH as described for oxygen and carbon dioxide fluctuations.

Nutritional Disorders

Vitamin deficiencies

Vitamin deficiences are less common in carp, due to its more natural nutrition, but intensive feeding can lead to problems. The minimal requirements for the most important vitamins are given in Chapter 8.

Phosphorus deficiency

Induces deformation of the frontal bone in carp, reduced bone growth and abnormalities of the vertebrae. The dietary requirement for phosphorus is 0.6–0.7% of food.

Sekoke disease

This syndrome is observed in carp fed with silkworm pupae. It is characterised by a destruction of Langerhans' islets in the pancreas, lipidosis of inner organs, cataract and degeneration of eye muscle, retina and chorioidea.

Clinical Diagnosis

Some diseases such as carp erythrodermatits, carp epithelioma or branchiomycosis may be diagnosed directly at necroscopy. Most parasitic diseases are detectable by light microscopy.

Cultivation methods for viral and bacterial agents are identical to those in other fish. In addition, there is widespread use of detection of the spring viraemia virus of carp and *Aeromonas salmonicida* subsp. *nova* with polyclonal specific antisera in direct or indirect test systems. Examination of neutralising antibodies against SVC-V may be helpful in overviewing the epidemiological situation.

The routine histological control of carp allows detection of nutritional and environmental disorders even at a very early stage.

Therapy

Therapy is often more difficult in carp than in other farmed fish. When the pond is in full production, carp prefer natural food and will not accept artifical medicated food. Bath treatments are impractical because of the amount of chemical required for the large body of water in a carp pond. The danger of pollution of the natural environment often prevents the administration of topical medications. Therefore chemotherapy is applied only if other prophylactic measures fail — such as pond disinfection, quarantine and very good husbandry.

Direct medication by the oral route or bathing is restricted to the earlier stages of development. In some cases, the parenteral injection of antibiotics is used when fish are transferred from one pond to another.

THERAPEUTIC AGENTS USED IN CARP		
Substance	**Development stage**	**Dosage**
Antibiotics		
Chloramphenicol	Bacterial infections	30–50 mg/kg i.p. 2–2.5 g/kg food for 8 days
Oxytetracycline	Bacterial infections	2 g/kg food
Sulfadimethoxine–Trimethoprim	Bacterial infections	2 g/kg food for 10–14 days
Fumagillin–DCH	Prophylactic treatment of myxosporean swim-bladder inflammation	1 g/kg food for 10–14 days (not registered in most countries)
Antiparasitics		
Sodium chloride	Ectoparasites in fry	1–1.5 kg/100 l water bath for 20 minutes
Formaldehyde	Ectoparasites	1 ml of 38% solution/l H_2O
Potassium permanganate	Ectoparasites, fungal infections	10 g $KMnO_4$/m^3 H_2O for 10 minutes
Trichlorphon	Ectoparasites, especially leeches and lice	1 g/2 m^3 H_2O in the pond, (caution: some fish species (e.g. pike) are very sensitive)
Malachite green oxalate	Ectoparasites, especially *Ichthyophthirius*	0.1 mg/l long-time bath (not allowed in some countries)
Niclosamide	Cestodes	100 mg/kg fish for 3 days

FIG. 17.8 Therapeutic agents used in carp.

Figure 17.8 summarises the most common therapeutics.

Prevention of Disease

Preventive control is essential on carp farms. The most important factor is regular monitoring of water quality, often performed routinely by experienced fish farmers. The control of pH and of plant growth is especially important. A useful preventive measure is the liming of the ponds.

To prevent the introduction and transmission of infectious agents, especially parasites, strict quarantine is necessary. Additionally, the water must be managed carefully. At fry and fingerling stages in particular, the pond water should be warmed but the reservoirs for warming must not contain other fish. After transfer of fish from one pond to another, the pond bottom should be cleaned, dried and disinfected by liming.

Vaccinations are not used for carp. A vaccine against SVC was developed but it was found that improved management was more effective.

Special measures are necessary before hibernation, including routine necropsies. Fingerlings are especially endangered. Even low parasitic infections such as by coccidia or cestodes need treatment to avoid high or total loss in early spring.

18

The Veterinary Approach to Eels

EVERT LIEWES AND OLGA HAENEN

There are 19 different species of eel (*Anguilla*) in the world. They can be found in Europe, East Africa, India, Australia and North America.

They are catadromous fish which spawn at specific oceanic locations, depending on the species involved. The development of the leptocephali (larvae) of the European eel, *Anguilla anguilla*, starts in the Sargasso Sea. During their voyage across the ocean, these transparent larvae actively feed and grow. At this stage they are shaped like a willow leaf but the process of metamorphosis into the familiar round and elongated shape associated with eels is initiated when the leptocephali reach the border of the Continental shelf. They become transparent glass eels, ready to enter the continental waters during a spring tide when the fresh river water has a temperature of 8–12°C.

In these tidal waters the tiny glass eels, weighing on average about 0.3 g, are captured and subsequently transported to the eel farms. Glass eels are not usually infected with parasites until they attract them when they enter fresh water, where they start feeding and after they have reached a certain stage of pigmentation.

Early feeding of the glass eels requires special highly palatable feedstuffs. The normal practice is to feed them at first with cod roe and later with a glass eel starter diet before they are weaned onto a commercial eel crumble. The correct feeding strategy is essential for the successful rearing of eels. The pigmentation process can be accelerated if the eels are kept in warm water but the heating of the water should be gradual.

When the glass eels are fully pigmented, they are known as yellow eels; they have a white or yellowish belly and a dark grey, brown or greenish back. This is the adolescent growth phase in continental waters and at this stage they may be reared on farms.

Eels of adult size, have a silvery-white pig-mentation on the belly and a dark-coloured back: they are referred to as *silver eels*. Silver eels have a thicker skin and are generally rather fat (the muscle may contain 25–30% fat) and sometimes their eyes become enlarged. Full-grown silver eels stop feeding and try by all means to migrate out to sea. In the ocean, silver eels develop mature gonads.

Males of the European eel become silver from a size of 80–150 g, females become silver from a weight of 250 g or more and may become as large as 0.5–2.5 kg. However, under intensive conditions only a small percentage grow larger than 130–150 g. Marked differences in growth between males and females are also apparent in other species. These differences in size, and the weight at which growth declines, differ between the species.

Figure 18.1 shows the general anatomy of the adult eel.

Farming Systems

The most important cultured species are the Japanese eel (*Anguilla japonica*) and the European eel (*A. anguilla*). In North America the American eel (*A. rostrata*) is sometimes farmed, and other species are found in Australia.

The world production of cultured eels amounts to approximately 100,000 t per annum, largely of the Japanese eel, of which Japan alone produces about 37,000 t. The production of European eels amounts to approximately 6,000 t, of which 30–35% is from recirculation systems.

There are marked inter-species differences in culture techniques, the size of the glass eel, adult sizes and preferred feeding methods. Sources of information on the wider aspects of eel culture are given in the Further Reading section and, for the sake of simplicity, this chapter gives only a brief

311

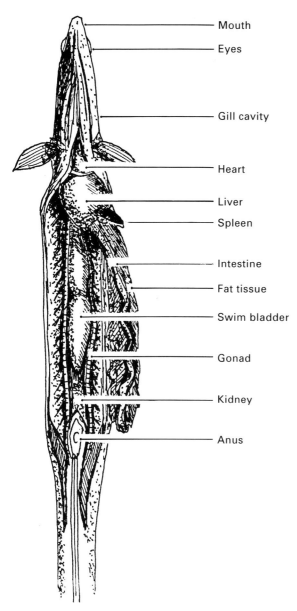

Mouth
Eyes
Gill cavity
Heart
Liver
Spleen
Intestine
Fat tissue
Swim bladder
Gonad
Kidney
Anus

FIG. 18.1 General anatomy of the internal organs of the eel (redrawn after Bertin, 1951).

review of the three different culture systems for the European eel.

Pond Culture

Eel culture in the Far East and in Italy is based mainly on pond culture systems. In Italy these are generally open-air ponds, although some are lagoons in *vallicultura* systems — a form of semi-extensive fish polyculture including eels. In Japan and Taiwan the so-called still water pond method is used: the ponds are frequently covered with greenhouse structures. They are equipped with temperature control systems and usually incorporate a paddle-wheel aeration system.

In pond culture eels are grown semi-intensively. Stocking densities in Europe vary from 3 to 10 kg/m². Traditionally the eels are fed with a paste diet, often supplemented with fresh fish. Feed conversion ratios using a paste diet vary from 2.0 to 4.0. Most pond culture systems in Italy are stocked with wild-caught fingerlings weighing 10–40 g.

Flow-through Systems

These systems are generally found in combination with power plant effluents or on sites where large amounts of suitable warm ground water are available (artesian wells). The stocking densities in flow-through eel farms vary generally from 20–40 kg/m². In most flow-through systems there is some form of water treatment: the water is aerated and often it is also recirculated after suspended solids have been removed with drum filters. The feeding systems varies from a paste diet composed of fresh fish to pellets distributed by automatic feeders.

Recirculation Systems

The European culture of eels in recirculation systems is concentrated in The Netherlands and Denmark. Recirculation units vary in production capacity from 5 to 500 t per annum. The stocking densities may be very high, varying between 40 and 200 kg/m². The units have drum filters to remove suspended solids with purpose-built biological filters for the oxidation of ammonia; liquid oxygen is added to the water to achieve supersaturation.

The eels are invariably given a low-pollution diet (crumble or pellets), generally by means of automatic feeders. Almost all the European systems are stocked with glass eels, or with fingerlings (10–15 g) reared from glass eels by other farms.

WATER QUALITY IN RECIRCULATION UNITS		
	Range	**Optimal**
NH_4–N	0.2–38.9 g/m^3	<1.0 g/m^3
NO_2–N	0.1–15.5 g/m^3	<0.5–1.0 g/m^3
NO_3–N	7–181 g/m^3	<75–100 g/m^3
Oxygen	—	6.5–8.0 g/m^3
pH	5.7–9.0	±6.8–7.2
Temperature	12.7–29.9°C	23–25°C
Water exchange	200–400 l/kg feed	—

FIG. 18.2 Water quality in recirculation units.

Husbandry Techniques

Water Temperature and Quality

Eels are able to survive in water of relatively poor quality but they do not necessarily thrive. The water quality parameters listed in Fig. 18.2, which were compiled during a survey of representative Dutch and Danish recirculated eel farms, are important in eel culture. Many of the problems in eel farming, especially in recirculation systems, are related to bad water quality conditions. The fish pathologist should therefore *always* check on the water quality parameters.

Production and Growth Parameters

The stocking densities in recirculation units may be very high. Some important production related parameters for recirculation systems are summarised in Fig. 18.3.

Feed and Growth

The European eel is a relatively slow growing species. It requires at least 18 months to grow from glass eel to a marketable weight of 130–150 g. In practice the overall specific growth rate (SGR) for the whole culture period does not exceed 0.75%. Farms realising higher growth rates do very well. Fingerlings up to 5 g have a maximum SGR of 2.5%; eels of 80 g have an SGR of about 1% and bigger eels about 0.4–0.5%. On average feed conversion in recirculation systems is about 1.9 but ratios as low as 1.2–1.4 are possible under optimal conditions.

Quality of Stocking Material

Many problems in eel farming are caused by the poor quality of the stocking material. These problems generally arise from three sources: origin, diseases and transport.

Care must be taken in selecting fingerlings for on-growing. It is important to ascertain the following information from the source of supply:

- Clinical history of the eel farm where the stock are purchased.
- Water quality at the source farm.
- Growth rate of the stock prior to transport. (A growth rate of $\geq$ 1% of eel fingerlings weighing 10–15 g is acceptable.)
- Standards of water quality during transport.

PRODUCTION-RELATED PARAMETERS FOR RECIRCULATION SYSTEMS		
Parameter	**Range**	**Optimal**
Average stocking density	40–200 kg/m^2	>50–80 kg/m^2
Annual productivity	100–200 kg/m^2	>120–150 kg/m^2
Stocking density:		
Eels weighing <25 g	30–85 kg/m^2	
Eels weighing >25 g	38–200 kg/m^2	
Liquid oxygen use	0.8 kg/kg feed	
Biofilter surface	80–120 m^2/kg feed day	120–140 m^2/kg feed day
Water-flow standing stock	12–15 m^3/t eels	15–30 m^3/t eels
Water exchange time basins	20–40 minutes	30–40 minutes

FIG. 18.3 Production-related parameters for recirculation systems.

(These must be high and the purchaser should negotiate to pay only for elvers which survive the first 24 hours.)

- Wild-caught fingerlings mostly carry disease and parasites. They should always be examined and certified by a fish disease laboratory before they are introduced on to a farm.

Ventilation of the Production Facility

High levels of carbon dioxide, which cause the fish to become sluggish and inappetent, are sometimes found in recirculation systems using liquid oxygen. This may be reduced by simply installing some aeration with ambient air in the culture tanks. The water treatment unit should be sufficiently capable of strippping CO_2, while the production unit and biofilters require good ventilation.

Some farms may suffer from persistent CO_2 problems due to the buffering capability of the water. In such cases advice from a specialist waste water treatment or chemical engineer should be sought.

On a recirculation farm, the daily measurement and recording of water quality parameters, feed dosage and mortalities are of utmost importance. Many growth-related problems can be traced back to poor water quality.

Regular Grading

Eels tend to grow at different rates much more than other fish species. Regular grading, usually with automatic graders and fish pumps, helps to control the problem.

Minimising Stress

Eels are very susceptible to stress. Changes in water temperature, grading, poor water quality or direct sunlight may induce disease; high levels of suspended solids and high water temperatures are more than likely to do so.

Ultraviolet Installations

A recent trend in recirculation technology is the use of UV sterilisers, which help to reduce overall bacterial counts in the system's water. Many eel farmers are enthusiastic about UV installations, claiming reduced mortality rates and enhanced growth rates.

General Hygiene and Quarantine

As recirculation units are closed systems, often using tap or ground-water supplies, they can be kept relatively free from eel diseases. Any new shipment of glass eels or fingerlings should be kept in quarantine, treated for ectoparasites and checked for any other disease. Pigmented elvers are frequently found in glass eel shipments and they often carry diseases as they have been feeding in a freshwater environment.

Many eel farmers use disinfection foot baths for visitors at the door. The biggest risks of contamination are from eel traders' lorries. It is advisable to have a separate room for storage of marketable eels (generally stored in water of 12–15°C), with a separate door and access road to the outside. No equipment, boots or other material from this storage room should be used elsewhere on the farm and ideally there should not even be a door connecting the production area to the storage room: the eels should be shipped into the storage tanks through a pipe.

Major Diseases

Resistance to disease varies according to the eel species and there are risks when a new species is first imported. For example, European eel stocks recently suffered a devastating infection with the nematode parasite *Anguillicola*, which is indigenous in eels in the Far East.

Viral Diseases

Viruses are not major causes of disease and mortality for the European eel. Recently, however, there has been some concern about the eel reovirus (EVE) and the eel rhabdovirus (EVEX) in cultured eels in Europe, especially as EVEX is also infectious to rainbow trout fry. EVE has been identified as an important disease agent in the Japanese eel (*Anguilla japonica*), causing significant losses.

Cauliflower disease

Cauliflower disease, or eel papillomatosis, does not normally occur in America, Japan or southern

Europe. Cases of eel papillomatosis in the latter may be related to the stocking of fingerling eels imported from northern Europe. The disease is widely distributed in the Baltic Sea and the North Sea, where it affects up to 25% of wild eels in the coastal regions, particularly the smaller fish.

Affected eels develop white to light brown cauliflower-like skin papillomas, especially around the mouth and the pectoral fins. When the papillomas are enlarged, they may interfere with feeding to such an extent that the eels starve and die. Tumour growth is inhibited by low water temperatures and by medium to high levels of salinity.

Viruses have been isolated from eels suffering from Stomatopapillomatosis. However, transmission experiments have not been successful and it is therefore no longer considered as a viral disease.

There is no cure for this phenomenon. It has not been seen in recirculation eel farms stocked with glass eels. In freshwater eel culture, where ponds are stocked with wild-caught fingerling eels, high incidences of eel papillomatosis have occasionally been recorded.

Eel Virus European (EVE)

This disease also known as viral kidney disease or branchionephritis, originally affects mainly the Japanese eel and can kill up to 50% of stock. In 1970 2,700 t of eels in Japan were lost due to this disease. It has also been isolated from the European eel.

In Japan, viral kidney disease generally occurs during the winter. Various lesions have been noted but the disease is characterised by swollen and congested gills and tubular, interstitial necrosis of the kidney. Infected gills show epithelial hyperplasia and clubbing of the gill lamellae and filaments. Histological investigation of the kidney glomerular nephritis shows hyaline droplet degeneration of the tubular epithelial cells and interstitial necrosis. The gills are not necessarily always affected in all reported incidences of this disease. Experimentally infected eels showed slight petechiation of the abdominal skin, congestion of the anal fin and muscular spasms.

In Europe the virus has caused mortalities of up to 10% on Dutch eel farms since 1990 following a stress trigger (Fig. 18.4), with clear clinical signs.

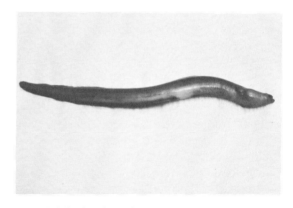

FIG. 18.4 Sub-adult farmed European eel with EVE. Petechial haemorrhages can be seen all over the body. The skin is swollen; the operculum is severely thickened. (CVI, Lelystad.)

Although it does not affect salmonids, EVE is very similar to IPNV type Ab of salmonids.

There is no cure for viral kidney disease but good hygiene will help to prevent it. Japanese eel farmers claim that keeping the salinity of the pond water during overwintering at 5–10% helps to improve survival rates through winter.

Eel virus of America (EVA)

A rhabdovirus has been isolated from the American eel (*Anguilla rostrata*) although it has not yet been proven that EVA was the cause of an epizootic condition. EVA is virulent to rainbow trout fry.

Eel virus European X (EVEX)

This is also a rhabdovirus. The role of the virus in eel disease is unknown although it is virulent to rainbow trout.

Bacterial Diseases

Most bacterial eel diseases are termed 'red disease', as many of them produce haemorrhages and ulcers. Only columnaris disease is an exception to this rule. In general some indication of the type of bacterial infection can be gained from studying the eels' gross pathological changes, but attempts should always be made to identify the causative agent. The Further Reading section at the end of this chapter provides sources for more details on bacteriology and diseases.

Aeromonas *infections*

Aeromonas hydrophila is distributed world-wide and affects many eel species, either as a primary pathogen or as a secondary invader of previously infected or stressed fish. It can cause significant economic losses.

Known as freshwater eel disease, red fin disease or eel furunculosis, this disease specifically occurs when eels are exposed to marginal water quality conditions such as high levels of organic matter, high temperatures, low oxygen levels etc. It can cause massive lethal epizootics following stressful events like catching, grading and transport at high water temperatures.

Typical signs of infection include loss of appetite or sudden death. Eels may swim near water inlets or on the water surface (Fig. 18.5a). As the disease advances, the eels become sluggish and hang in a peculiar curved way near the water surface.

Affected eels develop red spots on the abdomen and fins, especially in the anal region. The reddening of the skin and fins is due to congestion of the blood vessels. The skin of the eels may then start to develop bluish patches, and the epidermis may slough off, exposing the musculature. In serious cases, there may be boil-like swellings (which can burst open), especially on the head.

When the visceral organs are investigated, extensive haemorrhages can be observed around the intestines. The posterior liver lobes are often congested with blood and the kidney and spleen may be swollen. The heart does not usually show any gross pathological changes. The last part of the digestive tract and the anus may show severe reddening. Due to the haemorrhages the eels become anaemic, and there may be ascitic fluid.

The pathology of the disease is probably associated with the production of toxins by the causative agent. The course of the disease may be acute (2–3 days) or only progress slowly over a period of many weeks. The eels can be treated successfully with antibiotics, for example oxytetracycline.

Pseudomonas *infections*

'Red spot disease' caused by *Pseudomonas anguilliseptica*, creates great problems in the culture of the Japanese eel. It has also been isolated from European eels where it has caused mortalities of 10–15%.

Affected eels often have sub-epidermal petechial haemorrhages, especially seen on the abdomen in Japanese eels. The fins and the anus are not affected. The viscera show no gross pathological changes except a light distension of the stomach and some congestion of the hepatic vessels. In the European eel, haemorrhages and sometimes ulcers develop around the mouth, on the head and perhaps also in the anal region. The skin in these areas shows some necrosis.

The pathology of the disease is probably associated with the production of toxins by the causative agent. The disease frequently occurs at water temperatures of 15–18°C and is less pathogenic at water temperatures of 20–25°C, so that Japanese eel farmers try to reduce the disease problems by raising the water temperature to 26–27°C. The disease can be cured with antibiotics, for example oxolinic acid.

Vibriosis

Vibrio disease of eels generally occurs in eels which live in brackish or salt water with a salt content of 10‰ and more. Hence the disease is also called 'saltwater eel disease', 'saltwater furunculosis', 'saltwater red disease' or 'red pest'. Most frequently the causative agent is *Vibrio anguillarum*. Other *Vibrio* species which cause infections in eels include *V. alginolyticus*, *V. damsela* and *V. vulnificus*.

Acute septicaemic *Vibrio* infection. This is generally related to an infection with *V. anguillarum*, which can cause mass mortalities and has been isolated from eels in Europe, Japan and North America. It is estimated that up to 60% of the wild eels in the coastal regions of the North Sea, the Baltic and the Mediterranean may be suffering from this disease.

The acute phase may be characterised by inappetence or sudden death without external symptoms. Moribund eels may come to the surface at intervals and show septicaemic convulsions. There may be haemorrhages on the skin, fin margins and anus; swelling and reddening of the musculature around the heart; tetanic spasms producing contraction of the anus; and the development of red swellings (boils), which may be covered with translucent skin. The liver often shows petechial haemorrhages, and eels become anaemic. In the final stage of the disease the musculature and internal organs show extensive haemorrhaging, while the kidney and spleen show severe swelling.

The disease is especially dangerous when the water temperatures exceed 19–22°C. Low water temperatures stop the disease at once. The disease can be treated with antibiotics, for example chloramphenicol in countries where this drug is allowed to be prescribed.

Chronic *Vibrio* infection. In saltwater eel farms in Europe, sub-acute infections with *V. anguillarum*, *V. alginolyticus*, *V. damsela* and *V. vulnificus* have been diagnosed. In general the mortality rates are very low but can continue over long periods. It is thought that these sub-acute infections are favoured by high stocking densities, stress and poor water quality. The general signs include loss of appetite, low but continuous mortalities and petechiation of the abdomen, fins and gills. The anus may be red and a pale liver may show petechial haemorrhages.

Eels infected with *V. vulnificus* also show a typical pink–red discoloration of the fins and a strongly swollen spleen. Those infected with *V. alginolyticus* show a red anal fin, ulcers on the sides, haemorrhages in the mandibula, and no petechial haemorrhages.

The condition can be cured by treatment with antibiotics like oxolinic acid. Improvement of the rearing conditions and the reduction of stress are also important factors in minimising the incidence of this infection.

Edwardsiellosis

The bacterium *Edwardsiella tarda* (synonym *Paracolobacterium anguillimortiferum*) has been isolated from diseased Japanese eels and from diseased native Australian eels (*Anguilla reinhardtii*). The disease has also been isolated from European eel in Norway.

Clinical signs include bloody congestion of the anal fin, swelling and reddening of the anal and urogenital region, petechial haemorrhages on various parts of the body (especially on the abdomen) and muscular and dermal lesions showing extensive necrosis. Abdominal wall tissue adjacent to the infected tissue may be eroded, leaving a hole in the abdomen. There is focal necrosis of the haematopoietic kidney tissue, and the infected kidney is greatly enlarged; the foci develop into abcesses and subsequently into smaller or larger cavities or ulcers filled with a red purulent substance with a foul odour. The liver is occasionally affected in a similar way. The pathogen spreads from these lesions into the adjacent visceral organs or musculature.

Edwardsiellosis differs from an *Aeromonas hydrophila* infection in that it produces macroscopic putrefactive lesions. Experiments indicate that the extensive necrosis observed in this condition is not caused by a toxic substance excreted by the pathogen.

Edwardsiellosis mainly occurs in the summer months in the Far East. It can be treated with antibiotics, for instance oxytetracycline.

Columnaris disease

This bacterial condition produces typical damage of the tail and the fins and may also affect the gills in many eel species (Fig. 18.5b). The causative agent is *Flexibacter (Chondrococcus) columnaris*. The disease occurs at water temperatures of 16–22°C but not below 15°C. Isolation of the causative bacterium has revealed that highly pathogenic and nearly non-pathogenic strains exist. However, mortalities among infected eels can be high.

Infection of the gills (branchial flexibacter infection). Columnaris infection produces swollen gills, necrotic gill lamellae, and asphyxia. Infection of the gills of eels is often associated with viral kidney disease.

Infection of the integument. The disease affects mainly the tail-fin, which may be eroded. At first, the fins start showing damage and get a whitish appearance. The eels become slimy and collect detritus on their skin. The skin, and subsequently the muscle tissue, may erode away and ulcers can develop. A scondary infection with *Saprolegnia* can give the ulcers a roughened and enlarged appearance.

In general the internal organs do not show any signs of gross pathological changes but the haematocrit value is reduced. The disease can be cured with antibiotics, e.g. oxytetracycline.

FIG. 18.5 External symptoms of (a) *Aeromonas*, (b) *Columnaris* and (c) *Saprolegnia* infections, circles indicate affected areas (redrawn after Querellou, 1974).

(a) *Aeromonas* infection of eels

Side view

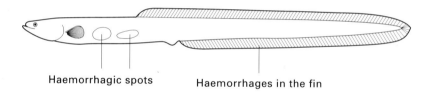

Ventral view

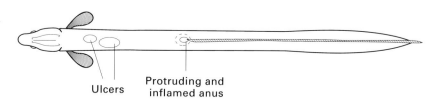

(b) Columnaris disease

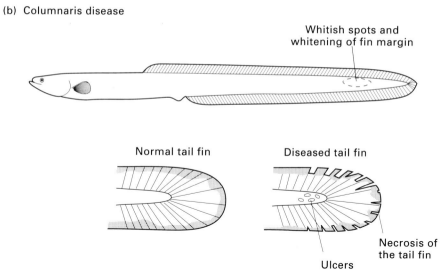

(c) *Saprolegnia*

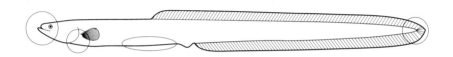

Non-specific fish pathogenic bacteria

Eels cultured in sea water have been found to be infected with *Acinetobacter lwoffi*. It is a normal water bacterium and is not known to be a primary pathogen of fish. Symptoms include loss of appetite, pink–red discoloration of fins, low but constant mortalities and strongly swollen spleens. Fast-growing fish are frequently infected. The bacterium can be isolated from spleen, liver and kidney.

Other non-specific eel pathogenic bacteria are

Aeromonas sobria and *Pseudomonas* spp. (e.g. *Ps. fluorescens*). Infections with these bacteria are often caused by stress and unfavourable water quality. It is possible to treat such infections with antibiotics, depending on the antibiogram obtained.

Fungal Infections

Saprolegnia

This ubiquitous fungal infection, caused by *Saprolegnia parasitica*, appears as white cotton-wool-like areas on the head, pectoral fins, abdomen or tail fin and can cause considerable mortalities among eels. The diseased fish swim around at the water surface and do not feed.

In larger eels (over 50–70 g) the fungus generally remains superficial and does not penetrate into the muscles. In elvers the fungal hyphae penetrate the skin, causing necrotic lesions and haemorrhages in the skin and muscles. In bad cases the infection may spread to the buccal cavity and cause symptoms similar to bacterial gill disease (Fig. 18.5c). In severe cases the tail and fins may erode away. The disease occurs at water temperatures of around 15°C, but disappears when the water temperature exceeds 20°C. In general Saprolegniasis is considered to be a secondary pathogen.

The disease can be treated with malachite green. Raising the water temperature also helps to overcome the problem, especially in elver rearing.

Diseases Caused by Protozoan Flagellates

Blood parasites

Infections with *Trypanosoma* are frequently found in wild eels. These flagellate blood parasites are transferred by leeches. Flagellate infections do not produce any apparent pathological changes in the eels.

Costia

Costia necatrix generally affects the skin and gills. The skin becomes very slimy and may show superficial lesions in severe cases. Smears from skin and gills should always be examined for this parasite. Even small numbers of *Costia* may severely irritate the European eel. The best

treatment results have been obtained with long-term baths with acriflavine–HCl or lactardine. Formalin baths do not eliminate the infection completely.

Sporozoan parasites

Eimeria

The coccidian parasite (*Eimeria anguillae*) has been reported in New Zealand, Europe and North America. It develops in the epithelial cells of the intestine. Infected New Zealand eels become severely emaciated and the only external feature of this infection is a slightly distended body wall, due to the swelling of the bladder (a common observation in emaciation). The liver is pale and the intestine is soft and weak. The dissected intestine shows whitish areas, especially in the anterior part, in which mature cysts are usually found. In heavy infections the mucosa and submucosa of the intestinal wall show extensive necrosis.

Dermocystidium

This organism is now classified under Sporozoa but is considered by some authors to be a fungus. In Europe it has caused massive infections in cultured eel stocks. On the gills many cysts can be observed, causing the operculum to distend outwards. *Dermocystidium* especially seems to infect elvers and small eel fingerlings, and it can be diagnosed in fresh gill smears. There is no known cure for the infection.

Haemogregarina

The parasite *Haemogregarina bettencourti*, which has been found in erythrocytes of the European eel, is most likely transferred by leeches, in which it multiplies asexually by means of schizogony. It is not known whether the condition gives rise to any pathological changes.

Cnidiosporidian Parasites

Eels are parasitised by a considerable number of Cnidiosporidians. The most important parasites in this group are *Myxidium giardi* and *Pleistophora anguillarum*.

Myxidium

There are a large number of *Myxidium* species known to infect eels. *Myxidium giardi* is the most frequently encountered and is one of the first parasites to appear in elvers. Infection rates can be very high, especially in the freshwater environment, though they are minimal in the marine environment. The infection appears as cysts in (a) the internal organs or (b) the skin:

(a) The parasite can be found in the kidney, stomach, gills and intestine, where it forms white circular to oval spots with a size of 0.1–2.0 mm. In elvers the cysts are also in the wall of the gall bladder.
(b) Heavily parasitised eel skins have been reported in American, New Zealand and European eel species. Small cysts form in the connective tissue layer below the epidermis and this can induce small ulcers or whitish raised areas on the skin (1–2 mm in diameter), covering the whole body except the head and the gills. The skin may show cloudy spots and become rough, gritty and sometimes ulcerated. The skin ulcers make the eels unsuitable for marketing.

Myxidium can easily be diagnosed when these cysts contain spores. The cysts in the internal organs often contain trophozoites, which can be made visible by staining a squash with Giemsa.

No large-scale outbreaks of this condition have been reported in European eel farms. Infections occur mostly in farms using wild-caught fingerlings. The economic significance of the disease in European eels is not clear. The parasite has caused serious losses in other eel species, such as the Japanese eel and the American eel, especially amongst elvers. At present there is no known treatment for this disease.

Other infections with Myxosporidia

Myxosoma dermatobia, *Myxospora anguilla* and *Myxobolus* form cysts in the skin and internal organs, especially the kidney, of the Japanese eel. In wild American eels *Ceratomyxa* has been found in the biliary vessels and gall bladder.

Pleistophora

Pleistophora anguillarum is a microsporidian infection of the Japanese eel. The parasite multiplies in the muscles, where it induces considerable deformation and lesions. Diseased eels swim in a strange curved fashion. The site where the infection occurs becomes indented. The parasite causes muscle paralysis, haemorrhages and sometimes fin degeneration. There is no cure for this disease and eel farmers therefore rely on good hygiene and the eradication of infected stock to avoid spreading of the disease.

Ciliate Parasites

Infection with ciliates are very common in eels. They have been reported from all over the world. Ciliates are responsible for many problems in eel culture as most of them thrive at the high water temperatures found on eel farms. Only *Chilodonella* occurs more frequently at low water temperatures and is thus more often associated with problems of eels in storage basins.

Ichthyophthirius

Infection by *Ichthyophthirius multifiliis* causes the disease known as white spot. It is very common in both wild and cultured eels and the irritation causes them to swim around wildly at the water surface. They often stop feeding.

Eels and elvers are very sensitive to this parasite even when only small numbers are found in smears. Infected eels show typical white spots and produce large amounts of mucus. There may be mortalities amongst small eels before these white spots appear. Smears of skin and gills should be examined.

The parasite often enters the system with elver or fingerling shipments. The condition can be treated with a bath of formalin, malachite green and methylene blue. In many eel farms salt is added to cure the infection but, due to the nature of its life-cycle, it is a very difficult parasite to eradicate from recirculation systems.

Trichodina *and* Trichodinella *spp.*

Trichodina infections are regularly encountered in wild and cultured eels. Those living in fresh water are generally infected with *Trichodina anguillae* and *Trichodinella epizootica*. The eels become slimy and heavily infected eels develop superficial skin lesions. Larger eels seem less sensitive to high numbers of the parasite. Elvers are particularly sensitive. Smears of skin and gills should be examined. The parasite can be treated with a bath mixture of formalin, malachite green and methylene blue.

Chilodonella

Chilodonella cyprini is frequently found on the gills and skin of European eels kept in freshwater storage basins at temperatures of 5–13°C. Eels with severe infections become very slimy and in some areas the superficial layers of the skin erode away. These areas become whitish and show light haemorrhages.

Chilodonella infections in cold water can be treated with a bath mixture of formalin, malachite green and methylene blue. Infections at water temperatures above 20°C do not respond well to this therapy and repeated treatments at higher dosages are required.

Ectocommensals

In fresh water, infections of *Scyphidia* and *Trichophyra* are found on the gills and skin of many eel species. These ectocommensals are generally a sign of poor water quality and high levels of suspended organic material. Infections with *Trichophyra* frequently occur in Japanese eel culture. Infections with *Scyphidia* and *Vorticella* have been found in saltwater eel culture. These infections can easily be treated with baths of a mixture of formalin, malachite green and methylene blue.

The biofilters in recirculation systems also harbour many other zooplanktonic organisms. In several recirculation farms large numbers of such organisms cause irritation to the eels and reduce their appetites. One is the mite *Histiostoma anguillarum*, which has been found in large numbers on eel gills.

Diseases Caused by Platyhelminths

Trematodes and cestodes are known to parasitise eels. Disease symptoms generally occur with infections of monogenean trematodes.

Monogenean trematodes

Monogenean trematodes are frequently found on European and Japanese eels, especially in eel stocks reared in intensive pond culture or recirculation systems. Infections have been found in fresh water as well as salt water.

The monogenean trematodes of eels are found mostly on the gills. Not all gill branches are equally infected, and so several gill branches have to be dissected and examined. The parasites attach themselves to the gills with a pair of hooks, causing severe irritation and excessive mucus production. In recirculation systems the direct life-cycle of the parasite can cause massive infections (sometimes up to 600 *Pseudodactylogyrus* on the gills of an eel). Such infections may cause mortalities. The most important monogenean trematodes on eels are species of *Pseudodactylogyrus* and *Gyrodactylus*.

***Pseudodactylogyrus* infections.** This is often a major problem of eel culture in Denmark. The most common species of the parasite in European eels are *Pseudodactylogyrus anguillae* and *P. bini*; *P. microrchis* infections are rare. All three species of *Pseudodactylogyrus* also parasitise Japanese eels.

P. anguilla can be found everywhere on the gills; *P. bini* is generally found on the outer margins of the gills. The adult parasites measure about 1.5 mm when they start producing eggs. The optimal temperature for the development of the parasite and its eggs is 22–25°C. At these temperatures the eggs hatch in 6–7 days. The eggs produce free-swimming oncomiracidia (0.2 mm) which then infect new hosts.

Eels infected with up to 25 *Pseudodactylogyrus* do not reveal any symptoms of disease. Infections from 50–100 parasites cause a serious reduction in appetite. Higher infection rates lead to mortality. Treatment is difficult but mebendazole is used.

Gyrodactylus. *Gyrodactylus* spp. have also been observed on the gills, although not in such large numbers as with *Pseudogyrodactylus* species. One of the first signs is inappetence. Treatment is with formalin.

Nematode Parasites

Eels suffering from nematode infections in intensive culture have been reported in Japan and

Europe, where the swim-bladder nematode has caused serious problems. There have also been reports of an eye disease in Japanese eels caused by *Philometra anguillae* (*Filaria anguilla*) but other nematode infections are rare in cultured eels. Cysts caused by *Goezia* spp. have been found in the stomach, intestines, skin and musculature of European wild-caught eels.

Anguillicolosis

The nematode *Anguillicola crassus*, known to be an unimportant parasite in the swim-bladder of Japanese eels, was probably introduced into European eel populations via live eels imported from East Asia. It then spread very rapidly among wild European eels populations in fresh water, reaching infection levels of 94% in some cases. Although the percentage of infected wild eels is still high, the number of parasites per swim-bladder has decreased over the years and the pathological effects have become less severe. The infection can only be transmitted in a freshwater environment.

The intermediate host is a crustacean copepod. In the swim-bladder lumen the adult nematodes, reaching a length of 18–70 mm, can easily be observed (Fig. 18.6). Juvenile nematodes (0.6–0.8 mm) can be detected with a binocular microscope in the normally translucent swim-bladder wall, often near blood capillaries.

The pathology is most noticeable in eel infected in their post-juvenile stages. In these larger eels

(a)

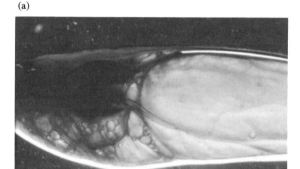

(b)

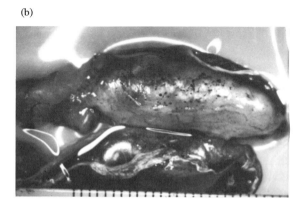

FIG. 18.7 Swim-bladders (a) uninfected and (b) heavily infected with *Anguillicola crassus*, from wild European eels in Lake IJssel, The Netherlands. Note the severe lesions caused by the nematode, with secondary inflammations, haemorrhages and severe fibrosis. (CVI, Lelystad.)

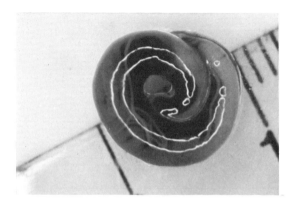

FIG. 18.6 Adult female *Anguillicola crassus*, about 2 cm long. The ovary (white) is filled with eggs and first and second stage larvae. The parasite has fed on eel blood (dark region). (CVI, Lelystad.)

the swim-bladder frequently contains a foamy fluid, which in later stages becomes brownish-red in colour. In severe infections the swim-bladder is dilated, its wall thickens and becomes opaque and may show signs of inflammation (Fig. 18.7). In such cases there is a reduction in growth of 20–30% and increased mortality rates of 10–20%, caused by secondary bacterial infections after rupture of the swim-bladder. When elvers or fingerlings become infected with low numbers of the parasite, the swim-bladder wall reacts by thickening and generally no severe pathological symptoms develop.

There is no 100% effective disinfection for this parasite on eel farms. Treatment of infected eels with long-term baths of L-levamisole has some curative effect, but does not completely cure the condition. Recirculation farms, therefore, stock their basins with *Anguillicola crassus*-free glass eels or fingerlings rather than with infected wild-caught fingerlings. However, small pigmented eels are frequently found in shipments of glass eels and, as such elvers have been feeding, they are frequently carriers of Anguillicolosis (and other infections). Because it is very difficult to remove the pigmented elvers from the shipments, several recirculation farms have become infected through this route. It seems that infected small eels show normal growth performance and development.

Crustacean parasites

Infections by crustacean parasites occur regularly in open air pond culture of eels in Europe and Japan. These parasites are not known to cause problems in intensive recirculation systems.

Argulus

This typical skin parasite has been causing serious problems in Italian valliculture. Occasional extensive infections have been recorded in other parts of Europe, North Africa, America and Asia. *Argulus foliaceus* and *A. laticauda* have been found on eels.

Parasitised fish show reddening of the skin, which becomes slimy and irritated and shows a whitish discoloration. The parasite causes necrosis of the skin, due to the toxic enzymes and substances it releases into the skin. It does not grow at temperatures over 28°C or below 10°C. *Argulus* infections should be treated with insecticides like trichlorphon or with salt baths. Infected ponds should be disinfected by drying.

Ergasilus

Infections with *Ergasilus gibbus*, *E. caeruleus* and *E. sieboldi* can be found on the gills. The parasite causes serious hypertrophy of the gills as it feeds on gill epithelial cells, releasing enzymes so that the production of these cells is increased. *Ergasilus* infections can be treated with insecticides like trichlorphon but the adult parasites are less susceptible than the juveniles.

Lernaea

Sudden outbreaks of anchor worm *Lernaea cyprinacea* disease occur in Japanese eel culture.

The parasite is typically red and attaches itself into the musculature. The attachment site is often surrounded by a red rim. The parasite develops optimally at water temperatures of 14–32°C.

Anchor worms can be treated with salt baths but the eggs and larvae survive low salinities. Another possible treatment is the use of insecticides like trichlorphon but these do not affect the eggs.

Gas-bubble Disease

Gas-bubble disease is caused by supersaturation of nitrogen gas in the water. There are three main causes of supersaturation in eel farming:

(1) Recirculation systems add liquid oxygen to the culture water under pressure. When very high oxygen levels are achieved (e.g. 150–200%) this causes an imbalance in the gas equilibrium of the water so that other gases, such as nitrogen, are forced to form bubbles. Gas-bubble disease may result if these bubbles are not removed properly.
(2) Supersaturation of water with nitrogen may also occur due to suction of ambient air through leaky pipe joints or pumps.
(3) When water is heated, the gas equilibrium changes. Warm water has a lower maximum dissolved gas content. Supersaturation with nitrogen may therefore also occur in heated power plant effluents and in ponds which are heated significantly by the sun during the day.

Elvers are very sensitive to gas supersaturation of the culture water: it causes the formation of large nitrogen gas bubbles in the tissue of the head and gills. The affected elvers float near the water surface and subsequent mortalities may be very high. Larger eels become sluggish and can be seen swimming at the surface; their fins become pinkish-red and sometimes the fin rims are whitish. On closer examination of the fins and gills, small gas bubbles may be observed in the capillaries. Subsequent mortalities may continue for some time even when the cause of the gas supersaturation has been removed.

Clinical Diagnosis

Clinical diagnosis is based intially on obtaining a good clinical history from the client:

(1) Where did the glass eels or fingerlings originate from?
(2) When did the problems first occur?
(3) Was any peculiar behaviour observed?
(4) What are the problems exactly?
(5) Which clinical signs can be observed?
(6) Have there been any problems related to water quality in the past few days or weeks?

Necropsy and Parasitology

Necropsy should be carried out in the following stages:

(1) External abnormalities observed.
(2) Skin smear.
(3) Examination of gills — gross, and by microscope.
(4) Examination inside the body cavity:

- the liver
- the spleen
- the gut
- the swim-bladder
- the kidney
- musculature.

Bacteriology

For bacteriology, a smear of the swollen spleen is Gram-stained. If there are many of the same bacteria present, a bacterial disease could be the case. For isolation of bacteria a sample of liver, kidney and spleen tissue is inoculated on tryptone soya agar plates and/or sheep blood agar. If the eels are kept in sea water, marine agar should also be inoculated. Skin smears for control of *Myxobacteria* should be inoculated on low nutrient agar plates, (such as cytophaga agar). Plates are incubated at 15, 22 or 28°C, depending on the water temperature at the fish farm. Subsequently the bacteria should be determined and an antibiogram should be made.

Virology

If a virus infection is suspected, whole live eel or pools of liver, spleen, kidney and brain are transported at 4°C to the fish disease laboratory. Here the virus can be isolated, by inoculating live sterile fish cell lines with homogenates of the pooled organs. When a cytopathogenic effect (CPE) results, the virus is determined by using specific antibodies. Serology has also become an important diagnostic tool. For instance, eels from farms infected with EVE show a high neutralising titre against this virus a few weeks after the outbreak.

Histopathology

For histopathological investigations, samples of the organs should be fixed in buffered formalin.

Therapy

Chemotherapy should be used with caution. Some therapeutants are eliminated very slowly

ANTIMICROBIAL COMPOUNDS USED IN EEL CULTURE		
Drug	**Method**	**Dose**
Tetracycline	feed	50–80 mg/kg fish/day for 7 days
	bath	20 mg/l for 1 day
TCN (tetracycline, chloramphenicol, and neomycin)	bath	50 mg/l for 1–2.5 hours
Sulphonamides	feed	100–200 mg/kg fish/day for 7–14 days
Furaltadone-HCl	bath	30 mg/l for 2 hours
Furazolidone	feed	25–80 mg/kg fish/day for 7–21 days
Flumequine	bath	25 mg/l for 3 hours
	feed	6–10 mg/kg fish/day for 6–10 days
Oxolinic acid	feed	3–12 mg/kg fish/day for 7–10 days
Chloramphenicol	bath	20 mg/l for 1 day
	bath	50–80 mg/l for 8 hours
	feed	50 mg/kg fish/day for 7 days

FIG.   18.8 Antimicrobial compounds used in eel culture.

ANTI-ECTOPARASITIC DRUGS USED IN EEL CULTURE		
Drug	**Method**	**Dose**
General treatment: Sodium chloride Formalin	bath bath	2000 ppm permanent 30–40 mg/l permanent 80–200 mg/l for 30 minutes
Ichthyophthirius or *Chilodonella* Malachite green	bath	0.05–0.1 mg/l permanent
Costia, Trichodina, Ichthyophthirius, Chilodonella FMC (formalin + malachite green + methylene blue)	bath	per 1000 l water: 10 ml 37% formalin + 37 mg malachite green + 37 mg methylene blue
Costia Acriflavin–HCl or lactaridine	bath bath	5–10 mg/l for 2-3 days 1–3 mg/l for 2 x 24 hours

FIG. 18.9 Anti-ectoparasitic drugs used in eel culture.

from the fish, leaving residues, so that there must be a waiting period after treatment (usually more than three weeks) before the eels can be sold for human consumption.

Anti-bacterial Compounds

Based on an antibiogram, a choice can be made from the antimicrobial compounds listed in Fig. 18.8, which is based on practical data. Diseased eels are generally inappetent and in such cases the only method of treatment is by bath. Individual eels are not normally injected with antimicrobial compounds.

Anti-fungal Compounds

An effective therapy against *Saprolegniasis* is a bath with malachite green (0.05–0.1 mg/l for 2 or more days). Considerable care should be taken with this straining substance, as it is known to be cytotoxic, teratogenic and mutagenic. Wear gloves and protect the face.

Anti-parasitic Compounds

Anti-protozoal (flagellates and ciliates)

Long-term bath treatments against ectoparasites (24–48 hours) are much more effective in curing the disease than short-term baths. During short-term baths, parasites in the gill cavity are not exposed thoroughly enough to the treatment

and often reappear soon afterwards. Some anti-protozoal treatments for eels are listed in Fig. 18.9.

Anthelmintic compounds

The treatments listed in Fig. 18.10 are intended to cure infections with ectoparasitic monogenean trematodes and endoparasitic nematodes.

Anti-crustacean compounds

Crustacean infections can be cured with a bath of formalin and trichlorphon at concentrations similar to those listed in Fig. 18.10. Trichlorphon is rather toxic to eels and should be used with care.

Sedation

Eels can be sedated with tricaine-methane-sulphonate (MS 222, 100 mg/l) or metomidate 1 ml per 5 l from a 50 mg/l solution).

Prevention of Disease

Prevention of fish diseases can be carried out by a combination of good management and stocking with healthy fish from the start. Fish farmers should be encouraged to contact their veterinarian as early as possible when a disease is suspected. There are effective commercial vaccines against *Vibrio* infections in some European countries. However, vaccination is usually less effective on marine eel farms because many different *Vibrio*

FIG. 18.10 Treatments against monogenea and nematodes.

TREATMENTS AGAINST MONOGENEA AND NEMATODES		
Drug	**Method**	**Dose**
General treatment: Formalin	bath	30–40 mg/l permanent 80–200 mg/l for 30 minutes
Pseudodactylogyrus Mebendazole	bath	200 mg/1000 l water, for several days, repeat after 1 week
Nematodes (difficult to cure) Trichlorphon L-Levamisole–HCl	bath bath	0.25–0.75 mg/l permanent (toxic!) 20 mg/l during 6 days, to be repeated after 2 weeks

spp. can attack the fish, one by one. At present there are no vaccines for pathogenic eel viruses.

Acknowledgements – We would like to thank Andries Kamstra (RIVO) for his useful comments and suggestions on the husbandry aspects of eel culture in recirculation systems.

Further Reading

Hine, P. M. and Boustead, N. C. (1974) *A Guide to Diseases in Eel Farms*. Fish Research Division Occasional Publication No. 6, Ministry of Agriculture and Fisheries, Wellington, New Zealand. 28 pp.

Hoffman, G. L. and Meyer, F. P. (1974) *Parasites of Freshwater Fishes*. T. F. H. Publications Inc., Neptune City, N.J., USA. 224 pp.

Kamstra, A. and Davidse, W. P. (1991) *An Evaluation of the Biological, Technical and Economic Aspects of Growing Eel in Recirculation Systems*. Rijksinstituut voor Visserijonderzoek, IJmuiden, The Netherlands — Landbouweconomisch Instituut, Den Haag, The Netherlands. R.I.V.O. Report AQ91–O4. 63 pp (in Dutch).

Liewes, E. W. (1991) Eel culture and management. *Arbeiten des Deutschen Fischerei-Verbandes* **51**, 60–73 (in German).

Matsui, I. (1980) *Theory and Practice of Eel Culture*. A. A. Balkema Books, Rotterdam, The Netherlands. 133 pp.

Ogami, H. (1970) *Practical Guide on the Diseases of Eel*. Shokugyo Times Company, Tokyo, Japan. 93 pp (in Japanese).

Querellou, J. (1974) Eel rearing in Japan. *Piscic. fr.* **37**, 9–57 (in French with English summary).

Rickards, W. L. (ed.) (1978) *A Diagnostic Manual of Eel Diseases Occurring Under Culture Conditions in Japan*. University of Carolina, Sea Grant Program (Raleigh, N.C. USA). Publ. no. UNG-SG-78-06. 89 pp.

Sano, T. (1976) Viral diseases of cultured fishes in Japan. *Fish Pathology* **10**(2), 221–226.

Tesch, F. W. (1977) *The Eel, Biology and Management of Anguillid Eels*. Chapman and Hall, London. 434 pp.

Usui, A. (1991) *Eel Culture*. (2nd edn.) Fishing News Books Ltd., Farnham, Surrey, U.K. 160 pp.

Willemse, J. J. (1979) Guide to the internal morphology of the European eel, *Anguilla anguilla* L. (Pisces, Teleostei). *Aquaculture* **17**, 91–103.

19

The Veterinary Approach to Turbot

RONNIE SOUTAR

Experimental culture of turbot (*Scophthalmus maximus*) followed on from trials with sole and plaice. Adult turbot are tough, sedentary fish with a piscivorous diet, making them apparently ideal subjects for aquaculture. Moreover, turbot is a high-value species and the wild catch is unreliable. However, larval rearing is more difficult than for the salmonids and this has been the major limitation on the development of turbot farming.

For this reason, most hatcheries developed where high levels of technical expertise and funding were available — generally in conjunction with Atlantic salmon farming and therefore centred on Northern Europe. Turbot prefer higher water temperatures than the ambient level in these areas, so that heated water had to be supplied. One economical method of providing this was to use the effluent water from power stations.

While artificially heated water has allowed the development of satisfactory larval rearing systems, there are problems associated with such developments. For this reason, on-growing is now being developed in areas with natural ambient sea temperatures within the optimal range. In particular, Galicia, in north-west Spain, has become the industry's major centre, with an estimated output of around 1500 tonnes in 1991. The introduction of turbot to Chile, where conditions are very similar, may see considerable growth there. These facilities relied initially upon the importation of juveniles hatched elsewhere but hatcheries are being developed by many of the on-growing companies in order to avoid the shortfalls in supplies of juveniles.

As such facilities are developed, the most likely area of veterinary involvement may be in the hatchery sector, although disease is already having an impact during on-growing. Unfortunately, as turbot farming is still developing rapidly and the market is keenly contested, many of the techniques which have proven successful for individual companies remain carefully guarded commercial secrets. In many cases, therefore, the veterinarian will have to apply basic principles of disease investigation when confronted with a problem which may already have been met and overcome elsewhere. Awareness of the problems encountered during the rapid expansion of salmon farming in Norway and Scotland may help to avoid the development of similar situations during turbot farming's boom period.

Farming Systems

Hatchery

Turbot eggs are planktonic and are incubated suspended in the water column of small tanks (usually made of PVC). Water should be filtered and preferably sterilised, and may be recirculated.

After hatching, juveniles are transferred into tanks with a water supply of equally high quality. Tanks of up to 4 m in diameter may be used. Flow rates may be limited by restrictions on the volume of suitable water and aeration or, more commonly, oxygenation will be required.

Hatchery units also include facilities for the culture of live foods. Such cultures are normally in tanks under sterile conditions, while the algae on which they in turn are fed are grown in large plastic bags under artificial light.

Nursery

At around 2–5 g (90 days old), juveniles are transferred from the hatchery to the nursery. Nursery tanks may be of fibreglass or PVC, either square (sides 1–2 m) or circular (1–4 m diameter). Both hatchery and nursery units will normally be enclosed within buildings, to permit environmental control and for security.

On-growing

Various cage systems for the on-growing of turbot have been tried, generally including some form of fixed, solid base on which the fish can rest. These systems are not entirely suitable for the species, largely due to the unsettling effect of movements of the cage bottom. Also, the requirement of turbot is for a sufficient surface area of bottom space rather than for a high total water volume, and this is difficult to achieve with cage systems.

On-growing is now carried out almost exclusively in on-shore tanks using pumped sea water. The tanks may be circular with a diameter of 4–10 m, or square with sides of 2–10 m, and are made of concrete, PVC or plastic-lined metal. A depth of 1–1.5 m is common but the capacity of a unit tends to be expressed in terms of surface area rather than volume. Raceways have been found to be unsuitable.

Water intakes should be as far from the shore as is practical and deep enough to avoid surface disturbance and high planktonic loadings. In the fertile waters off Galicia, for example, both micro- and macro-algae can be problematic. Intakes should include some facility for the removal of seaweed, otherwise blockages may have disastrous effects.

Steps must be taken to avoid the fouling of pipes by marine growths, which could severely restrict flow rates. However, care must be taken to ensure that such measures do not affect the stock. Fish kills have occurred where chlorine has been used to limit fouling and this may be a particular problem where power station effluents are used. For the avoidance of fouling, water distribution in open channels may be preferable to pipes.

Flow rates can be much less than for salmonids, with water exchange rates of 2–3 hours in tanks. Aeration or oxygen injection (minimum 5 mg O_2/kg fish/hour) will be required; oxygen levels should be monitored constantly and maintained near saturation. Provision should be made for systems failures, with back-up water pumps and generators.

Unlike some flat-fish, turbot feed during daylight, but high intensity light hampers feeding and it is important that the tanks be shaded, particularly during high summer. This can be achieved by siting the tanks within a building, which gives better environmental control and protection for workers, or by using solid or net covers on individual tanks, which is much cheaper and appears to be effective.

Broodstock

Broodstock are normally held in tanks up to 4 m in diameter in a unit associated with the hatchery, within light-proof buildings to allow photoperiodic manipulation.

General Husbandry

Broodstock and Hatchery

Turbot broodstock are normally stocked at a ratio of one female to two or three males, at a temperature of 10–16°C. Stocking density is around 3 fish per 10 m^2. The age at maturation varies; on average, a female will spawn first at around three years old. The broodstock are normally kept under artificial lighting to allow the manipulation of photoperiod and thus influence the season of spawning. Annual light cycle manipulation can lead to early maturation but is not normally practised.

Natural spawning is in April or May. By photoperiod manipulation, it has been possible to extend the spawning period from February to November. Eggs may be collected (Fig. 19.1) from an individual female every two days but this varies greatly with temperature. Around 12 collections might be expected from an average female within the spawning period. Hormonal induction of spawning, using pituitary extracts, has been attempted but is not commonly used; it will induce spawning within 24 hours in females in suitable condition.

In comparison with salmonids, turbot eggs are small and numerous. They are just over 1 mm in diameter and a female might produce around one million eggs per kg body weight. The eggs can be disinfected after collection to reduce the risk of

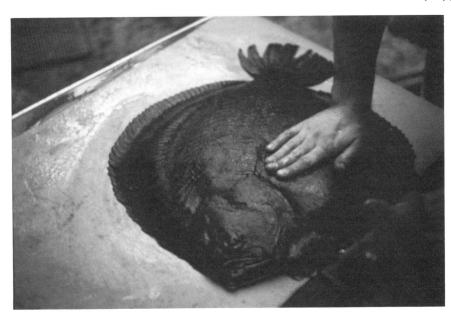

FIG. 19.1 Stripping a turbot broodfish.

vertical bacterial transmission; the exact methods of disinfection vary and hatcheries are unwilling to discuss them but general principles can be applied.

Eggs are incubated at 15°C and will hatch in around five days at this temperature. Viable eggs are pelagic, as are newly-hatched larvae. Feeding should commence 3–4 days post-hatching at 15°C and metamorphosis to the typical flatfish morphology should be complete by around day 30. After metamorphosis, when they will be around 20 mm long, the juveniles become bottom-dwelling.

For successful incubation and larval rearing, full-strength sea water which has been filtered and sterilised (normally uv treated) should be used. Artificial sea water has been used in static systems at this stage and has the benefit of purity and sterility. The water should be well oxygenated and stability of temperature is important. Light levels should be suppressed. The pH should not vary significantly from that of oceanic water.

In the early part of their life-cycle (Fig. 19.2), turbot require live food. For first feeding, this is supplied by rotifers (*Brachionus plicatilis*). These will be cultured on site and the quality of the cultures is of crucial importance. Recent work suggests that juvenile turbot survive and grow better when their rotifer food is pumped directly

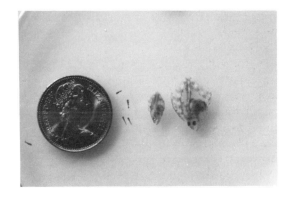

FIG. 19.2 Juvenile turbot — newly-hatched, early metamorphosis and fully metamorphosed.

from the culture on a continuous basis rather than a quantity of rotifers being placed into the tanks daily.

Vibrios, particularly *V. alginolyticus*, and aeromonads are commonly found in rotifer media but are unlikely to be significant if present in low numbers. As far as possible, however, the cultures should be bacteria-free, remembering that any bacteria present may bloom when the rotifers are introduced into the hatchery tanks. Certain bacteria may actually be beneficial to the juvenile turbot, either by producing trace nutrients or by inhibiting the growth or invasive ability of potentially pathogenic bacteria; *Lactobacillus* spp. may have a role here.

The algae on which the rotifers are fed are also cultured on-site and obviously influence the quality of the rotifers as turbot food. The algae should be of mixed species to ensure an optimal nutritional balance but *Isochrycis galbana* should be the major component as this is found to produce rotifers rich in long-chain polyunsaturated fatty acids (PUFAs). The addition of fish oil to the rotifer culture has been suggested as a means of improving their fatty acid profile. The pH and temperature of the rotifer medium are important; pH values of around 6 and a temperature range of 19–25°C have been successful.

From day 10, brine shrimp nauplii (*Artemia salina*) should be introduced to the diet; rotifers should be phased out by day 12. As with rotifers, cultures of *Artemia* are introduced directly into the hatchery tanks and it is again important that no contaminants or potential pathogens are introduced with them. *Artemia* of increasing size are fed until around day 30 (the end of the pelagic phase), by which time the juveniles will have been transferred into weaning tanks.

Juvenile turbot can take inert food when they reach 15–20 mm long. The change should be gradual, with *Artemia* given simultaneously or on alternate days during the weaning period. Specialised weaning diets have now been developed to precede the use of crumbs and pellets. There is a risk that overfeeding will foul the water at this stage, as the fish will not feed on food which is on the bottom of the tank. Particular attention to feeding rate and tank hygiene is required but it is difficult to state an exact food requirement; this will be a matter for good stockmanship, responding to the appetite of the fish. Cannibalism can become a problem and is addressed by careful grading of the stocks for size, which will also be of value in determining feeding rate and the timing of weaning.

Nursery

For transport to the nursery, juveniles may be shipped in plastic bags containing one part water to three parts pure oxygen, cooled to reduce the metabolic rate. If these bags are packed into insulated containers, the fish should withstand air transport and arrive in good condition.

The juveniles will weigh around 2–5 g when they enter the nursery and will stay there until they are around 30 g and 15 cm long, at three to four months old. During this phase they will become accustomed to pelleted food.

The optimum water temperature in the nursery is 19°C. If inflowing water is filtered and water quality parameters are carefully maintained in the correct range, this should be a relatively trouble-free stage. The turbot will be almost constantly graded for size by hand to maintain uniformity within tanks. Stocking rates should be 2–4 kg/m^2 during the nursery stage.

The importance of aeration will be obvious if it is remembered that the oxygen capacity of water falls with increasing salinity and temperature. A check should be kept on oxygen levels, although the requirement will be influenced by stocking levels and water flow rates.

On-growing

On arrival at an on-growing site, young turbot will be stocked at around 4 kg/m^2 of tank bottom. A temperature of around 16°C is optimal, with a range of 12–18°C through the year being typical. Water parameters should be as close to oceanic as possible and oxygenation or aeration will be required. Stocking densities increase as the individual fish grow: Fig. 19.3 gives an approximation of size and stocking density at various stages of on-growing.

Standard harvest size is 2 kg and the aim would be to reach this after about 2½ years of on-growing; it has been estimated that an on-growing unit must produce over 50 t annually to be profitable. Females grow faster than males; in this respect it

SIZE AND STOCKING DENSITY DURING ON-GROWING		
Age (months)	Average weight (kg)	Stocking density (kg/m^2)
4	0.04	5
6	0.08	8
12	0.3	15
18	0.7	25
24	1.3	35
30	1.8	40

Fig. 19.3 Size and stocking density during on-growing.

is worth noting that when turbot were crossed with brill (*Scophthalmus rhombus*), the progeny were all female.

Feed may be fresh fish, moist diets (35–40% moisture content) or, increasingly, dry pelleted foods. Feeding rates and FCR will obviously vary with the type of food used and the size of the turbot, but follows general salmonid principles.

Tank hygiene is important. Uneaten food must not be allowed to accumulate on the bottom, where it would rapidly lead to water fouling. Turbot appear to be naturally 'lazy' and will spend a large amount of the time lying on the bottom. If conditions are poor, this will result in the development of surface lesions and infections.

The placid nature of the fish allows them to be handled more easily than salmonids and often without the use of anaesthesia. Grading for size is normally done manually.

Various attempts have been made at polyculture of turbot with Atlantic salmon, in both cages and tanks. Results have generally been poor, due to the problems of maintaining a suitable environment for both species, and such ventures are unlikely to be economical.

Legislation

The legislation most likely to concern veterinarians covers the movements of turbot across national boundaries. Such traffic has been relatively common to date, with hatcheries in one country supplying on-growing facilities in another.

Within the European Community, or in countries trading with it, governing legislation changed at the end of 1992. Movements of juvenile turbot are likely to include intra-community trade (e.g. from Germany, France and the UK to Spain), export from the EC (e.g. EC countries to Chile) and import into the EC (e.g. from Norway to Spain). All such movements will require veterinary certification of the health status of the stock to be transported.

Certification has so far centred particularly on the absence of IPN virus but other conditions may be specified, depending on the countries involved. In certifying juvenile turbot as free from a given disease, it should be remembered that they are hardy fish and may be asymptomatic carriers of pathogens which may only become detectable when the fish are severely stressed.

An area of legislative difficulty for veterinarians in the UK, and of some importance elsewhere, has been the absence of licensed drugs for the treatment of turbot diseases. As a food animal, there are strict limitations on prescribing for turbot. For growers, it is likely to be acceptable under EC law to use in-feed drugs licensed for use in other farmed fish or, where these are unavailable, drugs licensed for in-feed use in other farmed animals.

The problem has been greater in attempting to treat juveniles. At the time of writing, there are no antibacterials licensed in the UK as bath treatments for fish of any species. EC laws will allow the use of a drug which is licensed for another means of administration but, if such a drug is used outside the limits of its licence, full responsibility falls on the prescribing veterinarian.

This may lead to additional problems involving effluent controls and the farmer's consent to discharge. Relatively large volumes of dilute antibacterial material will be discharged following bath treatments and the veterinarian may be held responsible for any perceived effect on the environment. Discharge from land-based aquaculture units is likely to be the subject of close scrutiny in the future and the use of effluent treatment plants of various types may be enforced.

Major Diseases

Hatchery and Nursery

Bacterial septicaemia

This is the most common disease of larvae. It is generally seen as depressed appetite and a sudden increase in daily mortalities. Affected fish may show abnormal swimming or may settle on the tank bottom. The typical signs of acute septicaemia may be seen on clinical examination and post-mortem — skin darkening, ascites, exophthalmos, external and internal haemorrhaging. However, sudden death is the most striking feature and may occur without the appearance of other clinical signs.

The causative organisms tend to be opportunists rather than primary pathogens. *Vibrio*, *Pseudomonas* and *Aeromonas* species appear to be most commonly involved but a variety of other bacterial species may be seen — many cases will involve mixed infections. The primary pathogen *Vibrio anguillarum* has also caused epizootic disease in juvenile turbot.

Septicaemia occurs in larvae from around day 7 and is uncommon in weaned juveniles. It may be precipitated by a number of stressors, particularly temperature and feeding abnormalities, but there are often no obvious predisposing factors. In the later stages of nursery production, septicaemia is more likely to be due to true vibriosis (*V. anguillarum*) unless environmental conditions are very poor.

External parasitism

From about day 12, larvae may suffer attack from ciliate protozoans. The exact identity of these organisms often remains undetermined, as does their source. Their presence is normally first signalled by appetite depression and then by an increase in mortalities. Protozoan parasites of the type seen in other farmed fish may also parasitise juvenile turbot. *Ichthyobodo* (*Costia*) and *Trichodina* spp. will present with typical symptoms.

Fin rot

This presents as in salmonids, with erosion of fins. Early lesions are small blisters; in advanced cases, fins may be reduced to ragged vestiges and ulcerated lesions may be present on other areas of the body. The primary cause of this condition is disputed; bacteria, particularly *Aeromonas*, *Pseudomonas* and *Vibrio* species are found but may be secondary invaders. Ciliates have also been associated with some cases. Water quality parameters may be important, as may water temperature (particularly high temperatures or sudden fluctuations).

Depigmentation

Although perhaps not strictly a disease, veterinary opinion may be sought as this condition has financial implications. Also termed 'pseudo-albinism', the condition presents as white patches on the dorsal (pigmented) surface. Virtually the whole surface may be white in some fish. This appears to have no deleterious effect on the health of farmed turbot (although it would presumably lead

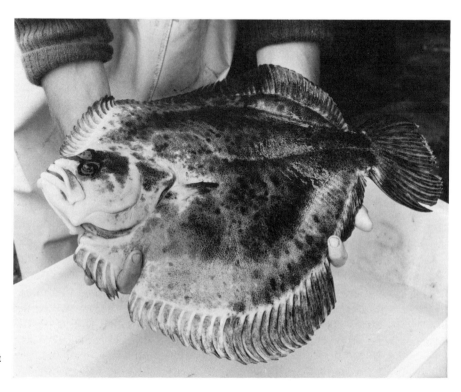

Fig. 19.4 Market-sized turbot showing depigmentation.

to increased risk of predation in the wild) nor does flesh quality appear to be affected. Depigmented fish have been and are marketed (Fig. 19.4); however, as the supply of juveniles has increased to fill demand, on-growers now tend to reject affected fish in favour of normally pigmented stock. The aetiology remains in doubt; nutritional deficiency, particularly in fatty acid and thiamine levels, appears to be involved but higher than normal light intensity during early larval rearing has also been implicated.

Deformities

A number of deformities are seen in juvenile turbot. A high incidence may generally be taken as indicative of sub-optimal hatchery conditions.

On-growing

Viral conditions

Herpesvirus scophthalmi virus (HSV) is known to be carried by wild turbot but has not, so far, been a significant commercial problem. Affected fish show lethargy and inappetence and tend to lie on the tank bottom in a typical position, with the head and tail raised. HSV results in the formation of 'giant cells' which may be detected in skin and gill smears; these show coarse granulation and have very large nuclei.

An epizootic IPN infection in turbot occurred in France when asymptomatic carriers were transferred from 11°C to water at 18°C. Diseased fish showed anorexia and lethargy, while anaemia, intra-muscular haemorrhage and necrosis of the kidney haematopoietic tissue were distinguishing features. The source of the infection was not determined. This case has implications for veterinarians carrying out disease certification and might suggest the value of stress testing any suspect stock before transport between facilities.

A reovirus was isolated from turbot growers suffering increased mortalities and showing abdominal distension and haemorrhages at the vent and fin-bases. A vibrio, possibly *V. splendidus*, was apparently also involved in this condition.

Experimentally, turbot have been shown to be susceptible to VHS virus, displaying the classical symptoms at lowered temperatures. This could have some importance if turbot were reared in polyculture with salmonids.

Bacterial infections

Vibriosis, caused by *V. anguillarum*, would appear to be the primary bacterial disease of turbot growers. However, the fish appear relatively resistant and most outbreaks have been in stressed populations, e.g. at elevated temperatures. Signs are typical of a haemorrhagic septicaemia, although corneal opacity may be a distinguishing feature.

In adverse conditions, or when fish are severely stressed, non-specific *Vibrio* spp. infections and septicaemias associated with other opportunist bacteria are seen. The list of those bacteria continues to grow and includes *Aeromonas*, *Pseudomonas*, *Alteromonas*, *Flavobacterium* and *Chondrococcus* species, while a number of others have been isolated from apparently healthy turbot.

Aeromonas salmonicida infection has been seen in turbot kept in polyculture with infected Atlantic salmon. Turbot would appear to be more resistant than salmon to furunculosis but to succumb when the bacterial challenge reaches high levels. Signs are typically septicaemic but with surface lesions. Skin lesions may be seen, particularly where environmental conditions are sub-optimal. Myxo-bacteria appear to have a predilection for the dorsal–lateral line and may be seen as a pale, shiny growth in this area. Secondary infections of traumatic lesions appear to be favoured by the sedentary nature of turbot.

Fungal infections

When untreated trash fish is used as food, *Ichthyophonus* infection is a potential risk. Symptoms in turbot are as for other species.

Microsporidial infection

An emerging problem in Galicia has been overwhelming infection of young growers with a microsporidian. This has been identified as *Tetramicra brevifilum*, which is known to occur as a natural infection of wild turbot. In typical cases, morbidity and mortality are high. The parasite is found throughout the musculature and internal organs. Characteristic microsporidian xenomata are formed with localised tissue destruction becoming generalised. Moribund fish present grossly with muscle tissue replaced by a jelly-like substance and with internal organs swollen and white-spotted. Destruction of the tissues rapidly leads to disability and death.

The source of infection is uncertain. Both water and food should be investigated; the former seems a more likely route given that infection does not appear to have been confined to turbot on diets of untreated fish. Within affected tanks, death of infected individuals will lead to release of large numbers of spores and the condition is likely to spread rapidly.

Internal parasites

Haemogregarines are believed to cause anaemia and have been implicated in a proliferative condition in young growers. Where wild-caught turbot are used as broodstock, the cestodes *Bothriocephalus scorpii* and *B. gregarius* may be found. They should be unable to complete their life-cycle under normal farm conditions but heavy infestations could result in failure to thrive and poor breeding performance. Nematodes, including *Hysterothylacium* and *Cucullanus* spp., may also be found in wild-caught fish being reared as broodstock.

External parasites

Protozoa, such as *Trichodina* spp., may build up in tanks; *Costia* have been problematic in cages. These should be readily detected and treated. *Lepeophtheirus* spp. and gyrodactylids have been reported from turbot and could be problematic if established in tanks.

Miscellaneous conditions

Hepato-renal syndrome (HRS) leads to chronic ill thrift. It is characterised by thickened bile ducts, with hepatic fibrosis in advanced cases, and swollen renal tubular epithelium, with focal calcium deposition and dilation of the renal ducts. It was a more common problem in the early development of turbot farming and the exact cause has not been determined. However, a nutritional aetiology seems certain and the disease has been linked to binders used in food preparation. Suggested factors range from vitamin deficiencies to heavy metal contamination.

Granulomatous hypertyrosinaemia, which may be found to affect the kidney of cultured turbot, appears to be caused by tyrosine crystal deposition. The condition, is associated with ascorbic acid deficiency, which may be a feature of food condition, particularly food storage conditions. Decreased growth rates followed by increased mortalities are the clinical signs and the condition will be exacerbated by deficiencies in other vitamins.

Yellow turbot are occasionally found in the on-growing phase. There is dispute over whether this is a true jaundice but affected fish appear to have liver pathology. Again, nutritional factors have been implicated.

Algal blooms (particularly *Gonyaulax tamarensis*) have been experienced in Galicia but so far there have been no associated mortalities.

Chlorine poisoning has been experienced in facilities using power-station effluent. Chlorine is added to the water to prevent fouling of pipes in the power station. Although this is buffered by the sea water and reduced by aeration, toxic levels can be experienced. Larvae and juveniles are more susceptible to chlorine toxicity and it would be unusual for these to be exposed to effluent water which had not been treated to reduce chlorine levels. Continuous exposure of growers to sub-lethal levels may be reflected in gill pathology and poor performance.

Neoplastic conditions may be encountered, generally as isolated cases, often confined to broodstock. Juvenile turbot are reported as suffering skin papillomata and visceral neoplasia on a Galician unit. *Vibrio* spp. were thought to be contributing to this syndrome.

Clinical Diagnosis

Skin and gill scrapes should provide diagnostic material for external parasites. With care, these techniques can be performed in conscious larger turbot without deleterious effects; juveniles will have to be sacrificed for sampling. Such examinations should be carried out regularly.

Bacteriological samples should be taken routinely from freshly dead fish or sacrificed moribunds, even where mortality rates are low. For the diagnosis of septicaemic conditions in growers,

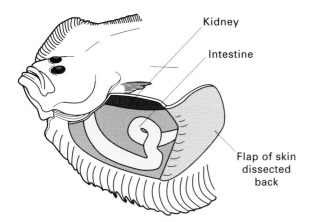

FIG. 19.5 Position of the kidney. A skin flap has been lifted and the abdominal organs moved aside. If the swim-bladder is carefully peeled away, the uncontaminated surface of the kidney (shaded) should be revealed and bacteriological samples can be taken.

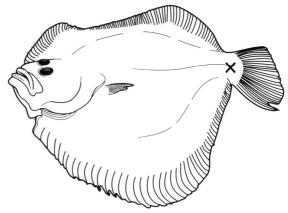

FIG. 19.6 Point of insertion (X) of needle for blood sampling. The needle should be directed cranially towards the midline in the vertical and horizontal planes.

samples can be taken from the kidney. This should be straightforward if due attention is paid to the anatomical features of flatfish (Fig. 19.5). Marine agar or TSA with added salt (2% NaCl) are suitable for plating out.

Where the size of the fish precludes kidney sampling, as in septicaemias of juveniles, diagnostic samples can be achieved from homogenised whole fish. Fresh-dead juveniles should be soaked initially in methanol, or something similar, to avoid contamination from surface bacteria. After 10–20 minutes they should be transferred into sterile water to rinse for a further ten minutes before being moved into a sterile mortar and thoroughly macerated. It should then be possible to take representative samples using a sterile loop and plate this material out.

Both fresh and fixed material should reveal the presence of typical microsporidian spores in *Tetramicra* infection. The characteristics of the organism are well described in the paper by Matthews and Matthews (1980).

Blood sampling of broodstock or larger growers is straightforward, with samples being drawn from the caudal vein (Fig. 19.6). If the fish are handled carefully, anaesthesia should be unnecessary and they should suffer no ill-effects. Sampling for virology follows basic principles, although the choice of cell line is limited. For certification purposes the standard salmonid cell lines should be used.

Histological examination can be valuable in the diagnosis of a wide variety of conditions and follows standard procedures. The importance of having fixed material examined by histopathologists used to dealing with turbot tissues is worth emphasising but, in the examination of nursery-stage juveniles, a paper by Cousin and Baudin-Laurencin (1987) may be found valuable in establishing the normal and abnormal histological pictures.

Therapy

Viral Diseases

There being no effective treatment, viral infections should be controlled by standard containment methods or selective culling, following general principles.

Bacterial Diseases

For juveniles on live foods, in-feed treatments are obviously precluded and antibacterial therapy has to be by bath. Although such therapy should, in theory, always be preceded by bacterial isolation and sensitivity testing, there are arguments for bypassing this protocol in the case of acute septicaemic disease:

- Mortalities will escalate rapidly if treatment is not given immediately clinical signs are noted.
- Many septicaemias will be mixed infections,

| ANTIBACTERIALS WHICH HAVE BEEN USED AS BATH TREATMENTS FOR TURBOT ||
Drug	Dose rate (mg/l)
Furanace	0.2–10
Chloramphenicol	10–50
Furazolidone	70
Halquinol	25
Neomycin	50–75
Nitrofurazone	20–50

FIG. 19.7 Antibacterials which have been used as bath treatments for turbot.

making isolation and determination of antibiogram difficult and time-consuming.
- The choice of therapeutant will, in practice, be very limited.

For these reasons, it may be preferable to treat presumptively and carry out the investigation of aetiology in parallel with therapy.

The drug which has been used with most success as a bath treatment for juvenile turbot is oxytetracycline (25–100 mg/l). Figure 19.7 shows some antibacterials which may also have some value.

The normal method is to add the initial dose to the whole tank and let it be diluted slowly by the normal water exchange. Doses will vary according to flow rates and the tabulated dose rates should be regarded as a guide only. Toxic effects may be experienced under certain conditions; when these or any other antibacterials are used, a trial should first be carried out on a small number of fish. The availability of the drugs for treatment will be subject to the laws of the country concerned.

In the treatment of larger turbot for bacterial diseases, in-feed medication may be used and will follow the same general principles as for salmonids. A wide variety of antibacterials has been used and the choice of drug for a given case will depend on antibiogram and availability.

Ectoparasitic Diseases

Formalin at 150–250 ppm for 1 hour can be used to treat protozoans such as *Trichodina*. Always check the condition of the gills before treating the fish and ensure there is adequate oxygenation in the water. Invasive ciliates in juveniles have proven resistant to a variety of chemical treatments, although formalin may be successful in early infections.

Endoparasitic Diseases

Therapeutants active against *Tetramicra* are being sought with limited success. Amongst those tried to date are:

Fumagillin (5–50 mg/kg fish for up to 20 days)
Furazolidone (5–75 mg/kg fish for 5–10 days)
Toltrazuril (no dose has been established).

Dose rates have varied and it must be stressed that these have been trials; management of this disease is in the very early stages.

The following drugs have been effective against *Bothriocephalus* sp. infestation:

Praziquantel (5 mg/kg)
Niclosamide (40 mg/kg)

In both cases the stated dose is given daily for three consecutive days.

Miscellaneous Conditions

Some success in the treatment of granulomatous hypertyrosinaemia has followed the injection of large doses of ascorbic acid.

Prevention of Disease

Hatchery and Nursery

By far the most important factor here is water quality — in particular, low bacterial loading within hatchery tanks. This can be achieved in a number of ways but filtration and sterilisation of the water supply will be the essential principles. Water-flow rate and pattern and feeding rate will have an effect on the tank environment and should be investigated where problems are suspected. Salinity and pH are critical and must be maintained within acceptable limits.

Food quality is also of obvious importance, perhaps more so here as live foods are involved. Systems of rotifer and artemia production may fall outside veterinary knowledge and specialist advice may be required if a problem in this area is suspected. However, it should be possible to ascertain whether the cultures have a high degree of bacterial contamination which might be transferred into the fish-holding tanks. Important factors here will be the source of the live-food cultures and the media on which they are fed, as well as the quality of the water in which they are reared. A good culture room will operate at laboratory standards of hygiene and should be quite separate from other farm facilities.

Hatchery hygiene should be of a high standard. Nets and cleaning utensils should be dedicated to individual tanks. Tanks should be cleaned and disinfected between batches of fish. Staff working with broodstock should change their protective clothing and carry out disinfection procedures before working with juveniles. Eggs should be disinfected before incubation if there is any doubt over the health status of broodstock.

Grading is important to reduce stress and physical damage in smaller fish. However, its effect on the spread of disease should be considered where individual tanks have endemic infections.

Vaccination against vibriosis can reduce the incidence of *Vibrio anguillarum* infection and may also help where other *Vibrio* sp. are involved. Commercial bath vaccines are available and work is being carried out on oral vaccines.

On-growing

Only certified disease-free juveniles should be brought into an on-growing facility. This is particularly important where the source is outside the on-growing country. Buying from an experienced hatchery/nursery should ensure that young turbot arrive in optimal condition. Transport facilities should be checked out and transport time kept to a minimum.

The nutritional needs of turbot and how to fulfil them are the subject of on-going investigation. Moving away from whole fish diets would appear to be safer from the view-point of disease transmission but it must be ensured that replacement foods are of the highest quality. In particular, the vitamin and fatty acid contents of feed would appear to be very important. The conditions under which food is stored on the farm should also be checked, particularly during periods of high temperature. If trash fish is being used in the diet, pasteurisation will reduce the risks.

Water source and quality are also important —

sudden changes in water quality parameters can be as damaging as extremes, so steps should be taken to avoid, for example, temperature fluctuations. Oxygen levels should be maintained near saturation and checks made that water flow is not being restricted (e.g. by organisms fouling intake pipes). Regular tests on pH, salinity and levels of metabolites, especially ammonia, should be made.

Hygiene should follow the same general principles as for the nursery. Tanks must be cleaned regularly, with cleaning equipment dedicated to individual tanks. Removal of mortalities can be difficult and extra attention should be paid to this very important task. Tanks must be emptied and disinfected between batches. Protective clothing and footwear for on-farm use should not be worn elsewhere. Staff who visit other units must undergo full disinfection procedures on their return. This will be particularly true for health staff, who handle sick fish and take samples; it should be foremost in the mind of the visiting veterinarian!

Acknowledgements — Sincere thanks to John Barrington and Dr Jonathan Shepherd of Ecoline (UK) Ltd, Andrew Barbour and Bill Cleeve of Golden Sea Produce Ltd and Hilary Duggua of Stirling University Library for invaluable help in the preparation of this chapter.

Further Reading

As turbot farming is relatively new, there are few reference works available. The most comprehensive is:
Liewes, E. W. (1984) *Culture, Feeding and Diseases of Commercial Flatfish Species.* 104pp. A. A. Balkema, Rotterdam, Netherlands.
Good background information can also be found in:
Shepherd, C. J. and Bromage, N. (1988) *Intensive Fish Farming.* 404pp Blackwell Scientific Publications, Oxford.

References

Austin, B., Morgan, D. A. and Alderman, D. J. (1981) Comparison of antimicrobial agents for control of vibriosis in marine fish. *Aquaculture* **26**, 1–12.
Buchanan, J. S., Richards, R. H., Sommerville, C. and Madeley, C. R. (1978) A herpes-type virus from turbot *Veterinary Record* **102**, 527–528.
Castric, J., de Kinkelin, P. (1984) Experimental study of the susceptibility of two marine fish species, Sea Bass and Turbot, to viral haemorrhagic septicaemia. *Aquaculture* **41**, 203–212.
Castric, J., Baudin-Laurencin, F., Coustans, M. F. and Auffret, M. (1987) Isolation of infectious pancreatic necrosis virus, Ab serotype, from an epizootic in farmed Turbot. *Aquaculture* **67**, 117–126.
Cousin, J. C. B. and Laurencin F. B. (1987) Histological alterations observed in Turbot from days 15 to 40 after hatching. *Aquaculture* **67**, 218–220.

Devesa, S., Toranzo A. E. and Barja J. L. (1985) First report of vibriosis in Turbot cultured in northwestern Spain. *Fish and Shellfish Pathology* (Editor Ellis, A. E.), pp. 131–140. Academic Press, London.

Devesa, S., Barja J. L. and Toranzo A. E. (1989) Ulcerative skin and fin lesions in reared Turbot. *Journal of Fish Disease* 12, 323–333.

Gatesoupe, F. J. (1990) The continuous feeding of Turbot larvae and control of the bacterial environment of rotifers. *Aquaculture* 89, 139–148.

Lamas, J., Anadon, R., Devesa S. and Toranzo, A. E. (1990) Visceral neoplasia and epidermal papillomas in cultured Turbot. *Diseases of Aquatic Organisms* 8, 179–187.

Lupiani, B., Dopazo, C. P., Ledo, A., Fouz, B., Barja, J. L., Hetrick, F. M. and Toranzo, A. E. (1989) New syndrome of mixed bacterial and viral aetiology in cultured Turbot. *Journal of Aquatic Animal Health* 1, 197–204.

Matthews, R. A., Matthews B. F. (1980) Cell and tissue reactions of Turbot to *Tetramicra brevifilum. Journal of Fish Disease* 3, 495–515.

Messager, J. L. (1986) Influence of ascorbic acid on granulomatous tyrosinaemia in cultured Turbot. Pamaq.1 pp. 381–390 *Spec. Publ. Eur. Aquacult. Soc.* No. 9.

Olsson, J. C., Westerdahl, A., Conway, P. L. and Kjelleberg, S. (1992) Intestinal colonisation potential of Turbot- and Dab-associated bacteria with inhibitory effects against *Vibrio anguillarum. Applied Environmental Microbiology* 58, 551–556.

Sanmartin Duran, M. L., Caamano-Garcia, F., Fernandez Casal, J., Leiro, J. and Ubeira, F. M. (1989) Anthelmintic activity of Praziquantel, Niclosamide, Netobimin and Mebendazole against *Bothriocephalus scorpii* naturally infecting Turbot. *Aquaculture* 76, 199–201.

20

The Veterinary Approach to Halibut

MARY BRANCKER

Atlantic halibut, *Hippoglossus hippoglossus*, appears to have excellent potential as a commercial proposition for farming either in cages in the sea or in tanks on land. They are pleasant to handle, have a good health record and are regarded as a fish whose flesh and flavour is in the luxury class. Farming of the halibut is not a commercial proposition at present but the indications are that it will be farmed successfully later in this decade. Research into the subject is being carried out in Scotland and Norway, and halibut appears to be suitable for farming in the colder northern waters of the UK.

Halibut is a flat fish that can grow to at least 3 m in length and 340 kg in weight (Fig. 20.1); they can live for 30 years. The underside of the body is white and the top side is dark and patterned. As with other flat fish, the halibut begins life similar in appearance to young round fish but after approximately 75 days the left eye moves to the same side of the head as the right eye and from then on the young halibut swims on its side. In a small proportion of cases it is the right eye that moves.

Farming Systems

The basic equipment required for farming halibut is very similar to that used on other fish farms but certain modifications are necessary. The time spent in the hatchery is long and complicated. Subsequently the fish spend a considerable amount of their time lying down rather than swimming.

The hatchery may be based on either a recirculation or a flow-through system. Whichever method is used, this is a time requiring skilled staff and efficient equipment as each animal is held in the hatchery for several weeks at a very critical period in its development. Unsatisfactory conditions will result in a high fall-out rate and various deformities in the developing larvae.

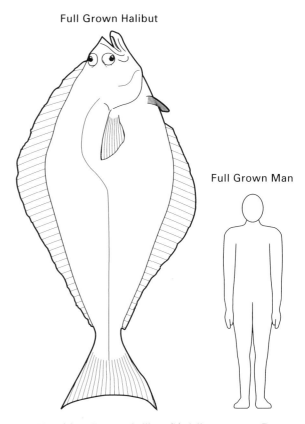

Full Grown Halibut

Full Grown Man

FIG. 20.1 (a) Full grown halibut, (b) full grown man. Drawn to scale.

Although time is usually measured in degree-days rather than standard 24-hour days in fish farming, this does not give accurate data for halibut hatchery work. At present there is a difference of opinion as to the ideal way of presenting the data so that in some cases degree-days will be given and in others standard 24-hour days.

The fertilised eggs (Fig. 20.2) are incubated for 14–15 days in water at a temperature of 3–6°C and a salinity of 34 ppt, in complete darkness and

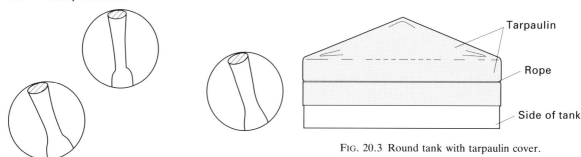

FIG. 20.3 Round tank with tarpaulin cover.

FIG. 20.2 Halibut eggs 3 days prior to hatching. Diameter 3 mm.

usually in relatively small tanks at a density of 300/litre. After hatching the larvae are transferred to a holding facility at a density of 20/l with water of the same salinity and temperature as in the incubator. Particular care is taken to shield them from noise and ensure that they are in complete darkness. The actual shape and size of the containers which have been used successfully at this stage vary enormously, some being a mere 460 l whilst others may be mesocosm tanks of 7–14 m³.

After 50 degree-days a flow rate is gradually introduced and the lighting is slowly increased. After 170 degree-days the temperature is raised by 1°C per day until it is comparable with the water in the larval rearing tank.

The larval rearing tanks usually have a capacity of 900 l and they may be 'greened up' by the addition of algae to the water prior to the arrival of the larvae. Food is introduced at this stage and the larvae remain in these tanks until they are feeding well, the eye has come round and they are ready to swim on their sides and lie on the bottom of the tank. They are then regarded as weaners and can be moved out of the hatchery and into the on-growing tanks.

The on-growers are housed in tanks of various sizes at a stocking density of 40 kg/m²; the water-flow rate is increased and sand is provided so that they can bury themselves completely. Subsequently this sand may be replaced by fine gravel. Full daylight is avoided but the light and the temperature are no longer so critical. Tanks held out-of-doors have to be covered, (Fig. 20.3) as fish of all ages appear to dislike light, and low-flying birds cause apprehension.

When the on-growers are large enough to be contained by a net they may be moved to a cage in the sea, where growth appears to be as good as or better than in those which remain in land based tanks. At present, 160 m³ salmon cages are being used at a stocking rate of 30 kg/m². The cages have been modified by the provision of a tarpaulin floor for the halibut to lie on, but they move off the floor when the sea is rough. It seems that it will be necessary to make further changes in an attempt either to absorb the wave energy or possibly to arrange for the whole structure to be submersible.

The broodstock should be housed in large tanks at a stocking rate of 1 fish/m² and kept as quiet as possible. If the tanks are outside they should be covered but this is not necessary if they are inside with very dim lighting. Unlike the on-growers, the broodstock do not need either sand or fine gravel as substrate as long as the floor of the tank is completely smooth. A portable table with folding legs is useful when halibut are being stripped: the legs at one end of the table are lowered so that the fish can be guided to swim up on to the table with minimal handling.

Transport of mature fish from one tank to another is best carried out by means of a sling made of a smooth material and kept moist throughout the operation (Fig. 20.4).

Various methods of identifying broodstock and potential broodstock have been tried. Some individuals may have unusual markings or possibly a very obvious scar but a proportion are difficult to tell apart. Tags are often used but equally often they become lost. Branding has to be repeated. The microchip appears to be the method with the most potential — it is not ideal, as the reader has to be held very close to the site of the chip, but at least it is permanent.

General Husbandry

Halibut are neither excitable nor delicate but they do appreciate careful, efficient and kindly

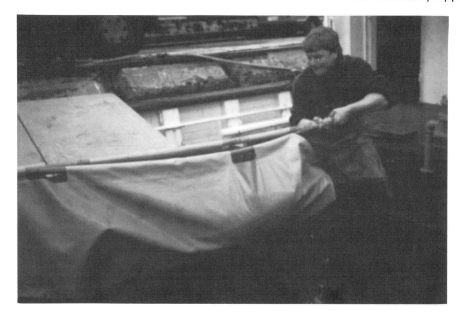

FIG. 20.4 Transporting a large halibut.

handling. A good stockman will be well repaid for his skill.

Eggs and larvae are not easy to culture but each female compensates by producing an enormous number of eggs. The rate of loss will certainly be reduced as techniques improve but it is probable that the hatchery will always be an area requiring a highly skilled workforce. There appear to be several important parameters in the hatchery and it is essential that at least five of these are correct, whilst the remaining conditions should be reasonably near the ideal. The most essential factor is that the eggs and larvae should be handled with the greatest care at all stages.

The most acceptable food for first feeding appears to be zooplankton but this is unlikely to be a sound commercial proposition unless it also is farmed. Naturally occurring zooplankton is erratic in supply, even in Norway, and can never be relied upon off the Scottish coast. Even when it can be obtained, there are problems with various parasites which are small enough to pass through the filter and eventually infect the young halibut.

Research is in progress to produce an inert encapsulated diet that is small enough to be taken, is acceptable to the larvae and contains the essential nutrients for growth. Meantime rotifers, copepods and artemia are fed, usually after being fed themselves on algae specially grown in the hatchery.

First feeding takes place in the hatchery. When the eye has come round, the fish are swimming on their sides, metamorphosis is complete, and the young halibut are feeding well they can be moved out of the hatchery into tanks with an increased flow rate and an ambient temperature. The changes in temperature, lighting and flow rates have to be carried out with care, preferably in the hatchery, and it is essential that any fish which are not ready for these conditions should not be moved. If weaners are moved before they are ready, they will suffer an irreversible set-back even if their condition is noticed quickly and they are returned to the hatchery.

It is necessary to grade the weaners (Fig. 20.5) at regular intervals as the growth of individual fish is not similar and the larger fish may not appreciate that small fish are not intended to be their food.

Food should be offered at frequent intervals and fed to appetite. Extra food will tend to lie on the bottom, even with good flow rates, and will pollute the water in the tank.

Once the mouths of the young fish are large enough, they appreciate chopped up mysids and can be introduced gradually to an adult diet. At present on-growers and broodstock are fed herrings,

FIG. 20.5 Weighing and measuring a young halibut.

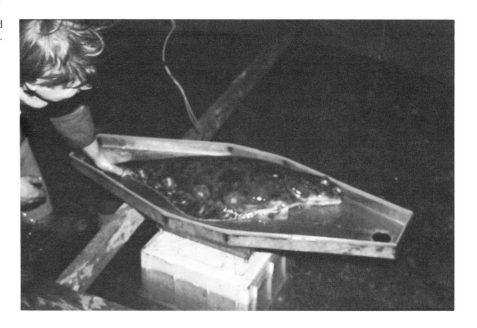

mackerel, sprats and sand eels and also freshly prepared sausages composed of a mixture of minced fresh fish, high quality fish meal and essential vitamins and minerals. Feeding is usually two or three times a week: a halibut has a large stomach and a short intestine, and food passes very slowly out of the stomach. If food is offered daily, the appetitie is not stimulated and the total intake per week is reduced. Home-bred fish on their first year out of the hatchery have a conversion rate of 1.46:1. The aim is to produce a market-size fish of 5 kg in 3.5–4 years.

The potential broodstock will reach maturity when they are 6 or 7 years old and weigh at least 4 kg. Females are usually heavier than males of the same age. During the autumn of that year they will eat less food and the development of the gonads will be apparent. This is the first stage at which it is possible to determine the sex: as the swelling becomes noticeable it can be seen that it extends considerably further back in the female than in the male. The exact date when spawning starts will vary from year to year, depending very much on the temperature of the water, but on the west coast of Scotland it is usually in February. By using photoperiod techniques it is possible to advance the commencement of spawning by one month each year.

The broodstock groups should be set up early in the autumn and it appears to be necessary to have a similar number of each sex in each group. It has been suggested (although this is not proven) that pair-bonding takes place. Very little food is taken during the run-up to ovulation. The best results are obtained if the fish are kept quiet and held in a subdued light.

The females will spawn naturally. Unless the water is of a very good quality and there is a high flow rate, the eggs tend to become infected and over-ripe by the time they are collected. There is also the risk that fertilisation by the male may not have taken place. For these reasons it is more usual to strip both the male and the female manually. This is accomplished by lowering the water level in the tank, encouraging the fish to swim up on to the table already described, and then applying gentle pressure to the area over the gonad. The eggs or the milt can then be collected in sterile jugs. Spawning continues every 3–4 days for 4–6 weeks and the average production is 50% of bodyweight, although the amount produced varies.

Legislation

There is no specific legislation applying to halibut farming but there is a great deal of general legislation which is relevant, relating to the siting of cages, tanks and farm buildings, the potential pollution of the environment, and the health status of the stock.

Major Diseases

The history of halibut in captivity is too recent for much information on disease to be available. It can be said, however, that these fish appear to have a well developed immune system and a will to live, and that wounds show a good healing response.

Trematodes (*Entobdella hippoglossi*) attach themselves to the skin of halibut on both the upper surface and the lower surface of the body. Although they do not appear to cause much inconvenience in small numbers it is advisable to remove them. In certain circumstances they can become a serious infestation and then it is essential that treatment is carried out. The salmon louse (*Lepeophtheirus salmonis*) does not attack halibut but the less host-specific *Argulus* has been seen on them.

Recent trials have indicated that healthy halibut are not susceptible to furunculosis (*Aeromonas salmonicida*) but further investigation is required to determine whether their immunity is complete. There are conflicting reports regarding IPN but it appears that halibut are not easily infected.

The most worrying situation is the apparent predisposition of the larvae to develop anatomical abnormalities (Fig. 20.6). This is comparatively common in the majority of fish species and as fish produce great quantities of eggs it is not of paramount importance. However, it will need further research as a sudden increase in the numbers affected could be catastrophic.

Another condition which requires further research is the lack of skin pigmentation which is seen in a number of the farmed fish. It does not appear to affect the health of the fish but it is of importance commercially. Usually the absence of skin pigment is not total and in many cases there may be only a few small non-pigmented areas. In the latter there often appears to be a familial pattern.

A few of the broodstock have become totally blind, whilst others are blind in one eye. This appears to be a progressive disease and similar in many respects to gas bubble disease in salmon, but the actual cause is not yet known. It is the subject of current research.

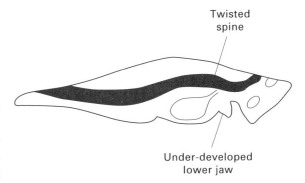

FIG. 20.6 Deformed larvae.

Clinical Diagnosis

Because there is so little detailed information regarding the health status of halibut, it is difficult to make a rapid diagnosis when faced with a pathological condition in these fish. The usual considerations should be taken into account — such as the temperature and quality of the water, the vicinity of other fish farms, the quality of food and the presence of any potential carriers of disease including predators and human visitors. The temperature of the water appears to affect halibut adversely and they will eat less food when the temperature goes over 14°C. Appetite is also adversely affected by increased day length even in covered tanks. Sexually mature fish lose their appetite as they come up to the spawning season and usually do not eat at all throughout the spawning period.

A change of colour tends to be an indication of disease. A dark fish lying on the bottom and not coming up at feeding time is almost certainly not healthy. The usual specimens should be submitted to a laboratory and the remaining stock monitored closely.

Ultrasound equipment (Fig. 20.7) has been used on halibut broodstock and it appears to have considerable diagnostic potential. The skin surface of these fish makes for good contact and portable equipment makes the application of this technique on remote fish farms a practical option.

Therapy

Treatment follows the lines recommended for farmed fish, although the broodstock may need

FIG. 20.7 Ultrasound examination of the gonads of a
mature halibut.

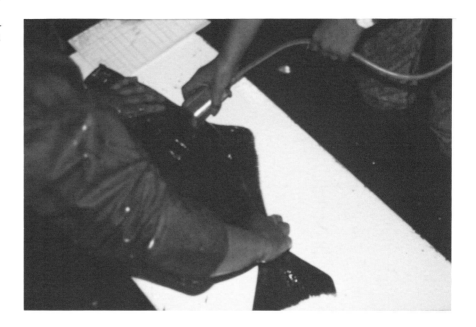

special consideration because of their size and because during the pre-spawning and spawning periods they are easily stressed.

Treatment for trematodes is by immersion in either fresh water or a formalin solution.

Attempts have been made to aspirate the contents of the cysts which are associated with the eye condition described earlier. However, the cyst reforms during the following weeks and this treatment does not appear to have any beneficial effect.

Individual nursing care for valuable broodstock should always be considered and the fish in question should be housed at a low stocking density in a dark tank, with a good flow rate and the water at around 10°C. Force-feeding can be employed if appropriate, although it is time-consuming.

If anaesthesia is necessary, phenoxetol appears to be a satisfactory choice and both induction and recovery are smooth.

Prevention of Disease

High standards of cleanliness are essential on a fish farm and great care should be taken to ensure that no infection is brought in through infected water, contaminated clothing or the introduction of stock without either certification or quarantine. External and internal parasites should be eliminated completely if possible. Careful post-mortem of fish that die or are culled (quite apart from any being examined because of suspected disease) can be valuable.

21

The Veterinary Approach to Cod

OLE TORRISSEN, INGEGJERD OPSTAD and ODD MAGNE RØDSETH

Production of cod larvae in ponds for sea ranching started at the Flødevigen Hatchery as early as in 1884, and large scale hatching of cod eggs was initiated at the Wood Hole Station in 1985. The purpose of the early production of Atlantic cod larvae was either to maintain or to strengthen wild stocks by releasing unfed larvae into the sea. The idea that aquaculture production of Atlantic cod might be a possibility was initiated by the success of the farming of Atlantic salmon in Norway in the late 1970s. The intensification of cod farming has been hampered by the lack of a regular supply of fry, the price level, and low productivity due to cannibalism and uncontrolled mortalities. However, cod and Atlantic halibut are the marine species regarded as having the greatest potential for commercial cold-water farming.

General Biology

There are large populations of cod (*Gadus morhua*) in the North Atlantic ocean. In the west they are common from Cape Hatteras in the south along the coast to the edge of the northern ice. Abundant populations are also found along the coasts of Greenland and Iceland. In the eastern Atlantic cod are distributed off the European continent from the northern part of the Barent Sea into the Bay of Biscay.

There are large environmental variations within this distribution area. In the warmer parts cod may live and feed in water temperatures up to 20°C, while in the colder areas they survive and graze in water temperatures colder than 0°C. The salinity of the environment varies from about 35 ppt in the oceanic area to about 10 ppt in the Baltic Sea and in fjords and ponds. Eggs and larvae tolerate temperatures between 4 and 8°C and salinities between 20 and 35 ppt.

The biology of the cod is characterised by a great flexibility and adaptability to different environments and sources of nourishment. The life-cycle of the cod is usually divided into four stages:

(1) Eggs.
(2) The pelagic stage.
(3) The benthic stage.
(4) The mature stage.

The fish spawn from February to April, and then the eggs develop. In the first part of the pelagic stage the larvae utilise the yolk-sac, but need to start exogen feeding before the yolk-sac is fully consumed (Fig. 21.1). This change from endogen to exogen nutrition is a critical period: if nourishment is not optimal at the time the larvae start feeding, the result may be massive mortality and a weak year class.

During the pelagic stage the eggs, larvae and fry drift with the current. The duration of this stage depends upon the environmental conditions and the availability of suitable feed. From June throughout the rest of the year, the fry change from a pelagic life to a benthic life. On the west coast of Norway the benthic stage begins in June; while in the Barent sea it starts in October. The abundancy of a year class is not only dependent upon the survival during the pelagic stage but is also greatly influenced by growth and mortality during the benthic stage. As cod are cannibals, large fish may feed on smaller fish when there is limited food available.

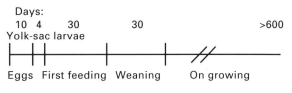

FIG. 21.1 The different stages during the life-cycle of the cod in farming.

The age at sexual maturation varies from 2 to 10 years. When cod first mature, they spawn every year until death unless deterred by extreme malnutrition or environmental changes. They spawn in batches, which means that only a portion of the eggs become mature at one time. Unlike the eggs, the sperm are mature from the beginning of the spawning season. During spawning the male and the female swim side by side with their abdomen against each other, spraying the eggs and the milt, and mixing them with vigorous movements of the fins. After a few days a new portion of eggs become mature and is ready to be fertilised. When the eggs have been fertilised they float in the upper water column and hatch there. Outside Norway, cod will spawn in water temperatures from 2 to 6°C in a salinity range of 35–10 ppt.

Diet changes with age, living area and the season. Prey size increases with the increasing size of the fish and this reduces competition among the different size groups. During the pelagic stage the prey is various sizes of *Calanus*. In the benthic stage the prey is more diverse but is mainly different kinds of bottom-living animals such as prawn, krill and other crayfish. With increasing size other fish become more suitable prey. Generally, the cod is an opportunist and will eat whatever is available, including other cod.

Farming Systems

Broodstock and Egg Production

A closed-pen system is normally used for the spawning and collection of eggs. A suitable volume for the spawning pen is 170,000 l with a depth and a diameter of 6 m (Fig. 21.2).

The water supplied to the pen should be sand filtrated, aerated and transported from a source with a stable salinity and temperature (often from a depth of about 50 m). The water inlet is located at the bottom of the pen. The overflow passes through a flexible tube and into the egg collector, which is 1m × 1m × 1m and is made from 500 μ plankton gauze (Fig. 21.2).

The broodstock should be selected in the preceding year, when each fish should be sexed and tagged. They should be transferred to the spawning pen at the beginning of February. The manual handling of the fish is stressful and may

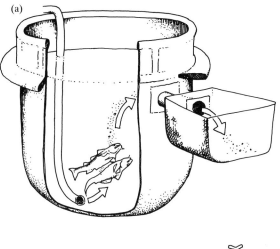

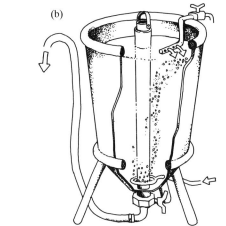

FIG. 21.2 (a) Spawning pen for cod. (b) Incubator for cod eggs.

cause wounds and diseases, with a negative effect on the spawn quality and an increase in the risk of the transference of infectious agents to the offspring. Each breeding fish should weigh at least 3 kg to avoid selecting for small fish and early maturation. Those kept in captivity and fed well will provide at least one litre of eggs per kg of fish during one spawning season.

The normal incubator has a volume of 70 l and can stock 0.5 l eggs (600,000–800,000 eggs/l). The seawater inlet is a perforated tube at the water surface, and the overflow is through a perforated central tube covered with 350 μ plankton gauze in the middle of the tank which flows through a level tube located outside the incubator. To prevent the eggs from clogging the gauze gentle air bubbling can be used. The water supplying the incubators (0.5–1 l/min) should have the same salinity as the spawning pen.

The incubators should be cleaned and disinfected before use. The eggs from the spawning pen should be collected early in the morning to avoid harmful effects from direct sunlight. Before incubation, the eggs should be disinfected with Buffodine (1 dl Buffodine per 10 l sea water in 10 minutes). The eggs are rinsed afterwards with clean sea water.

Dead eggs should be removed daily from the incubators by blocking the water-flow and the aeration for about 15 minutes. Dead eggs sink to the bottom; they are siphoned out and their numbers estimated. Then water-flow and aeration are restored.

After fertilisation, eggs hatch after 9–10 days at 7°C (or 13–14 days at 5°C). As the eggs are sensitive to stress during the first five days (at 7°C), handling or vigorous water-flow and air-bubbling must be avoided.

Extensive System for Fry Production (Pond Culture)

The extensive production of cod fry in ponds is at present the most cost effective production method for commercial purposes. The larvae are offered an environment and plankton community comparable to that in nature — a mesocosmos. Figure 21.3 illustrates one of the ponds used for cod production in Norway, the Parisvatnet.

This system of production is limited by the availability of suitable ponds which can be easily closed with a barrage. The ponds must be located in areas where the water temperature is acceptable, with a minimum of 5–6°C during March and a maximum of 18–20°C. There must also be access to good quality sea water. Phytoplankton production is usually limited to the upper 10 m. Ponds with greater depths may become anoxic. The recommended pond size is 200,000–500,000 m³; larger ponds increase harvesting problems and exacerbate the difficulties of weaning the fry to formulated diets. The production potential for cod in a pond is defined as the number of surviving fry 60–90 days after the cod were stocked as newly hatched larvae. The length of the fry at this age is 3–5 cm and the wet-weight is 0.2–1 g, which is the normal size for weaning to formulated diets.

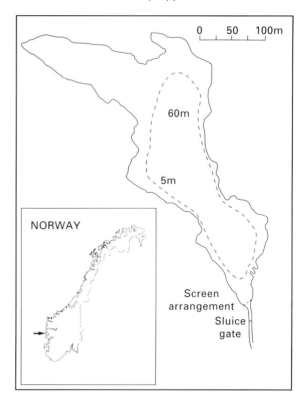

Fig. 21.3 Map of Parisvatnet showing depth of contours. Geographic location of the pond is indicated by the arrow (From: Blom *et al.*, 1991.)

A year cycle in a pond starts and ends with a Rotenone treatment to eliminate unwanted aquatic predators or competitors. A concentration between 0.5 and 1.0 mg/l is required. Rotenone, which kills phytoplankton as well as zooplankton, is mixed with sea water in a tank and distributed over the pond surface. The insecticide disintegrates over 3–4 weeks at water temperatures of 7–10°C and should therefore be used in the autumn (November) when the temperature is sufficiently high to ensure complete disintegration. Large amounts of decaying fish have a deleterious influence on the pond's environment: it is crucial that dead fish are collected and removed immediately after treatment. One month later the barrage may be opened and a grate installed. The perforation in the grate should be no larger than 4 mm. The deep-water pump should also be started at this time.

Fertilisation of the water will increase phytoplankton production and provide the basis for increased zooplankton production. About 7–10 days before the larvae are ready to be released into the pond, 1 kg inorganic fertiliser is dissolved in 2,000 l fresh water and spread over 5,000–6,000 m². The chemical composition by weight for the important elements is: 21.0% N, 3.5% P, 10.5% K and 0.5–1.0% Si. (The silica enhances the production of diatoms.)

Because cod larvae are raised in stagnant water, the pond is closed and the deep-water pump stopped before the larvae are released during March (on the west coast of Norway). The amount of prey (microzooplanktonic rotifers and nauplii) ought to be more than 5/l in the pond to ensure a sufficient feed supply. (Limitation in the amount of zooplankton after metamorphosis will encourage cannibalism among the cod and greatly reduces the number of fry surviving in the system.) The salinity should be 31–32 ppt and the water temperature above 5°C. The amount of larvae released ranges from 20 to 30 per 1000 l pond volume.

After the larvae have metamorphosed, a formulated feed can be given by automatic feeders but supplementation with larger zooplankton is recommended. At a size of 1 g wet-weight, the fry are harvested and transferred to an intensive feeding system in tanks or sea pens.

The production rate for a pond is usually 2 fry 1000 l water volume. However, feed availability and feeding success are important factors determining survival and growth. As metamorphosis approaches, the amount of live prey required increases by several magnitudes. Securing acceptable feed supplies is the main obstacle in the production of cod fry in pond systems.

Intensive Fry Production

Fibre glass tanks with conical bottoms and a capacity of 250 l are used for intensive fry production. They are supplied with sea water which has been sand-filtrated, micro-filtered (5 µ) and UV-treated. The water supply rate is 350–500 ml/min/l tank volume and the overflow exists through a central tube covered with plankton gauze (200 µ). A regime of 16 hours light:8 hours dark is used.

There has been no success so far in producing formulated diets for cod larvae, and live zooplankton are required for feeding the larvae beyond metamorphosis.

Rotifers are produced in 250 l conical tanks with aeration. The tank water is filtered through a 0.2 µm mesh. The culture temperature is kept at 24°C and the salinity at 20 ppt. The rotifers are fed mainly on baker's yeast (0.1 mg/rotifer/day). Once a week they are fed with phytoplankton (*Isochrysis*) and once a week most of the water in the culture is changed by filtration.

The nutritional value of rotifers and *Artemia* is low. In order to increase the nutritional value for the larvae it is necessary to fill the digestive tract with a dense nutrient mixture, to enrich it. The enrichment mixture might either be purchased commercially or produced locally from fish eggs. The amount of enrichment is 0.5 g enrichment mixture to 2.4 million rotifers.

At 4 days old the cod larvae are transferred from the hatchery to the tanks and are fed twice a day with enriched rotifers (*Brachionus plicatilis*). The amount of larvae per litre is in the range 5–10, and the amount of rotifers in rearing tanks is 2–3 ml. The temperature should be 8–10°C. The best larval growth is achieved when they are fed rotifers enriched with dried cod roe. The expected production potential is 2 metamorphosed larvae per litre water volume.

To increase fry production and decrease mortality, it is important to start the formulated diet early. Just after metamorphosis (at a weight of 0.13 g and a length of 12 mm) the survival and growth are highest with moist feed (40–50% water). Dry formulated feed can be offered to cod of an average length of 19 mm and a wet weight of 0.5 g with good results. The greatest problem during weaning is cannibalism. A second problem is the texture of the small sized feed particles.

Culture in Net Pens

Fingerlings larger than 1 g can be transferred to sea pens. The production systems for cod are copied from those for Atlantic salmon, using cages of 20–30 m³ for the fry and pens from 600 m³ (10 m × 10 m × 6 m) to 8,000 m³ (diameter 30 m, depth > 30 m) for large fish. Cod shorter than 30 cm encourage cannibalism, and it is therefore crucial to maintain a uniform size with frequent size grading.

The gonadosomatic index (i.e. weight of gonads × 100/body-weight) for mature cod reaches values of up to 20%. As the fish reduce feed consumption during the last stage of maturation and as eggs and sperm are considered to be waste products with low market values, it is not economical to feed the cod throughout a spawning season. The fish should be slaughtered before the final growth of the gonads, 3–4 months before expected spawning time.

Nutrition

The muscle of cod is lean with less than 1% fat, and the fat level seems not to be influenced by the nutritional status to any significant extent. Cod deposit lipids in the liver; they are stored almost exclusively as triacylglycerols and the fat content of the liver may exceed 70%. A hepato-somatic index (liver weight × 100/total body-weight) above 10% is considered normal in farmed cod compared to 3–6% in wild caught cod.

Under favourable conditions with sufficient feed supply and high growth rate, cod tend to mature sexually at about 22 months — before reaching a marketable size. Controlling the growth of farmed cod in order to allocate the energy expenditure to somatic growth rather than liver lipid storage and sexual maturation is considered a major challenge. As the liver and gonads are considered to be waste, it is obvious that reducing the amount produced is of great economic importance.

Two factors are predominant in determining lipoid liver deposition: dietary fat level and feeding intensity. A ratio of lipid energy to total diet energy higher than 0.3–0.4 will give a hepato-somatic index higher than 10–12%. Atlantic cod have a limited ability to utilise carbohydrates as energy and a positive effect of low levels (5–7%) of dietary starch on appetite and growth has been shown. Higher levels give increased plasma glucose levels and urinary and gill excretion of glucose. The requirements for dietary micronutrients (trace minerals and vitamins) or minerals have not been determined for cod and it is assumed that they are comparable to those of Atlantic salmon.

Diet Formulation

So far there has been no success in the development of formulated diets for cod larvae, and the production of cod fry depends on naturally occurring zooplankton or produced rotifer and *Artemia* nauplia. High survival is achieved when weaning the cod fry to formulated diets when they have reached a weight above 0.5 g. Wet or moist diets based on micronised squid mantle and supplemented fat, vitamins and minerals seem to be superior to dry pellet diets during the weaning from live feed organisms to formulated feeds. Commercial diets for cod are based on high quality fish meal, extruded carbohydrate sources and hydrolysed proteins supplemented with marine fat attractants such as squid meal or crayfish meal, vitamins, carotenoids (astaxanthin, >5 mg/kg), minerals and betain ® (T. Skretting Ltd, Stavanger; Felleskjøpet, Sandnes). The chemical composition of feeds for cod is shown in Fig. 21.4. The amounts of carbohydrate in commercial diets are all above the recommended level probably because of the price of fish meal and the pellet binding capacity of carbohydrates.

CHEMICAL COMPOSITION OF DIETS FOR COD			
	Pellet size (0.3–0.6 mm)	Pellet size (1.0–3.0 mm)	Pellet size (2.5–10 mm)
Water	9.5	9.5	9.5
Protein	46.5	45.5	45.5
	(55.5)	(53.5)	(53.0)
Fat	9.0	10.0	10.0
	(22.0)	(24.0)	(24.0)
Carbohydrates	23.0	23.5	27.0
	(22.5)	(22.5)	(23.0)
Fibre	1.0	0.5	0.5
Ash	11.0	11.0	7.5

FIG. 21.4 The values in brackets are the percentage of metabolisable energy. (T. Skretting Ltd., Stavanger, Norway: Marine feeds, 1990.)

National Legislation

The farming of cod is regulated under the same laws as Atlantic salmon and other fish species. In Norway there is specific legislation regarding fish farming, farm size, ownership, location and other technical matters but the welfare of the fish is under the administration of a general law for all living animals. These laws have been discussed in Chapters 11 and 12.

Major Diseases

Viral Diseases

Viral erythrocytic necrosis (VEN)

This infection of marine fish is caused by the erythrocytic necrosis virus (ENV). VEN has a wide host range (e.g. Anguillidae, Clupeidae, Gadidae and Salmonidae) and extensive geographical distribution. Prevalence rates of up to 90% have been recorded in wild populations. The infection manifests only as pathological alterations in circulating erythrocytes. Typical signs in Atlantic cod include small eosinophilic inclusions in the cytoplasm or as a blemish on the nucleus and vacuolisation of the nucleus with various degrees of necrotic degeneration or karyolysis.

Although VEN has been observed in cultured cod, the infection has not been associated with massive mortalities. However evidence of its negative consequences has been found, including anaemia, greater susceptibility to vibriosis, decreased tolerance to oxygen depletion, and a decreased ability to regulate serum sodium and potassium. This indicates that while VEN itself may not directly cause mortalities, it may weaken and predispose infected fish to secondary infections, reducing their ability to survive in the wild.

Ulcus syndrome

This environmentally dependent infectious disease occurs mainly in cod aged 1.5–2.5 years old. Initial signs are multiple papules and vesicles on the lateral surface of the body which develop further into erosions and ulcers. Typically, the skin ulcers are round, reddish in the centre, and surrounded by white necrotic tissue (Fig. 21.5). Rhabdovirus and iridovirus particles have been isolated from diseased cod. Secondary bacterial infections, especially *Vibrio* spp., invade skin ulcers and reinforce the development of the disease.

The ulcus syndrome is observed regularly in populations of cultured cod, without so far causing

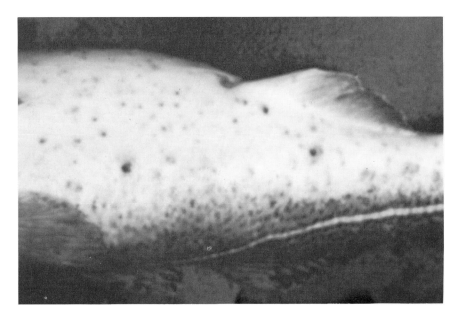

FIG. 21.5 This picture shows a cod with Ulcus syndrome. Picture courtesy of Odd-Magne Rødseth.

serious epizootics. However, low frequencies undoubtedly represent an important predisposing factor of more serious secondary infectious diseases.

Bacterial Diseases

Vibriosis

Epizootics of vibriosis have been reported for a number of wild marine species. In Asia, North America and Europe vibriosis is economically the most serious infectious disease of cultured marine fish and it accounted for the mortality of up to 40–45% of the total production of juvenile cod in Norway in 1986–1988.

One of the latest additions to the list of *Vibrio* species pathogenic for fish is *Vibrio salmonicida*, which causes cold-water vibriosis. The disease was first described in 1979 in salmonid farms on the north-west coast of Norway, and for many years it was believed that the disease only affected sea-farmed Atlantic salmon. However, 15 cod farms in northern Norway suffered high mortalities due to cold-water vibriosis in 1988, since when epizootics due to *Vibrio* spp. have been restricted to *V. anguillarum*.

Clinical signs vary with age and temperature. In the period from metamorphosis until the fry have reached 5–8 g, a peracute outbreak is often observed. Death occurs with no visible gross pathological changes except for the darkening of the skin and peri-orbital oedema. Skin lesions are normally absent. After recovering from a peracute epizootic, it is common for the affected population to contain chronically diseased carriers, acting as a reservoir of infection. If carrier fish are stressed, the carrier state may develop into clinical disease with the infection spreading to healthy fish in the population. Following a peracute outbreak in spring, repeated acute outbreaks often occur in late summer and autumn as a result of handling stress and changes in water temperature. External signs in an acute outbreak are similar to those caused by other Gram-negative bacteria. Primary lesions include erythema at the base of fins and tail and in the head region. Gross internal lesions are rarely observed.

In cod 1–3 years old, vibriosis is often manifest as a chronic infection, causing low steady mortality over a long period. The most characteristic disease signs are inflamed, swollen and reddened fins (Fig. 21.6). Many fish may have unilateral or bilateral exophthalmos with either serous haemorrhagic fluid in the eye or keratomalacia. Blind or partially blind fish usually have signs of malnutrition because they have not been able to feed properly.

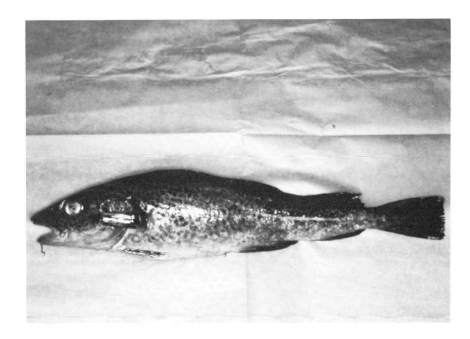

FIG. 21.6 This picture shows cod with vibriosis, caused by the bacteria *Vibrio anguillarum*. Picture courtesy of Kari Andersen.

Cold-water vibriosis has many characteristics in common with vibriosis. Typical disease signs include loss of appetite, disordered swimming, darkening and external petechiation. Internally, haemorrhages in the abdominal wall, swim-bladder and intestine are easily observed. As the name indicates, cold-water vibriosis appears during the winter when the water temperature is low.

Fin rot

Fin rot is frequently encountered in cultured fish. In general its occurrence is an indicator of adverse environmental conditions. In cultured cod, tail rot is first manifest as a grey, patchy, discoloured area on the caudal peduncle. As the disease progresses, the skin between the fin rays becomes frayed and eroded. In advanced stages, clinical signs may include open lesions and erosion of the skin on the caudal peduncle, complete erosion of the musculature of the peduncle, and loss of the caudal fin.

No aetiological agent can be identified as the primary cause of the disease. It is thought that externally induced wounds are invaded by bacteria that disintegrate the skin tissue. The wounds may be caused by ectoparasites, aggressive behaviour or handling. The secondary infections of the wounds include bacteria from the genera *Pseudomonas*, *Aeromonas*, *Chondrococcus* and *Vibrio*. The disease process is primarily due to an insanitary environment, especially in crowded populations combined with high water temperature and eutrophic water with a high bacterial load.

Furunculosis

Aeromonas salmonicida is a well known pathogen of freshwater and anadromous salmonids and freshwater non-salmonids. Infections of *A. salmonicida* subsp. *acromogenes* have been described, in wild caught Atlantic cod held in a seawater tank in Canada. In Norway, atypical furunculosis has not yet been isolated from cultured cod, but the bacterium has caused mortalities among wrasse (Labridae) used as cleaning fish against salmon lice (*Lepeophtheirus salmonis*) and cultured wolffish (*Anarhichas minor*). Regarding furunculosis caused by *Aeromonas salmonicida* subsp. *salmonicida*, the possibility of transmission from farmed

salmon to marine fish has been investigated. Field studies from a farm where cod were reared in net pens adjacent to salmon showed that the cod population were unaffected although several outbreaks of furunculosis in the salmon population were reported. However, in a series of laboratory cohabitant challenge experiments, *A. salmonicida subsp. salmonicida* was detected in one moribund cod (out of 25). No carrier state was demonstrated when a latent carrier test was performed on the survivors.

Fungal Diseases

Mycotic infections are of considerable concern in fresh water, where facultative pathogens of the class Oomycetes can develop infections at all stages of the fish life-cycle. In the marine environment, *Ichthyophonus hoferi* is one of the few recorded fungal diseases of fish. In contrast to the fresh water Oomycetes, *I. hoferi* is both an internal and an obligate pathogen.

I. hoferi is best known as the cause of periodic mass mortalities among North Atlantic herring (*Clupea harengus*). However, there is little evidence of host specificity shown by the fungi. Distribution of the disease appears to be worldwide, affecting wild and cultured fish. There have also been epizootics on freshwater fish farms, but in most cases the sources have been directly associated with the marine environment by use of infected marine fish as feed. Although the disease has not been diagnosed in cod farms these must be considered to be vulnerable. Field data from the waters of Greenland, the north-west Atlantic, the North Sea and the Baltic Sea show that cod are susceptible to infection by *I. hoferi*.

Disease signs depend on the severity of the infection. Generally infected fish exhibit little or no external signs but the fungus induces the formation of grey–white lesions in the internal organs. The lesions, which may have a cheesy or hard consistency, are easily observed on gross macroscopic examination. However, since many disease conditions involve a similar response, the diagnosis should not rely upon macroscopic inspection alone.

Ectoparasites

The most common ectoparasites in reared cod are protozoa such as *Trichodina* spp. (Fig. 21.7)

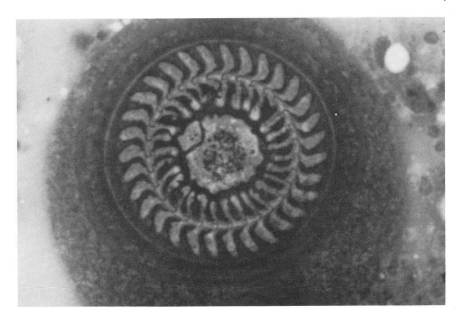

FIG. 21.7 This picture shows *Trichodina* sp., which are the most common ectoparasites on farmed cod. Picture courtesy of Ingrid Uglenes.

and *Ichthyobodo necatrix*. Acute protozoan outbreaks have been observed, especially under crowded conditions with high water temperatures and organic loads. The parasite attacks host epithelium, resulting in large skin lesions and damage to gill epithelium. If no action is taken, there may be high mortality as a direct result of the parasite infection or as a result of secondary bacterial infections.

Another parasite which causes mortality in cultured cod is *Gyrodactylus* spp. (Fig. 21.8). This monogean trematode attaches to gills and skin, causing damage similar to that described for the parasitic protozoa.

In pond conditions, there is a high risk that the life-cycle of different parasites will become condensed within the rearing system. In ponds where snails of the genus *Littorina* release cercariae of *Cryptocotyle lingua* during the summer, cod fry may be covered with black spots caused by the encapsulated metacercariae of the parasite. On adult fish this parasite represents only an aesthetic problem, but fish larvae and juveniles may be killed by a few cercariae if they penetrate the brain or heart.

Another parasite which affects cultured cod is the copepod *Learnocera branchialis*. Its copepodids settle on the gill tips of flatfish, preferably on the first dorsal gill arch. The adult female of *L. branchialis* attached to the base of the gill arch of cod and is easily observed when the gill cover is spread out. The parasite pushes its head deep into the host tissue, sucking blood near the heart.

The salmon louse *Lepeophtheirus salmonis*, has become a serious problem in the culture of Atlantic salmon in sea water. Another caligid copepod, *Caligus* spp., is found on the skin of cultured cod. The copepods feed on cutaneous and subcutaneous tissue of the host and may cause extensive damage. To date, *Caligus* infections of cod have not caused serious mortalities. Based on experience from parasitic copepods and intensive aquaculture, it is important to be aware of this potential problem.

Endoparasites

Most individual cod in wild populations are infested with endoparasites, but in the great majority of cases there appears to be no significant harm to the host fish. In the North Sea, heavy infestations of *Abothrium gadi* (cestoda) larvae of *Contracaecum* and *Anisakis* (nematoda) and *Echinorhynchus gadi* (acanthocephala) have been noted. The same endoparasitic species have been observed in cultured cod without any adverse effects on the fish or impairment of their normal growth and development.

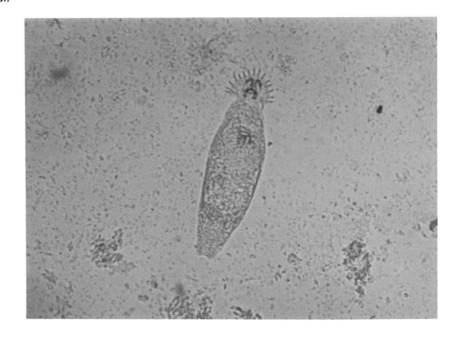

Clinical Diagnosis

Viral Diseases

Although various fish cell lines have been tried, all attempts to culture ENV have so far been unsuccessful. Presumptive diagnosis of VEN is made by observation of small (1–4 µ) eosinophilic cytoplasmic inclusions or degenerative changes in the nucleus. The diagnosis can be confirmed by identification of cytoplasmatic icosahedral virons in transmission electron microscopy analysis of erythrocytes with nuclear damage and inclusions.

A presumptive diagnosis of IPN can be based on clinical signs and supporting histopathological findings. Confirmation is obtained by isolation and serological identification of the virus. However, a qualitative isolation and identification of IPNV is not sufficient to assign to it the cause of mortality. When IPNV is the primary cause of mortality, the virus titre is usually 10^5 or greater. IPNV is replicated in a variety of cell lines; rainbow trout gonad (RTG), fathead minnow (FHM) and chinook salmon embryo (CHSE) are usually the cell lines of choice. If the virus is the causal agent, cytopathological effect can be observed within 24–36 hours.

Two viruses have been isolated from cod suffering from ulcus syndrome, but neither agent has been shown to be present in all cases. The diagnosis of ulcus syndrome is based on clinical signs and histological features of the lesions.

Bacterial Diseases

Diagnosis of vibriosis is by disease signs, isolation and identification of the aetiological agent. A presumptive diagnosis can be based on disease signs and observation of vibrio shaped bacteria from stained tissue imprints (spleen, kidney, necrotic muscle tissue). The causative bacterium can easily be isolated in pure culture from the anterior part of the kidney. Kidney tissue is aseptically streaked on a general-purpose bacteriological media such as trypticase soya agar or brain/heart infusion agar supplemented with 1% NaCl. Plates should be incubated aerobically at 20–25°C for 24–48 hours. A verified diagnosis is based on cultural and biochemical properties or by using specific antisera.

The same procedure should be followed for cold-water vibriosis. However, since *V. salmonicida* has an optimum temperature for growth at 15°C, the incubation temperature should be lowered.

Fungal Diseases

Infection by *Ichthyophonus hoferi* can be diagnosed from the occurrence of the characteristic post-mortem germination of spores. Pieces of infected organs are squashed with a cover glass and examined with a phase-contrast microscope. The presence of spherical spores with double refractive walls and germination of spores producing branched hyphae can be used to provide field identification of the fungi. Specific identification and verified diagnosis of the disease should include histopathological examination and growth on Hagem's modified fungus medium or Sabouraud dextrose agar with 1% bovine serum added.

Ectoparasites

Generally diagnosis of ectoparasites is based upon disease signs and observation of the parasite in slide preparations of gills or skin mucus. Signs of ectoparasitic infection include a thickening of the mucus on the most heavily infected parts of the body. Infected fish appear grey in colour and may roll in the water and rub against the bottom or the sides of the tank. Excessive parasitism of the gills may cause extensive accumulation of mucus on the gills but there may be no other external signs except increased breathing frequency.

Therapy

There is no effective therapy for viral diseases in marine animals. Nor are there any practical therapeutic procedures to cure systemic mycosis affecting marine fish, although it has been reported that fungicide and antibiotic drugs such as phenoxethol and penicillin are effective in the early states. For fungal and viral problems, therefore, prevention and avoidance are essential.

Therapeutants used against bacterial infections and parasites in cod are given in Fig. 21.9. The efficacy of these treatments relies on early recognition of disease signs and diagnosis. Therapeutic procedures for ectoparasites usually depend on the severity of the infestation: outbreaks can sometimes be controlled by the small adjustments described for the prevention of disease. No treatment is usually given in the case of endoparasites but, if necessary, medications in Fig. 21.9 can be given via the feed.

Prevention of Disease

Viral Diseases

Avoidance is the universal control measure for viral diseases of marine animals. In view of the endemic prevalence of VEN, broodstock originating from wild populations should be kept in quarantine until shown to be free of disease. The most effective measure for the control of IPN is avoidance, but this approach requires that the water supply and the broodstock are both free of IPNV. Reduction in water temperature may decrease the viral replication and may be of some help in controlling the mortality. There are no effective methods for treating ulcus syndrome.

Bacterial Diseases

Vibrio spp. constitute part of the normal microflora of the marine ecosystem and may also constitute part of the natural microflora of fish, so that the fish are continually exposed to the potential pathogen, which may cause disease under certain stressful conditions. Based on the facultative nature of the pathogen and the importance of environmental factors in the initiation of the disease cycle, control measures should focus

THERAPEUTIC AGENTS USED AGAINST INFECTIONS OF COD		
Drug	**Dose mg/kg fish**	**Indication**
Oxolinic acid	25 l x 10 days	Bacteria
Flumequine	25 l x 10 days	Bacteria
Formalin	1:4000; repeat after 5–6 days	Ectoparasites
Praziquantel	5 mg/kg fish x 1–2 days	Ectoparasites
Albendazole	5 mg/kg fish x 1 day, rpt 3 days later	Ectoparasites
Fenbendazole	5 mg/kg fish x 1 day, rpt 3 days later	Ectoparasites
Di-*n*-butyl tin oxide	250 mg/kg fish x 5 days	Ectoparasites

FIG. 21.9 Efficacy of therapeutants relies on early recognition of disease signs and diagnosis.

on basic hygiene, optimalisation of farm husbandry practices, and immunoprophylaxis.

As well as the reduction or elimination of the pathogen from the environment, it is important to improve the disease resistance of the host.

Conditions usually found to be decisive in the development of vibrio epizootics include overcrowding, reduced dissolved oxygen, high and fluctuating water temperatures, increased quantities of excretory products and organic pollution in the water.

Vibrio anguillarum has been a successful candidate for vaccine development for salmonids. Commercial formalin-inactivated vaccines based on isolates from cod are now available in Norway; they are bivalent products, containing cells of *V. anguillarum* serovar 02a and 02b. Vaccine trials under controlled laboratory conditions and in the field trials have demonstrated a high degree of protection against vibriosis.

Fungal Diseases

Prophylactic measures should focus on preventing introduction of mycotic disease into cultivated fish stocks. This includes the sterilisation of trash fish used as feed and the quarantine isolation of broodstock originating from wild populations.

Ectoparasites

Outbreaks of ectoparasitic infections can be controlled by small adjustments like increasing the water-flow, eliminating the sources of skin and gill irritants and reducing the biomass and organic pollution in the rearing system.

Endoparasites

Control measures for endoparasites of cultured cod should focus on reduction or elimination of a link in the transmission cycle. Elimination of the most important intermediate hosts, the crustaceans, is impossible in pond culture, but in on-growing facilities the use of fresh fish as feed should be avoided.

Further Reading

Dahl, E., Danielsen, D., Moksnes, E. and Solemdal, P. (Editors) (1984) *The Propagation of Cod, Gadus morhua*, Vol. 1. L. Flødevigen Rapp.

dePauw, N., Jaspers, E., Ackerfors, H., Wilkins, N. (Editors) (1989) *Aquaculture — a biotechnology in progress*, pp. 133–138, European Aquaculture Society, Bredene, Belgium.

Holm, J. C., Suåsand, T. and Wennevik, V. (Editors) (1991) Håndbak i Torskeoppdrett. Havforskning-sinstitutlet. (Institute of Marine Research, Bergen, Norway.)

22

The Veterinary Approach to Ornamental Fish

RAY BUTCHER

Ornamental fish-keeping is a popular hobby in the United States and western Europe and also in the UK, where 14% (3.5 million) of all households are thought to keep ornamental fish. In 1990, the value of fish imported into the UK was approximately £12 million, and the value of the trade worldwide was approximately £4 billion. The majority (90%) of fish supplied to the trade are bred in fish farms and imported by air. Of the fish imported into the European Community in 1990, 24.4% went to the UK, 24.3% to Germany, and 18.4% to France. The principal source is Singapore and the Far East (71%), although significant numbers are also imported from the USA (8%), South America (6.4%), Israel (6.2%), Japan (3.8%), and Africa (2%).

These figures give an indication of the importance of the trade to the economy of the exporting countries. The popularity of the hobby in the West also highlights its potential importance in companion animal veterinary practice.

Ornamental Fish Systems

The classification of ornamental fish-keeping can be divided broadly between pond and aquarium systems. The latter can be further sub-divided into freshwater and marine, and also cold-water and tropical (heated).

There are many different ornamental fish species, each of which has evolved in specific conditions of its natural habitat. An essential feature of successful fish-keeping is to maintain water quality parameters within the optimum range for the species. Often a range of different species may be kept in the same tank (as in a typical community tank) and it is important to select fish that can thrive in similar conditions so that they do not become predisposed

EQUIPMENT AVAILABLE	
For aquaria	**For ponds**
Heater/thermostats	Aerators: waterfalls
Pumps for water	fountains
circulation	venturi devices
Aerators	Pumps for water circulation
Filters	Filters
Protein skimmers	
Ultraviolet irradiation	
Ozone	
Lighting	

FIG. 22.1 A summary of available equipment.

to disease. The veterinarian needs a good encyclopaedia on aquarium fish which will indicate the optimum environmental parameters for each species.

A variety of plants and invertebrates may also be kept in aquaria. These, too, have specific water quality requirements and it is important to check that these, as well as the fish, are compatible.

To meet the interest in keeping ornamental fish, a whole battery of equipment has been developed. A full discussion of this aspect is beyond the scope of this book, though Fig. 22.1 gives a summary of what is available and Fig. 22.2 illustrates ranges of equipment for aquaria and ponds. Some of the many excellent publications in this field are given in the Further Reading section at the end of this chapter.

Aquaria

The water in an aquarium usually circulates within a completely closed system, though fresh water is added periodically as partial water changes. The maintenance of correct water quality is

Fig. 22.2 Typical equipment for the home aquarium — powered undergravel filter, heater thermostat, air pump and air stone. (Photograph by David Ford.)

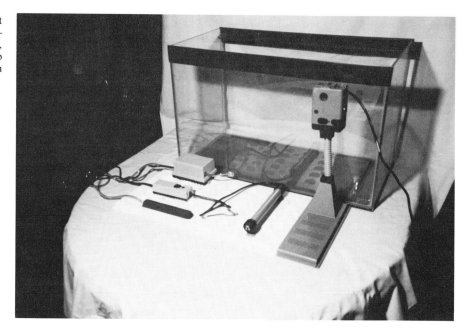

entirely in the hands of the aquarist, who is assisted by the development of a whole battery of equipment dealing with heating, lighting, filtration and aeration. The most difficult systems to maintain are those for marine fish, which require complex accessory equipment.

Ponds

The majority of garden ponds contain a range of fish species, most commonly goldfish, carp, koi, tench and orfe. The ponds are often relatively well planted, and local wildlife (e.g. aquatic insects and amphibians) is often encouraged to produce a 'natural' ecosystem. These systems are rarely self-maintaining, however, and usually require aeration equipment and external filters to remove waste products. Much depends on the size of the pond and the stocking density. Ponds stocked solely with koi are often devoid of vegetation and require elaborate filtration systems to maintain water quality.

General Husbandry

Ornamental fish are kept for the length of their natural life span, and considerations of weight gain and food conversion ratios are not appropriate.

The overriding factor in developing husbandry systems is to provide and maintain optimum water quality parameters and the correct nutritional balance for each species.

In any closed water system the build up of parasites or other pathogenic organisms is likely and may eventually predispose to disease. The use of prophylactic remedies to reduce parasite numbers is therefore another important consideration in ornamental fish keeping.

The principal factors which need to be considered in relation to general husbandry conditions are summarised below.

Position

An aquarium must be positioned away from room heaters, draughts and direct sunlight as these may result in fluctuations of water temperature. Natural sunlight may also stimulate unwanted algal growth. A convenient power source is necessary to drive the associated equipment and it must be remembered that the support structure should be strong enough to take the weight of the water contained within the aquarium.

Ponds are situated ideally on level ground with some shade, although overhanging trees or shrubs may pollute the water when they shed their leaves in the autumn. To avoid contamination by pesticides or herbicides, thought should be given to the position of the pond in relation to other garden features.

Size

The old-fashioned goldfish bowl is far from ideal, and tanks with a relatively high ratio of surface area to volume should be used. The larger the volume of water in the tank, the easier it is to maintain constant environmental conditions. A 54-litre tank can be regarded as the minimum for tropical fish, whilst 90 litres is the smallest tank size recommended for marine fish keeping.

Similarly, ponds with a large volume of water are easier to maintain than smaller ones. The depth should be at least 0.9 m to allow for possible freezing of the superficial layer in the winter, and the surface should have minimum dimensions of 2 × 1.5 m to allow for adequate gaseous exchange.

Heater/Thermostats

These are not required for most cold-water species although they are used in tropical and marine tanks to maintain a steady temperature of around 23–26°C. In general, two smaller units are better than one large one as this helps to distribute the temperature evenly, and also reduces the risk of complete failure of the heating system. Even if there is a reliable heater/thermostat, the routine use of an aquarium thermometer to check the water temperature is important.

Small, low power heaters may be floated on ponds in winter to prevent total freezing of the surface water. They make no significant difference to the temperature of the main volume of water.

Filtration

Since the systems for keeping ornamental fish are generally 'closed', mechanical or biological filters are usually necessary (except in small cold-water aquaria containing very few fish) to deal with nitrogenous waste products, especially as the stocking rate increases. Regular maintenance of any type of filter is important. The three most commonly used methods include foam cartridges, under-gravel and power filters.

In under-gravel systems the air from an air pump draws the water through a 5–8 cm layer of coarse gravel situated above a filter plate on the tank floor.

Power filters are best suited for large tanks and in general should turn over the tank volume

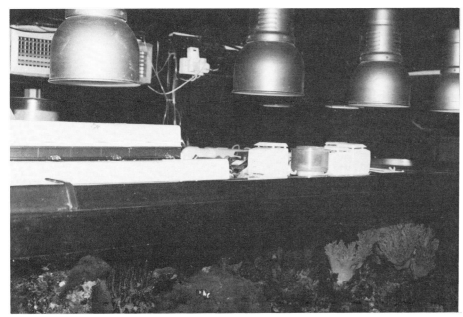

FIG. 22.3 Filtration system and protein skimmers mounted on a large display marine aquarium.

several times during a 24 hour period. They can be situated inside or outside the aquarium, and utilise small pumps to pull water through a filter body containing a foam cartridge.

In marine aquaria, under-gravel filtration is often supplemented by external power filters containing carbon and/or protein skimmers (Fig. 22.3). Ozone and ultraviolet radiation my also be used.

In small garden ponds with a low stocking density, the level of toxic waste products can be reduced by partial water changes alone. As the number of fish increases, the level of toxic waste also rises and biological filters become essential. In their simplest form these consist of a tank filled with gravel, or a similar substrate, through which the pond water is circulated by pumps. The gravel not only acts as a mechanical filter but also provides a large surface area for the growth of *Nitrosomas* spp. and *Nitrobacter* spp., the bacteria which are responsible for the nitrification process.

These simple filters tend to clog easily, and so for larger ponds, especially those for koi, there are usually multi-chambered systems containing different materials that allow the water to be filtered mechanically before it passes through the biological filter (Fig. 22.4a,b). In addition, zeolite may be used in the filter specifically to remove nitrites and ammonia, and ultraviolet irradiation may be used to reduce the level of algae.

Aeration

Aeration of aquaria is usually provided by the filters although it is possible to supplement this by using air stones. Aeration is important to improve oxygen uptake by the water and also to drive off excessive carbon dioxide. It is essential in marine tanks since the level of dissolved oxygen in sea water is reduced.

Lighting

Artificial lighting is essential to maintain a constant environment, since fluctuation in normal daylight may encourage unsightly algal growth as well as variations in temperature.

Stocking Density

The stocking levels at which fish can be kept very much depends on the quality of the environmental

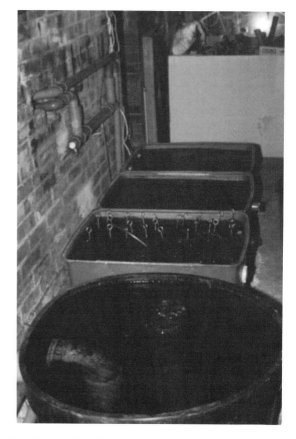

FIG. 22.4 (a) A multi chamber filtration system for a moderate sized garden Koi pond.

parameters. The following can only therefore be regarded as a guide.

- *Cold-water aquaria*: allow 62 cm^2 of water surface for each centimetre of fish.
- *Tropical freshwater aquaria*: allow 26 cm^2 of water surface for each centimetre of fish.
- *Cold-water and tropical marine aquaria*: allow 155 cm^2 of water surface for each centimetre of fish.
- *Ponds*: allow 150 cm^2 of water surface for each centimetre of fish.

Note that fish over 5 cm in length require even more space in proportion to their body size.

Water Quality

Tolerance levels for water quality parameters vary greatly with the species and it is not possible

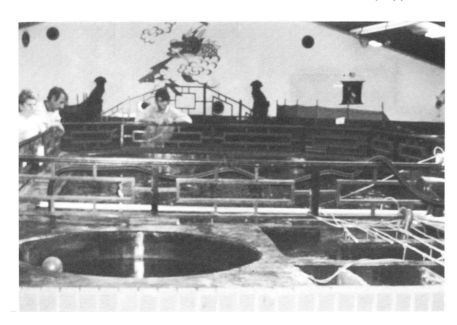

FIG. 22.4 (b) A multi chamber filtration system for a commercial Koi outlet.

to give here a range of values for all ornamental fish. These can be found in a good aquarium encyclopaedia.

In a fully equilibrated closed system the aquarist may only need to check water quality parameters on a weekly basis. If, however, there have been any changes to the system (e.g. new fish added or filters cleaned) more frequent testing would be advisable until equilibrium has been restored. A list of the parameters that are generally checked is given in Fig. 22.5. Test kits are readily available to measure many of these parameters, and more accurate (and more expensive) electronic meters are available to measure pH, hardness, and dissolved oxygen.

WATER QUALITY PARAMETERS

Total ammonia nitrogen (TAN)
Un-ionised ammonia
Nitrite
Nitrate
Dissolved oxygen
Chlorine
pH
Alkalinity
Hardness
Salinity
Copper

FIG. 22.5 A list of measured water quality parameters.

Diurnal or seasonal changes can affect water quality. Dead leaves falling into a pond in the autumn will cause a significant rise in ammonia and nitrite levels, whereas algal blooms in the summer may radically reduce dissolved oxygen levels, especially at night when photosynthesis ceases. Treating algal blooms with chemicals can precipitate a rise in ammonia concentrations.

Partial Water Changes

In an aquarium with a very low stocking level it may be possible to control the levels of ammonia and nitrite simply by performing regular partial water changes. Even in systems with a bacterial filter, such water changes are to be recommended.

In freshwater and marine aquaria, about 25% of the tank volume should be removed every 2–4 weeks and topped up with conditioned water of a similar temperature and quality. Tap-water conditioners are available. In ponds, 25% of the volume should be removed once or twice a year by trickling a hose into the pond and letting the excess overflow.

Feeding

Fish need a balanced diet but the specific requirements vary with individual species. Farmed fish are generally fed a high protein diet to maximise growth rates, but it is better to give ornamental fish a lower amount of high quality protein. The energy sources are then taken from the carbohydrate content of the food, which breaks down to non-polluting carbon dioxide and water.

Good quality commercial diets are the safest: they include additional essential nutrients to allow for losses during the manufacturing process.

Live foods may also be fed, and in some cases (e.g. conditioning fish for breeding) this is thought to be essential. However, live aquatic foods, such as *Daphnia* or *Tubifex* worms, may introduce parasites including *Ichthyophthirius*, *Lernaea*, *Chilodonella*, and *Camallanus*. It is possible to cultivate some types of live food in a way that isolates them from sources of infection (e.g. hatching brine shrimp eggs for first-feeding to fry) but in general non-aquatic live foods such as garden earthworms, aphids and flies are preferable.

The practice of feeding 'table scraps' should be discouraged. These generally contain saturated fats which are not suitable for fish.

Legislation

Legislation relating to the keeping of ornamental fish will vary between different countries, and is also subject to changes with time. It is therefore important to consult the appropriate references for the current situation pertaining to each country as required. In general, the legislation might relate to:

(1) The import and export of fish in relation to the welfare aspects of transport.
(2) The import of fish relating to preventing the introduction of new diseases.
(3) Welfare aspects with regard to fish kept at wholesale or retail premises.
(4) The control and supply of drugs for medication.
(5) The ethical considerations of vet/client relations.
(6) The health and safety aspects of handling potentially toxic chemicals.
(7) The disposal of clinical waste.
(8) The pollution of the environment from the use of toxic materials.

Chapters 11 and 12 explain the legislation affecting farmed fish in the EC and Norway

respectively. In relation to ornamental fish it is perhaps worth stressing the following points.

The Dispensing of Medicines

Different countries may have legislation that restricts the dispensing of medicines to veterinarians or other competent people. As an example, the UK's Medicines Act (1968) states that a veterinarian can dispense prescription-only medicines (POMs) only to animals within his care. This may require a home visit, an examination of the fish at the surgery, or simply a discussion with the owner if the problem and management system is familiar to the veterinarian. The choice will depend on individual circumstances, but in all cases the fish must be truly in the veterinarian's care. Accurate case records with details of all medications supplied are important in this context.

All medications should be dispensed in suitable, correctly labelled containers that comply fully with national guidelines. Withdrawal periods are not applicable to ornamental fish but it is important to warn clients of any health hazards that may result from accidental exposure to medications supplied.

The treatment of small numbers of fish may involve the dispensing of small amounts of chemicals. In some cases (as with formalin) the concentrated form may be toxic, and where practice staff are involved with measuring this out prior to dispensing, the appropriate safety procedures should be followed to comply with any national health and safety legislation.

Preventing the Introduction of Disease

The fact that the majority of ornamental fish kept in the West are bred in fish farms in the Far East, America, or Israel and are then imported by air presents the possibility of introducing disease organisms into the country. National legislation relating to the prevention of introduction of disease may make provision for the licensing of imported fish, or may restrict areas from which fish may be imported.

Where such measures fail, and a disease is introduced, further legislation may come into effect to prevent the spread of the disease. The only example of such a notifiable disease with relevance to ornamental fish in the UK at present is spring viraemia of carp (SVC).

Welfare Aspects

The large-scale transport of fish in high densities has significant welfare implications. The International Air Transport Association (IATA) has developed a code of practice for the transport of animals (including fish) by air, and recommendations relate to the types of container, stocking density, etc.

The welfare of fish in retail outlets is also important, and national legislation relating to animal cruelty may be applicable. There may be a requirement for retail outlets to be licensed. The Ornamental Fish Industry (OFI) UK has suggested minimum water quality standards that may be adopted by local authorities.

Major Diseases

Environmental Aspects

Environmental conditions outside the optimum range for a species may directly result in the development of specific diseases. Smaller variations or rapid fluctuations within the normal range may stress the fish sufficiently to predispose it to disease from other causes. The main environmental factors are:

- Abnormal levels of dissolved gases — oxygen, nitrogen, hydrogen sulphide, methane etc.
- Increased levels of metabolic waste products — ammonia, nitrite and nitrate.
- Additional water quality parameters — pH, hardness, conductivity, temperature and suspended solids.
- Toxins — heavy metals, chlorine, pesticides, herbicides.
- Miscellaneous factors — sunburn, trauma, predation (e.g. cats or herons).

Viruses

Only a small number of viruses are considered at present to be of importance in ornamental fish.

Carp pox

This results in an epidermal hyperplasia and is found in a number of carp species. It is thought to be the result of infection with a herpes virus, and presents as characteristic discrete 'candle-wax' lesions. It is seasonal in incidence, epidemics occurring in spring but disappearing in late summer as the temperature drops. Immunity to the infection is not thought to be strong and there may be recurrence in subsequent years.

Spring viraemia of carp (SVC)

SVC is the most important viral disease of ornamental carp. It is caused by *Rhabdovirus carpio* and is notifiable in the UK under the Diseases of Fish Act 1937 (as amended).

At infected sites, the disease usually develops as water temperatures begin to rise in spring. Clinical acute disease will occur only when these are above 8°C, and losses may be significant. Clinical signs include lethargy, darkening of the skin, respiratory distress and loss of balance. Abdominal distension (dropsy) and exophthalmos (popeye) are usually pronounced, and there may be petechial haemorrhages of the gills and skin. Internal visceral haemorrhages and the presence of serosanguinous fluid within the abdominal cavity are the most frequently reported post-mortem findings.

SVC is often included as a component of the complex of diseases known as the carp dropsy syndrome (or infectious dropsy). Fish affected by SVC are often also suffering from a primary or secondary bacterial septicaemia.

Swim-bladder inflammation (SBI)

This has been described as another component of the carp dropsy syndrome and is thought to be a separate entity to SVC. It usually affects cyprinids in their first summer, symptoms being abdominal distension and exophthalmos. In more acute cases, darkening of the skin and loss of balance may be the only symptoms observed prior to death. At post-mortem, pathology is usually restricted to degenerative changes of the swim-bladder, with haemorrhages and necrosis of the epithelium.

Lymphocystis

This viral infection has been described in many species of freshwater and marine fish. The disease is chronic in nature and results in the development of small circumscribed skin nodules (described as 'pearl-like'). These may be single or multiple, and may give a 'sandpaper' effect when present in very large numbers on the skin. Eventually an inflammatory reaction produces necrosis and sloughing leaving an intact epidermis. The condition, although unsightly, is rarely fatal.

Cichlid virus (Ramirez dwarf virus)

This virus is thought to be responsible for the acute disease in the South American *Apistogramma ramirez*, imported as a tropical aquarium fish into the USA. Clinical symptoms are inappetence, pallor, respiratory distress and haemorrhages of the skin and iris. The mortality is between 40 and 80%.

Bacteria

As well as acute systemic and chronic granulomatous diseases, some bacteria may directly invade the epithelium causing damage to the fins, skin ulceration or gill damage, whereas others may infect areas already damaged by other means. Skin ulceration can progress to systemic invasion and can result in severe osmoregulatory imbalance.

Acute systemic disease

This can be caused by a primary pathogen, but is more commonly due to secondary infection of a fish that is weakened by intercurrent disease, stress or immunosuppression. The clinical signs reflect the generalised septicaemia with inappetence and lethargy, together with erythema and petechiation of the skin and fins. There may be ulceration of the skin. The internal organs may be congested and show haemorrhages, and ascites (dropsy) and exophthalmos (popeye) may occur. Peracute infections can occur in which there are sudden deaths without prior clinical signs.

The organisms most commonly associated are the Gram-negative rods such as *Aeromonas*, *Pseudomonas*, *Vibrio*, *Flavobacteria*, *Yersinia* and *Edwardsiella* spp. Specific identification requires the isolation of the infective organism, usually from the fish's kidney. Some of these organisms are associated with specific diseases — *Yersinia*

ruckeri is the causative agent of enteric red mouth (ERM) that can affect goldfish, whereas 'hole-in-the-head' in young catfish results from an infection by *Edwardsiella ictaluri*. *Aeromonas* spp. are often seen in carp with spring viraemia.

Streptococcal septicaemia can occur as epizootics in warm water. *Pasteurella piscicida* may cause acute systemic disease or a chronic granulomatous disease (pseudotuberculosis).

It is possible for any of these bacteria to produce a more chronic disease which presents as skin ulceration.

Carp erythrodermatitis

Also called goldfish ulcer disease or simply ulcer disease it is caused by *Aeromonas salmonicida achromogenes*, a variant of the bacterium that causes furunculosis in salmonids. This is an obligate pathogen and carriers can exist. It can occur as part of the carp dropsy syndrome in association with spring viraemia, or with swim-bladder inflammation. The ulcers are said to have a characteristic 'punched out' appearance, having a red centre surrounded by a white rim, the latter itself being surrounded by an erythematous area.

Myxobacterial disease

This disease is caused by the Cytophagaceae (slime bacteria). These are generally secondary pathogens or opportunist invaders, and the commonest example is *Chondrococcus* (previously *Cytophaga* or *Flexibacter*) species. Various disease conditions are attributed to these organisms, but in general they are classified as:

Environmental (bacterial) gill disease. This is generally a sequel to initial gill damage resulting from environmental factors (such as raised ammonia levels) and is often compounded by parasitic infestations. The damaged tissue then becomes invaded by myxobacteria, and as the disease progresses there is hyperplasia of the gill lamellae, which severely compromises gill function.

Columnaris disease. This is usually associated with stress, nutritional imbalances or other husbandry problems. It is also called cotton-wool disease or mouth fungus, the latter being especially common in live-bearers (such as Black Mollies). It seldom occurs below 10°C, and can occur as an explosive epidemic above 18°C.

Cold-water disease (fin rot, peduncle disease). This requires the presence of predisposing factors, although once established the bacteria will spread to healthy tissue. The lesions generally begin as fin rot, but progressively spread to involve the base of the tail (the peduncle). It is a chronic condition, usually seen in cold water from 4–10°C. The causative organism is usually *Cytophaga psychrophila* and this does not grow above 12°C. A form of peduncle disease may, however, occur in warm water above 25°C.

Chronic granulomatous disease

These diseases are generally insidious in onset with the formation of granulomata in the tissues. The pathological effects depend on the organ that is affected, and granulomata in the skin may ulcerate at the surface.

The commonest organisms involved are *Mycobacterium* sp. which produce a chronic to subacute disease in all water conditions. The disease is especially associated with over-stocking. Oral transmission is the most usual, although infection through wounds or via ectoparasites may occur. The incubation period is about 6 weeks and all imported fish are potential carriers. Affected fish are generally listless and may become emaciated. Abdominal swelling together with exophthalmos are not uncommon, and grey-white nodules can be seen in the internal organs at post-mortem.

A similar disease can result from infection by *Nocardia asteroides*, although in this case infection is thought to be principally via wounds or injuries. *Flavobacterium* spp. have been associated with a chronic granulomatous disease in Black Mollies and other aquarium fish, and *Pasteurella* spp. are involved in the chronic condition known as pseudotuberculosis.

Fungi

Various fungi have been associated with disease in fish, and the symptoms range from superficial lesions to those of a fulminating systemic disease. Generally, however, most fungal disease is

secondary, precipitated by poor environmental conditions, malnutrition or other primary disease. Once an infection is present within an aquarium or pond, however, the level of infective material may increase dramatically to the point when even apparently healthy fish succumb.

Saprolegnia spp. and *Achyla* spp. occur worldwide in fresh and brackish water and can affect both fish and their eggs. They have long branched hyphae that usually colonise already damaged tissue, but once infection is established the production of proteolytic enzymes causes further damage so that the fungus can spread. The lesions appear as tufts of cotton-wool-like material (the mycelium) which start superficially, but may progress with deeper invasion of the tissues. Death may occur rapidly if the gills become involved. Dead fish are an ideal breeding ground for the fungus and their presence will enormously increase the number of infected spores in the water.

Branchiomyces spp. produce a disease of gill tissue (gill rot). It is seen especially in cyprinids, although probably most freshwater species are susceptible. It is confined to Europe, Japan, India and parts of the USA. The spores attach to the gill surface where they germinate. The hyphae then penetrate the gill tissue causing necrosis which gives a typical 'marbled' appearance.

Ichthyophonus hoferi results in a systemic granulomatous disease. Heavy infection can result in a 'sandpaper' effect of the skin. These lesions may become melanised or may rupture leaving small ulcers. Extensive growth can result in abscess formation with the presence of grey, white or yellow nodular lesions in the internal organs. Mortality levels depend on the degree of infection and the organs affected.

Dermocystidium spp. can form cysts anywhere in the body, but are commonly seen in the skin or gills. These yellowish-white cysts are usually smooth and can be up to 1 cm in diameter. Low levels of infection cause little harm although heavy infestations may be debilitating, especially if present on the gill.

Verticillium piscis has been associated with granulomata in goldfish, whereas *Exophiala pisciphila* has been isolated from skin lesions in a variety of marine aquarium fish. *Aureobasidium* spp. have also been isolated from necrotic lesions in the liver of marine species, and *Aphanomyces*, *Rhizopus* and *Phoma* spp. have all been associated with ulcerative lesions in fish.

Protozoan Parasites

Flagellates

Ichthyobodo spp. (*Costia*) are found world-wide on freshwater fish, they are obligate parasites with both free swimming and attached forms on the host. Fish eggs and amphibians may be affected, and cysts may form in adverse conditions.

The disease (slime disease) shows the typical symptoms of ectoparasite infestation. The marked irritation of the skin results in behavioural changes including 'flashing', rubbing against objects, and breaking the surface of the water. An excess of mucus is produced giving the fish a dull grey coloration and a slimy feel. Damage to the fins or gills (either directly by the parasite, or due to rubbing) can lead to secondary infection by fungi or bacteria. Long-standing disease may result in the exhaustion of the mucus secreting cells so that the skin becomes very dry.

Cryptobia spp. are similar in appearance to *Ichthyobodo* and are mainly associated with cichlids and cyprinids. They are generally considered to be commensals on the skin and gills, although severe gill damage has been reported in carp. Invasion of the stomach with haematogenous spread in cichlids may be associated with Malawi or Cichlid bloat. The organisms are thought to occur in the blood stream as trypanoplasms.

Amyloodinium spp. (marine) and *Oodinium* spp. (freshwater) are found in warm waters and hence are only a problem in tropical aquaria. The parasitic stage is the trophont which attaches to the skin and the gills, causing necrosis. It contains chlorophyll, and sufficient numbers give the skin a velvety gold or rust-coloured appearance. The common names of the disease are Velvet, Gold Dust, or Rust Disease.

Hexamita spp. are found in the alimentary tract and have been reported in a variety of species world-wide. Disease is more commonly seen in freshwater species. Infection is probably via the oral route and becomes established in the intestine or caeca. Haematogenous spread to other organs may occur. The spread of the disease is by the release of encysted forms in the faeces.

Large numbers of parasites may be present in normal healthy fish, and it is thought that predisposing factors are necessary to precipitate the disease. A number of disease entities have been associated with these organisms, including:

- Necrotic ulcerative gastritis in Siamese fighting fish, with an associated granulomatous peritonitis.
- Sudden death of young cichlids, such as angel fish and gouramis.
- Severe enteritis in angel fish (in association with *Capillaria* nematodes).
- Hole-in-the-head disease in cichlids, although a strict causal relationship has not been demonstrated in this case, and nutritional factors are probably involved.

Trypanosomes are not uncommon in both fresh and salt water, where they are transmitted by a leech vector. Although few appear to be pathogenic, anaemia has been described in the goldfish.

Eimeria is the most common genus of coccidia found world-wide in fish. The lesions involve the intestinal or caecal epithelium and may result in emaciation, lethargy and general poor health. Reports of disease predisposing factors are generally required before the disease is established.

Ciliates

Ichthyophthirius multifiliis is common world-wide and produces the disease known as white spot or 'Ich'. The infective stage is the tomite, which penetrates the epidermis of the skin or gills and develops into the trophont. The mature trophonts may reach 1 mm in diameter producing the characteristic and readily visible 'white spot'. Once mature, the trophont leaves the fish, encysts and produces 2000 tomites. The speed of the life-cycle is temperature dependent, taking 6 days at 27°C, but 15 days at 15°C. *Cryptocaryon* spp. produce a marine equivalent of the disease.

Tetrahymena corlissi occurs in warm waters, where guppies and other live-bearers are the most susceptible to 'Tet disease' — hence the common name of 'Guppy killer'. The parasites may swarm in particular areas of the fish, producing discrete white patches. There may be no obvious predisposing cause, but generally only stressed or debilitated individuals are affected. Females show a higher incidence than males. The parasite can invade most tissues and organ systems, leading to rapid mortality. Deep ulcers may be visible with invasion of the organism into the musculature. *Uronema* causes a marine form of this disease.

Chilodonella spp. can affect all species of freshwater fish and produce the symptoms typical of ectoparasites as discussed above. *Brooklynella* is a marine equivalent.

Trichodinids (including *Trichodina*, *Trichodonella* and *Tripartiella* spp. are found world-wide and can affect the skin and the gills of all marine and freshwater fish. The symptoms are those of a typical ectoparasite.

Scyphidia include a variety of organisms such as *Scyphidia*, *Epistylis* and *Vorticella* spp. These are generally regarded as commensals, but rapid multiplication can occur when there is a high organic loading in the water leading to skin irritation.

Trichophyra spp. are found most commonly on the gills of freshwater fish, where they are usually considered to be commensals. Asphyxiation may occur, however, if they are present in large numbers.

Microspora

These intracellular parasites produce chronic boil-like lesions, usually in individual fish. When they occur below the skin they appear as grey swellings which may rupture leaving an open wound. Terminal cases may become emaciated, lethargic and show abnormal coloration. *Pleistophora hyphessobryconis* is the causative agent of Neon Tetra disease which normally presents as a loss of colour with milky white areas under the skin along the dorsum.

Myxozoa

The infective stage is the spore, which is characterised by the presence of strongly Giemsa-staining polar bodies. This is then thought to release a motile form into the blood which enters the target tissue to form a trophozoite.

Henneguya spp. may produce microscopic or larger masses in various organs including the skin and gills of carp. These may be symptomless, but debility might be a sequel to a widespread infection. *Myxobolus* spp. occur not uncommonly in carp.

Mitraspora cyprini infection causes severe kidney pathology in goldfish and other cyprinids, while another myxosporean is associated with swim-bladder inflammation in carp.

Metazoan Parasites

Monogenean flukes

These have a world-wide distribution, although they are probably more common in fresh water. Most species are host specific but some cross infection may occur.

Dactylogyrus spp. are known as the gill fluke. Eggs are produced which fall from the host and hatch into free swimming larvae. *Gyrodactylus* sp. (known as the skin fluke) are more commonly found on the skin. They are viviparous with juveniles developing within the body cavity which are then released directly onto the host. Often these juveniles themselves contain further juveniles and so parasite numbers can build up very rapidly under the right conditions.

The symptoms shown depend on the area affected. Infection of the skin results in slime disease, with all the signs typical of ectoparasites as discussed above. Damage to the gills will produce respiratory distress and possibly osmo-regulatory imbalance, and is likely to predispose to secondary bacterial or fungal infection.

Digenean flukes

These organisms have complex life-cycles and fish may be involved as primary or intermediate hosts depending on the parasite species. Invasion of fish by large numbers of cercariae may result in death due to osmotic imbalance. In general, however, the symptoms will depend on the host site and the particular species of parasite involved. In cases where an abnormal host is involved, there may be a massive inflammatory reaction.

The metacercariae of *Neascus* spp., seen most commonly in cyprinids, produce cysts in the skin up to 0.5 mm in diameter. These become melanised, and hence the common name of the condition is black spot.

Diplostomum spp. (eye fluke) encyst in the eye and may cause cataract and blindness. *Clinostomum* spp. (yellow or white grubs) produce large nodules

(0.5 cm in diameter) which may ulcerate if they are near the surface.

Sanguinicola inermis is potentially a serious problem in carp. The organisms enter the host as cercariae and continue to migrate around the body, usually remaining within the blood vessels of the skin. They eventually pass to the blood vessels of the gill, where they mature and lay eggs. Serious gill damage may result at the time the eggs hatch.

Tapeworms

Cestodes occur world-wide and are generally host specific. Fish can be the final, intermediate or transport host depending on the species. Adult cestodes are usually found in the gut, whereas intermediate stages may occur in any tissue or body cavity.

Ligula spp. are seen most commonly in cyprinids, where the intermediate stage is found within the abdominal cavity. They may reach up to 20 cm in length and may cause severe organ atrophy and localised peritonitis. Sexual maturity may be inhibited in infected fish.

The intermediate of *Triaenophorus* spp. encysts in the liver and damage can occur during the migratory stage. Similarly the intermediate of *Diphyllobothrium* spp. is usually found in the abdominal cavity where generally little damage is caused, although damage may occur during the migratory phase.

Bothriocephalus sp. (Asian tapeworm) is found in the adult form in the gut of carp where it can reach up to 20 cm in length. Infected fish have a swollen abdomen and may become sluggish and emaciated. Intestinal obstruction can result in fish losses.

Nematodes

Nematodes are found world-wide and may occur in fish as the adult or larval stages, although actual disease is rare. Fish with heavy infestations may show anaemia, emaciation and unthriftiness, and may become susceptible to other diseases. Intermediate stages may cause cysts in muscles or other organs, and severe tissue reactions may occur if the organisms are present in unnatural hosts.

Larval stages of *Eustrongyloides* sp. are red in colour, may reach up to 8 cm in length and are found coiled up in fibrous capsules. *Philometra* species, often called blood worms are thin and red and up to 16 cm long. The adult females are found in the skin, fins, or lying free in the body cavity. They migrate to the surface and protrude the posterior part of their body through the skin releasing live larvae directly into the water.

Capillaria spp. are generally thought of as pathogens of aquarium fish, causing gut ulceration and emaciation. Affected fish stop feeding, often lie on their side and may die. Their faeces may appear translucent due to excessive mucus production. Angel fish and cichlids, as well as young armoured catfish, appear to be especially susceptible.

Camellanus spp. are common parasites of many live-bearing tropical fish. They are thin red worms up to 1 cm in length which may be seen protruding from the vent. Larvae may be carried in the tissues of aquatic organisms, such as *Daphnia* spp., although some species produce live larvae which do not need an intermediate host, and so heavy infestations can build up quickly. Damage to the intestine with ulceration can occur.

Acanthocephala

Pomphorhynchus spp. attach to the epithelium of the alimentary tract by means of their spiny heads. Ulceration and necrosis can occur, although large numbers of the worms need to be present to produce clinical disease.

Mollusca

The larval stages (glochidia) of freshwater mussels are parasitic, and may become a problem in fish held in ponds fed from streams containing mussel beds. They become encysted on the gills and the skin and in large numbers they can cause significant gill damage.

Crustacea

Lernaea cyprinacea is the anchor worm found on carp, but it is not host specific. It is more important in warm water and is unable to complete its life-cycle below 15°C. The female anchor worm is fertilised on the host's body, to which it attaches by means of a penetrating cephalic process. Egg sacs are formed on the posterior part of the body which trail in the water releasing eggs which hatch into nauplii. Even small numbers of parasites will cause serious damage to the host. As well as the general signs of ectoparasitism, the attachment sites are usually very inflamed and may develop into granulomata with necrotic centres. These may be very slow to heal after removal of the parasite.

Ergasilus spp. (gill maggots) occur in both fresh and salt water. These are much smaller than *Lernaea* and they attach to the gills, causing severe damage at the attachment sites.

Argulus spp. (fish lice) are found world-wide, but in Europe are most often associated with freshwater problems. Egg production ceases below 16°C, and hibernation on the body of the host occurs below 8°C. The female leaves the host to lay eggs on aquatic plants. These hatch to form free-living larvae which then find a new host to continue the life-cycle, the whole process taking 40–100 days, depending on the temperature. The parasites are easily visible with the naked eye, and the clinical signs are those typical of ectoparasitism. They may be involved in the transmission of viruses, such as spring viraemia of carp.

Annelida

Piscicola spp. (fish leeches) may cause skin damage during feeding, and this may result in debility and predispose to secondary infection. They are known to act as intermediate hosts for certain blood parasites, such as trypanosomes and trypanoplasms, and may transmit the causative virus of spring viraemia of carp.

Toxins

Many of the symptoms shown in relation to toxins are common to a wide range of substances. Acute poisoning frequently results in a complete fish kill, the fish showing few clinical signs prior to death. (Infectious agents rarely cause 100% mortality.) Sub-lethal levels of many toxins may affect the gills, producing respiratory distress, and the fish may show avoidance behaviour if the toxin is not equally distributed throughout the water. Chronic exposure to some toxins, particularly

heavy metals, can result in retarded growth, loss of reproductive ability and deformity.

There are five main groups of substances which are potentially toxic to ornamental fish:

Metals

The most commonly cited as harmful are aluminium, copper, lead, iron, zinc and cadmium. Lead, iron and zinc may leach into the water from older domestic water supply systems and it is important that water which has been in such a system for some time is flushed through before any is used for fish. Similarly, copper could be a hazard in newer domestic systems. Alum is sometimes added to the domestic water supply to remove colour and suspended material from the water, particularly in peaty areas.

The toxicity of metals varies with water quality parameters such as pH, hardness and the presence of organic material or other elements.

Gases

Chlorine is the principal exogenous gas which is toxic to fish. All tapwater used for fish should be allowed to stand for at least 24 hours, preferably with aeration, to allow any dissolved chlorine to dissipate. Commercially available tapwater conditioners can also be used.

Hydrogen sulphide and methane result from the anaerobic breakdown of organic material within the pond or aquaria. Problems may arise in stagnant ponds or during the winter when ice covering the surface prevents the dissipation of these gases into the atmosphere.

Organic compounds

Many wood preservatives are toxic and so decorative material introduced into an aquarium (e.g. ornamental bog oak) must be treated with a non-toxic compound. Many household polishes, paints and DIY materials are toxic and should not be used in the vicinity of aquaria or garden ponds. Care should be taken in the choice of materials for pond construction.

Biocides

The majority of these compounds are directly toxic to fish and care should be taken to avoid contamination of aquaria or ponds. This includes domestic and veterinary insecticides, such as sprays and slow-release fly strips, and also garden herbicides.

Therapeutic agents

Many of the agents used may be toxic if overdosed or if the fish are suffering from inter-current disease. Great care must be taken when calculating dosages to take account of the variable water quality parameters such as pH, hardness and temperature. Not all fish species have the same tolerance to drugs, and this should be borne in mind when a variety of fish species are treated together.

Neoplasia

Although there are a few exceptions, the incidence of neoplasia in general becomes more common with the increasing age of the individual, and hence tumours are probably encountered more frequently in ornamental fish than in the food-fish species.

The most commonly reported tumours are those on the surface, simply because they are more easily identified. Papillomata are common in many species of freshwater and marine fish. The tumour is benign, and can vary in form from a slightly raised area of hyperplastic epidermis to very obvious papillary projections. Carp pox is frequently classified as a neoplasm, although strictly it is a virus-induced hyperplasia of the epidermis. Neurofibromas and fibromas are found relatively frequently in goldfish, presenting as single or multiple sub-cutaneous masses. Tumours of the pigment cells (melanomas) are also quite common.

Intra-abdominal tumours may be suspected in fish with long-standing abdominal swelling, although a specific diagnosis can only be made at post-mortem. Tumours of the liver, pancreas, kidney, gonads and gastrointestinal tract have all been described in a variety of species of ornamental fish.

Lymphosarcomata have been described, often taking the form of ulcerating sub-cutaneous lesions, with metastases to other organs. Teratomas have been described in tropical fish, most often guppies, in which they usually take the form of a prominent ventral abdominal swelling.

Nutritional Diseases

Nuritional disease can occur for a variety of reasons:

SPECIFIC NUTRITIONAL PATHOLOGIES			
Pathological condition	Possible causes		
	Deficiencies	Dietary excesses	Toxicity
Cataract	Zinc Copper Selenium Tryptophan Methionine Riboflavin Vitamin A	Calcium	Choline
Vertebral deformity	Phosphorus Tryptophan Vitamin C		Calcium Lead
Fatty digestion of the liver	Fatty acid Tryptophan	Fat	Oxidised fat
Fin erosion and susceptability to myxobacterial disease	Riboflavin Vitamin C		
Skin/fin haemorrhages	General vitamins		

FIG. 22.6 Specific nutritional pathologies.

- Insufficient food resulting in starvation.
- An imbalanced diet leading to deficiencies of certain essential nutrients. This may be associated with specific essential dietary requirements in individual species.
- Poorly formulated diets.
- Incorrect storage leading to oxygenation of fats and degeneration of vitamins etc.
- Toxic factors in the diet.

These problems can be avoided by using a good quality commercial diet.

A full discussion of specific nutritional diseases is given in Chapter 8 but a summary is given in Fig. 22.6.

Clinical Diagnosis

The manifestation of a disease in fish often involves a complex interaction between pathogens and various predisposing factors, such as environmental changes or intercurrent disease. Any investigation should take account of this and the veterinarian should adopt a standard approach which allows a full appraisal of the husbandry/management system and the water quality, as well as of the fish themselves.

The management system is best assessed by a visit to the site. If this is not feasible, careful questioning of the owner is essential. A checklist of management factors to be considered is given in Fig. 22.7.

Ideally this appraisal should be made when the system is functioning normally, before any disease outbreak occurs. In the presence of a disease problem, the investigation might usefully follow the steps suggested in Fig. 22.8.

This is the sort of approach that would be adopted for the investigation of any fish disease

A CHECKLIST OF MANAGEMENT FACTORS	
Fish	Species
	Numbers / size
	Frequency of introducing new fish
	Quarantine procedure
Plants	Types
	Frequency of introducing new plants
	Quarantine / pretreatment procedure
Feeding	Type of food
	Frequency of feeding
	Storage
Pond/aquarium	Volume of water
	Surface area
	Source of water
	How long established
	Frequency and method of cleaning
	Siting within room or garden
Water circulation	Pumps — types and capacity
	Water changes — proportion / frequency / source
	Average loss through leaks / evaporation
	Waterfalls / fountains / airstones
	Material used in pipe manufacture
Filtration	Types
	Capacity
	How long installed
	Frequency and method of cleaning
	u/v filters — size and position
Heating	Types
	Thermostats / monitoring
Lighting	Natural
	Artificial — types of tube
Water quality	Parameters tested
	Frequency of testing
Routine treatments	Medications used
	Dosage
	Frequency

Fig. 22.7 A checklist of management factors.

outbreak. Ornamental fish, however, do pose some special problems. They are truly companion animals, and the emotional feelings of some aquarists mirror those of dog and cat owners. They may be unwilling to sacrifice a dying fish for a full examination in case some miracle cure may save it. They are even less likely to agree to the sacrifice of a group of apparently normal fish to assess the underlying health status of the whole population. An added problem in the case of koi or marine fish is that the monetary value of the individual fish may be relatively high.

All of the post-mortem and laboratory techniques discussed elsewhere in the book with regard to food-fish can obviously be utilised where appropriate, but in addition techniques involving the examination and sampling of live/anaesthetised fish are of prime importance.

Examination of the Fish in the Water

Ideally the fish should be viewed in the water, both from above and from the side if possible. An assessment of the movement and respiratory rate should be made, together with a comparison of the individual's behaviour in relation to the other fish. Those that remain solitary or swim in a lethargic fashion may be unwell. Those that mouth at the surface or congregate at sources of oxygenated water may be suffering from gill problems or anaemia. Flashing or rubbing against objects in the water may indicate the presence of ectoparasites.

For closer inspection of a fish in water, transfer it into a polythene bag. This allows examination from all angles and also permits a more accurate assessment of colour changes, which

BASIC STEPS FOR INVESTIGATING A DISEASE PROBLEM	
History	An appraisal of the underlying system and management (as in Fig. 22.9) History of current problem: • Numbers / species of fish affected • timescale • presenting symptoms • mortalities Possible changes in management acting as a trigger: • filter changes • pond / aquarium cleaning • changes in feeding regime • introduction of new fish / quarantine • faulty heating, lighting, or pumping equipment • power cuts Possible environmental changes acting as a trigger: • fluctuating temperatures • algal blooms • predators (cats, herons) • sudden leaf fall Self medication: • compounds used (many aquarium remedies do not have active ingredients listed but it is essential to try to discover the basic composition of the compound) • dosage and treatment protocol Possible exposure to toxins: • aerosols, solvents, weed killers etc.
Examination of the environment/water testing	Examination of all in-contact fish
Examination of the fish	Examination of affected fish within pond / aquarium Clinical examination of fish out of the water
Laboratory examination	Post-mortem procedure Further laboratory tests

FIG. 22.8 The basis steps needed for investigation of a disease problem.

may not be seen easily once the fish is out of the water.

Anaesthesia or Sedation

For examination out of the water, it is generally necessary to anaesthetise or sedate fish. The two common agents used are tricaine methanesulphate (MS222) and ethyl-4-aminobenzoate (benzocaine), although MS222 is the only licensed product available in the UK. These drugs are added to the water, but great care should be taken when calculating the dose to allow for species variations in tolerance as well as the fact that efficacy and toxicity are influenced by variations in water quality. Recovery from anaesthesia should be in water that is identical to that to which the anaesthetic agent was added, and this requirement should be considered if fish are brought to the surgery for examination.

Sampling from Live Fish

Under anaesthesia a close examination of the skin, gills and eyes can be made, and the abdomen can be palpated. Impression smears can be taken from the gills. Biopsies taken from skin lesions can be submitted for histological examination. Skin scrapings can also be taken from an anaesthetised fish to identify the presence of ectoparasites, although sampling from a conscious fish is preferable since the anaesthetic agent may adversely affect the parasites, making them more difficult to identify. Blood samples can be taken from larger species but the interpretation of the results is difficult.

Post-Mortems and Further Laboratory Tests

Post-mortem techniques and further laboratory analysis are discussed in Chapter 5. A potential problem with ornamental fish species is their relatively small size. It may be more practical to take samples for bacteriology from the spleen rather than from the kidney. Similarly, histological analysis may be best performed if 0.5 cm 'steaks' (i.e. transverse sections cut from head to tail) are fixed and submitted, rather than attempting to dissect out individual organs.

SUMMARY OF PRESENTING SIGNS

Sudden death
Skin problems
• Grossly visible parasites or agents
• Discrete coloured lesions
• Generalised changes in colour
• Generalised changes in skin texture
• Hyperaemia or haemorrhages of the skin
• Ulceration of the skin
• Nodules on the skin
• Subcutaneous nodules
Fin problems
Eye problems
Gill problems
• Pallor
• Excessive mucus
• Discrete lesions
Faecal changes
Problems within the abdominal cavity
• Ascites
• Haemorrhages on viscera
• Grossly visible parasites or parasitic cysts
• Tumours or granulomata
• Miscellaneous conditions
Behaviour problems

FIG. 22.9 A summary of presenting signs.

Presenting Signs

A summary of presenting signs is given in Fig. 22.9.

Therapy

A full discussion of the therapeutic agents used to treat fish diseases is given in Chapter 7, although there are a few particular points with regard to ornamental fish that are worth stressing.

As in the case of anaesthetic drugs, the calculation of dosages is difficult since individual fish species may have different tolerances to the drugs, and the efficacy or toxicity of the drugs themselves will vary in different water quality conditions.

Because residues are not a concern in ornamental fish, it is possible to use unlicensed products in the UK if no equivalent effective licensed products are available. Even so, the current review of 'water treatments' is likely to lead to legislation which may dramatically affect the availability of many of the common proprietary medications.

Economic constraints, although important, are less of a factor when dealing with ornamental fish. In general, they can be treated as individuals since they can be netted easily and then, with the aid

DOSAGES OF ANTIBIOTICS ADMINISTERED VIA THE WATER°	
Oxytetracycline	13–120 mg/l (chelated by hard water)
Doxycycline and Minocycline	2–3 mg/l
Chloramphenicol	20–50 mg/l
Potentiated sulphonamide	(80 mg trimethoprim and 400 mg sulphadiazine per ml) used at 1ml/100–120 l
Nifurpirinol	0.1 mg/l
Metronidazole	7 mg/l (double for *Oodinium*)
Dimetridazole	5 mg/l (said to inhibit spawning)
Neomycin	50 mg/kg (used in sea water)
Gentamycin	4–5 mg/kg (used in sea water)
Kanamycin	50–100 mg/l
Nitrofurazone	1–3 mg/l

of anaesthetic agents, topical treatments of lesions can be performed or injections given. Individual fish are also more easily observed by aquarists so that more prompt treatment should be possible. However, it also encourages 'self-medication', which might significantly affect diagnosis or further treatment.

Antibiotics

These can be administered via the water, by inclusion in the food or by injection. Ideally the choice of antibiotic used should be based on 'sensitivity testing', but in practice it is usually empirical.

Administration via the water

This is the least effective and yet probably the most widely used method for ornamental fish. The widespread, uncontrolled use of antibiotics in the Far East has led to the development of antibiotic resistance. The method should not be used in systems dependent on bacterial filtration, although it may be necessary if the fish are not feeding. In that case a separate treatment tank is required in which water quality can be controlled by regular water changes. Calcium present in hard-water areas will often chelate certain antibiotics, reducing their availability.

The suggested doses of antibiotics administered in water are given in Fig. 22.10.

Administration via the food

The four most common antibiotics used are oxytetracycline, oxolinic acid, amoxycillin and the potentiated sulphonamides. These are generally mixed with the food, although manufactured medicated foods are preferable since the availability of the drug is more uniform. Medicated flake foods containing oxolinic acid or oxytetracycline are available. Specialist manufacturers of flake or pelleted foods will supply medicated foods on receipt of a Veterinary Written Direction.

Dosages for marine fish may be different from those for freshwater fish as there is a reduced uptake of oxolinic acid and oxytetracycline in the former. Sulphonamides may be dangerous due to the potential formation of crystals in the more concentrated urine of marine fish.

DOSAGES OF ANTIBIOTICS BY INJECTION	
Ampicillin	10 mg/kg daily
Chloramphenicol succinate	40 mg/kg daily
Gentamicin	3 mg/kg every other day
Oxytetracycline	10 mg/kg daily
Potentiated sulphonamide (48%)	1 ml/16 kg every other day
Enrofloxacin	5–10 mg/kg daily

ANTHELMINTICS USED IN ORNAMENTAL FISH			
Medication	**Intestinal parasite**	**Dosage**	**Method of administration**
Praziquantel	Tapeworms	5–100 mg/kg	Stomach tube In feed i/m injection
Mebendazole	Tapeworms	25–50 mg/kg	In feed
Piperazine citrate	Nematodes	25 mg/10 g food	In feed
Levamisole	Nematodes	10 mg/l	Via water

FIG. 22.12 Anthelmintics used in ornamental fish.

Administration by injection

This is the best method when fish are of a sufficient size. The sites for injection are a matter of personal preference. Suitable drugs and dosages are given in Fig. 22.11.

General Antibacterial Agents

Several agents have been used widely as water treatments and may be useful supplements to antibiotic therapy.

Benzalkonium chloride. A blend of quaternary ammonium compounds and is used as a permanent bath at 0.1–0.5 mg/l, although the dose should be halved in soft water. It is useful against myxobacterial infections, especially bacterial gill disease, where the detergent action gently lifts the mucus from the gill surface.

Chloramine-T. Also useful for myxobacterial infections, it has an effect against *Costia*, white spot and *Gyrodactylus* spp. Its action is based on a slow breakdown of hypochlorous acid, releasing

COMMON ECTOPARASITIC TREATMENTS		
Medication	**Ectoparasitic**	**Dosage and administration**
Formalin	Protozoa and flukes	250 mg/l — 30–60 minute dip or 15–25 mg/l — continuous bath
Malachite green	Fungi and some protozoa	2 mg/l — 30 minute dip or 0.1 mg/l — permanent bath
Formalin with malachite green (Leteux–Meyer mixture)	Protozoa	25 mg/l formalin — 60 minute dip +0.05 mg/l malachite green — 60 minute dip or 15 mg/l formalin — continuous bath +0.05 mg/l malachite green — continuous bath
Potassium permanganate (difficult – not recommended)	Protozoa (also BGD)	1–5 mg/l — 60 minute dip
Methylene blue (harmful to filters)	Protozoa	1–2 mg/l
Copper sulphate (Important to monitor copper levels)	Protozoa in marine and freshwater aquarian	0.1 mg/l
Trichlorphon	*Lernaea* spp. *Argulus* spp. Flukes	0.2 mg/l — permanent bath
Salt water	Leeches	20–30 g/l — 15–30 minute dip
Fresh water	Ectoparasites on marine fish	2–10 minute dip

FIG. 22.13 Common ectoparasitic treatments.

oxygen and chlorine, and it should not be used at the same time as other chemicals.

Acriflavine. A fairly popular disinfectant used in koi. Other species have a variable tolerance to it, and plants are often adversely affected.

Anthelmintics

The drugs or medications used for ornamental fish are summarised in Fig. 22.12. Chapter 7 gives a more detailed discussion.

Treatments for Ectoparasites

Various medications have been used, generally in a concentrated solution as a short dip, or a more dilute solution as a permanent bath. Care should be taken in the latter case if the system incorporates a biological filter. These chemicals are relatively toxic and it should be remembered that weak, debilitated fish are more susceptible to their adverse effects. Great care should also be taken when handling the chemicals in their concentrated forms, and adequate protective clothing should be worn. A list of the more commonly used treatments is given in Fig. 22.13.

In addition to the traditional water treatments, Ivermectin (MSD) has been used by intramuscular injection for the treatment of *Lernaea* spp. in goldfish.

Salt

Salt has already been mentioned in relation to the treatment for leeches. Its most useful role, however, is to reduce osmotic stress, and hence metabolic requirements, in freshwater fish with gill damage or ulcers. Concentrations of 0.15% (1500 mg/l) are increased over 3 days to 0.3% (3000 mg/l).

Local Applications

Ornamental fish have the advantage that it may be possible to anaesthetise them and treat lesions individually. Adult *Lernaea* are best removed in this way, although treatment of the water is still necessary to kill the larvae.

Ulcers require thorough debridement followed

by application of antibacterials such as povidone iodine or topical antibiotics. The ulcer is then packed with a barrier cream, such as Orabase® (Squibb), to reduce the osmotic stress on the fish. Parenteral antibiotics may be given at the same time.

Care should be taken to disinfect nets and other equipment between handling each fish. Benzalkonium chloride is useful in this respect.

Prevention of Disease

Good Husbandry and Management

As mentioned throughout this book, the manifestation of clinical disease often requires predisposing factors, which may reflect on the management of the system. Good husbandry methods, frequent observation of the fish and regular testing of water quality parameters are of prime importance in the prevention of disease.

Prophylactic Treatments

A low level of parasites may be another predisposing factor to disease. It is impossible to eliminate these completely and, since a closed aquarium or pond favours parasite multiplication, it is wise to treat periodically as a prophylactic measure — perhaps 3 or 4 times per year.

In aquaria, the environmental conditions are fairly constant. In ponds, however, seasonal fluctuations are unavoidable: spring and autumn are times when the fish are particularly stressed and hence susceptible to disease. Special vigilance is needed at these times, and prophylactic antiparasitic or antibacterial treatments are worthy of consideration.

Quarantine

Perhaps one of the greatest risks of introducing disease to an established system is via new fish or aquatic plants. Strict quarantine is essential, and a period of at least 4–6 weeks should be considered. Even in that time some diseases (e.g. mycobacterial infections) may not become apparent.

A completely separate quarantine unit with its own filtration system and disinfected equipment is required. In general, tropical fish should be quarantined at 22–25°C, and cold-water fish at not less than 12–15°C, since the speed of the pathogens' life-cycles is temperature dependent.

Prophylactic treatments are of value during the quarantine period, although care should be taken with recently imported fish since these are probably already stressed and so may be more susceptible to the toxic effects of the treatments.

Vaccination

A vaccine has recently become available for the protection of cyprinids against erythrodermatitis and ulcer disease caused by *Aeromonas salmonicida*.

Acknowledgements — I would like to acknowledge all the authors of the *Manual of Ornamental Fish* (1992) published by BSAVA, Cheltenham. I had the pleasure to edit this manual, and owe much of the knowledge on which this chapter is based to their efforts. Figures 22.4, 22.5, 22.6, 22.8 and 22.9 are taken from this text.

Further Reading

Andrews, C., Excell, A., Carrington, N. (1988) *The Manual of Fish Health*. Salamander Books, London.

Brewster, B., Chaple, N., Cuvelier, J., Davies, M., Evans, D., Evans, G., Phipps, K., Scott, P. W. (1989) *The Interpet Encyclopaedia of Koi*. Salamander Books, London.

Butcher, R. L. (Editor) (1992) *The BSAVA Manual of Ornamental Fish*. BSAVA Publications, Cheltenham.

Carrington, N. (1985) *A Fishkeeper's Guide to Maintaining a Healthy Aquarium*. Salamander Books, London.

Mills, D. (1987) *The Marine Aquarium*. Salamander Books, London.

Riehl, R. and Baensch, H. A. (1987) *Aquarium Atlas*. H. A. Baensch Publishers. Melle, Germany.

Scott, P. W. (1991) *The Complete Aquarium*. Dorling Kindersley, London.

Van Ramshorst, J. D. (1978) *The Complete Aquarium Encyclopaedia of Tropical Freshwater Fish*. Elsevier-Phaidon, Oxford.

23

The Veterinary Approach to Sea-bass and Sea-bream

PANOS CHRISTOFILOGIANNIS

The commercial production of sea-bream and sea-bass is expanding rapidly in the Mediterranean countries. A better understanding of the biology, nutritional requirements and optimal environmental conditions for these species has led to viable production levels but a persistent obstacle is the presence of several pathogens which induce severe mortalities and major economic losses.

Gilthead sea-bream (*Sparus aurata*) (Fig. 23.1). A euryhaline, eurythermal species which reproduces from October to December in the open sea. It is distributed discontinuously in the Mediterranean Sea (but is rare in the Black Sea) and also in the Atlantic from the British Isles to the Cape Verde Islands and the Canary Islands. Sexual maturity develops in males at 2 years of age (20–30 cm) and in females at 2–3 years (33–40 cm). The sea-bream is a protandrous hermaphrodite and is the first species to leave the lagoons for the open sea in early autumn. Its feeding range includes molluscs, crustaceans, small fish and plants. It is sensitive to low temperatures and low levels of dissolved oxygen.

Sea-bass (*Dicentrarchus labrax*). Another highly euryhaline and eurythermal species, is distributed discontinuously around the Atlantic from 30°N (Moroccan coast) to 55°N (Irish, North and Baltic seas). It is ubiquitous along Mediterranean coasts, where it enters coastal inlets and river mouths. Adults leave the Mediterranean lagoons from

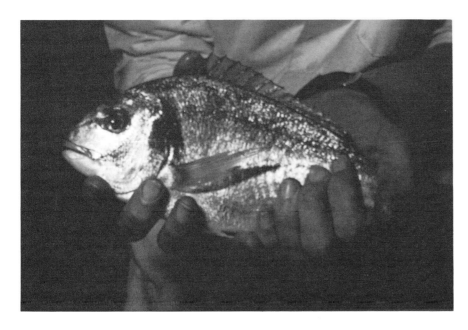

FIG. 23.1 Gilthead sea-bream (*Sparus aurafa*).

October to December in order to reproduce in the open sea. Sexual maturity develops in males at 2 years of age (23–30 cm) and in females at 3 years (31–40 cm). The sea-bass's feeding range includes small fish, prawns, crabs and cuttlefish.

Farming Systems

Extensive Lagoon Systems

The traditional (extensive) method of lagoon management in Greece is by placing special barriers (Fig. 23.2) in opportune lagoon sites to capture fish during their autumn migration to the open sea. The areas of brackish water managed in this way are called *divaria*. Barriers made of reeds, nets or cement stay open from February until May for the lagoon's natural enrichment with fry.

Semi-intensive Lagoon Systems

Semi-intensive techniques in lagoon management involve artificial enrichment with fry, fertilisation of the lagoons, and improvement projects. Specialist fishermen collect fry from coastal waters during May and June. The fry are transported in oxygenated tanks for a first stage of growing in special ponds, until they reach a size which enables them to survive in the lagoon.

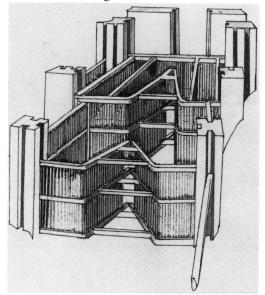

FIG. 23.2 Modern fish barriers used for lagoons management in Mediterranean region.

Projects for improved productivity involve the development of sufficient canals and openings to the open sea for intercourse, water exchange and enrichment with plankton and fry. Peripheral ditches (with fresh or salt water) are dug for salinity control, and also wintering ditches at least 2 m deep in several areas of the lagoon. Finally, vegetation control is important in order to avoid suffocation of the fish.

Losses in fish production in the lagoons are due to insufficient enrichment with fry, predation, lowered fresh water (due to lack of rain) and lack of sufficient improvement projects.

Intensive Systems

In the intensive production of sea-bass and sea-bream in Greece, on-growing units are supplied with fry by hatcheries. In 1990, up to 80% of these supplies were from Greek sources and the rest were imported from France, Spain, Italy and Cyprus.

General Husbandry

The management of captive broodstock in the breeding stations includes natural maturation, the induction of ovulation by hormonal injections, fertilisation in spawning tanks, and incubation in open-water circulation systems.

Hatchery techniques involve complete environmental control. Live food (rotifers and brine-shrimp nauplii and metanauplii) is given during the first 45 days post-hatching. Weaning and adaptation to an artificial pelleted diet (600–800 mm) is a crucial stage in the larval production line. At the end of the weaning period, juveniles weigh 1.5–2.0 g and are 75 days old. They are grown further until they reach a suitable size (1.5–2.5 g) for sale to farmers as on-growing stock in floating sea cages (Figs 23.3 and 23.4).

The on-growing juveniles reach 400–450 g in 16 months over one winter, or in 18–20 months over two winters. Feeds are distributed by automatic feeders every 10–15 minutes for small fish (2–15 g) or by hand for larger fish. Nets have to be changed every 15–20 days in summer, and grading is necessary at least two or three times in order to avoid growth differentiation and cannibalism. Stress from handling often induces high mortality levels. Preventive treatments are given to avoid outbreaks of disease.

In 1990, Greece's 11 breeding stations produced 11 million young sea-bream and sea-bass weighing 1–2 g; the 95 on-growing units had a total production of 1600 tonnes.

Legislation

The legislative background of aquaculture development in Greece is based on the new Act 18922/90 which was passed in the Greek Parliament in July 1990. The industry must also comply with EC legislation.

Major Diseases

Viral Diseases

Lymphocystis

Lymphocystis is a benign chronic infection caused by an iridovirus. It results in characteristic cell hypertrophy (50,000–100,000-fold increase in cell volume) typically in the skin and fins of the most advanced orders of fish. Lymphocystis virus is the largest known icosahedral virus with specific tropism for fibroplastic cells.

The external signs of disease are whitish-grey nodules (aggregates of hypertrophic cells) which cover a large portion of the body and often the entire surface of the caudal and pectoral fins of the gilthead sea-bream. Lymphocystis cells are sometimes in the muscle, peritoneum and membranes covering internal organs, mainly among marine fish.

Major features of the lymphocystis cells are their thick hyaline capsule, the central enlarged nucleus and predominant basophilic DNA cytoplasmic inclusions where the virus is replicated.

The disease can be diagnosed by visual examination and should not be confused with superficial cysts of trematodes (which show internal movement). Diagnosis can be confirmed by histological sections. Distinction between lymphocystis and epitheliocystis is based on the nucleus position, which is typically peripheral in epitheliocystis.

In the transmission of the disease external surfaces, including the gills, are the major portal of entry. The oral route does not seem to be

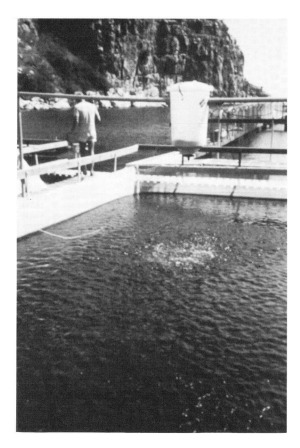

FIG. 23.3 Typical cage operation for on growing sea-bream.

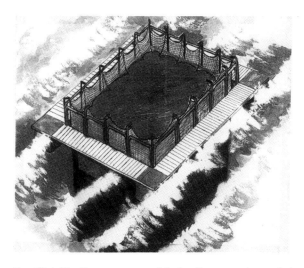

FIG. 23.4 Floating sea cage used during the ongrowing period in sea bass and sea bream culture.

involved and no evidence exists for vertical transmission.

Lymphocystis seldom causes significant mortalities, but it has commercial implications: growth is reduced and affected fish are rejected for human consumption. It can also spread to healthy fish.

Lymphocystis has been reported in sea-bream from Israel, Portugal, Italy and Spain. It tends to occur in young fish around 8 months of age, usually in overpopulated sea-cage farms and inshore holding tanks. It may regress within a month or two; it seems that an age-dependent resistance develops. Mortalities in Greece and Turkey during the disease's outbreaks are thought to be caused by secondary infections.

At present there is no known method of therapy or evidence of immunisation against the disease. In the USA, suggested control measures include holding the fish until the lesions are shed, marketing the apparently clear specimens and disinfecting the holding facilities, resuming operation with clean stock.

Viral erythrocytic infection (VEN)

VEN in sea-bass is an erythrocytic infection caused by a hexagonally shaped virus of 150–360 nm (presumably Iridoviridae). The virus causes cytoplasmic inclusion bodies and nuclear degeneration. It seems to induce anaemia and also to increase susceptibility of the infected fish to secondary infections. There is a higher prevalence of the disease in adult cultured sea-bass in overcrowded farms, and also under higher ambient water temperature conditions.

Infectious pancreatic necrosis (IPN)

IPN virus has been isolated from apparently healthy sea-bass larvae. Experimental inoculation of trout with the isolated virus induced mortalities.

Viral haemorrhagic septicaemia (VHS)

Sea-bass are readily infected with the VHS virus by injection or by natural infection at temperatures below 15°C, although no pathogenic effects are seen at 20°C.

High infection doses cause more than 90% mortalities in injected fish and around 50% in water-route contamination.

MAJOR VIRAL DISEASES
Lymphocytis
Viral erythrocytic infection (VEN)
Infectious pancreatic necrosis (IPN)
Viral haemorrhagic septicaemia (VHS)
Distended gut syndrome (DGS)
Nervous syndrome in sea-bass
Sea-bream papilloma agent

FIG. 23.5 Major viral diseases of sea-bass and sea-bream.

Diseased fish display the classical features of VHS (darkening, exophthalmia, severe anaemia, haemorrhages in the abdomen and the musculature), and high yields of the virus are recovered from several organs. Anti-VHS neutralising antibodies are found in the sera of sea-bass which overcome the infection.

Sea-bass birnavirus

A birnavirus has been associated with mass mortalities in sea-bass larvae in French hatcheries, usually 20 days post-hatching at 19°C. The moribund larvae display a spiral swimming motion, distended swim-bladder and gall bladder, white faecal casts and exophthalmia. Histopathologically, delamination of the intestinal epithelium and hypertrophy of the swim-bladder and the gall bladder are seen.

In Martinique, cultured sea-bass, during the first year of life, are susceptible to a contagious disease characterised by whirling and hyperexcitability, associated with severe brain lesions (spongiosis and small round basophilic inclusion bodies). Icosahedral viral particles were found to cause damage in the nervous cells. Mortalities in mass rotifer culture caused by a birna-like virus, have been seen. It is possible that viral transmission to certain fish species may occur, explaining poor fish larval survival rates in some hatcheries.

Distended gut syndrome (DGS)

Sometimes sea-bream larvae are unable to digest rotifers and *Artemia* nauplii, and develop a swollen abdomen. They exhibit a disoriented spinning motion and are swept passively with the current. A viral agent is suspected and virus-like particles, 80 nm in diameter, have been found in the cytoplasm of necrotic cells in the mid-gut wall.

Sea-bream papilloma

A virus-like form in the cells of a benign maxillary neoplasm of gilthead sea-bream in Spain has been suggested as the agent of the 'sea-bream papilloma'. The tumour-like lesions are papillomatous in appearance and fibroepithelial histologically, with an intact basement membrane. There is no evidence of metastasis or interference with feeding.

Bacterial Infections

The major bacterial pathogens are shown in Fig. 23.6.

Vibrio spp.

Vibriosis is one of the more serious problems in marine fish. To date seven species of *Vibrio* have been considered as fish pathogens: *V. anguillarum*, *V. ordalii*, *V. alginolyticus*, *V. carcharidae*, *V. cholerae* no. 01, *V. damsela* and *V. vulnificus*. Diseases they cause manifest themselves as an ulcerative haemorrhagic septicaemia. In sea-bream in warm-water conditions (20–28°C), injury from handling is the primary factor in the aetiology of acute septicaemia by non-specific *Vibrio* spp.

In lower temperatures, chronic integumental or systemic infections cause adverse growth conditions in sea-bream and sea-bass. These chronic infections (unlike the acute form) are often associated with specific clinical symptoms. Infected fish are inactive, lethargic, torpid, dark in colour, and

MAJOR BACTERIAL PATHOGENS	
Vibrionaceae	Vibrio anguillarum, V.ordalii, V. alginolyticus, V.damsela Aeromonas spp.
Pasteurellaceae	Pasteurella piscicida
Enterobacteriaceae	Edwardsiella ictaluri
Pseudomonadaceae	Pseudomonas spp.
Cytophagaceae	Chondrococcus spp.
Mycobacteriaceae	Mycobacterium marinum

FIG. 23.6 Major bacterial pathogens of sea-bass and sea-bream.

suffer scale loss. Ecchymoses, petechiae and dermal haemorrhages are visible between the scales on the head, the ventral side of the body, the base of the fins and mainly around the injuries. Skin lesions quickly form ulcers that lead to distinct gradation of the skin and expose the underlying skeletal muscle, while tail and fins begin to fray.

Internally, congestion and haemorrhages of the liver, spleen, kidney, peritoneum, swim-bladder and intestinal wall capillaries could lead to the formation of necrotic lesions. Plasmid-mediated toxins are responsible for the swollen viscera and the haemorrhages. The intestine (mainly the rectum) are often extended and full of clear mucoid liquid. The gall bladder is also extended and full of bile. Finally, anaemia is usually in evidence.

V. alginolyticus has been isolated from the fish meal used to make pelleted feed, which may be significant for the disease's epidemiology. *V. anguillarum* (strain V62) has caused mortalities in hatcheries and in on-growing units on the Mediterranean coast of France, while sea-bass and turbot are very susceptible to vibriosis by *V. anguillarum* (strain 408), which is used for vaccine production. *V. damsela* has been isolated from mortalities in stressed sea-bream juveniles in Spain.

Aeromonas spp. and Pseudomonas spp.

These species cause dermal and sub-dermal lesions, like deep ulcers filled with yellowish exudate, in the interorbital region of moribund mature sea-bream. Histopathologically, a typical chronic inflammatory response is present with extreme proliferation of macrophages and lymphocytes, haemorrhages and focal necrosis.

Chronic infections by non-specific *Vibrio* spp. and *Pseudomonas* spp. also seem to cause a distinct syndrome with white coloration of the head (white head disease) in Israel. Haemorrhagic inflammation of the cephalic branches of the lateral line and integumental necrosis are the main clinical signs.

It has been reported that Vibrionaceae predominate in the necrotic tissue of the Mediterranean marine fish while Pseudomonadaceae predominate in the necrotic tissue in Atlantic marine fish.

Pasteurella piscicida

Pasteurellosis or pseudotuberculosis has recently become a serious problem in sea-bass culture and it develops in an acute and a chronic form. The acute form of the disease affects fish in the first year, causing darkening, anorexia and high mortalities. During the chronic form, lower mortalities occur and white granulomata visible to the naked eye are found mainly in the spleen. There is evidence that carriers under stressful conditions could suffer from reinfection.

Edwardsiella sp.

High mortality levels due to *Edwardsiella ictaluri* have been reported in Spain in sea-bass 2–3 months old.

Myxobacteria (flexibacter *spp.*)

Myxobacteria are long, thin, flexible bacteria showing oscillating or gliding movement and can only be diagnosed by examination of fresh smears. They demonstrate the typical movement in fish-muscle/seawater broth, but grow poorly on solid and semi-solid media.

Myxobacteria have been found in focal necroses of the gill filaments, coupled with dermal lesions, in high mortalities among juveniles and adult sea-bream, in Israel. This is usually after netting operations, although spontaneous infections occur occasionally. In some cases the gill rot due to Myxobacterial infection is associated with heavy infections of the monogenean parasite *Furnestia echeineis*.

Gills lose their smooth appearance and the gill filaments become frayed and covered with whitish mucous nodules or necrotic material, which develops 2–3 days after handling. Remaining filaments assume a dark brown colour.

There is an increased prevalence of myxobacterial gill infection in sea-bass with deformed opercula. Infected fish remain near the surface of the water, moving to the edge of the holding facility; they swim aimlessly and slowly and the opercula may not close normally.

Fungal Diseases

Ichthyophonus hoferi

Ichthyophonus hoferi is an obligate parasite of marine and freshwater fish with a complicated life-cycle. It grows between 3 and 20°C and its optimum growing temperature is 10°C.

Infection by this parasite is seen in wild and cultured sea-bass on the Spanish Mediterranean coast. Generally fish become infected orally, by swallowing the multinucleate resting spores of the fungus. In the stomach the spores release amoeboid stages that penetrate the intestinal wall and are transported to various internal organs via the blood stream. In the tissue, the parasite grows and propagates by multiple division. Well vascularised organs (liver, kidney, spleen, heart, muscles) are most frequently infected.

The host reaction depends on the fish species. Generally the parasite is encapsulated by the host tissue and its growth ceases but sometimes it releases multinucleated plasmodia that undergo division and invade the surrounding tissues, leading to the death of the host.

Signs of heavy infections are tumbling swimming movements, emaciation of the body muscle and swelling of the visceral organs.

Usually the disease is detected on necropsy, when characteristic spherical cyst stages are observed microscopically in the smears of granulomatous lesions of different organs. Granulomas involving macrophages, fibrocytes and eosinophilic granular cells are the most common lesions seen in infected sea-bass, while several stages of the fungus (endospores, resting spores, germinating spores) may be observed.

A seasonal pattern of the infection of sea-bass seems to be related to temperature. The frequency of the disease is higher in adult fish and is more prevalent in cultured fish than in the wild population.

Prevention is by removing the infected fish and avoiding contaminated fish products.

Parasitic Infections

The major parasites of sea-bass and sea-bream are classified in Fig. 23.7. Most of them are

MAJOR PARASITES	
PROTOZOA	Class: Digenea
Phylum: Sarcomastigophora	*Pycnadenoides senegalensis*
• *Amyloodinium occelatum*	*Pseudopycnadema fischathali*
• *Cryptobia* spp.	*Acanthostomum imbutiforme*
• *Colponema* spp.	*Labratrema minimus*
Phylum: *Apicomplexa*	Phylum: Aschelminthes
• *Haemogregarina* spp.	Class: Nematoda
• *Eimeria* spp.	*Contracaecum* spp.
Phylum: *Microspora*	
• *Pleistophora* spp.	**ARTHROPODA**
Phylum: *Myxozoa*	Phylum: Crustacea
• *Ceratomyxa* spp.	Order: Copepoda
• *Chloromyxum* spp.	*Ergasilus* spp.
• *Henneguya* spp.	*Colobomatus labracis*
• *Myxobolus* spp.	*Caligus minimus*
• *Kudoa* spp.	*Lernatropus kroyeri*
Phylum: Ciliophora	*Lernaelophus sultanus*
• *Cryptocaryon irritans*	*Peroderma* spp.
• *Trichodina* spp.	Order: Isopoda
• *Tripartiella* spp.	*Nerocila orbiguyi*
Phylum: Platyhelminthes	Phylum: Acanthocephala
Class: Monogenea	*Colvanacanthus blennii*
• *Microcotyle chrysophrii*	Phylum: Annelida
• *Microcotyle labracis*	Class: Hirudinea
• *Polylabris tubicirrus*	*Tracheobdella lubrica*
• *Diplectanum aequans*	
• *Furnestia echeneis*	
• *Epibdella melleni*	
• *Lambellodiscus* spp.	

Fig. 23.7 Major parasitic infections of sea-bass and sea-bream.

considered in more detail here, in the order shown in the table, beginning with the protozoa.

Amyloodinium occelatum

This thermophilic, euryhaline diflagellate is one of the most pathogenic fish parasites. Its proliferation has resulted in high levels of mortality for post-larvae and adult sea-bream in France and Israel. There are also reports of numerous mortalities in sea-bass in Israel and in the North Adriatic region of Italy.

Heavily infected fish 'scratch' their skin on solid objects. In heavy gill infections, fish congregate at the water surface gasping for air.

Cryptobia *spp.*

Chronic mortalities caused by this flagellate have been described in sea-bream in saltwater concrete tanks in France. The parasites are attached to the gill filaments by their posterior flagellum,

producing focal erosion on the gill epithelium. Infestations are located predominantly on the gills and on the mucosal integument of fingerlings, yearlings and breeders; but the infection shows only skin prevalence in larvae and post-larvae of sea-bream in hatcheries.

Vacuolar degeneration of the cells penetrated by the parasites, with cloudy swelling of the surrounding epithelial cells, is followed by hyperplasia of the entire epithelium of the gill filaments, with consequent fusion of the lamellae.

Colponema spp. are also flagellate parasites which infect the gills of both wild and farmed populations of sea-bass and sea-bream in France and Israel, but are not widely seen.

Eimeria *spp.*

Among the coccidians, two new species of *Eimeria* have been reported in sea-bass: *E. bouxi* and *E. dicentrarchi*. General signs of coccidiosis include emaciation, lethargy and perhaps mortalities;

internal signs include white blisters on the intestinal walls, swollen intestines full of fluid, light-coloured faeces and oocysts. Diagnosis is based on oocyst observations in intestinal scrapings or faecal smears viewed at magnifications of 200–400×. The only available treatment for fish coccidia is with coccidiostats used for higher vertebrates.

A benign *Haemogregarina* has been described in sea-bream and the cystozoite stage of the parasite has been identified in the viscera of the fish.

Microspora

Pleistophora senegalensis parasitises sea-bream off the coast of Senegal. The lesions are small, whitish nodules on the gut wall, full of oval pyriform spores. There is no therapy for microsporidiasis but quarantine and restriction of movements will reduce the possible spread of the pathogen.

Myxosporea

Infection by *Kudoa* spp. in the kidney of sea-bream causes massive structural damage on 85% of the glomeruli but no changes in the surrounding haematopoietic tissue. Additional cysts are present in the peritoneum and in the gut mesenteries.

Infection by *Chloromyxum* spp. is seen in the cardiac and pyloric region of the stomach of sea-bream. The coelozoic and histozoic stages of the parasite cause hypertrophy, degeneration and deformity of the epithelial cells of the gastric mucosa.

Infections by *Myxobolus* and *Henneguya* spp. have been reported in sea-bass; there is no encystment reaction.

It is believed that these myxozoan infections (which also include *Ceratomyxa* spp.) are introduced into the culture system by wild fish.

Cryptocaryasis

Cryptocaryon irritans is widespread in subtropical and tropical seas and has been found infecting farmed on-growing sea-bream but not in hatchery fish. It is the marine counterpart of *Ichthyophthirius multifiliis* and is the cause of white spot disease.

The growing stage (trophont) burrows under the skin and gill surface of the fish, feeding on tissue debris and body fluids and forming white nodules up to 1 mm in diameter, visible to the naked eye. Under the microscope, the permanent rotating movement and characteristic horseshoe-shaped macronucleus of the parasite can be seen.

The organism drops off the fish, encysts and produces several hundred swarmers (tomites) by binary fission. The tomites actively attach to new hosts. Mass infection can lead to extensive skin necrosis.

Recent studies in the eastern Mediterranean have identified a new ciliate species distinct from *C. irritans* in its ecology and pathogenesis. It causes mass mortalities in sea-bream and tends to migrate more actively, digging tunnels within the epithelium and encysting individually without forming the former's characteristic tomont 'carpets'.

Trichodiniasis

Trichodinids are a major ectoparasitic problem in fry and fingerlings of sea-bass and sea-bream in Israel, France and Italy. Infected fish often have a greyish sheen due to excess mucus production, while the fins may become frayed and there may be epithelium erosion. Common indications of the disease include loss of appetite, listlessness, or signs of anoxia (badly affected gills), darkening, gill and dermal irritation with epithelial hyperplasia. Diagnosis is based on microscopic observation of mounts of material from the skin, fins and gills.

Epitheliocystis

This widespread chronic infection can be very pathogenic, mainly to juveniles in nurseries. Epitheliocystis organisms are intercellular prokaryotes affecting skin epithelial and gill chloride and epithelial cells, causing cell hypertrophy and the formation of distinct transparent capsules (0.3–0.5×0.5–1.0 μ) on the gill filaments and within the skin epithelium. The gills swell and lose their lamellae structure. It has been suggested that the aetiological agent is a chlamydial organism and its pleomorphic developmental cycle has been described.

Two degrees of severity are recognised. In the

chronic 'benign' condition, which is widespread under natural and cultured conditions, gill infection leads to limited tissue response with thin epithelial envelope around the developing capsule. The 'proliferative' condition is an extreme epithelial hyperplasia that leads to impairment of the gill's respiratory capacity and is accompanied by heavy mortalities.

Young hatchery-propagated sea-bream are retarded in growth, with some showing opercular cover deformations. Clinical signs of moribund fish are lethargy, lying near the surface, distended opercular cover and rapid respiration.

A defence mechanism (probably of an immunological nature) seems to prevent hyperinfection in wild fish populations but in hatchery-bred fish this mechanism seems to be debilitated (due to hereditary or environmental factors during egg or post-natal stages) and this leads to high levels of mortality. The disease can be transmitted by contamination of nets and other fish culture appliances.

In order to avoid confusion with lymphocystis, it should be noted that the latter disease results in enlarged cells; it seldom, if ever, involves the gills and it does not occur in salmonids, ictalurids or cyprinids, all of which are susceptible to epitheliocystis.

Monogenea

Gill fluke infections by monogenean parasites are considered to be of major importance in fry and fingerling culture, leading to lethargy and loss of appetite, with the fish swimming near the surface. The parasites, which can be observed with the naked eye, are of several species.

Gyrodactylus spp. (small viviparous flukes, rarely more than 0.4 mm in length) are usually located on the skin rather than the gills. They have caused epizootics in the early life stage of wild sea-bream and sea-bass fry and fingerlings in Israel. *Dactylogyrus* spp. are the true gill flukes and have been reported as major ectoparasites of sea-bream and sea-bass in Italy.

Furnestia echeineis has been reported in both wild and cultured populations of sea-bream in Israel and in cultured sea-bream in France. Heavy infections on the gills and the inner opercular integument of juvenile fish lead to myxobacterial

infection (gill rot) and mass mortalities in the final stage. This parasite in combination with epitheliocystis often causes high mortalities in hatcheries; with trichodinids it causes epizootics in nursery fish.

Diplectanum aequans is another monogenean gill parasite causing mortalities in sea-bass yearlings in Israel and France. It has a winter seasonality and causes proliferative reactions of epithelial cells in the infected gills. It is difficult to treat and prophylactic measures must be adopted. Formalin treatment (375 ppm) for one hour has been found effective against only the juvenile stages of the parasite.

Microtyle chrysophrii has been reported as a gill parasite of sea-bream in France, Israel and Italy, and *M. labrachis* in France and Italy (generally parasitising adult sea-bass only in the open sea).

Epibdella melleni, a tropical monogenean parasite with low specificity, has infected sea-bass reared in sea cages in Martinique. Recent research indicates the importance of parasite transference to a cultured species which is not a natural host in wild populations; for example, in Corsica in 1982 heavy mortalities in sea-bream were reported to be due to *Polylabris tubicirrus*, a species previously reported only on sparidae of the genus *Diplodus*.

Digenea

Digenetic trematodes are often abundant parasites of the alimentary canal. They have indirect life-cycles, with a mollusc as an intermediate host. The infective stage swims actively and enters the final host orally or through the integument. Large numbers of the metacercariae of bucephalid trematodes and heterophyids survive for a long time in the liver, mesenteries and muscles of sea-bream fingerlings. Adult trematodes, when abundant in the gut, cause inflammation of the intestinal wall. Infection of the mid-gut of sea-bass by *Acanthostomum inbutiforme* has caused enteritis. Distomatosis occurs commonly in the Mediterranean lagoons. There have been reports of *Labratrema minimus* metacercariae in the liver of sea-bream.

Metacercariae look like black spots in the skin (due to melanin deposition) while in the viscera they look like whitish-yellow spots, less than 1 mm in diameter, and their identification is extremely difficult.

Wild populations are known to be important in parasitic infections by digeneans. For example, the digenetic helminth *Pycnadenoides senegalensis*, a parasite of the wild sparidae of the western Mediterranean, has infected cultured sea-bream in France.

Acanthocephala

Besides being infected by trematode metacercariae, wild fry entering the lagoons are often found to be infected by ubiquitous larvae helminths such as *Colvanacanthus blenii*. These acanthocephalids are elongated cylindrical worms ('spiny' worms) with an indirect life-cycle.

Crustacea

Most of the important crustacean species infecting sea-bass and sea-bream belong to the subclass Copepoda.

Ergasilus spp. are one of the more important ectoparasites of the euryhaline species in Italy. Despite their small size, they can become very harmful by colonising the skin and fins. Their typical habitat is the gills; the females cause damage and erosion of the gill epithelium due to their attachments and feeding activities, but the males are not parasitic. *E. labrachis* infects seabass mainly in brackish waters.

Caligus minimus and *Colobomatus labrachis* are gill parasites of sea-bass in cage culture in France, Israel, Tunisia and Italy. *Caligus* is an almost exclusively marine organism and one of the most dangerous copepod fish parasites.

Lernatropus kroyeri, a haematophagus copepod gill parasite of sea-bass, has been reported in France.

Some of the crustacean parasites are isopods, such as the haematophagus *Nerocilia orbiguyi* which has been reported in Corsica as causing gradual emaciation and hyperochromic macrocytic anaemia in sea-bass. As well as their haematophagus action, isopod gill parasites destroy the host tissue and seriously reduce the respiratory surface of the gills.

Several organophosphate compounds are effective against copepod and isopod parasites. Aeration during the treatment is essential.

Hirudinea

These annelids are leeches: they are segmented parasites with anterior and posterior suckers. In Italy, high mortalities caused by *Tracheolobdella lubrica* have been described in sea-bass in brackish water. The leech attaches to fins, branchial opercula, eyes and head, and even inside the mouth. Its control is very difficult in large areas of brackish water. It has been suggested that the primary factor is very low salinity levels in the water.

Miscellaneous Diseases

Non-functional swim-bladder

The inflation of the swim-bladder occurs in two stages. Initial inflation in 5 mm sea-bass larvae (7 days old) and in 4 mm sea-bream larvae (around 5 days old), coincides with oil globule resorption. When initial inflation fails, swim-bladder development stops. The second stage is expansion: the swim-bladder stretches backwards until it becomes stable in 40–50 mm fish (20–30% of the total length).

The initial inflation of the swim-bladder in gilthead sea-bream is triggered by gulping air at the surface. The presence of an oily surface film or excessive turbulence in the rearing tank inhibits inflation by blocking the larvae's access to the surface.

Lack of inflation can result in up to 80% postlarvae having non-functional swim-bladders; and also weighing 20–30% less than the normal fry.

A selective mortality of fry with non-functional swim-bladders can occur during weaning due to stress during handling or hypoxic conditions. Radiography of dead fry has shown that 86–100% of these had non-functional swim-bladders.

Swim-bladder hypertrophy

A critical phase in sea-bass culture is the transformation from post-larva to juvenile. Mass mortality in this phase is associated with swimbladder hypertrophy, which is related to nutritional deficiencies (ascorbic acid, B6 deficiencies) and environmental stressors, and is combined with problems during weaning.

Deformities

The cause of larval and post-larval deformities in sea-bream and sea-bass has yet to be determined. Nutritional, genetic and environmental aetiologies have been suggested. The increased rate of abnormalities under optimal culture conditions is primarily due to complete elimination of natural selection. The majority of abnormalities that appear in larvae (0–40 days) are lethal, while those apparent in post-larvae (after 40 days) do not interfere with survival.

The most common abnormalities or deformities are:

* Spinal cord abnormalities (lordosis, scoliosis).
* Mouth deformities.
* Operculum and gill arch abnormalities.
* Dysfunction of swim-bladder.
* Exophthalmus ('eye ball disease').

Asymmetric deformities of paired organs may be due to prenatal causes, a stress effect on incubated eggs, or the adverse effect on broodstock fish during vitellogenesis. Neonatal abnormalities potentially originate from polyploidy or aneuploidy, due to thermal shocks, radiation, chemical factors or by interspecific hybridisation.

Lordosis

Lordosis is an irreversible deformity of the vertebral column which occurs from the 40th day post-hatch. Possible causes include lack of swim-bladder, dietary deficiencies during the zooplanktonic phase, congenital aetiology and excessive levels of heavy metals (cadmium, copper) in the fry diet. Affected fish are dark in colour, have difficulty in swimming, remain on the surface and die in a short period.

White stripe disease

Traces of chlorine in tap water in hatcheries seem to play a significant role in the formation of an integumental dysplasia in the dorsal and anal fins of sea-bream larvae. This condition is termed 'white stripe disease' due to the pale white coloration of the fins.

Tumours

Ameloblastic-fibro-odontoma is an enlarged rounded tumour with a sand-paper surface on the anterior end of the lips of sea-bream.

Spontaneous branchial osteochondroma is a benign tumour of adult sea-bream that involves the gill arch and numerous gill rays. Death is caused by the tumour's interference with breathing, respiration, osmoregulation and excretion of nitrogenous waste products.

Swim-bladder abnormalities due to teratomic tumour of the gas gland have been linked with skeletal abnormalities in sea-bream. This tumour, appearing after hatching, is yellow and occupies the entire space within the swim-bladder.

Cannibalism

Cannibalism is a major problem causing considerable mortalities in post-metamorphosis sea-bass. It seems to be induced by overcrowding of fingerlings, inadequate food supply and delayed morning feeding. Rapid transfer from *Artemia* to commercial feeds promotes cannibalism and differential growth. Feeding method, quantity, quality, particle size and distribution are important factors.

Competition in fingerlings leads to a feeding hierarchy which promotes size differences. Cannibalism is size-related: the predator must be twice the length of the victim. With such size differentiation, any decrease in food supply triggers dramatic cannibalistic behaviour with high losses.

In order to reduce cannibalism in sea-bass fingerlings, special attention has to be paid to feeding techniques and distribution. Size grading must be carried out as early as possible (by 50–60 days) and then frequently thereafter. The smallest fingerlings have to continue on a live diet, gradually adapting to artificial feeds.

Sunburn

Sunburn can occur during summer in surface swimming fish (especially a problem in floating cages) but can be induced even in bottom dwellers feeding on photodynamic drugs such as phenothiazine, despite the fact that ultraviolet light penetrates poorly into water. The problem can be solved by avoiding these agents in the feeds, and providing artificial shade over the sea cage.

Diet-related Diseases

Systemic granuloma

Systemic granuloma is an acute and chronic granulomatous disease that causes high mortalities in cultured sea-bream. Although the agent has yet to be identified, the disease has dietary and biochemical metabolic aetiology. Usually it occurs in O+ group fish fed certain types of fish meal, or frozen fish, subject to prolonged storage. Possibly the high fatty acid content of the diet has a significant role.

Initially the pathological signs develop in the kidney. The main pathological signs of the acute form of disease are tyrosinaemia and degeneration and necrosis in the epithelium of the renal tubules due to crystalline tyrosine accumulation in the kidney. Macrophage-like cells accumulate in the collapsed tubules, forming an epitheloid granuloma. The melano-macrophage centres have a significant role in this inflammatory response. Biochemical analysis indicates no evidence of failure of the tyrosine catabolic enzyme system.

Fish that survive the early acute stage develop an extreme visceral granuloma with extreme hypertrophy, gradual fibrosis and necrosis of the kidney and spleen, while blood tyrosine levels decline and crystalline deposits in the kidney disappear, suggesting a different aetiology of the chronic phase. However, autoimmune or hypersensitivity response mechanisms have yet to be proved.

In severe conditions granulomatous lesions spread to the liver, mesenteries, pericard and epicard. White nodules are found at the base of the fins or on the fin rays.

A characteristic sign of the chronic stage is a crystalline cloudy sedimentation in the anterior eye chamber, resulting in irreversible and extreme deformity of the iris, pupil and lens. At this stage death usually occurs, either due to secondary bacterial septicaemia or, more frequently, due to cannibalistic attacks.

Prevention of the disease is possible by avoiding 'spoiled' feeds and changing to 'fresh' fish, which significantly reduces incidence of the disease.

Lipoid liver degeneration (yellow disease)

In cultured red sea-bream in Japan, feeds spoiled by prolonged storage and full of rancid fats seem to cause a syndrome which is characterised by accumulation of lipofuscin or ceroid on the hepatocytes. The liver appears swollen and bronzed with rounded edges while extreme anaemia with concomitant pallor of the gills are significant clinical signs.

Fatty livers

'Fatty livers' are often seen in farmed sea-bream and sea-bass because of improperly balanced diets. This syndrome is caused by over-storage of lipids in the hepatocytes which leads to vacuolisation, atrophy and degeneration of these cells with partial displacement of the liver by adipose tissue. There is also biliary congestion, retarded growth, gradual emaciation, lethargy and, occasionally, dermal lesions. It is important to discover whether liver modifications, due to artificial feeding, are simply a reaction to imbalanced feeding or a true nutritional pathological process.

Intestinal steatosis

Artificial feeds seem to cause a form of intestinal steatosis in cultured sea-bass mainly in the postvalvular intestine (which is involved in protein macromolecule absorption). Abundant lipid droplets accumulate in the intestine's epithelial cells, and lipid granules are found in the interenterocytic spaces and in the lamina propria. Lipid overloading within the mucosa leads to injuries ranging from a simple impairment of enterocytic striated border to cellular necrosis and abrasion.

Broken neck syndrome

This new syndrome in sea-bass is of uncertain aetiology. The dominant symptom observed is the separation of the head from the body in the isthmus region, which leads to mass mortalities.

Affected fish, 1–2 years old, display a spectrum of symptoms within a month. The first symptoms are darkening and inappetence, usually accompanied by lipoid liver degeneration due to hepatic lipase inactivation. A period of erratic and unco-ordinated swimming at the surface is followed by sinking to the bottom of the net. At this stage external signs include fin erosions, and haemorrhages at the fin's base, on the skin, the opercula and at the base of the head. Anaemic gills indicate severe anaemia.

Finally there is a total loss of equilibrium with the fish lying on the bottom of the holding facility with atrophy and disconnection of the muscles in the isthmus region. This myopathy, accompanied by an increase in transaminase activity, is a progressive tetanic condition and is probably a consequence of hepatic damage. At this stage high mortalities occur.

The internal pathological signs include: abundant visceral fat; lipoid degeneration of the liver, spine and kidney; hyperaemia; empty alimentary canal; ascites; internal haemorrhages; aneurysms and epithelial hypertrophy of the gills. Radiological spine distortion with the first four cervical vertebrae bending upwards is not due to structural damage but to muscular contraction in the cephalic region.

Negative results of parasitic, bacteriological, viral and toxicity tests and the variability of symptoms suggest that the syndrome is a consequence of malnutrition or some form of deficiency. The presence of heavy metals in the feeds (lead, zinc, chromium, copper) together with vitamin C deficiency seem to be potential aetiological agents.

Vitamin Deficiencies

Ascorbic acid (vitamin C)

Ascorbic acid deficiency leads to reduction in wound-healing capacity and skeletal malformation syndrome with spinal lordosis, scoliosis, spinal fracture and opercular and gill lamellar deformity. There is a significant tendency to haemorrhages and increased susceptibility to secondary infections, all because of the related failure of collagen synthesis.

In sea-bass fingerlings, deficient diets cause reduced growth, and the affected fish display dark coloration, loss of equilibrium, sluggishness, increased susceptibility to fin rot, bleeding from the gills, short operculum, short snout, 'pop eye', short body and fragile gill filaments. Mass mortalities occur after 6 weeks.

Vitamin E

Vitamin E is linked with selenium and plays a significant role in formulated fish diets, mainly dissolved in a high concentration of unsaturated lipids. Auto-oxidation and breakdown of lipids in the diets, due to atmospheric oxygen, generates active free radicals with toxic properties. Vitamin E is a component of a complex protective system against the toxic effect of free radicals and controls the cell membrane architecture.

Supplementation of vitamins E and C in the diets of farmed sea-bass in Martinique suppressed the symptoms of darkening, skin ulceration, lethargy, anorexia, emaciation, hepatic lipoid degeneration, pancreatitis, muscular degeneration and renal atrophy caused by the feed's lipid peroxidation.

Vitamin B_6 (pyridoxine)

The main symptoms of pyridoxine deficiency in gilthead sea-bream are retarded growth, poor food conversion, hyperirritability with erratic swimming behaviour, degenerative changes in peripheral nerves, focal necrosis in the brain and in the spinal cord (scoliosis) and, consequently, high mortality levels.

Clinical Diagnosis

The methods used to diagnose diseases in sea-bass and sea-bream are the same as those described in salmonid species. Where special techniques for specific diseases of sea-bass and sea-bream are required, they have been mentioned in the Major Diseases section.

Therapy

Dose rates are not given for the majority of therapeutants in this section as there appear to be no specific recommendations for sea-bass and sea-bream. Veterinarians specialising in these species are advised to follow dosages recommended for other warm-water species and to prescribe with caution until an optimal therapeutic range is established for each antimicrobial agent.

Antibiotics

The most commonly used antibiotics are:

oxytetracycline
oxolinic acid
flumequine
trimethoprim/sulphadiazide
erythromycin.

The nitrofurans (e.g. nitrofurantoin) are potentially some of the most active drugs against fish pathogens. Quinolones (flumequine, oxolinic acid) are effective against all bacteria except *Pseudomonas* spp.

Flush treatments with nitrofurans are commonly used against acute septicaemias and gill myxobacteriasis, while in chronic conditions medicated feeds (tetracyclines or chloramphenicol) are applied. Chlamydia, for example, are sensitive to penicillin, chloramphenicol and tetracyclines. Although suitable control methodology is not available for epitheliocystis, attempts to control it by the use of chloramphenicol are described in the literature.

Sulphonamides, oxytetracycline and oxolinic acid have been used for the treatment of pasteurellosis but usually an antibiogram is necessary in order to estimate any possible strain resistance.

Antibiotic application requires continuous surveillance and the use of antibiograms prior to treatment in order to avoid drug resistance (sometimes coded by R-plasmids). There are also legislative restrictions on drug residues in fish flesh.

Fungicides

Although there are no therapeutic procedures for *Ichthyophonus hoferi* infection, the use of phenoxethol is promising for aquarium fish but only in the early stages of the disease. It should be noted that infected fish will carry the infection for life.

Parasites

Traditional treatments of parasitic diseases are based on compounds such as formalin, malachite green and acriflavine. It should be noted that the conventional flush treatment with formalin, copper sulphate or malachite green, employed to control ectoparasitic infections, is *not* effective for *Amyloodinium occelatum*: the required doses (formalin 200 ppm, or malachite green 0.5 ppm) necessary to eradicate this parasite are toxic to post-larva fish.

The tomont stage of *Amyloodinium occelatum* is very resistant to high concentrations of parasiticides: only the sporulating tomonts or the emerging offspring have been found to be susceptible to chemical treatment. Prevention of re-infection and eradication of the disease in hatchery tanks are possible with continuous treatment. Trials with 0.75 ppm copper sulphate for 14 days or 0.5 ppm for 6 days have been effective. Although copper sulphate and acriflavine are both well tolerated by fish, copper sulphate is preferred because it is cheaper and readily available.

Other antimicrobial compounds employed are

COMPOUNDS USED AGAINST FISH PARASITIC INFECTIONS	
Formalin	Main chemical for control of external parasites, although it can be toxic to fish
Organophosphates	Effective against parasitic copepods but not against monogeneans
Trichlorphon	Effective against trichodinids, crustaceans and monogeneans (*Dactylogyrus*)
Praziquantel	Tapeworms and digeneans
Toltrazuril	Coccidiostat agent effective against trichodinids, myxobolus, microsporidia, monogeneans (*Gyrodactylus* and *Dactylogyrus*)
Chloramine B, chloramine T and aureomycin	Against trichodinids
Dipterex	Against ergasilids
Ivermectin	Potentially against ergasilids

Fig. 23.8 Compounds used against parasitic infections in fish.

shown in Fig. 23.8, which suggests some of their applications. No control method has yet been found against epitheliocystis or visceral infections by myxosporans and haemogregarines.

Cryptobia

Eradication of cryptobia infection is possible within a week after fish have been treated three times in two days by lowering water salinity to 0% for 50 minutes, then gradually increasing it back to 35% over the next 2 hours.

Cryptocaryasis

The tomont stage of *Crytocaryon irritans* is also vulnerable to a rapid decrease in water salinity. Trials used for eradication of the disease have involved the following alternatives:

- Salinity reduction (0–10‰) for 3 hours, four times at 3-day intervals.
- Movement of fish to floating cages in the open sea.
- Continuous exposure to copper sulphate, which could often be toxic in therapeutic concentrations (0.5–1 ppm) is sedimented in sea water by magnesium carbonate.

Similar controls have been suggested for *Amyloodinium ocellatum*.

Trichodiniasis

Trichodinids are difficult to eradicate with chemical treatment. Improvements in husbandry are essential for successful control — prevention is the best method of control. The avoidance of overcrowding, a sufficient water flow and aeration, and a decrease in water pollutants are vital in order to prevent outbreaks of the disease. Immersion treatment for 10 minutes in sodium chloride (30 ppm) or the use of acetic acid (0.001 ppm) or formalin (0.005 mg/l) have been found effective for the eradication of trichodinids.

Monogenea

Control of monogenean parasites is possible under good husbandry conditions, balanced nutrition and the elimination of the primary cause of an increased monogenean population. Compounds used for parasite treatment include acetic acid, ammonium hydrochloride, formalin, mebendazole, trichlorphos, potassium permanganate and sodium chloride. Control of *Furnestia echeineis* infection is possible with 200 ppm formalin bath treatment for 1 hour, with supplementary application of nitrofurazone in order to avoid myxobacterial infection.

Digenea

There is no chemotherapeutic agent against digenean metacercariae. Any attempt to control the disease is based on the elimination of the intermediate hosts by the use of copper or phenolic compounds, and the removal of the adult parasites from the intestines using di-*N*-butyl tin oxide.

Prevention of Disease

The control of disease should vary with the aetiological agent, and it can be achieved in several ways:

- *Quarantine*, in order to avoid introduction of pathogens.
- *Optimal husbandry and management policies*, in order to reduce handling stress and unsuitable conditions that increase susceptibility to several pathogens and induce immunosuppression. Husbandry conditions play a major role in the manifestation of parasitic disease: under stressful conditions, ubiquitous parasites become major pathogens. However, the range of parasites introduced by wild fry into the culture system may be minimised by quarantine, by selecting the least infected class of wild fry and by disinfecting fish through flush treatment prior to their introduction. Quarantine and flush treatment are also recommended when wild spawners are employed.
- *Immunisation*. Vaccination trials against vibriosis in sea-bass by intraperitoneal injection and by bath administration have shown promising results.
- *Increase in the genetic resistance* of the fish and the use of disease-resistant stock. This is a major field of research, with considerable potential.
- *Use of chemicals* for chemoprophylaxis.

Further Reading

Journals containing articles on sea-bass and sea-bream include:
  Aquaculture
  Bulletin of the European Association of Fish Pathologists
  Journal of Fish Diseases

24

The Veterinary Approach to Game Fish

RUTH FRANCIS-FLOYD

The term 'game fish' refers to a group of fresh-water and riverine fish which are valued by sports fishermen. This group of fish includes families such as the centrarchids (bass, sunfish and crappie), striped bass and its hybrids, perch and pike (Fig. 24.1). There is some geographical variation as to where different species are grown. The centrarchids and striped bass are more common in the southern United States while the pike and perch are more common in the northern United States and Europe.

Game fish can be cultured under a variety of circumstances with different objectives by the aquaculturist. In the southern United States many landowners manage recreational ponds which are stocked for game fishing. Different stocking regimes result in different types of fishing; for example, some lakes are managed to produce trophy bass, where others might be managed to produce pan fish (e.g. sunfish). A number of federal and private ventures produce fingerlings (4–8 cm) of various species for private sale or for release into natural waters in stock enhancement programmes. Finally, the striped bass and its hybrids are gaining enormous popularity in the southern United States as food fish; they are managed intensively for maximum production of marketable food animals (0.5–1.0 kg).

Farming Systems

Recreational Pond Management

Recreational ponds are typically privately-owned ponds which have been stocked with game fish for purposes of recreational fishing (Fig. 24.2). In the southern United States recreational fishing ponds are commonly stocked with largemouth bass (*Micropterus salmoides*), bluegill (*Lepomis macrochirus*) and channel catfish (*Ictalurus punctatus*). The most prized game fish are often predators at the top of the food chain. These fish do not adapt well to prepared diets and so in many

TAXONOMIC CLASSIFICATION OF CULTURED FISH WHICH HAVE BEEN CATEGORISED AS GAME FISH			
Taxonomic family	**Common name or group**	**Common name of fish**	**Genus and species**
Centrarchidae	Bass	Largemouth bass	*Micropterus salmoides*
		Smallmouth bass	*M. dolomieui*
		Spotted bass	*M. punctulatus*
	Sunfish (bream)	Bluegill	*Lepomis macrochirus*
		Red-ear sunfish	*L. microlophus*
		Green sunfish	*L. cyanellus*
	Crappie	Black crappie	*Pomoxis nigromaculatus*
		White crappie	*P. annularis*
Percichthyiade	Temperate bass	Striped bass	*Morone saxatilis*
		White bass	*M. chrysops*
		White perch	*M. americana*
		Yellow bass	*M. mississippiensis*
Percidae	Perch	Walleye	*Stizostedion vitreum vitreum*
Esocidae	Pike	Northern pike	*Esox lucius*
		Grass pickerel	*E. americanus vermiculatus*

FIG. 24.1 Taxonomic classification of cultured game fish.

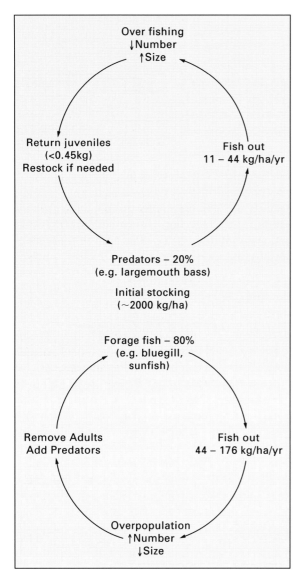

FIG. 24.2 Schematic representation of game fish management in a pond for recreational fishing.

which includes light stocking and feeding rates designed to minimise the problems of water quality and disease.

Largemouth Bass Fingerling Production

Largemouth bass will be used as the main example of game fish fingerlings produced commercially for sale to private recreational pond owners. Largemouth bass and other game fish fingerlings are also reared by fishery's biologists in federal or state hatcheries for use in stock enhancement programmes. The fingerlings may be reared either extensively or intensively (Fig. 24.3) depending on the producer's goals, facilities and resources. Extensive systems involve minimal manipulation and handling of fish; the fry are left to grow out in the same pond as broodstock. Intensive rearing involves removal of fry from the brood pond to grow out in a hatchery or rearing ponds. The advantages and disadvantages of the two systems are shown in Fig. 24.4.

Commercial Hybrid Striped Bass Production

Striped bass (*Morone saxatilis*) are riverine fish which live in marine, brackish or freshwater environments. The fish are anadromous and spawn in flowing water. Culture techniques for rearing of hybrid striped bass are summarised in Fig. 24.5. A fundamental difference in the culture of striped bass and its hybrids (Fig. 24.6) compared to many freshwater game fish is that captive spawning must be induced by hormone injection. Larval fish and fry must be provided with live food, usually brine shrimp nauplii. Once fish are classified as Phase I fingerlings (approximately 45 days of age) they can be grown out in a production pond and fed a commercial diet using methods similar to those for growing out channel catfish.

General Husbandry

Recreational Pond Management

Successful recreational pond management results from careful consideration of stocking rate and species combinations (Fig. 24.2). Stocking rates should be light enough to minimise water quality

instances smaller fish which are capable of rapid reproduction are provided as food. For optimal fishing, a balance must be maintained between predators and forage fish.

Recreational ponds are often owned and managed by individuals with little or no experience of aquaculture or pond management. Before recommending stocking rates and species combinations, it is important to determine precisely the objective of the pond owner. These ponds are often best suited for a 'hands-off' management approach problems. Oxygen depletion can be minimised by light stocking rates ($\leq$ 2000 kg/ha), the avoidance of heavy algal blooms (Secchi disc $\leq$ 45 cm), and having supplementary aeration available. Problems caused by the accumulation of nitrogen by-products, ammonia and nitrite, can be minimised by light stocking and appropriate feeding rates. Nitrite toxicity is of great concern in channel catfish but is substantially less toxic to largemouth bass.

Game fish which are most prized by sportsmen (e.g. largemouth bass) are predators at the top of the food chain. Unless they are specifically trained to accept a pelleted diet, supplemental feeding is neither necessary nor recommended. Instead, forage fish are stocked into recreational ponds as a food source for carnivores and also as 'pan fish' (i.e. suitable for frying). Common examples of forage fish in the southern United States include bluegill, sunfish and fathead minnow (*Pimephales promelas*). Proper management of zooplankton in the pond ensures an adequate food supply for them.

A recreational pond can be stocked so that approximately 60–80% of the biomass consists of forage fish. If the balance between forage species and predators is disrupted, the forage fish will increase in numbers and decrease in size, while the predators will decrease in total numbers but increase in size. Ideally, bluegill should be greater than or equal to 15 cm long, and bass should be between 0.45 and 0.90 kg. The most common reasons for imbalance between forage fish and predator populations are either improper initial stocking ratios or the removal of large predators by anglers without taking any of the forage species. The removal of 55–220 kg/ha per year is recommended from recreational ponds but no more than 20% (by weight) of these fish should be bass. Large bluegill should be removed from the pond when caught as they have a high reproductive potential and are too big to be eaten by predators. Small bass should be returned to the pond after capture.

If an increase in fish productivity is required, the pond may be fertilised to stimulate zooplankton production, increasing the food supply and therefore the biomass of bluegill. Red-ear sunfish (*L. microlophus*) can be used as an alternative or as a supplement to bluegill. Red-ear sunfish have

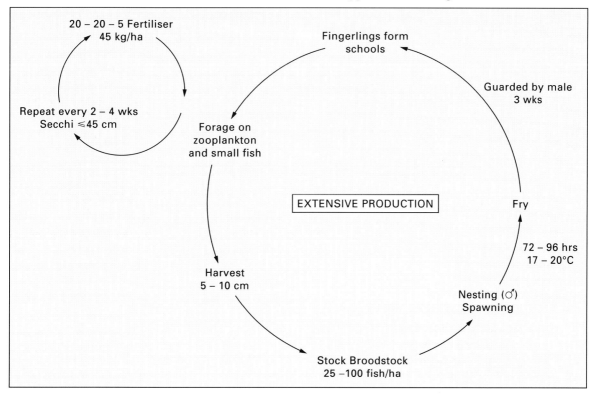

FIG. 24.3 (a) *Caption overleaf*

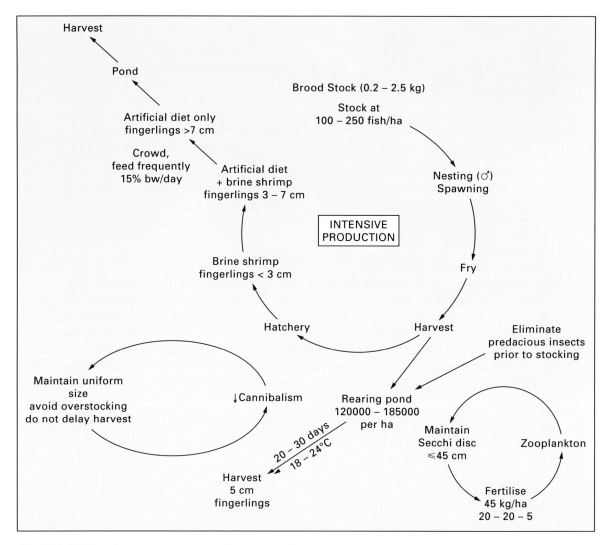

Fig. 24.3 (a) Extensive management system for largemouth bass fingerling production. Fry remain in the brood pond with the adults. (b) Intensive management system for largemouth bass fingerling production. Fry are removed from the brood pond and reared separately.

a lower reproductive rate than bluegill and consequently problems with overpopulation are less common. Bluegill fecundity declines in ponds with clear, alkaline water, ponds with low water levels, and ponds in which they are subject to excessive predation.

White and black crappie are highly prized game fish in the southern United States. They thrive when stocked into large ponds (> 0.5 ha), particularly if there is some turbidity in the water. Crappie feed on forage fish of intermediate size. If crappie are overstocked in a small pond they will overpopulate, resulting in a large population of stunted fish.

Other species used as forage fish in bass ponds include threadfin shad (*Dorosoma petenense*) in south Texas and Florida, tilapia in sub-tropical and tropical countries outside the United States, tench (*Tinca tinca*) in South Africa, and roach (*Leucisecus ritilus*) and rudd (*Scardinius erythrophthalmus*) in Europe.

Channel catfish and blue catfish (*Ictalurus furcatus*) are popular additions to game fish ponds in the southern United States. Catfish fingerlings should never be stocked into a pond containing bass of any size as few will survive to a harvestable weight. If adult catfish are already present in a

ADVANTAGES AND DISADVANTAGES OF EXTENSIVE AND INTENSIVE REARING SYSTEMS FOR LARGEMOUTH BASS FINGERLINGS		
System	**Advantages**	**Disadvantages**

Extensive	Minimal effort
	Minimal capital
		No management control over
		  number of fry produced
		Survival of young fish variable,
		  due to cannibalism by larger fish

Intensive	Ability to produce maximum
	  number of fingerlings from
	  available bloodstock
	Each stage of production is
	  completely controlled
		Cannibalism
		Intensive management of zooplankton
		  as primary food for larval fish
		Difficulty in training juvenile fish to
		  accept prepared food instead of live
		  food

FIG. 24.4 Advantages and disadvantages of extensive and intensive rearing systems for largemouth bass fingerlings.

game fish pond, spawning containers may be provided. Young catfish will provide an additional source of forage fish for bass. Brown bullhead (*Ictalurus nebulosus*) are not recommended as a forage species in game fish ponds because of their tendency to overpopulate and they may even prey upon juvenile bass.

Although largemouth bass is one of the most popular game fish in the southern United States, other species may be better suited for colder climates. Smallmouth bass (*M. dolomieui*) and chain pickerel (*Esox niger*) are good replacements for largemouth bass in the northern United States and Europe.

The most significant water quality problem which occurs in recreational sport fishing ponds is oxygen depletion. Catfish die when dissolved oxygen concentrations fall below 1.0–1.5 mg/l for any period of time. Striped bass are less tolerant of low levels of dissolved oxygen than catfish and die when oxygen concentrations reach the range of 1.3–3.7 mg/l. The largest fish in a pond are usually killed first, most frequently in the early morning. Common causes of oxygen depletion in recreational ponds include stratification and heavy algal blooms. Investment in supplemental aeration equipment should be encouraged but may not be possible in all cases.

Largemouth Bass Fingerling Production

Fingerling production of largemouth bass (Fig. 24.3) begins with broodstock management. Broodstock are moved into spawning ponds in the spring. They should be at least one year old and 200 g

but no larger than 2.5 kg. Above this size they are difficult to handle and may be less efficient in terms of egg production per unit of body-weight.

Largemouth bass may be produced extensively or intensively. Figure 24.4 compares the advantages and disadvantages of each system.

For extensive production, brood fish are stocked lightly (25–100 fish/ha) into spawning ponds. Broodstock can be sexed by insertion of a probe into the urogenital pore. In male fish the probe will stop at the urinary bladder, a short distance into the urogenital pore, and perpendicular to the ventral body wall of the fish. In females the probe can be inserted gently all the way into the ovary. Although this is the easiest and quickest method to sex broodstock it is not always reliable, particularly when fish are not in spawning condition.

Male largemouth bass create a nest in the bottom of the pond in spring when the water temperature is in the range 17–20°C. Gravel can be provided for nest construction. In Europe, partitions have been placed between piles of gravel to create individual spawning sites. These partitions act as a visual barrier and therefore decrease fighting while increasing the number of fish which can spawn in an area. Following completion of nest preparation the male encourages a female to spawn in the vicinity of the nest. After fertilisation of the eggs, he chases her from the nest and guards the eggs, which are sticky and adhere to the nesting material. Fry hatch within 72–96 hours and the male continues to guard the young fish for up to 3 weeks until they form schools and begin foraging throughout the pond.

For intensive rearing of largemouth bass fry and fingerlings, broodstock are initially stocked at

FIG. 24.5 Commercial hybrid striped bass production. A unique feature of culturing these fish is that brood-stock must be induced to spawn utilising hormone manipulation.

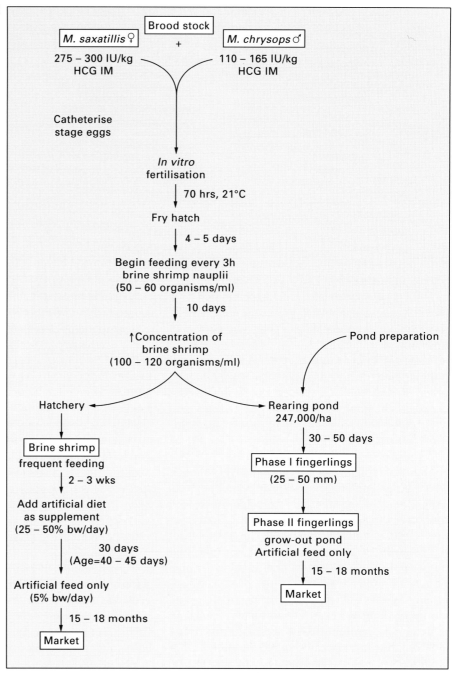

100–250 fish/ha. Nest preparation and spawning occur as described above. When fry are free-swimming they can be removed from the spawning pond with a small mesh seine or traps.

If fry are moved to a rearing pond it is important that the pond is properly prepared before stocking. The pond is fertilised by adding organic or inorganic nutrients to stimulate phytoplankton and zoo-plankton populations which are the primary food for fry and small fingerlings. A 20–20–5 fertiliser can be applied at 2–4 week intervals, or as needed, to maintain a Secchi disc reading ≤ 45 cm.

TAXONOMIC CLASSIFICATION OF STRIPED BASS HYBRIDS		
	Common name	**Species**
Temperate bass species:	Striped bass	*Morone saxatilis*
	White bass	*M. chrysops*
	White perch	*M. americana*
	Yellow bass	*M. mississippiensis*
Striped bass hybrids:		♀ ♂
Original hybrid		*M. saxatilis* x *M. chrysops*
Reciprocal hybrid	Sunshine bass	*M. chrysops* x *M. saxatilis*
White perch hybrid	Virginia bass	*M. saxatilis* x *M. americana*
Reciprocal white perch hybrid	Maryland bass	*M. americana* x *M. saxatilis*
Yellow bass hybrid	Paradise bass	*M. saxatilis* x *M. mississippiensis*

FIG 24.6 Taxonomic classification of striped bass hybrids.

Fertilisation should be initiated at least 10 days prior to the anticipated stocking date.

Because predation by carnivorous insects is an important cause of poor production, the next step is to eliminate such insects before fry are placed into the pond. Historically, a thin layer of diesel fuel was applied to the surface of a pond a few days before stocking to control predacious insects, many of which are air-breathers and were suffocated by the oil. As diesel fuel is not approved for this use in the United States, this practice is no longer recommended.

Another cause of the disappearance of fry or small fingerlings in intensive pond-rearing is cannibalism. This is exacerbated by overstocking, stocking mixed sizes of fry, inadequate food supply and delayed harvest.

Hatchery-rearing of largemouth bass fry is challenging because of the difficulty of getting young fish to accept prepared foods. Bass are carnivores. Fry and young fingerlings (<6 cm) rely on aquatic invertebrates as their primary food source; larger fingerlings (6–8 cm) prey on small frogs, crayfish and small fish. Under hatchery conditions, young fish must be trained to accept an artificial diet. Best results have been achieved in training young bass 3.0–7.0 cm long, which are crowded and fed frequently at a feeding rate of about 15%. If necessary, small amounts of ground fish can be added to the pelleted ration to encourage initial acceptance of the prepared diet. Once fish have accepted an artificial diet they may be moved to a pond.

Stocking rates for bass fry vary based on the anticipated fingerling size at harvest. Stocking rates of 120,000–185,000/ha should result in a harvest of 5 cm fingerlings within 20–30 days at water temperatures of 18–24°C. An alternative programme for the production of larger fingerlings is to stock a rearing pond with forage fish such as fathead minnow (5000/ha) followed by juvenile bass in 3–4 weeks at a stocking rate of 2500/ha. Minnow:bass ratios must be monitored if this method is to be used with maximum success. If the minnow population becomes depleted more minnows should be added. If some bass grow rapidly they should be removed to prevent losses from predation.

Commercial Hybrid Striped Bass Production

Historically, male and female striped bass have been collected from the wild just prior to spawning, and eggs and milt stripped from the fish for *in vitro* fertilisation under hatchery conditions. The larvae were often stocked into natural waters at 5–10 days of age for stock enhancement programmes. Evolution of a commercial food fish industry with these species is a relatively recent phenomenon.

Female fish can be induced to spawn by intramuscular injection of 275–300 IU human chorionic gonadotropin (HCG)/kg body-weight. Male fish can be injected with 110–165 IU/kg HCG to stimulate milt production and flow. The male and female may be left together to spawn (tank spawning method) or egg samples can be collected by catheterisation of the female to determine the best time to strip fish and fertilise eggs *in vitro*.

Tank spawning

The tank spawning method is the easiest management strategy for induced spawning of striped bass, but cannot be used to produce hybrids as the female striped bass will not voluntarily spawn in the presence of the male white bass (*M. chrysops*). To spawn striped bass using this method, the male and female are injected as described above. The fish are then placed into circular tanks (1.2–2.4 m diameter) which have a peripheral current (10–15 cm/sec). To increase the chance of a successful spawn and viable egg production, two female fish and four male fish can be placed in each tank. The adult fish should spawn 26–62 hours post-injection, after which they can be removed from the system. Eggs or larvae can be collected and placed into a smaller holding area for 2–5 days, then stocked into a rearing facility or natural waters.

In vitro *fertilisation*

In vitro fertilisation is necessary for the production of striped bass hybrids. Figure 24.6 shows the taxonomic classification of striped bass hybrids. Success is dependent upon accurate 'staging' of the eggs of the female to determine the proper time for stripping, by extracting a sample of eggs for evaluation. A catheter is placed into the ovary of the female fish (under anaesthesia) 20–30 hours after HCG injection. Gentle aspiration with a syringe attached to the end of the catheter will draw a few eggs into the tip of the instrument. They can then be examined under the microscope at low power: the nucleus of ripe eggs is centrally located.

When eggs are ready for ovulation, they can be stripped into a dry pan or bowl using gentle abdominal pressure. Milt can be added by gently squeezing the abdomen of a ripe male. Water is added, the eggs are gently mixed, and are ready for incubation. Striped bass or striped bass hybrid eggs hatch within 70 hours at water temperatures of 21°C. Fry can be stocked into rearing facilities at 2–5 days of age.

Larval fish

Larval striped bass or striped bass hybrids are raised in a hatchery until 5–10 days of age. Feeding should be initiated 4–5 days after hatching and be frequent (every 3 hours). Initially, young striped bass are fed brine shrimp nauplii in a solution of 50–60 organisms/ml, but the concentration should be increased to 100–120 organisms/ml by the time the larval fish are 15 days old.

Pond-rearing

If larval striped bass are to be pond-reared they should be stocked into a properly prepared pond at 5–10 days of age. Striped bass and striped bass hybrids are carnivorous. The larvae feed on zooplankton and as the fish grows the diet shifts to larger prey items. Larval striped bass can be stocked at rates of 247,000/ha.

Fingerlings

Within 30–50 days the fry should reach a size of 25–50 mm (0.3–1.5 g), at which stage they are termed phase I fingerlings and can be stocked directly into natural waters or stocked into grow-out ponds. They can be started on trout or salmon feed at this time and do not require a special training period to accustom them to the artificial diet.

If fingerlings are maintained in the same environment until they reach a size of 170 mm (usually late autumn or early winter) they are termed phase II fingerlings. Fish should reach market size between 15 and 18 months of age.

Intensive rearing

An alternative to pond production of striped bass and its hybrids is intensive rearing in tank or raceway systems. The principal advantages of intensive systems are that the fish farmer has precise control over the rearing system, water quality and production. Disadvantages include the need for an appropriate water supply (dependable flow, adequate quality) or an appropriate recirculating system. Intensive rearing systems require greater management skill and labour than pond production systems. Fish health management can be complicated by water quality or nutritional problems and disease outbreaks can result in catastrophic loss if mismanaged.

Feeding

Larval striped bass and phase I fingerlings require frequent feedings of live food such as brine shrimp. At 2–3 weeks of age supplemental food (either a flake or salmonid food) may be added to the diet. By 3–4 weeks of age the young fish can be weaned off the brine shrimp. Prepared food should initially be offered at very high feeding rates (25–50% body-weight/day) and divided into many feedings. When the fish reach an age of 40–45 days the feeding rate can be decreased to 5% body-weight/day.

Water quality

Water quality requirements of striped bass and its hybrids are similar to those of other warm-water fish although they are more sensitive to low oxygen conditions than some species. Low oxygen ($\leqslant 4$ mg/l) in hatching jars can result in mortality and developmental abnormalities of fry. There have been reports of restlessness, erratic swimming, bottom sitting, loss of equilibrium and death in striped bass fingerlings exposed to low oxygen conditions (1.3–3.7 mg/l): fish which succumb assume a unique posture, characterised by an arched back, open mouth and flared gills (Fig. 24.7).

Striped bass and their hybrids are euryhaline, being able to survive in fresh, brackish or sea-water systems. Larvae, however, will not tolerate salinities greater than 20 ppt until after metamorphosis. A salinity of 10 ppt is preferred for handling or shipping fish.

Striped bass are similar to other warm-water fish with regard to ammonia tolerance. They are more tolerant of ammonia when housed under brackish conditions than under either freshwater or marine conditions.

Striped bass are also similar to other warm-water fish with regard to pH tolerance, total alkalinity and total hardness. They are not as tolerant of acid conditions as some freshwater pond fish and pH below 6.6 should be avoided. Total alkalinity and total hardness should be $\geqslant$ 150 mg/l.

Light

It is important to remember that these fish are intolerant of sudden changes in light intensity. If

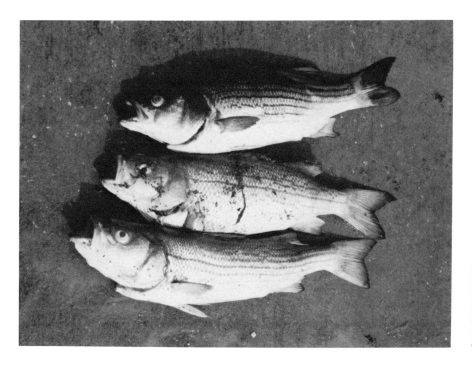

Fig. 24.7 Hybrid striped bass which have died from hypoxia. Note the unique posture characterised by arched back, open mouth, and flared gills. (Photo courtesy Dr C. E. Chichra.)

they arrive in a shipping box, the box should never be opened under direct sunlight. Fish should be stocked early in the morning (assuming adequate dissolved oxygen is present) when light intensity is low. For fish housed in indoor systems, timers should be set to bring up light intensity slowly rather than changing instantly from black dark to bright light.

National Legislation

In the United States regulations which govern ownership, production and sale of game fish differ substantially between states. In Florida, for example, it is legal to produce and sell game fish fingerlings to stock private ponds but it is unlawful to sell these animals for food. Commercial growers of striped bass or striped bass hybrids in this state must purchase a special licence to sell fish for human consumption. Carcasses must be tagged or specially packaged prior to sale. Largemouth bass, chain or red fin pickerel cannot be sold as food animals in the state of Florida.

Game fish regulation in Florida is under control of the Florida Game and Freshwater Fish Commission. Similar agencies in each state should be contacted to determine individual state laws. The Lacey Act, a federal law in the United States, in essence makes it a violation of federal law to violate state law, and this can apply to producers (sellers) of fish and buyers, even if they are in different states. Inquiries concerning federal regulations in the United States should be directed to the United States Department of the Interior, Fish and Wildlife Service.

Major Diseases

External Infections

Red sore disease

The most common disease problems encountered on game fish by recreational pond owners can be grouped under the general term 'red sore disease'. Several organisms tend to be involved in this syndrome. On bluegill the disease often begins as small foci of proliferative, haemorrhagic tissue on the tips of dorsal fin rays. A wet mount of tissue scraped from this area and examined with a light microscope under 100× and 400× often reveals colonies of the stalked protozoan, *Heteropolaria* spp., and occasionally fungal hyphae typical of *Saprolegnia* spp. The stalks of *Heteropolaria* spp. are branching and non-contractile. A similar protozoan, *Vorticella* spp., is distinguished by its contractile stalk. If lesions are limited to the tips of fin rays and there is no mortality, treatment may not be necessary. In Florida, infestations with *Heteropolaria* spp. are common on bluegill in recreational farm ponds. Usually these infections are self-limiting with little or no mortality. 'Red sore disease' occurs primarily in the spring and autumn when water temperatures are changing.

Initial lesions on the fin rays may spread to the lateral body wall, particularly the area immediately anterior to the dorsal fin or the area surrounding the insertion of the pectoral fin. Lesions in these areas tend to develop into shallow ulcers with protozoan colonies along the periphery of the ulcerated tissue. Fungal elements may infest dead or dying tissue in the centre of the lesion.

Heteropolaria spp. can cause significant problems in striped bass reared under aquaculture conditions. The problem is most serious in the summer, when water temperatures and organic material are high.

Bacterial infections

Secondary infections with opportunistic bacteria are common sequelae to protozoan infestations and can be an important component in the 'red sore disease' syndrome. *Aeromonas hydrophila* is the bacteria most commonly associated with ulcerative 'red sore disease'. *Pseudomonas fluorescens* or *P. putrefaciens* are encountered occasionally in dermal ulcers. *Chondrococcus columnaris* should be ruled out as a contributing pathogen. If *C. columnaris* is contributing to the ulcerative lesions, the ulcers are often deeper and 'dirtier' than if only *Aeromonas* or *Pseudomonas* are involved. *Edwardsiella tarda* has also been associated with ulcerative skin lesions in largemouth bass.

If bacteria are isolated only from the lesion, and if the mortality rate is low (only a few fish per day), a single treatment with potassium permanganate may be adequate to control the problem. If bacteria are isolated from viscera of dying fish, systemic treatment with an appropriate antibiotic is indicated.

Ectoparasites

Amyloodinium ocellatum is one of the most important ectoparasites which infect striped bass reared in brackish water systems (salinity $\geqslant$ 3 ppt). The organism attached to gills or skin and may give infected fish a shiny appearance which has resulted in the lay term of 'velvet disease'. Infected fish are lethargic and anorectic; mortality rates are usually high. The problem is identified by examining a wet mount of gill tissue, skin, or fin at 100× with a light microscope.

Although *Heteropolaria* and *Amyloodinium* are among the most common and significant external infections of game fish, most protozoans and ectoparasites associated with diseases of warm-water fish have been identified in game fish. Lice (*Argulus* spp.) are commonly found on the skin and *Ergasilus* spp. are commonly found on gills of largemouth bass in ponds or lakes. These seem to be of minimal clinical significance when present in low numbers and fish are not excessively crowded. Leeches are also observed occasionally in freshwater game fish. Leech infestations are usually self-limiting and associated with little or no mortality.

Internal Parasite Infections

There are several internal parasites of game fish which deserve mention.

Digenetic trematodes

Digenetic trematodes are commonly found in muscle tissue of free-ranging game fish, and occasionally in muscle tissue of striped bass or its hybrids. The two species most commonly encountered are *Clinostomum complanatum*, the yellow grub, and *Posthodiplostomum minimum*, the white grub. A less common digenetic trematode which is found in muscle tissue of largemouth bass is *Uvilifer* sp., which appears as small black spots in muscle fillets. Larval digenetic trematodes are also found in the viscera. From a production perspective the principle concern regarding the presence of these parasites is their impact on carcass quality.

Another digenetic trematode, the eye fluke *Diplostomum flexicaudum*, has been reported in the eyes of striped bass in a North Carolina hatchery. Affected fish had obvious exophthalmia, but no mortality was directly attributed to the presence of the parasite.

The life-cycle of these digenetic trematodes involves a wading bird which is the definitive host, a snail which is the first intermediate host, and the fish which is the second intermediate host. As the encysted parasite cannot be eliminated from the fish, and as wading birds are protected species (in the United States), control of the parasites involves control of snail populations. This can be achieved partially by draining, drying and harrowing the pond, and treating the soil with hydrated lime at 1000–2000 kg/ha. Snail control in full ponds which contain fish is difficult. Snail populations in Florida have been partially controlled by treating fish ponds at night (when snails are active) with an appropriate concentration of copper sulphate, which is very toxic in water of low alkalinity. Calculate the rate of application by dividing the total alkalinity (T Alk) by 100; for example, if T Alk = 100, the rate of application is 100/100, i.e. 1 mg/l.

Nematodes

Several nematodes occur in game fish. *Goezia* spp., an intestinal parasite, has been associated with mortality of cultured striped bass fed raw fish. Other nematodes observed in game fish include *Cucullanis* spp. *Philometra* spp. and *Spinitectus* spp. *Contracaecum* spp. is an encysted nematode commonly encountered in the abdominal cavity of largemouth bass. Although it may be present in large numbers, the pathogenic effect appears to be minimal.

Cestodes

A cestode, *Proteocephalus ambloplites*, commonly referred to as the bass tapeworm, has been associated with sterility of female largemouth bass. The adult tapeworm lives in the intestine of fish but the larval stages go through a copepod (first intermediate host) and the ovary of a female bass (second intermediate host). Larval migration through ovarian tissue causes sterility and the reproductive potential of female animals declines as the incidence of parasite infestation increases in a population. Direct control of the parasite is not practical, although praziquantel has proven efficacious for control of intestinal cestodes in aquarium fish. A more practical means of control is to sterilise ponds to eliminate the first intermediate host (copepod) and rear replacement stock in a hatchery where they cannot be infected as juveniles.

Acanthocephalans

Leptorhynchoides thecatus and *Neoechinorhynchus cylindratus* have been found in free-ranging largemouth bass in Florida. *Pomphorhynchus laeve* has been reported in wild caught striped bass broodstock. The clinical significance of these gut infestations is uncertain.

Systemic Diseases

Natural epizootics of *Edwardsiella tarda* and *Streptococcus* spp. have been observed in free-ranging populations of game fish in Florida. *Pasteurella piscicida* has been associated with mortality of free-ranging white perch in the Chesapeake Bay. In addition, individual fish infected systemically with *Aeromonas hydrophila* and *Pseudomonas fluorescens* have been recovered from freshwater lakes in Florida.

Systemic bacterial infections (unrelated to red sore disease) are most likely to be a cause of significant mortality when game fish are crowded or stressed by poor water quality, handling or transport. Epizootics of *Aeromonas hydrophila*, *Chondrococcus columnaris*, *Pasteurella piscicida* and *Edwardsiella tarda* have been reported in game fish reared under aquaculture conditions. Outbreaks of *Aeromonas hydrophila* are often manifested by moderate mortality, often with an acute onset following a stressful event. The disease is often characterised by the presence of ulcerative skin lesions, but skin lesions are not always seen when fish are dying from a systemic infection. Diagnosis is based on bacterial isolation from viscera.

Vibriosis

Vibriosis is reported to be one of the most significant causes of mortality of cultured striped bass. It is usually a problem in fish reared in marine or brackish water systems, although it can occur in freshwater systems. Clinical signs of vibriosis are similar to other systemic bacterial diseases. Affected fish may die in large numbers and haemorrhagic lesions may be visible externally. Diagnosis is based on isolation and identification of bacteria.

Pasteurellosis

Pasteurellosis has been reported as a devastating disease of cultured and free-ranging striped bass. Clinical signs exhibited by sick fish include changes in skin pigmentation and a swollen spleen. Catastrophic loss (80% mortality within 3 weeks) has been reported with initial mortality severe enough to justify inclusion of oxygen depletion on a differential diagnosis. Definitive diagnosis is based on isolation of the bacterium *P. piscicida*. Factors which are believed to contribute to the outbreak include high water temperatures (24–29°C), high salinity (16–22 ppt), high stocking rates (standing crop of approximately 2250–3350 kg/ha or 62,500–137,500 fish/ha), and introduction of the infection through inflowing coastal waters.

Columnaris disease

Columnaris disease, caused by the myxobacterium *Chondrococcus columnaris*, is one of the most important diseases of cultured striped bass. Early stages of the disease are external and can develop into a systemic infection if uncontrolled. Lesions associated with columnaris infections often begin on the dorsal aspect of the body and are characterised as progressive ulcerations which have irregular margins and a yellow–brown colour. Columnaris infections can be limited to gill tissue, in which case the fish appears normal except that the gill epithelium is necrotic or missing altogether. Severe cases of columnaris may be manifest by ulcers deep enough to expose the vertebral column or, if the infection is limited to the gills, the presence of bare cartilaginous gill arches.

The presence of the bacterium can be determined from wet mounts of diseased tissue and observation of typical 'haystack' colonies at 1000×. The diagnosis should be confirmed by isolation of the bacterium on Ordal's medium. Control of external infections can be achieved with potassium permanganate; however, systemic infections require antibiotic therapy, with oxytetracycline as the antibiotic of choice.

Viral diseases

Systemic viral diseases have not been problematic in cultured game fish. Lymphocystis, an iridovirus, has been reported in striped bass from the eastern United States. The author observed lesions typical of lymphocystis on the pectoral fin of a crappie caught by a sports fisherman in Mississippi. Lymphocystis lesions appear as blister-like masses on the skin or fins of affected fish. The disease is spread by ingestion of infected tissue. If lymphocystis is suspected in a population of cultured fish, affected individuals should be culled.

Infectious pancreatic necrosis (IPN) is a serious disease of salmonids. Striped bass may serve as asymptomatic carrier fish and should be tested for IPN (via a serum neutralisation test), before being stocked into natural waters or culture facilities where they are in direct contact with salmonids.

Clinical Diagnosis

Clinical evaluation of game fish can be similar to that for other warm-water fish. Skin and gill biopsies are very effective for identifying external parasites, bacteria and fungal infections.

Bacterial cultures of ulcerative skin lesions and viscera, particularly posterior kidney, are essential for identification of bacterial agents. It is important to culture both lesions and viscera in cases of 'red sore disease' to determine whether systemic antibiotic therapy is warranted. Media selected should include an all-purpose medium such as blood agar (5% ovine or bovine blood) and selective media including Ordal's for myxobacteria and Rimler–Shotts for *Aeromonas hydrophila*. Isolated bacteria can be identified using standard biochemical tests. Antibiotic sensitivity tests can be run on Mueller–Hinton agar.

Evaluation of gross and microscopic pathology should contribute to disease diagnosis in game fish as they would in any animal. Granulomas should always be tested for the presence of Mycobacteria by using an acid-fast stain, and for the presence

of fungal hyphae using an appropriate fungal stain. If branchiomyces (or other systemic fungal disease) is suspected, fungal cultures can be taken using potato dextrose agar.

Therapy

Therapy of game fish is similar to that of other warm-water fish. Bath treatments (Fig. 24.8) are effective for control of external infections. Copper sulphate, formalin and potassium permanganate seem to have similar efficacy against protozoal infestations on skin, gills and fins. Potassium permanganate seems to have a broader spectrum in its activity as it seems to be very efficacious against external fungal and bacterial (i.e. columnaris) infections which are common sequelae to parasitic damage.

Variation in salinity is an excellent means of controlling external parasitic infections if it can be done. *Heteropolaria* spp. occur in game fish housed in fresh water and are very intolerant of increases in salinity. *Amylodinium* spp., which occur in striped bass and its hybrids in marine environments, are intolerant of decreases in salinity.

Treatment of bacterial diseases should be based on antibiotic sensitivity tests if possible. In the United States there are still no antibiotics specifically approved for use in game fish. Terramycin, which contains the antibiotic oxytetracycline, is effective against many Gram-negative pathogens and is the treatment of choice for systemic columnaris infections. Romet, a potentiated sulphonamide containing sulphadimethoxine and ormetoprim, is also a broad spectrum antibiotic which is effective against many Gram-negative pathogens. Because these are the only two antibiotics presently approved for use in any food fish in the United States, it is imperative that therapy be based on sensitivity tests whenever possible to minimise the development of resistant infections.

Therapeutic decisions should be based on efficacy against the pathogen(s) identified, economic considerations and legal constraints. In many cases a change in some management practice or system design may be necessary for the permanent solution of a disease outbreak. The lack of approved drugs for game fish in the United States represents a difficult problem. Regulations which affect the use of therapeutants in aquaculture are changing

					Short-term bath		
Chemical	**Approved species**	**Approved use**	**Efficacy**	**Dip (mg/l)**	**(mg/l)**	**Duration**	**Prolonged bath**
Copper sulphate	None specified	Algicide	External parasites	500	4	30–60 minutes	Total alkalinity + 100 15–25 mg/l
Formalin	Trout Salmon Catfish Largemouth Bluegill	Parasiticide	External parasites	400	250	30–60 minutes (reduce concentration to 150 mg/l for water temperatures > 21°C)	
Potassium permanganate	None specified	Oxidiser* Detoxifier	External bacteria, fungi, parasites	1000	20	1 hour	2 mg/l
Salt	None specified	Osmo-regulatory enhancer	External parasites	30,000 for 1 hour (3%)	10,000 (1%)	1 hour	200 mg/l (0.02%)

SUMMARY OF APPROVED CHEMICALS

* No longer approved for this use in United States. Status under review by FDA.

FIG. 24.8 A summary of approved chemicals which can be applied as dips, short-term or prolonged baths.

rapidly and it is the veterinarian's responsibility to stay informed of these changes and be familiar with regulations which are in effect for the relevant industry and geographic area.

Prevention of Disease

Game fish are more sensitive to production stressors than some other food fish species which are more established. Whenever these fish are handled, care should be taken to ensure that they are maintained with adequate levels of dissolved oxygen and minimal levels of ammonia. Fish should be transported in a brackish water solution ($\sim$ 1% salt). Following handling or transport, a potassium permanganate bath may help to minimise secondary infections with columnaris or fungus, as well as remove incidental protozoal infestations. Potassium permanganate is not approved for this use in the United States.

A vibriosis vaccine has been used in salmonids to prevent vibriosis in cultured striped bass. Although this proved effective, it is not licensed for this use in the United States.

Further Reading

Amos, K. H. (Editor) (1985) *Procedures for the Detection and Identification of Certain Fish Pathogens, 3rd edn. American Fisheries Society (Fish Health Section), Bethesda, MD. 114 pp.*

Harrell, R. H., Kerby, J. H. and Minton, R. V. (1990) *Culture and Propagation of Striped Bass and its Hybrids,* pp. 79–98. American Fisheries Society, (Striped Bass Committee, Southern Division), Bethesda, MD.

McCraren, J. P. (Editor) (1984) *The Aquaculture of Striped Bass: A Proceedings,* pp. 177–204. Maryland Sea Grant Publication UM-SG-MAP-84-01. University of Maryland, College Park, MD.

Schnick, R. A., Meyer, F. P. and Gray D. L. (1989) *A Guide to Approved Chemicals in Fish Production and Fishery Resource Management.* University of Arkansas Cooperative Extension Service, Little Rock, AR. 27 pp.

Shotts, E. B., Jr and Rimler, R. (1973) Medium for the isolation of *Aeromonas hydrophila.* Applied Microbiology **26,** 550–553.

Stickney, R. R. (1979) *Principles of Warmwater Aquaculture.* John Wiley and Sons, New York, NY. 375 pp.

Stickney, R. R. (1986) *Culture of Non-salmonid Freshwater Fishes.* CRC Press, New York, NY. 440 pp.

Williams, J. E., Sandifer, P. A. and Lindbergh, J. M. (1981) Net-pen culture of striped bass × white bass hybrids in estuarine waters of South Carolina: a pilot study. *Journal of World Mariculture Society* **12**(2), 98–110.

Appendix I
Norwegian Legislation

A number of regulations and circulars are published by the Norwegian government. The numbers refer to codes used in the Norwegian Veterinary Manual. The Provisional Act of 22 June 1990 — Diseases of Aquatic Organisms — has the code 727.000.

701.00 Regulations concerning notification procedures to be followed by veterinarians for Groups A, B and C diseases.

702.290 Circular on the requisition of medicines for fish.

702.291 Circular on the stocking of medicated feed and medicated concentrates by veterinarians.

727.020 List of diseases covered by the Diseases in Aquatic Organisms Act.

727.041 Circular concerning guidelines for the monitoring of fish health status on premises cultivating fish for stocking purposes.

727.045 Circular concerning certificates of health and origin for live freshwater fish and eggs from premises cultivating fish for stocking purposes.

727.100 Diseases in aquatic organisms regulations.

727.110 Regulations delimiting the region to be designated as affected by furunculosis, and preventive measures to be applied.

727.120 Circular concerning the prevention and control of furunculosis.

727.200 Regulations concerning the vaccination of freshwater fish.

727.300 Regulations concerning the slaughtering of fish.

727.310 Regulations concerning the handling of fish waste.

727.400 Regulations concerning the disinfection of fish farms etc.

727.405 Code of hygienic practice for fish farms.

727.420 Regulations concerning the disinfection of inlet water supplying premises on which aquatic organisms are raised.

727.421 Instructions to the designated competent body approving the disinfection plant for inlet water supplying premises on which aquatic organisms are raised.

727.500 Regulations concerning the catching of freshwater crayfish.

727.700 Regulations concerning the transport of freshwater fish.

727.800 Circular concerning the killing of fish which are to be destroyed.

In addition, code 750.000 (The Animal Welfare Act) will apply to fish.

Appendix II

APPENDIX 2: USEFUL CONVERSIONS OR EQUIVALENTS	
Volume equivalent units	
1 cubic centimetre (cm^3)	= 1 ml
	= 1 g water at 4°C
1 cubic metre (m^3)	= 219.9 gallon (gal)
	= 1000 litres
1 millilitre (ml)	= 1 cm^3
	= 0.001 litres
1 litre (1)	= 1000 ml
	= 1000 cm^3
	= 0.264 gallon
1 percent solution (1%)	= 10 ml per litre
	= 1 g per 100 ml
	= 38 g per gallon
1 cubic foot (ft^3)	= 28.316 litres
	= 7.48 gallons
1 gallon (Imp gal)	= 4.55 litres
1 acre foot	= 1 acre of surface area 1 foot deep
	= 43,560 ft^3
Weight equivalent units	
1 microgram (µg)	= 0.001 mg
1 milligram (mg)	= 0.001 g
1 gram (g)	= 1000 mg
1 kilogram (kg)	= 1000 g
1 tonne, metric	= 1000 kg
1 ounce (oz)	= 28.35 g
1 pound (lb)	= 453.6 g
Linear equivalent units	
1 centimetre (cm)	= 0.394 inch (in)
1 metre (m)	= 100 cm
1 inch (in)	= 2.54 cm
1 square foot (ft^2)	= 930 cm^2
1 hectare (ha)	= 2.47 acres
1 acre (A)	= 0.405 hectare
Rates of flow	
1 litre per second	= 13.2 gallons per min
1 gallon per hour	= 1.26 ml per sec
1 million gallons per day	= 694 gallons per min
1 gallon per minute	= 0.00268 ft^2 per sec
1 cubic foot per second	= 449 gallons per min
Temperature conversions	
Celsius (°C)	= (Fahrenheit - 32) x 5/9
Fahrenheit (°F)	= (Celsius x 9/5) + 32

Index

Abdominal cavity, dissection   76
Abdominal swelling, common sign of disease   91
Acanthocephala parasites   126–127, 406
Acanthostomum inbutiforme infection, sea-bass   387
Acid rain   62–63, 93, 181, 182
Acid–base balance, gill involvement   6
Acinebacter spp. infection, eels   318
Acriflavine treatment   319, 376
Additives, to feedstuffs   174–175
Administration methods
   for anaesthetics   162
   for antibacterials   145–147, 212–213
   in sea cages   137
   for treatment compounds   132–133, 211–213
   for vaccines   143, 144
   via the food   144–151, 374–375
   via the water   131–143, 135–143, 292–293, 374
Aeration
   in anaesthesia   162, 164
   aquarium systems   360
   during transport   171, 219, 254–255
   in eel recirculation systems   314
   equipment   50
   need for   58
   in prawn culture   278, 280, 295
   seasonal variation   194
   in treatment   131, 132, 134, 137, 336
   turbot culture   330
Aeromonas spp.
   cause disease other than furunculosis   233
   clinical diagnosis   308
   and furunculosis   102
   identification   83–84
   MIC data   147, 149, 150, 152–153, 153
   opportunist pathogens   104
   virulence   234
Aeromonas spp. infection
   in Atlantic salmon in Scotland   200
   bacteriology   259
   in carp   301–302
   in channel catfish   259
   clinical signs   259
   co-trimazine treatment   148
   in cod   352

   control   104
   in eels   316, 318, 319
   in game fish   404, 406
   in ornamental fish   364
      vaccination   377
   in prawns   287
   in rainbow trout   233
   Romet treatment   150
   in salmonid hatcheries   31
   sarafloxacin hydrochloride treatment   150
   in sea-bass and sea-bream   383–384
   stress testing   38
   stress-induced   66
   testing for   210
   in turbot   333
Aflatoxin   96, 98, 109, 241
Airlift system, for mortality removals   34
Alarm systems   55
Albendazole   186
Alevins, development   44
Algae
   direct toxicity   59
   as prawn feed   294
   as starter feed   155
Algal blooms   32, 59, 95, 205, 228
   in aquarium systems   361
   in Atlantic salmon culture   199
   in Norwegian fish farms   183
   in prawn culture   283, 295
   in recreational ponds   399
   and temperature stratification   64
   in turbot culture   334
Algal derivatives, as immunostimulant   153
Alimentary tract examination   75
Alkalinity, diurnal variation   63
Alteromonas spp. infection, turbot   333
Aluminium   65, 93, 181, 182, 227
Amino acid requirements   96, 156
Ammonia
   causes gill damage   57, 60, 106
   and channel catfish   265
   effect on oxygen uptake   59
   as metabolic waste product   6, 30, 60–61, 94
   as nitrogen source for plants   60
   and parasitic disease   110

Ammonia—*continued*
  safe levels   61, 218, 227
  and striped bass   403
  toxicity   182
    for carp   307
Ammunition cans, as spawning containers   253
Amoebae, parasitic   111, 115
Amoxycillin
  dosage   147, 213
  MIC data   147
  in ornamental fish treatment   374
  resistance to   147
  in yellowtail treatment   147
Amyloodinium spp. infection   112
  in game fish   405, 407
  in ornamental fish   366
  in sea-bass and sea-bream   385
    treatment   392, 393
Anadromy   13, 223
Anaemia   59, 77, 263–264, 366
Anaesthesia   161–167
  in eels   325
  in halibut   344
  need for   161, 170, 218, 220
  non-chemical methods   166
  in ornamental fish   373
  recovery   162, 166, 373
  stages   163
Anaesthetics
  administration   162
  commonly used   163–166, 186
  desirable characteristics   162
  dosages   220
  economic considerations   162
  for slaughter   72, 206–207, 219
  variable response to   162
  withdrawal times   162
Anatomy
  eel   312
  flatfish   335
  and physiology
    of crustaceans   27–30, 273–275
    of teleosts   1–27
Anchor worm *see Lernaea*
Angel fish   137, 366
Anguilla spp. *see* Eels
Anguillicolis spp. infection, eels   322–323
Anguilliform motion   4
Animal experimentation legislation   173
Anisakis infection   125
Annelids, parasitic   115, 120, 369
Antibacterials *see* Antibiotics
Antibiotic sensitivity tests   84, 210
Antibiotic treatment
  administration by injection   213

administration by mouth   67
administration via food   144–151
administration via the water   142, 374
  dosage   145, 146
  of eels   316, 317, 324, 325
  for enteric redmouth (ERM)   105
  for fin rot   187
  of food fish   407
  for furunculosis   103
  of game fish   404, 407
  general principles   144
  for gill infections   187
  of grass carp (*Ctenopharyngodon idella*)   142
  of ornamental fish   142, 374–376
  of prawn diseases   292, 293
  prophylactic   216–217, 246, 285
  of rainbow trout   107, 245
  for red sore disease   407
  for *Renibacterium salmoninarum*   107
  of sea-bass and sea-bream   392
  for *Streptococcus* infection   107
  of tench   142
  of turbot   336
  for vibriosis   105
  of wels (*Siluris glanis*)   142
Antibiotics
  and biological filters   142
  dosage   374
  drug resistance   374
  levels in fish serum   153
  licensed
    in UK   213
    in US   266
Antifungal treatment, of eels   325
Antihelminthic treatment, of ornamental fish   375, 376
Antimalarials, use against protozoan parasites   143
Antioxidants, in diet   96, 158, 239, 391
Antiparasitic treatment
  of eels   325
  of sea-bass and sea-bream   392
Approved zones and farms   174
Aquaculture
  basic husbandry   31–41
  of channel catfish   249–251
  of cod   346–349
  code of practice   171, 175
  and disease   91–129
  effluents   228–229
  environmental aspects   57–67
  of game fish   395–396
  of halibut   339–340
  legislation   173–177
  nutritional aspects   153–159
  of prawns   275–281
  of rainbow trout   227–228

Aquaculture—*continued*
    rotational   31
    of sea-bass and sea-bream   380
    systems   43–55
    treatments   131–152
    varying conditions   131
    welfare aspects   169–171
Aquarium systems, for ornamental fish   357–361
Arctic char, drug doses   147
Argulus (freshwater louse)   119–120
    in carp   307
    in eels   323
    in game fish   405
    in halibut   343
    in ornamental fish   369
    in rainbow trout   236
    treatment   119–120, 133–134, 137
Aristichthys nobilis (bighead)   297
Artemia nauplii *see* Brine shrimp; Feed, live
Ascorbic acid, in treatment of turbot granulomatous
        hypertyrosinaemia   336
Asian tapeworm   126, 368
Aspergillus infection   109
Astaxanthin   158, 175, 290, 349
Astronutus ocellatus see Oscar
Atlantic salmon
    algal blooms   199
    aquaculture in Scotland   193–221
    bacterial diseases   199–200
    broodstock   196, 198
    cage farming   47
    Caligus elongatus   203
    cannibalism   204
    disease control   196
    disease syndromes   127–128
    drug doses   147
    drug resistance   153
    egg incubation   193
    endemic diseases   197
    enteric redmouth (ERM)   105, 199, 200
    erythrocytic inclusion body syndrome   100
    eye damage   204
    fading (failed) smolt syndrome   128, 199, 205
    feeding   155, 180, 196
    fibrosarcoma virus   100
    fin rot   199, 203
    fungal diseases   200–201
    furunculosis   199, 203
    gas bubble disease   199, 203
    Gyrodactylus infection   116
    Hitra disease   105
    Ichthyobodo infection   199, 201
    Ichthyophthirius multifiliis   202
    infectious pancreatic necrosis (IPN)   199

infectious salmon anaemia (ISA)   128
    Lepeophtheirus infection   117–119
    location of farms, in Norway   180
    mineral requirements   158
    myxobacterial skin infection   199
    Norwegian aquaculture   179–191
    oxytetracycline treatment   150
    pancreatic disease   98, 99, 127–128, 196, 199,
        204–205
    papilloma   97–98
    parasitic diseases   201–203
    peduncle disease   203
    Saprolegnia infection   199, 200–201
    sea lice   66, 67, 197, 199, 202
    Sphaerospora infection   199, 200–201
    stocking density   182, 189–190, 197
    swim bladder fibrosarcoma   98
    tapeworms   199, 203
    treatment methods
        in Norwegian farming   186–187
        in sea cages   134
    Trichodina infection   199, 201
    vibriosis   199
    viral diseases   199
    vitamin requirement   157
    water quality   196–197
    white spot disease   199, 202
Australia, fish health legislation   229–230
Autolysis, occurs rapidly post-mortem   69, 291–
    292
Avermectins   67
Axine spp.   116
Azaperone   165–166

Bacterial diseases   101–108
    of Atlantic salmon
        in Norway   185
        in Scotland   199–200
    of carp   301–302
    of cod   351–352, 354
    of eels   315–319
    of game fish   404
    of ornamental fish   364–365
    of rainbow trout   231–234
    of sea-bass and sea-bream   383–384
    treatment   243, 335–336
    of turbot   333, 335–336
    visible signs   74
Bacterial fouling, of prawns   287
Bacterial fry anaemia   231
Bacterial gill disease (BGD)
    of Atlantic salmon in Scotland   199
    benzalkonium chloride treatment   135

Bacterial gill disease (BGD)—*continued*
  clinical signs   199
  potassium permanganate treatment   141
  of rainbow trout   231–232
  and water quality   199
Bacterial kidney disease (BKD)
  of Atlantic salmon
    in Norway   184, 185
    in Scotland   198, 199
  clinical signs   199
  disease-free stock   198
  notifiable disease   174
  of rainbow trout   232, 246
  and *Renibacterium salmoninarum*   107, 199
  seasonality   107
  transmission   199, 246
  treatment   148, 185, 188
  and water temperature   232
Bacterial loading, reduced by benzalkonium
      chloride   135
Bacterial mass, in *Chondrococcus* infection   106
Bacterial necrosis, of prawns   286
Bacterial resistance *see* Drug resistance
Bacteriology
  culture media   210
  eels   324
  examination   80–85
  laboratory equipment   80
  in marine invertebrates   85, 291, 292
  sampling   207
Baculovirus disease, of prawns   285–286
Bait fish, culture   297
Bankruptcy disease, of rainbow trout   107
Basophils   19
Bass *see* Sea-bass; Striped bass
Bath treatments   65, 67, 211–212, 407
Behavioural changes, in clinical diagnosis   242
Benedenia infection, yellowtail   116
Benzalkonium chloride
  administration   135
  dosage   135, 186, 212
  for ornamental fish   375
  for rainbow trout   243
  stressful treatment   212
  as substitute for malachite green   135
Benzocaine   72, 163–164, 186, 220, 373
Bighead, *Aristichthys nobilis*   297
Bile   17
Binders
  carbohydrate   158, 349
  toxicity   96, 334
Biochemical tests, for bacteriological identification
      83
Biocides, toxicity   65, 95, 369–370

Biological filters   60–62, 360
  damaged by treatments   141, 142
Biological oxygen demand (BOD)
  and excess food   170
  and oxygen depletion   58, 59
  in rainbow trout farms   228
  and waste products   196
Birds *see* Predation
Black death, of prawns   290
Black gill disease, of prawns   290
Black mollies   365
Bleeding, during slaughter   53, 198, 219
Blood
  composition   18–19
  crustacean   29
  gas transport   19–20
  osmotic balance   12
Blood flow, in gills   7–8
Blood fluke   125–126
Blood pressure   14
Blood sampling   86–87, 209
Blood worms, ornamental fish   368
Blue catfish (*Ictalurus furcatus*)   251–252, 398–399
Blue-sac disease   128
Bluegill   395, 397, 398, 404
Body surface abnormalities   71
Body surface sampling   75, 82
Bohr effect   10, 19
Boil disease, of Pacific salmon   122
Bone, microscopic structure   3
Bothriocephalus spp. (tapeworm) infection   126, 368
  in carp   305–306
  praziquantel treatment   142
  in turbot   334, 336
Botulinum toxin   96, 107
Brain   21
Brambell Committee   169
Branchiomycosis   108
  in carp   302–303
  clinical diagnosis   308
  clinical signs   302
  control   108
  in ornamental fish   365
  in sheatfish   302
  in tench   302
  transmission   302
  in whitefish   302
Branchionephritis, in eels   315
Branchiura   119–120
Breeding patterns, wide variety   26
Brine shrimp, as live feed   51, 276, 279, 329, 348, 380
Brine shrimp *see also* feed, live
Brockman bodies   26
Broken neck syndrome, sea-bass   390–391

Broodstock
   antibiotic treatment   213
   Atlantic salmon   196, 198
   channel catfish   252–253, 256
   cod   346–347
   feed   156, 256
   halibut   340, 342
   prawns   294
   quarantine   355
   rainbow trout   227
   salmonid   36, 156
   stripping   220, 227
   turbot   328
Brook trout
   Salmonicola infection   117
   ulcer disease   103–104
Brooklynella spp. infection   112–113, 367
Brown bullhead   399
Brown trout
   Diphyllobothrium spp. infection   239
   disease resistant   230
   drug doses   147
Buccal pump mechanism, for gill water flow   8–9
Buffering capacity, of fresh and salt water   62, 63, 93, 180–181
Bullhead (*Ictalurus nebolosus*)   252
Buoyancy, normal   9–10
Butyl tin   393

Calanus, cod prey fish   346
Calcium
   effect of high levels   65, 96, 158
   essential for crustacea   28, 63
   homeostasis   25
Calculation of drug dosage   134–135
Caligulus spp. *see* Sea louse
Camellanus spp., ornamental fish   143, 368
Canada, legislation   174, 229
Cannibalism   95–96, 169
   in Atlantic salmon   204, 218
   in catfish   252
   in cod   345, 348
   in largemouth bass   401
   in sea-bass   389
Canthaxanthin   158–159, 175
Capillaria spp. infection, in ornamental fish   143, 368
Capillaries, permeability   15
Capillary congestion   74
Carangiform motion   4
Carassius auratus see Goldfish
Carbohydrates
   as binders   158, 349
   in commercial diets   349
   as pollutants   158
   storage and metabolism   17–18, 158
Carbon dioxide
   effect on oxygen uptake   59
   narcosis   219
   recommended levels   59
   transport in blood   20
   used for sedation   53–54
Carcass, gross lesions, in diagnosis   78
Cardiac myopathy syndrome (CMS)   127
Carnivorous fish   16, 169
Carophyllaeus spp. infection, carp   305–306
Carp
   Aeromonas infection   301–302
   alarm substance   4, 5
   ammonia intoxication   307
   anatomy   300
   aquaculture systems   297–300
   Argulus spp. infection   307
   Asian tapeworm   126
   bacterial disease   301–302
   blood fluke   125–126
   Bothriocephalus spp. infection   305–306
   branchiomycosis   108, 302–303
   broodfish, ectoparasite treatment   40
   Carophyllaeus spp. infection   305–306
   Chilodonella spp. infection   112, 305
   Chlamydia infections   107
   Choromyxum spp. infections   304
   clinical diagnosis   308
   coccidosis   126, 303
   Cryptobia infection   112
   cultivated species   297
   Dactylogyrus infection   116
   development   299
   Diplostomum spp. infection   305
   disease prevention   309
   egg mass   44
   Eimeria spp. infection   303
   Ergasilus spp. infection   306–307
   eye diplostomatosis   305
   feed
      commercial   298
      live   40, 297
      medicated   308
   fungal diseases   302–303
   gas bubble disease   307
   gill rot   302–303
   Hemiclepsis spp. infection   306
   hepatopancreas   17, 18
   husbandry   39–40, 298–300
   Ichthyophthirius multifiliis infection   305
   Khawia spp. infection   305–306

Carp—*continued*
  Lernaea infection 117
  marketable size 298
  mineral requirements 158
  Myxobolus spp. infection 121, 304
  myxosporean infections 303–304
  nutritional disorders 307–308
  overwintering 40, 298, 300–301
  oxygen requirement 40
  papilloma 97–98
  parasitic diseases 303–307
  pharyngeal teeth 16
  Philometra infection 125, 306
  phosphorus deficiency 308
  Piscicola spp. infection 306
  pond systems 297–299, 301, 307, 358
  praziquantel treatment 142
  pyloric caeca 16
  quinaldine sulphate anaesthesia 165
  Sanguinicola spp. infection 305
  saprolegniasis 303
  Sekoke disease 308
  Spaerospora renicola infection 303–304
  spring viraemia virus (SVC) 100, 174, 300, 308,
    362–363
  swim-bladder inflammation 303–304
  tapeworms 305–306
  Thelohanellus spp. infections 304
  tolerant of suspended solids 64
  treatment materials 308
  Trypanoplasma (*Cryptobia*) infections 303
  vaccination 143, 309
  veterinary approach 297–309
  viral disease 100, 300–301
  vitamin requirements 157, 307–308
Carp dropsy syndrome 100, 363, 364
Carp epithelioma 301, 308
Carp erythrodermatitis 103–104, 301–302, 308
  in ornamental fish 364
  vaccine 143
Carp lice 307
Carp pox 97–98, 301, 370
Carriers
  of *Aeromonas salmonicida* 200
  of enteric redmouth (ERM) 105, 144
  of furunculosis 102, 103
  of vibriois 144
Carriers *see also* wild fish
Caryophyllaeus, tapeworms 126
Catadromy 13, 311
Catfish
  cannibalism 252
  species 251–252
  viruses 100

Catfish *see also* blue catfish; channel catfish
Cauliflower disease (eel papillomatosis) 98, 314–315
Centrarchids 393
Ceratomyxa shasta 122, 238
Cestode parasites 124
  of carp 305–306
  of game fish 405
Chain pickerel 399
Channel catfish
  aeration equipment 50
  Aeromonas infections 259
  and ammonia 265
  anaemia 263–264
  anaesthesia 164, 166
  aquaculture systems 249–251
  bacterial diseases 257–259
  broodstock 252–253
  cannibalism 269
  Chilodonella infection 112
  Chondrococcus columnaris 257–259
  columnaris disease 257–259
  disease prevention 267–268
  earth pond culture 39, 45, 249–252
  Edwardsiella infection 105, 254, 257
  egg and fry production 44, 253
  enteric septic septicaemia 257
  feed 255–256
  feeding table 154
  as food fish 253–254, 269
  as game fish 395, 398–399
  harvesting 53, 270
  hatchery management 268–269
  Henneguya spp. 121–122
  husbandry 39, 251–256
  Ichthyobodo infection 260
  Ichthyophthirius multifiliis 260
  jaw teeth 16
  methaemoglobinaemia 265
  mineral requirements 158
  nitrite toxicity 397
  nutrition 255–256
  oxygen requirement 39, 45, 264–265
  parasitic diseases 259–262
  proliferative gill disease 261–262
  red spot (red fillet) syndrome 262
  Romet treatment 150
  Saprolegnia infection 263
  single crop vs. continuous production 254, 269
  spawning 252–253, 399
  Sphaerospora infection 261–262
  stress-induced disease 256, 262–263
  tolerance of contamination 57, 64
  transportation 254–255
  treatment 266

Channel catfish—*continued*
    Trichodina infections   260
    Trichophyra infection   261
    vaccination   269
    veterinary approach   249–270
    viral diseases   256–257
    vitamin requirement   157
    water quality   250–251, 264–265
    winter kill (winter fungus, winter mortality)   256, 263
    yellow flesh pigmentation   159
Channel catfish virus disease   100–101, 256–257
Characins, toxicity of treatment compounds for   138
Chemotherapy *see* treatment
Chilodonella spp. infection   112–113
    in carp   305
    in eels   321
    formalin treatment   138
    in ornamental fish   367
    in rainbow trout   236
    sodium chloride treatment   141–142
Chinook salmon, *Ceratomyxa shasta* infection   238
Chitin   28
Chlamydia infections   107–108
Chloramine-T   135–136, 186, 212
    administration   136
    dosage   136, 212
    and gill damage   65
    for ornamental fish   375
    possible impurities   136
    for rainbow trout   243, 244
    in treatment of *Gyrodactylus*   136
    in treatment of *Ichthyobodo*   135
    in treatment of myxobacteria   135
    in treatment of *Trichodina*   135
    in treatment of white spot   135–136
Chloramphenicol
    derivatives   150
    dosage   142
    for eels   317
Chlorbutanol   186
Chloride, counteracts nitrites   65, 265
Chlorine
    and gill disease   93–94
    in tap water   60, 369
    toxicity   60, 95
        in turbot culture   328, 334
    and white stripe disease   389
Chlorormyxum spp. infection, sea-bream   386
Chondrococcus spp.   106
    marine   106
    MIC data   149, 150
    and rainbow trout fingerling syndrome   106–107
Chondrococcus spp. infection
    in channel catfish   257–259

diagnosis   106
    in eels   317
    in game fish   404, 406
    in ornamental fish   364
    in rainbow trout   106–107, 231
    Romet treatment   150
    in turbot   333
Choroid body   26
Choromyxum spp. infections, carp   304
Chromaffin cells   11, 21, 25
Chromatophores, in the dermis   6
Chubb (*Leuciscus cephalus*), toxicity of treatment
        compounds for   138
Cichlid bloat   366
Cichlid virus, in ornamental fish   364
Cichlids, hole in the head disease   366
Ciliate parasites   111
    of carp   305
    of eels   320–323
    of ornamental fish   366–367
    of shrimp   138
Circulation control   15
Circulatory system
    crustacean   29
    teleost   13–15
Cleaning procedures   32, 54
Clinical diagnosis
    in marine invertebrates   85–86
    procedure   69–70, 89, 188, 205–206
Clinical medicine, of farmed fish, viii–ix
Clinical signs, and common causes   91–93, 241, 364
Clinostomum spp.   124
Clinostomum spp. infection
    in game fish   405
    in ornamental fish   367–368
Clostridium botulinum see botulinum toxin
Co-trimazine   147–148
    dosage   142, 147, 213
    ineffective against *Pseudomonas*   148
    in treatment of *Aeromonas*   148
    in treatment of *Yersinia ruckeri*   148
Coccidian parasites   126, 303
Coccidosis *see* Tapeworms
Cod
    Aeromonas spp. infection   352
    aquaculture   47, 345–349
    bacterial diseases   351–352, 354
    broodstock   346–347
    cannnibalism   345
    clinical diagnosis   354
    cold-water vibrosis   351–352
    Cryptocotyle lingua infection   353
    disease prevention   355–356
    eggs   346–347

Cod—*continued*
  feed
    chemical composition   349
    live   346, 348, 349
  fin rot   352
  fry production   347–348
  fungal diseases   352, 354–355, 356
  furunculosis   352
  general biology   345–346
  grading   348
  Gyrodactylus spp. infection   352–354
  Ichthyobodo spp. infection   352–353
  Ichthyophonus spp. infection   352
  Ichthyophthirius multifiliis infection   354–355
  Learnocera spp. infection   353
  legislation   350
  mortality removals   347
  nutritional requirements   349
  Pacific   230
  parasitic diseases   352–353, 355–356
  pond culture   347–348
  prey species   346
  rotenone treatment   347
  sea cages   47, 348–349
  sea louse (*Caligulus*)   353
  spawning pen   346
  treatment   355
  Trichodina spp. infection   352–353
  ulcus syndrome   350, 354
  veterinary approach   345–356
  Vibrio anguillarum   104
  vibriosis   351–352, 354–356
  viral diseases   350, 354
Coho salmon
  erythrocytic inclusion body syndrome   100
  viral haemorrhagic septicaemia (VHN)   230
Coho syndrome   108
Cold shock   166
Cold-water disease   106, 231, 365
Cold-water vibriosis   190, 351–352
Colobomatus spp. infection, sea-bass   388
Colour
  abnormal   71, 91
  normal   5–6
Colour vision   23
Colponema spp. infection, sea-bass and sea-bream   385
Columnaris disease   106
  bacteriology   259
  of channel catfish   257–259
  clinical signs   258, 364
  of eels   317–318
  of ornamental fish   364
  oxytetracycline treatment   407
  potassium permanganate   406–407

  of rainbow trout   231
  of striped bass   406
Concrete tanks   53, 110
Conductivity of water   64
Constant-head siphon, use in treatment   132
Containers, for examination   71–72
Contracaecum infection   125
Control
  of bacterial diseases   101–108
  of fungal diseases   108–109
  of parasitic diseases   109–127
  treatments   176–177
  of viral diseases   99–101
Control systems, in automated hatcheries   55
Copepod parasites   116–119, 353
Copper sulphate
  dosage   136
  toxicity   137
  in treatment of channel catfish   260, 266
  in treatment of game fish   407
  treatment for *Oodinium* infection   112
  treatment for parasitic diseases   136, 260, 392
  treatment for snails   405
Coronary blood vessels   14
Corpuscles of Stannius   11, 21, 25, 209
Costia see Ichthyobodo
Cotton wool appearance
  in columnaris disease   106, 364
  in *Saprolegnia* infection   108, 200, 319, 365
Cotylurus spp.   124
Cough response   9, 64
Courtship rituals   171, 219
Cranial nerves   22
Crappie   393, 398, 407
Crayfish plague, in Norway   184
Crustacea
  anatomy and physiology   27–30, 273–275
  bacteriology and histopathology   85–86
  parasitic   75–76, 115–120, 306–307, 323, 368–369, 388
  require calcium   63
  toxicity of treatment compounds for   138
Crustacea *see also* lobsters; prawns; shrimps
Cryptobia spp. infection   112, 125
  in ornamental fish   366
  in sea-bass and sea-bream   385
  treatment   393
Cryptocaryasis   112
  in ornamental fish   366
  in sea-bream   386
  treatment   393
Cryptocotyle spp. infection   124
  in cod   353
Ctenoid scales   6

Ctenopharyngodon idella see Grass carp
Culture media, for bacteriology   82–83, 210, 292
Cutaneous haemorrhage   74
Cutaneous senses   24
Cuticle   4
Cyanide poisoning   65, 95
Cycloid scales   6
Cyprinus carpio see Carp
Cytophaga see Chondrococcus

Dactylogyrus spp. infection   116
   dichlorvos treatment   137
   formalin treatment   138
   in ornamental fish   367
   in rainbow trout   236
   in sea-bass and sea-bream   387
   treatment   116, 137, 138
Dactylogyrus spp. infection *see also* gill fluke
Daphnia, as intermediate host   368
Dead fish *see* Mortalities
Dead sock   34, 54, 197–198
Debility parasitism   112, 118, 126
Deficiency diseases *see* Mineral deficiencies;
      Vitamin deficiencies   156, 157
Defoaming agents, in transportation of live fish   255
Deformities
   congenital   128
   of halibut   343
   of sea-bass and sea-bream   389
   of turbot   333
Dehydration, in marine environment   13
Demand feeders   52
Denmark
   eel culture, diseases   321
   fish health legislation   229
   rainbow trout production   46, 107, 223, 224
Depigmentation
   of halibut   343
   of turbot   332
Dermis, anatomy   5–6
Dermocystidium spp. infection
   of eels   319
   of ornamental fish   365
Dichlorvos treatment   137–138, 186
   for *Argulus* spp.   137
   for *Caligulus*   137
   for *Dactylogyrus*   137
   dosage   212
   environmental considerations   138
   for *Gyrodactylus*   137
   for *Lepeophtheirus*   137
   for *Lernaea* spp.   137
   for sea lice   137, 212

statutory controls   138
stressful   205, 212
toxic to characins   138
Diet *see also* feed   95–97
Digenean parasites   123–124
   of game fish   405
   of ornamental fish   367
   of sea-bass and sea-bream   387
   treatment   393
Digestion
   in crustaceans   29–30
   in teleosts   15–18
Digestive function test   88
Dihydrostreptamycin sulphate   188
Dimetridazole   142
Dip treatment   134
Diphyllobothrium spp. tapeworms   124
   in brown trout   239
   in ornamental fish   368
Diphyllobothrium spp.tapeworms, in rainbow
      trout   238–239
Diplectanum aequans infection, sea-bass   387
Diplostomum spp. infection   123–124
   in carp   305
   in ornamental fish   367–368
   in rainbow trout   238
   in striped bass   405
Direct tissue smears   84–85
Discharge licence   58, 67, 211, 331
Discharges *see* effluents
Discus (*Symphysodon discus*), *Capillaria* infection   143
Disease
   in aquaculture   91–129
   environmental considerations   66, 91–95, 214
Disease diagnosis *see* Clinical diagnosis
Disease prevention   215–217
   in carp   309
   in channel catfish   267–268
   in cod   355–356
   in eels   325–326
   in game fish   408
   and good husbandry   31, 91, 189, 193
   in halibut   344
   legislation   173–174
   in ornamental fish   376
   in prawns   293–295
   in rainbow trout   244–245
   in sea-bass and sea-bream   393
   in turbot   336–337
Disease-free stock   170, 218, 245
   and bacterial kidney disease (BKD)   198
   and infectious pancreatic necrosis (IPN)   99, 198
   turbot   337
Diseased fish, gross external features   73–74

Disinfection
  of clothing etc.   37, 216
  of earth pond systems   245
  in eel culture   314
  of eggs   142, 186, 245, 347
  iodophor disinfectant   36–37, 73, 142, 186, 245,
    294
  systemic   139
Dissection procedure   76–77
Distended gut syndrome, sea-bream   382–383
Diurnal variation
  of alkalinity   63
  in aquarium systems   361
  of oxygen levels   58–59, 131, 307
Divers, in removal of mortalities   33, 197–198
Dosage calculation   134–135
Dosage calculations   373–374
Doxycycline   142
Drainage system, for prawn hatcheries   278
Drug licensing *see* Treatment licensing
Drug residues, safe levels in food   175
Drug resistance
  to amoxycillin   147
  to antibiotics   152, 374
  to dichlorvos   137
  to organophosphates   188
  to oxolinic acid   149, 150, 213
  to oxytetracycline   213
  to quinolones   152–153

Earth pond systems
  for channel catfish culture   39
  drying and disinfecting   245
  and parasitic disease   110
  for rainbow trout   223, 224
  for shrimp culture   138
  and whirling disease   121
EC, legislation   173–177, 229
Ecdysis   28–29
Economic considerations
  and anaesthetics   162
  and feeding   35, 155, 156
  and legislation   173
  and ornamental fish   357
  in prawn culture   288, 293
  and stocking density   32–33
  and viral disease   98
Ectocommensals, of eels   321
Ectoparasite infection
  of carp   302
  of carp broodfish   40
  of cod   352–353, 355, 356
  copper sulphate treatment   136

examination for   74–75, 207, 219
  formalin treatment   138, 187
  of game fish   405
  malachite green treatment   187
  of ornamental fish   375–376
  sodium chloride (salt) treatment   141–142, 187
  of turbot   332
Edwardsiella spp.   105
  MIC data   147
Edwardsiella spp. infection
  in channel catfish   254, 257
  in eels   317
  in game fish   404, 406
  Romet treatment   150
  in sea-bass   384
  treatment   105, 150
Eels
  Acinebacter spp. infection   318
  Aeromonas spp. infection   316, 318, 319
  anaesthesia   325
  anatomy   312
  Anguillicolis spp. infection   322–323
  anti-ectoparasitic drugs   325
  antibiotic treatment   316, 317, 324, 325
  aquaculture   39, 311–314
  Argulus spp. infection   323
  bacterial disease   315–319
  bacteriology   324
  branchionephritis   315
  Chilodonnella spp. infection   321
  chloramphenical   317
  Chondrococcus infection   317
  clinical diagnosis   323–324
  columnaris disease   317–318
  Dermocystidium infection   319
  disease prevention   325–326
  ectocommensals   321
  Edwardsiella spp. infection   105, 317
  Eimeria spp. infection   319
  Ergasilus spp. infection   323
  examination   324
  farmed species   311
  feed   312, 313
    artificial   39
  flow-through systems   312
  fungal diseases, treatment   325
  furunculosis   316
  gas bubble disease   323
  gas levels   314
  gill disease   317
  glass eels, feeding   311
  grading   39, 314
  growth rate   313
  Gyrodactylus spp. infection   321

Eels—*continued*
  Haemogregarina infection   319
  haemorrhagic septicaemia   105
  Histiostoma infection   321
  histopathology   324
  husbandry   39, 313–314
  Ichthyobodo spp. infection   319
  Ichthyophthirius multifiliis infection   320
  Lernaea spp. infection   323
  levamisole treatment   322
  lymph heart   15
  migration   311
  mineral requirements   158
  Myxosporidia infection   320
  necropsy   324
  papillomatosis   98, 314–315
  parasitic diseases   126, 319–323
    treatment   325–326
  Pleistophora spp. infection   320
  pond culture   312
  Pseudodactylogyrus spp. infection   321
  Pseudomonas spp. infection   316, 319
  recirculation systems   49, 312, 314
  red disease   315, 316
  Saprolegnia infection   318, 319
    treatment   325
  Scyphidia infection   321
  silver eels   311
  stock quality   313
  stocking density   313
  stomatopapillomatosis   315
  Streptococcus infection   107
  stress   314
  stress-induced viral disease   315
  swim-bladder infection   322–323
  tail infection   317
  transport   313
  treatment   324–325
  Trichodina spp. infection   320–321
  Trichophyra infection   321
  Trypanosoma infection   319
  vaccination   325–326
  veterinary approach   311–326
  vibriosis   104, 316–317
  viral diseases   314–315
  virology   324
  Vorticella infection   321
  water quality   313
  water temperature   313
  world production   311
  yellow eels   311
Effluents
  from aquaculture   228–229
  and oxygen depletion   94, 228

  statutory control   58, 228–229
  treatment   50, 57, 331
Eggs
  Atlantic salmon   179
  channel catfish   253
  cod   346–347
  disinfection   142, 186, 245, 347
  halibut   339
  incubation   43–44, 193, 227–228
  international trade   54
  malachite green used in incubation   193
  number produced   26
  Saprolegnia infection   108, 234
  turbot   327, 328
Eimeria spp.   126
Eimeria spp. infection
  in carp   303
  clinical signs   303
  control   126
  in eels   319
  in ornamental fish   366
  in sea-bass and sea-bream   385–386
Electric shock, as anaesthetic   165, 219
Electron microscopy, in virology   88
ELISA tests   88
Endocrine system   11, 13, 24–26
  crustacean   30
Endoparasite infections
  of cod   353, 356
  of game fish   405–406
Enrofloxacin   150
Enteric redmouth (ERM)   105
  in Atlantic salmon   199, 200
  benzalkonium chloride treatment   135
  carriers   144
  clinical signs   105
  diagnosis   105
  notifiable disease   174
  in rainbow trout   231
  treatment   105, 135
  vaccination   143, 217, 246
  and *Yersinia ruckeri*   231
Enteric septic septicaemia, in channel catfish   257
Entobdella spp. infection, in halibut and sole   116, 343
Environmental considerations
  in aquaculture   57–67, 284
  in disease   70–71, 91–95, 363
  in feeding   156
  and fish welfare   169
  in parasitism   110
  in treatment   66–67, 138, 176
Environmental control
  in halibut production   340
  and physiological impact of changes   161

Environmental control—*continued*
  sea-bass and sea-bream production 380
  in turbot farming 328
Eosinophils 19
Epibdella spp. infection, sea-bass 387
Epidemiological considerations, in clinical
diagnosis 241
Epidermis 4–5
Epistylis, formalin treatment 138
Epitheliocystis, of sea-bream 386–387
Ergasilus spp. infection
  of carp 306–307
  of eels 323
  of ornamental fish 369
  of sea-bass and sea-bream 388
Erythrocytes 19
Erythrocytic inclusion body syndrome 100
Erythromycin 147, 213
  in treatment of bacterial kidney disease 148, 185,
    188, 243
Esox lucius see Pike
Essential amino acids 96, 156
Essential fatty acids 96, 156–157, 239
Eubothrium spp. tapeworms 126, 188, 213
Euryhaline fish 13, 15, 403
Eustrongyloides spp. infection 125
  ornamental fish 368
Euthanasia *see* Slaughter
Examination
  of eels 324
  post-mortem 73–79, 207–208, 292
  of prawns 291
  procedures 372, 373
  of slaughtered fish 206–207
Excretion, normal 6, 11–13
Excretory kidney *see* Kidney
Excretory system, crustacean 30
Exophilia infection 109
Exoskelton, of crustaceans 27–28
Exotic species, and new pathogens 110, 297, 305–306,
  362
Eye, normal structure and function 22–23
Eye damage, in Atlantic salmon 204
Eye diplostomatosis, in carp 305
Eye fluke 123–124
  clinical signs 238
  control 124
  in ornamental fish 367–368
  in rainbow trout 238
  in striped bass 405
Eye involvement
  in cod vibrioisis 351
  common sign of disease 91
  examination 74

  in parasitic infection 123–124
Eye pathology, in rainbow trout 241
Eye stalk ablation 30

Fading (failed) smolt syndrome, of Atlantic salmon
  119, 128, 205
Faecal casts 74, 205
Faecal material *see* Waste products
Fallowing
  of carp ponds 40
  importance of 31
  of salmon farms 180, 215–218
Fathead minnow 397
Fats *see* Lipids
Fatty acid deficiency 106
Fatty liver, sea-bream and sea-bass 390
Feed
  additives 174–175
  analysis 88–89
  artificial
    for first feeders 35
    for glass eels 311
    for halibut 341
    improved quality 58, 153, 229
    optimised composition 190
    for rainbow trout 228
    for turbot 329
  for Atlantic salmon 196
  for broodstock 156
  for channel catfish 255–256
  for cod, chemical composition 349
  consumption 153
  dry pellets 155
  for eels 312, 313
  excess 153, 216, 228
    biological oxygen demand (BOD) 170
    build-up under sea cages 57–58, 70
    in halibut culture 341
    removal 31–32, 41
  live 155
    for carp 40, 297–298
    for channel catfish 256
    for cod 348, 349
    for glass eels 311
    for halibut 341, 341–342
    for ornamental fish 362
    for prawns 276, 279, 281
    risks of contamination 40
    for salmonid larvae 44, 50–51
    for sea-bass and sea-bream 380–381
    for turbot 40, 327, 328–330, 336
  mechanical distribution 280

Feed—*continued*
  medicated   144–151, 175, 212–213
    for Atlantic salmon   189
    for carp   308
    for ornamental fish   374
  physical characteristics   95, 155, 170, 216
  quality and quantity   218
  for shrimp   156
  for striped bass   403
  types   155–156
  wet   155, 196
Feed conversion rate   153
Feeding
  abnormal   71
  automatic   51–52, 194, 196, 215, 228
  of channel catfish   154, 255–256
  control   154
  of crustaceans   29
  economic considerations   35, 155
  environmental considerations   156
  of glass eels   311
  manual   52, 153–154, 196, 228
  non-constant requirement   169–170
  of ornamental fish   361–362
  of prawns   281
  to ration not appetite   196
Feeding equipment   50–52
Feeding hierarchies   46–47, 95–96, 128, 156, 196, 228,
      389
Feeding methods   35, 153–155, 215–216
Fenbendazole   186, 213
Fertilisation methods   26
Fibrosarcoma, Atlantic salmon   98, 100
Filters *see* Biological filters
Filtration   50, 57
Fin lesions   73–74
Fin rot
  antibiotic treatment   187
  in Atlantic salmon   199, 203
  benzylalkonium chloride treatment   186
  chloramine-T treatment   186, 212
  and *Chondrococcus psychrophila*   106
  in cod   352
  in ornamental fish   365
  and *Saprolegnia* infection   108
  secondary infection   203, 352
  in turbot   332
Finland, fish health legislation   229
Fish, anatomy and physiology   1–30
Fish farming *see* aquaculture
Fish meal, in feed   58, 255, 285
Fish waste, in feed   155–156, 158
Five freedoms   169–171, 217–219
Flagellate parasites   111, 126, 366

Flashing, sign of parasitic infection   71, 116, 201, 235,
      366, 372
Flatfish
  anatomy   335
  papilloma   98
Flathead catfish, *Pylodictus oliveris*   252
Flavobacterium spp. infection, turbot   333
Flexibacter see Chondrococcus spp.; columnaris disease
Floating cages *see* sea cages
Flow rates, in turbot farming   328
Flow-through systems, for eel culture   312
Flumequine   147, 187
Flush treatment   211
Food *see* Feed
Food conversion ratio   35
Food fish production
  approved antibiotics   407
  channel catfish   269
Food regulations   174–175
Footbaths *see* Disinfection
Forage fish   397
Formalin treatment
  administration   138
  of channel catfish   260
  for *Chilodonella* infection   138
  combined with malachite green   139, 212
  for *Dactylogyrus* infection   138
  dosage   138, 212, 244
  of eels   320, 321
  for *Epistylis* infection   138
  in fumigation   141
  of game fish   407
  and gill damage   65
  for gill flukes   138
  for *Gyrodactylus* spp. infection   138
  for *Ichthyobodo* spp. infection   138, 319
  for parasitic diseases   138, 187, 260, 344, 392
  for skin flukes   138
  stressful to fish   132
  toxicity   138
  Trichodina   138
  of turbot   336
Freedom
  from fear and distress   170–171, 218–219
  from pain, injury or disease   170, 218
  from stress or suffering
    when slaughtered   171, 219
    when transported   171, 219
  from thermal or physical discomfort   170, 218
  from thirst, hunger or malnutrition   169–170,
      217–218
  to express normal patterns of behaviour   171, 219
Freshwater aquaculture
  construction of cages   225

Freshwater aquaculture—*continued*
   of rainbow trout   225–226
   in Scotland   193–194
   water purification   60–61
Freshwater eel disease   316
Freshwater louse *see Argulus*
Fry mortality syndrome (fry anaemia syndrome),
     rainbow trout   231
Fry rearing   44
   cod   347–348
   rainbow trout   223, 228
Fry troughs, use in treatment   132
Fumagillin   148, 336
Fumigation   141
Fungal disease   108–109
   of Atlantic salmon   200–201
   of cod   352, 354–355, 356
   of ornamental fish   365
   of prawns   287–288, 289
   of rainbow trout   234
   of sea-bass and sea-bream   384
   treatment   243–244
     with malachite green   139–140
   visible signs   74
Furazolidone   144, 148, 336
   administration   145
   dosage   145, 147, 148, 213
Furnestia echeineis infection
   sea-bream   387
   treatment   393
Furunculosis
   acute and chronic   200
   and *Aeromonas salmonicida*   102
   antibiotic treatment   103, 185
   of Atlantic salmon   199, 200
   benzalkonium chloride   135
   clinical signs   102, 200, 233
   of cod   352
   diagnosis   102
   of eels   316
   endemic   197
   of halibut   343
   in Norway   184, 185
   notifiable disease   174
   prevention and control   102–103, 185
   in Scotland   198
   stress testing   103, 198, 211, 220
   stress-induced   190
   suceptibility   200
   transmission   31, 102, 103, 181
   treatment   103, 135
   of turbot   333
   vaccination   103, 143, 185, 217, 246
Fusarium disease, of prawns   289

Gadus morhua see cod
Gaffkaemia, vaccine   143
Gall bladder, necroscopy features   77
Game fish
   Aeromonas spp. infection   404, 406
   Amyloodinium spp. infection   405, 407
   antibiotic treatment   404, 407
   aquaculture systems   395–396
   Argulus spp. infection   405
   bacterial infections   404
   bath treatments   407
   Chondrococcus spp. infection   404, 406
   clinical diagnosis   407
   Clinostomum spp. infection   405
   definition   393
   disease prevention   408
   Edwardsiella spp. infection   404, 406
   Ergaslus spp. infection   405
   Heteropolaria spp. infection   404, 405, 407
   husbandry   396–404
   parasitic diseases   405–406
   Posthodiplostomum spp. infection   405
   potassium permanganate treatment   404, 408
   Pseudomonas spp. infection   404, 406
   red sore disease   404
   Romet treatment   407
   Saprolegnia spp. infection   404
   Streptococcus spp. infection   406
   terramycin   407
   transportation   408
   treatment   407–408
   velvet disease   405
   veterinary approach   393–408
   viral diseases   407
   Vorticella spp. infection   404
Gas bubble disease   31, 59, 93
   of Atlantic salmon   199, 203
   of carp   307
   of eels   323
   of halibut   343
   in hatcheries   50
   in recirculation systems   203
Gas gland   10
Gases
   in blood   19–20
   dissolved   58–60
   in swim-bladder   10
   toxic   32, 60, 363, 369
Gastric mill, crustacean   30
Gastro-intestinal hormones   26
Gastro-intestinal tract, tissue sampling   79
Genetic abnormalities   128
Genetic disease resistance and susceptibility   190,
     267–268

Gentamycin 142
Giemsa staining 85, 87
Gill arch 6–7
Gill damage
    acute and chronic 94
    and algae 59
    and aluminium 65
    and ammonia 60, 106
    and blood fluke eggs 126
    and chloramine-T 65
    and formalin 65
    and low pH 62
    and malachite green 65
    and secondary infection 199
    and suspended solids 62, 64, 66, 94, 182
    symptoms 58–59
Gill disease
    antibiotic treatment 187
    benzylalkonium chloride treatment 186
    chloramine-T treatment 186
    and chlorine 93–94
    Chondrococcus infection 106
    in eels 317
    in ornamental fish 364
    and suspended solids 89
    and water quality 89
Gill flukes 115–116, 116
    formalin treatment 138
    in ornamental fish 367
    in sea-bass and sea-bream 387
Gill maggots 117, 369
Gill preparations 74–75, 211, 292
Gill rakers 6–7, 16
Gill rot
    Branchiomyces infection 108
    in carp 302–303
    in ornamental fish 365
    in sea-bream 384, 387
Gills
    crustacean 29
    necroscopy features 77
    normal anatomy and function 6–8
    in osmoregulation 6, 11
    post-mortem changes 78
    tissue sampling 78
Gilthead bream *see* Sea-bream
Glass eels *see* Eels
Glucans, as immunostimulant 153, 190
Glugea spp. 123
Goitre, in salmonids 96
Gold dust disease 366
Goldfish
    anaemia 366
    culture 297

Ivermectin treatment 142
    pond systems 358
    treatment for *Mitraspora cyprini* 139
    trichlorphon/mebendazole treatment 137
    ulcer disease 364
Gonads 26
Gourami 137, 366
Grading
    of eels 39, 314
    equipment 52–53
    of halibut 341
    methods 33
    need for 33, 52, 96, 197
    of rainbow trout 228
    of sea-bass 389
    stressful to fish 33, 196, 218
    of turbot 41, 337
Gram-negative rods, common pathogens 83, 101–102, 364
Gram-positive bacteria, as fish pathogens 101–102, 107
Granulomatous disease, of ornamental fish 365
Granulomatous hypertyrosinaemia, of turbot 334, 336
Grass carp
    antibiotic treatment 142
    Diplostomum spp. infection 305
    in eutrophic ponds 297
Green gland, crustacean 30
Grey and white matter, of spinal cord 22
Grilse, Atlantic salmon 198, 215
Gross surface features, of prawns 292
Gross surface pathology, in clinical diagnosis 91, 242
Growth promoters 175
Growth rate, of turbot 330
Growth table, Atlantic salmon 153
Guppies 366, 370
Gut wall, water and ion transport 11
Gyrodactylus spp. 115–116
Gyrodactylus spp. infection
    chloramine-T treatment 136
    of cod 352–354
    control 116
    dichlorvos treatment 137
    of eels 321
    epizootics 116
    in Norway 184, 185–188
    notifiable disease 174
    of ornamental fish 367
    of rainbow trout 236
    of sea-bass and sea-bream 387
    treatment 116

Haematocrit (packed cell volume) 87
Haemocytes, crustacean 29

Haemocytic enteritis, prawns   290
Haemoglobin, and gas transport   19–20
Haemogregarina spp. infection
　in eels   319
　in sea-bream   386
　in turbot   334
Haemolymph, crustacean   29
Haemopoietic tissue   11, 20
Haemorrhages, necroscopy features   77
Haemorrhagic septicaemia, in eels   104–105
Halibut
　anaesthesia   344
　Argulus spp. infection   343
　broodstock   340, 342
　clinical diagnosis   343
　congenital deformities   343
　culture systems   47, 339, 339–340, 340
　depigmentation   343
　development   339
　diseases   91, 343
　　prevention and treatment   343–344
　eggs   339
　Entobdella spp. infection   116, 343
　environmental control   340
　essential fatty acids   157
　feeding patterns   170
　furunculosis   343
　gas bubble disease   343
　grading   341
　hatchery   339
　husbandry   340–342
　identification methods   340
　infectious pancreatic necrosis (IPN)   343
　legislation   342–343
　spawning   342
　transportation   340–341
　trematode parasites   343
　　formalin treatment   344
　ultrasound diagnosis   343–344
　veterinary approach   339–344
　zooplankton in diet   341
Hamburger gill disease *see* Proliferative gill disease
Handling
　and disease   101, 108, 205, 215
　facilitated by anaesthesia   161
　stressful to fish   95, 162, 170, 197, 245
Harvesting systems   36, 53–54
Hatchery procedures   43–45
　for channel catfish   268–269
　environmental control   31–32
　for halibut   339
　incubation techniques   37
　for prawns   275–277, 281–282
　rainbow trout   227–228

for salmonids   36–37
　turbot   327
　for turbot   328–330
　use of malachite green   37
Hatching trays   43–44
Heart
　structure and function   13–14
　tissue sampling   78
Heavy metals
　safe levels in food   175
　toxicity   63, 64, 65, 94, 369
Helminth parasites   75–78, 126, 388
Hemibdella spp.   120
Hemibranchs   6, 7
Hemiclepsis spp. infection, in carp   306
Hemilcepsis spp.   120
Henneguya spp.   121–122
Henneguya spp. infection
　in ornamental fish   367
　in sea-bass   386
Hepatocytes   17
Hepatoma, rainbow trout   98
Hepatopancreas, of carp   17, 18
Hepatopancreatic parvo-like virus disease, of prawns   288
Hepatorenal syndrome, of turbot   334
Herbivores, digestive tract anatomy   15
Herpesvirus scophalmi virus, turbot   333
Herring, *Ichthyophonus* spp. infection   352
Heteropolaria spp. infection, game fish   404, 405, 407
Hexamita spp.   126
Hexamita spp. infection
　furazolidone treatment   148, 187
　in ornamental fish   366
　in rainbow trout   236, 243, 244
High temperatures *see* Water temperature
Hippoglossus hippoglossus see Halibut
Histiostoma infection, eels   321
Histopathology   78
　of eels   324
　of marine invertebrates   85
　of prawns   291–292
　sampling   209
History taking   66, 69–71, 206, 290–291, 323–324
Hitra disease   105, 143
Hole in the head disease
　of channel catfish   257
　of cichlids   366
Holobranchs   6, 7
Homarus americanus see Lobster
Homeostasis   12
Hormones
　endocrine   24–26
　gastrointestinal   26

Hormones—*continued*
  pituitary 24
  produced by chromaffin cells 25
Husbandry
  of Atlantic salmon 180–181, 189–190
  of carp 39–40, 298–300
  of channel catfish 39
  and disease prevention 91, 169, 180, 185, 189, 193,
      393
  of eels 39, 313–314
  of game fish 396–404
  general procedures 31–41
  of halibut 340–342
  of non-salmonids 38–41
  of ornamental fish 358–362
  of prawns 281–285
  of rainbow trout 226–229
  and reduction of antibiotic use 153
  of sea-bass and sea-bream 380–381
  of turbot 40–41, 328–331
Hydrogen peroxide 67, 118
Hydrogen sulphide 60, 95, 369
Hygiene
  and disease 216
  in recirculation systems 314
Hyperventilation 71
Hypodermis 6
Hypophthalmichthys molitrix (silver carp) 297
Hypothermia 166, 219
Hypoxia, in anaesthesia 162

Ichthyobodo spp. 111–112
Ichthyobodo spp. infection
  acriflavine–HCl treatment 319
  in Atlantic salmon 199, 201
  in channel catfish 260
  chloramine-T treatment 135
  clinical signs 235
  in cod 352–353
  in eels 319
  formalin treatment 138, 319
  lactardine treatment 319
  in ornamental fish 366
  in rainbow trout 235
  sodium chloride treatment 141–142
  treatment 111–112
  in turbot 332
Ichthyophonus spp. 108
Ichthyophonus spp. infection
  in cod 352
  in herring 352
  in rainbow trout 234

  in turbot 333
Ichthyophthirius multifiliis 112–113
  marine counterpart 386
Ichthyophthirius multifiliis infection
  in Atlantic salmon 202
  in carp 305
  in channel catfish 260
  clinical signs 112
  in cod 354–355
  in eels 320
  in ornamental fish 366–367
  phenoxethol treatment 392
  in rainbow trout 235
  in sea-bass and sea-bream 384
  and stocking density 305
  treatment 112, 212
Ictalurus catus (white catfish) 252
Ictalurus furcatus see Blue catfish
Ictalurus nebolosus (bullhead) 252
Ictalurus punctatus see channel catfish
Identification methods, for halibut 340
Immobilisation, by anaesthesia 161
Immunostimulants 153, 190
Impression smears 85
In-feed medication *see* Feed, medicated
Inappetance, common sign of disease 91
Incubation techniques
  hatchery routines 37
  rainbow trout 223
Indian polyculture systems, *Lernaea* infection 117
Industrial waste 94–95
Infectious haemotopoietic necrosis (IHN)
  clinical signs 99, 230
  control 99
  eradication 174
  notifiable disease 174
  of rainbow trout 230
  of salmonids 99
  triggered by vaccination 143
Infectious hypodermal and haemopoeietic necrosis, of
      prawns 288
Infectious lax anaemia (ILA) 128
Infectious pancreatic necrosis (IPN) 99
  of Atlantic salmon 199
  clinical signs 99, 199
  control 99
  disease-free stock 198
  endemic 199
  of halibut 343
  mortality 99
  in Norway 184
  notifiable disease 174
  and pancreatic disease 127
  of rainbow trout 99

Infectious pancreatic necrosis (IPN)—*continued*
 of salmonids   99
 in Scotland   198
 of sea-bass and sea-bream   382
 stress testing   333
 stress-induced   143
 of striped bass   407
 transmission   199
 of trout   230
 of turbot   333
Infectious salmon anaemia (ISA)   128, 184, 185
Injection, of treatment materials   67, 375
Injection sites   214
Inoculation, of culture media   82
Insects *see* Predation
Integument, of crustaceans   28
Inter-renal tissue   11, 21, 25
International trade
 in fish eggs   54
 in live shellfish   54
 in ornamental fish   54, 300
Interstitial fluid, protein concentration   15
Intestinal steatosis, sea-bream   390
Intestine   16
Iodophor disinfectant   36–37, 73, 186, 245, 294
 for egg disinfection   142
Islets of Langerhans   18, 26, 308
Isopoda, parasitic   120
Ivermectin
 dosage   142–143
 in treatment of ornamental fish   142, 376

Jaw teeth   16
Jaw tone, as measure of anaesthesia   162–163
Jumping, excessive   71

Kanamycin   142
Khawia spp. infection, of carp   305–306
Kidney
 haemopoietic tissue   20–21
 localised lesions   77
 structure and function   11–13
 tissue sampling   79
Koi
 acriflavine treatment   376
 aquaculture   297, 300
 high monetary value   372
 pond systems   358, 360
 sodium chloride treatment   142
Kudoa spp. infection, of sea-bream   386

Laboratories, specialised   69, 78, 87–89, 91, 101, 189,
  373
Laboratory equipment
 for bacteriology   80
 for veterinary examination   72–73, 210–211
Labratrema minumus infection, sea-bream   387
Labyrith (inner ear)   23
Lactardine, and *Ichthyobodo* spp. infection   319
Lactase   16
Lactate levels, in anaesthesia   165
Lactobacillus spp, in turbot culture   329
Largemouth bass
 acanthocephalan parasites   406
 cannibalism   401
 diet   401
 fingerling production   396, 399–401
 as game fish   395–396
 rearing systems   399
 Uvilifer spp. infection   405
Larval bacterial septicaemia, of prawns
  286–287
Larval mycosis, of prawns   287
Larval rearing, of salmonids   44, 50–51
Lateral line   2, 11, 23
Learnocera spp. infection, of cod   353
Leeches   120
 of carp   306
 control of infection   120
 of game fish   405
 as intermediate hosts   303, 306, 319, 366, 369
 of sea-bass and sea-bream   388
Legislation
 and aquaculture   173–177, 229–230
 Canadian   174
 and carp culture   300
 and cod culture   350
 and disease prevention   173–174
 EC   173–177
 economic considerations   173
 and game fish culture   404
 and halibut culture   342–343
 Norwegian   183
 and ornamental fish culture   362
 and prawn culture   284–285
 and sea-bass and sea-bream culture   381
 and treatment   173, 211
 and turbot culture   331
 UK, on fish diseases   198, 229
 and welfare considerations   173
Lens (eye)   22
Lernaea spp. (anchor worm)   117
Lernaea spp. (anchor worm) infection
 in carp   307
 dichlorvos treatment   137

Lernaea spp. (anchor worm) infection—*continued*
  in eels   323
  in ornamental fish   368–369
  in rainbow trout   236
Lernatropus spp. infection, in sea-bass   388
Leteux–Meyer mixture   139, 212
Leuciscus spp. (chubb and orfe), toxicity of treatment
      compounds for   138
Leucocytes   19
Leucothrix mucor infection, in prawns   287
Levamisole   143, 153, 322
Light intensity
  in aquarium systems   360
  in hatchery   32
  in striped bass culture   403–404
  in turbot farming   328
  welfare considerations   218
Ligula spp. tapeworms   124, 368
Lipase   16
Lipids
  dietary requirements   18, 96, 156–157
  excess   18, 96
  rancid   96, 157, 239–240
  storage and metabolism   17, 18, 96, 349
Lips   2, 16
Live feed *see* Feed, live
Live fish, transportation   89
Live-bearers   143, 364–366
Liver
  necroscopy features   77
  normal structure and function   17
  tissue sampling   78
Liver lipoid disease   96, 157, 239, 390
Lobsters
  oxytetracycline treatment   149
  sensitivity to malachite green   140
  vaccines available   143
Localised swellings   73
Loch-rearing, advantages and disadvantages   38
Lordosis, of sea-bass and sea-bream   389
Low temperatures *see* Water temperature
Lucioperca lucioperca (pike-perch)   297
Luminous vibriosis, of prawns   286
Lymph   15, 18
Lymphocystis
  of ornamental fish   363–364
  of sea-bass and sea-bream   101, 381–382
  of striped bass   407
  transmission   101, 382
Lymphocytes   19

Macrophages   19
Magnesium, effect of high levels   65

Maintenance diet   156
Malachite green   243–244
  administration   140
  available forms   139
  benzalkonium chloride as substitute for   135
  combined with formalin   139
  diagnostic use   292
  dosage   140, 212, 244, 325
  gill damage   65
  in hatchery procedures   37, 193
  for parasite treatment   187, 320, 321, 392
  for proliferative kidney disease   122, 132, 133,
      139–140
  for *Saprolegnia* infection   108, 234, 319
  sensitivity of lobster (*Homarus americanus*) to   140
  teratogenicity   141, 243
  toxicity   140–141
Malpighian cells   4–5
Management procedures
  damaging   95
  and disease diagnosis   70
  and disease prevention   31, 170
  for ornamental fish   371
  recommended   245
  stressful to fish   110, 197
  and treatment   153–154
Mangrove zone   284
Marine aquaculture methods *see also* Sea cages   47–49
Marine invertebrates, disease diagnosis   85–86
Marine prawns *see* prawns
Masou salmon, liver pathology   101
Mast cells   19
Mauthner axons   21, 22
Mebendazole   137, 321
Medicines *see* Drugs; Treatment
Melanomacrophage centres   20, 21
Metabolic waste products *see* Waste products
Metaenaeus spp. *see* Prawns
Metazoan parasites   115–120, 123–125, 367–369
Methaemoglobinaemia   61, 141, 265
Methane   60, 369
Methylene blue
  dosage   141
  for eel infections   320, 321
  toxic to scaleless fish   141
  treatment for nitrite toxicity   141
Metomidate   165–166
Metronidazole   142, 244
MIC data
  Aeromonas spp.   147, 149, 150, 152–153
  amoxycillin   147
  Edwardsiella tarda   147
  Flexibacter columnaris   149, 150
  oxolinic acid   149

MIC data—*continued*
  oxytetracycline 150, 152–153
  Pasteurella piscicida 147, 149
  Pseudomonas fluorescens 150
  quinolones 152–153
  Streptococcus spp. 147
  Vibrio anguillarum 147, 149, 150
  Yersinia ruckeri 149, 150, 153
Microscopic examination 73
  of prawns 291
Microsporidial infection 122–123
  of ornamental fish 367
  of sea-bream 386
  of turbot 333–334
Microtyle infection, sea-bream 387
Mineral deficiencies 96, 155
Mineral requirements 158
Minnows
  feral 297
  as forage fish 256
Minocycline, dosage 142
Mitraspora spp. infections, ornamental fish 139, 367
Moist feeds 155–156
Molluscs
  bacteriology and histopathology 85–86
  parasitic 115, 120, 368
Molly, trichlorphon/mebendazole treatment 137
Mondodon, baculovirus disease, prawns 285
Monocytes 19
Monogenean parasites 115–116, 137
  of carp 305
  of cod 353
  of eels 321
    treatment 325–326
  formalin treatment 138
  potassium permanganate treatment 141
  of sea-bass and sea-bream 387
  treatment 393
Moribund fish, slaughter 219
Morone saxatilis see Striped bass
Mortalities
  hygienic disposal 54
  removal 32–34, 70, 183, 189–190, 194, 197–198, 216, 218, 337, 347
Mortality patterns, in clinical diagnosis 241
Motile aeromonad septicaemia 233–234, 259
Moulting, of crustacean cuticle 28
Mouth fungus, of ornamental fish 364–365
Mouth teeth 16
Movement, abnormal 71
Movement restrictions 198, 199
MS-222 *see* Tricaine methanesulphonate
Mucus
  excess production in gill disease 74, 111, 116, 135

  excess reduced by treatment 141–142, 212
  normal secretion 4, 5
Muddy flavour, reduced by salt treatment 142
Mullet
  Axine infection 116
  Benedenia infection 116
  Oodinium infection 112
  Salmonicola infection 117
Muscle, types 3
Muscle necrosis, prawns 290
Mussels, contamination 67
Mycobacterium infection 85, 107
Mycotoxins 96, 109
Myomeres 3–4
Myxidium spp. infection 122, 320
Myxobacteria *see also Chondrococcus*
Myxobacterial infection
  chloramine-T treatment 135
  of ornamental fish 364
  of sea-bass and sea-bream 384
Myxobacterial skin infection, Atlantic salmon 199–200
Myxobolosis *see* Whirling disease
Myxobolus spp. 121
Myxobolus spp. infection
  of carp 304
  clinical signs 304
  of ornamental fish 367
  of sea-bass 386
Myxosoma cerebralis 120–121, 236–237
Myxosporidia 120–121
Myxosporidial infection
  of carp 303–304
  of eels 320
  of sea-bream 386
Myxozoal infection, of ornamental fish 367

Nanophyetus spp. 124
Necroscopy
  of eels 324
  gross features 76–85
Nematode parasites 125–126, 306, 321–323, 334, 368, 405
  treatment 143, 325–326
Neomycin 142
Neon tetra disease 367
Neoplasia 97–98
  in ornamental fish 370
  in sea-bream 389
  in turbot 334
Nephrocalcinosis 59, 94, 96, 158
Nerocilia spp. infection, in sea-bass 388

Nervous system
  crustacean   30
  teleost   21–24
Nets
  fouling   34–35, 197
  management   34–35, 64, 205, 216
  shape   194
Neutrosils (polymorphs)   19
Niclosamide   336
Nifurazolidone   187
Nifurpirinol   142, 148
Nitrites   60, 94
  and methaemoglobinaemia   265
  methylene blue treatment   141
  and nitrates   61
  safe levels   61
  toxicity to channel catfish   397
Nitrofurans   148, 243
Nitrogen cycle   60–61
Nitrosomonas and *Nitrobacter* spp.   60
No-blood disease   263–264
Non-salmonids, husbandry   38–41
Norway
  aquatic diseases   184
  cod production   347
  disease control   184
  legislation   183, 229, 350
  licensing of fish farms   185
  salmon farming   179–191
Notifiable diseases
  EC   174
  in Norway   183, 189
  of ornamental fish   362–363
  spring viraemia of carp   300
  in UK   198, 229
Nutritional aspects, of aquaculture   153–159
Nutritional diseases   95–97
  of carp   307–308
  of ornamental fish   370–371
  of prawns   290
  of rainbow trout   239–241
  of sea-bream   390
  of turbot   334
Nutritional factors, in pancreatic disease   127
Nutritional requirements   156–159, 349

Observation and examination of fish   71–73, 206–207,
      218, 228
Octimitis   126
Oedematous changes   74
Oesophagus   16
Oilseeds, in channel catfish feed   255

Olfactory organ   23–24
Oncorhyncus kisutch see Coho salmon
Oncorhyncus masou virus   101
Oncorhyncus mykiss see Rainbow trout
Oncorhyncus tshawytscha see Chinook salmon
Ongrowing systems   45–49
Onions and garlic, as chemical repellents   119
Oodinium spp. infection   112
  clinical signs   112
  metronidazole treatment   142
  in ornamental fish   366
Operator safety
  in prawn farming   293
  and treatment chemicals   138, 176, 193, 211, 212,
      244, 376
Opportunist pathogens
  bacterial   101
  fungal   108
  of prawns   287
  of turbot   331–332
Oral treatment materials   67
Oreochromis spp. *see* Tilapia
Orfe
  pond systems   358
  toxicity of treatment compounds for   138
Organic toxins   24, 65, 94–95, 369
Organophosphorus compounds
  environmental considerations   67
  operator safety   244
  in treatment of parasite infections   117–119, 388
Ornamental fish
  Aeromonas spp. infection   364
  Amyloodinium spp. infection   366
  anaesthesia   373
  antibiotic treatment   142, 374–376
  antihelminthics   375, 376
  aquarium systems   357–358
  Argulus   369
  bacterial diseases   364–365
  benzalkonium chloride   375
  blood worms   368
  branchiomycosis   365
  Brooklynella spp. infection   367
  Camellanus spp.   368
  Capillaria spp.   368
  carp erythrodermatitis   364
  Chilodonella spp. infection   367
  chloramine-T treatment   375
  Chondrococcus spp. infection   364
  chronic granulomatous disease   365
  cichlid virus   364
  clinical diagnosis   371–373
  Clinostomum spp   367–368
  cold-water disease   365

Ornamental fish—*continued*
columnaris disease 364
as companion animals 372
Cryptobia spp. infection 366
Cryptocaryon spp. infection 366
culture 297
Dactylogyrus spp. (gill fluke) 367
Dermocystidium spp. 365
Diplostomum spp. infection 367–368
disease prevention 376
dosage calculations 373–374
economic considerations 357, 372
ectoparasitic treatment 375–376
Eimeria spp. infection 366
environmental aspects of disease 363
Ergasilus spp. infection 369
Eustrongyloides spp. 368
eye fluke 367–368
feeding 361–362
fin rot 365
fungal disease 365
gill disease 364
gill flukes 367
gill maggots 369
gill rot 365
Gyrodactylus spp. (skin fluke) 367
Henneguya spp. infections 367
Hexamita 366
husbandry 358–362
Ichthyobodo spp. infection 366
Ichthyophthirius multifiliis infection 366–367
individual treatment 373–374, 376
international trade 54, 300, 357
ivermectin 376
laboratory analysis 373
legislation 362
Lernaea spp. infection 368–369
live feed 362
lymphocystis 363–364
management procedures 371
metal toxins 369
Mycobacterium infection 85, 107
myxobacterial disease 364
Myxobolus spp. infections 367
myxozoa infections 367
neoplasia 370
nifurpirinol treatment 148
nutritional diseases 370–371
Oodinium spp. infection 366
papilloma 370
parasitic diseases 362, 366–369
peduncle disease 365
Philometra spp. infection 368
Pleistophora spp. infection 367

Pomphorhyncus spp. infection 368
pond systems 357, 358
post-mortem examination 373
predation 363
prophylactic treatment 376
protein requirement 362
quarantine 376–377
Ramirez dwarf virus 364
record keeping 362
Sanguinicola spp. infection 368
Saprolegnia infection 365
Scyphidia infection 367
skin flukes 367
slime disease 366
sodium chloride (salt) 376
spring viraemia of carp 363
sunburn 363
swim-bladder inflammation 363, 364
tapeworms 368
Tetrahymena spp. infection 366
toxic gases 369
toxins 363, 369
transportation 363
treatment by injection 375
treatment licensing 362, 373–374
trichlorphon/mebendazole treatment 137
Trichodina complex infections 367
trypanosomes 366
Uronema spp. infection 367
vaccination 377
vandalism 66
veterinary approach 357–377
virus diseases 363–364
Vorticella infections 367
welfare aspects 362, 363
Oscar, trichlorphon/mebendazole treatment 137
Osmoregulation
crustacean 30
failure in diseased salmon 202, 203
normal 1, 6, 11–13
Otolith organ 11, 23
Oval, of swim-bladder 10
Ovary 27
Overfeeding 35, 66, 127, 170
Overfishing, of wild stocks 58, 284
Overwintering
of carp 40, 298, 300–301
of channel catfish 256, 263
and *Dactylogyrus* infection 116
lowers disease resistance 110
and *Myxobolus cyprini* infection 121
and pancreas disease 127
and parasitic disease 112
Oxidised fat *see* Rancidity

Oxolinic acid
  dosage   142, 147, 148–149, 187, 213
  drug resistance   149, 150, 213
  MIC data   149
  in treatment of eels   316, 317
  in treatment of ornamental fish   374
  withdrawal period   149
Oxygen deficiency, symptoms   58–59
Oxygen depletion
  by effluents   94
  potassium permanganate treatment   141
  in recreational ponds   399
Oxygen levels
  diurnal variation   58–59, 307
  seasonal variation   196, 265
  and water quality   31, 58–60, 182–183, 218
Oxygen requirement
  of carp   40
  of channel catfish   39, 45, 264–265
  normal   7–8, 18
  of rainbow trout   226–229
Oxygen transport, in blood   20
Oxygen uptake, normal   7–8
Oxygenation *see* Aeration
Oxytetracycline   149–150, 187
  dosage   142, 147, 149, 213
  drug resistance   213
  MIC data   150, 152–153
  in treatment for bacterial kidney disease (BKD)
      185
  in treatment of channel catfish   266
  in treatment for columnaris disease   407
  in treatment of eels   316, 317
  in treatment of ornamental fish   374
  in treatment of turbot   336
  withdrawal periods   150

Pacific salmon
  boil disease   122
  essential fatty acids   157
  Henneguya spp.   121–122
  infectious haematopoietic necrosis (IHN)   99
  Mycobacterium infection   107
Pain, perception by fish   161, 170, 218
Pancreas   17–18, 26
  test of exocrine activity   88
  tissue sampling   79
Pancreatic disease
  Atlantic salmon   98, 99, 127–128, 196, 199
  of Atlantic salmon   204–205
  control   128
  and infectious pancreatic necrosis (IPN)   127
  possible causes   127, 204

Pansteatitis, rainbow trout   241
Papilloma
  of Atlantic salmon   97–98
  of carp   97–98
  causes   98
  of eels   98
  of flatfish   98
  of ornamental fish   370
  of sea-bream   383
Paramoeba infection, in rainbow trout   236
Parasites
  annelid   115, 120, 369
  cestode   124, 305–306, 405
  classification   109
  coccidian   126, 303
  crustacean   75–76, 115–120, 306–307, 323, 368–369,
      388
  flagellate   111, 126, 366
  helminth   75–78, 126, 388
  identification and preservation   75–76
  metazoan   115–120, 123–125, 367–369
  microsporidian   122–123
  molluscan   115, 120, 368
  nematode   125–126, 306, 321–323, 334, 368, 405
  protozoan   78, 111–115, 120–123, 126
Parasitic cysts, necroscopy features   77
Parasitic diseases   109–127
  of Atlantic salmon   201–203
  of carp   303–307
  of channel catfish   259–262
  control   110–111
  of eels   319–323
  examination for   75, 210
  and individual treatment of fish   131
  of ornamental fish   362, 366–369
  of rainbow trout   234
  of sea-bass and sea-bream   384–388
  and secondary infection   111
  treatment   244
  of turbot   334
Passing through a film, treatment method   134
Pasteurella spp.   105–106
  MIC data   147, 149
Pasteurella spp. infection
  clinical signs   106
  of sea-bass   384
  of striped bass   406
  of white perch   406
Pathology
  of *Edwardsiella* infection   105
  of furunculosis   102
  of infectious haematopoietic necrosis (IHN)   99
  of infectious pancreatic necrosis (IPN)   99
  of pancreas disease   127

Pathology—*continued*
  of swim-bladder inflammation 100
  of vibriosis 104–105
  of viral haemorrhagic septocaemia (VHS) 99
Peduncle disease
  of Atlantic salmon 203
  and *Chondrococcus psychrophila* 106
  of ornamental fish 365
  of rainbow trout 231
Penaeus spp. *see* Prawns
Perch 106, 393
pH
  changes stressful to fish 62, 93
  and gill damage 62
  optimum 62–63
    for rainbow trout 227
  of Scottish water 196
  and toxicity of heavy metals 64
Pharyngeal teeth 16
Phenoxethol 392
Phialophora infection 109
Philometra spp. infection 125
  in ornamental fish 368
Philometrides spp. infection, carp 306
Phorma infection 109
Phosphates, limiting nutrient in fresh water 65
Phosphorus content, of waste products 228
Phosphorus deficiency, of carp 308
Photoperiod manipulation 24, 32
Photosynthesis 58, 64
Physical damage
  and disease 106, 110
  to fish 66, 95
Physoclists 9
Physostomes 9
Phytoplankton 348
Pigments 158–159, 175
Pike 297, 393
  benzocaine treatment 164
  Triaenophorus infection 124
Pike-perch, *Lucioperca lucioperca* 297
Pin-heads 205
Pineal gland 24
Piscicola spp. 120
Piscicola spp. infection, of carp 306
Piscine tuberculosis *see Mycobacterium* infection
Piscirickettsia salmonis 108
Pituitary 24
PKX cell 122, 237
Plankton, as feed 155, 341
Plasma, protein levels 18
Pleistophora spp. infection
  of eels 320
  of ornamental fish 367

of sea-bream 386
Poaching 65
Poecilia velifera see Molly
Pollution
  and *Branchiomyces* infection 108
  by fish farms 180
  and *Edwardsiella tardiella* 105
  from fish feed 156, 158
  implicated in papilloma 98
Polylabris tubicirrus infection, of sea-bream 387
Pomphorhynchus spp. 126–127
Pomphorhyncus spp. infection, in ornamental fish 368
Pond systems
  for channel catfish 249–252
  for cod 347–348
  construction 250–251
  for eels 312
  equipment 358, 359
  for koi 360
  for ornamental fish 357, 358
  for prawns 283, 295
  and *Pseudomonas* spp. infection 105
  site selection 250
  for striped bass 402
Post-larval stage, of prawns 275
Post-mortem examination 207–208, 242, 292, 373
Posthodiplostomum spp. infection, in game fish 405
Potassium permanganate
  administration 141
  in channel catfish treatment 260, 266
  in columnaris disease 406–407
  dosage 141
  in game fish treatment 404, 407, 408
Power stations, warm water effluents 312, 327, 328, 334
Pox *see* Papilloma
Prawns
  Aeromonas spp infection 287
  aquaculture 275–281
    economic considerations 293
    environmental considerations 284
    legislation 284–285
    operator safety 293
    record keeping 295
    site selection 279, 293
  bacterial fouling 287
  bacterial necrosis 286
  bacteriology 292
  baculoviral mid-gut gland necrosis 285–286
  batch production 294
  black death 290
  black gill disease 290
  broodstock 294
  chronic soft shell syndrome 290

Prawns—*continued*
  disease   285–290
    bacteriology   291
    clinical diagnosis   290–292
    prevention and treatment   292–295
    water quality   291
  feeding   279, 280, 281, 284
  formalin treatment for parasites   138
  fungal disease   287–288, 289
  Fusarium disease   289
  gill preparations   292
  haemocytic enteritis   290
  hatchery   275–277, 281–282, 285, 294–295
  hepatopancreatic parvo-like virus disease   288
  histology   291, 292
  husbandry   281–285
  hypodermal and haemopoeietic necrosis   288
  larval bacterial septicaemia   286–287
  larval mycosis   287
  larval rearing tanks   278–279
  Leucothrix mucor infection   287
  life-cycle   275
  luminous vibriosis   286
  maturation tanks   278
  microscopic examination   291
  Mondodon, baculovirus disease   285
  muscle necrosis   290
  nursery tanks   279
  nutritional diseases   290
  opportunist pathogens   287
  pond systems   274, 279–280, 283, 295
  protozoan fouling   287–288
  Pseudomonas spp. infections   287
  Rickettsia infections   288
  shell disease   288
  spawning tanks   278
  species used in aquaculture   272
  stocking density   294
  stocking of ponds   283
  tank systems   276–279
  transmission of pathogens   294
  vaccination   293
  veterinary approach   271–295
  vibriosis   286–288
  viral diseases   292
  vitamin deficiency   290
  waste products   285
  water quality   281, 294–295
  world production   271
Praziquantel   142, 186, 188, 336, 406
Predation
  by animals   47, 66, 95, 209, 218, 363
  by birds   47, 66, 95, 170–171, 218, 298, 363
  by insects   401

control   55, 194
Predator damage
  to anaesthetised fish   163
  and vibrioisis   200
Predators, as parasite intermediate hosts   66, 95, 110
Predatory fish, distinctive anatomy   15, 16
Proliferative gill disease, of channel catfish   261–262
Proliferative kidney disease (PKD)
  clinical signs   122, 237
  control   122
  fumagillin treatment   148
  malachite green treatment   132, 133, 139–140
  management aspects   153–154
  prophylaxis   246
  of rainbow trout   122, 153–154, 236–237
  treatment   148
Prophylactic treatment
  of ornamental fish   376
  of sea-bass   393
Protective clothing   216, 294, 337
Protein
  dietary requirements   18, 96, 156, 362
  economic considerations   156
Proteocephalus tapeworm   405–406
Protozoa
  epiphytic   110
  parasitic   78, 111–115, 120–123, 126
    of channel catfish   259–262
    of cod   352–353
    of eels   319
    of game fish   404
    treatment with antimalarials   143
    treatment with formalin   138
    treatment with malachite green   139–140
    treatment with potassium permanganate   141
    of turbot   332, 334
Protozoan fouling, of prawns   287–288
Pseudo-albinism, of turbot   332
Pseudobranch   9, 26
Pseudodactylogyrus spp. infection, eels   321
Pseudomonad sepicaemia   234
Pseudomonas spp., MIC data   150
Pseudomonas spp. infection
  co-trimazine ineffective   148
  of eels   316, 319
  of game fish   404, 406
  and haemorrhagic septicaemia   105
  of prawns   287
  Romet treatment   150
  of turbot   333
Pterophyllum scalare see Angel fish
Pycnadenoides senegalensis infection, in sea-bream   388
Pylodictus oliveris (flathead catfish)   252

Pyloric caeca 16, 18
Pyrethroid baths 118–119

Quarantine, in disease prevention 386, 393
Quinaldine sulphate 165
Quinolones 152–153, 243

Raceways
   for rainbow trout 224, 225
   for salmonids 46–47
   use in treatment 132
Rainbow trout
   aflatoxicosis 241
   amenability to captivity 223
   antimicrobials 245
   aquaculture systems 223–228
   Argulus infection 236
   bacterial diseases 231–234, 246
     treatment 243
   bankruptcy disease 107
   benzalkonium chloride 243
   broodstock 227
   cage systems 225–226
   Childonella 236
   chloramine-T 243, 244
   Chondrococcus spp. infection 231
   clinical diagnosis 241–242
   cold-water disease 231
   columnaris disease 231
   congenital deformity 128
   Dactylogyrus 236
   Diphyllobothrium spp. 238–239
   Diplostomum spathaceum 238
   disease prevention 244–245
   drug dosages 147
   earth pond rearing 46, 223, 224
   enteric redmouth (ERM) 105, 231
   erythromycin 243
   essential fatty acids 157, 239
   eye fluke 124, 238
   eye pathology 241
   feeding 228
   feeding hierarchy 228
   freshwater cages 225–226
   fry mortality syndrome (fry anaemia syndrome)
     231
   fry rearing 223
   fry tanks 228
   fungal disease 234
     treatment 243–244

   furazolidone treatment 148
   furunculosis 232–233
   grading 228
   Gyrodactylus 236
   hatchery procedures 227–228
   hepatoma 98
   Hexamita infection 236, 243, 244
   husbandry 226–229
   Ichthybodo spp. infection 235
   Ichthyophirius multifiliis 235
   Ichthyophorus infection 234
   incubation 223
   infectious haematopoietic necrosis (IHN) 230
   infectious pancreatic necrosis (IPN) 99
   Lernaea spp. infection 236
   lipoid liver degeneration 239
   marketing 223
   motile aeromonad septicaemia 234
   Myxosoma cerebralis 236–237
   natural location 223
   nutritional diseases 239–241
   oxygen requirements 226–229
   pansteatitis 241
   paramoeba 236
   parasitic disease 234
     treatment 243–245
   peduncle disease 231
   proliferative kidney disease (PKD) 122, 153–154,
     236–237
   pseudomonad septicaemia 234
   raceways 224, 225
   Saprolegnia infection 234
   sea cages 47, 228
   shock sydrome 157
   slaughter 53
   Streptococcus infection 107, 232
   stress reduction 244–245
   susceptibility to furunculosis 102
   susceptibility to pollutants 226, 227
   tank systems 225
   tolerance of salinity 228
   Trichodina infection 235–236
   vaccination 245–246
   vibriosis 234
   viral disease, treatment 242
   viral haemorrhagic septocaemia (VHS) 99
   vitamin requirements 239, 240
   water quality 226–229
   water temperatures 227
   water volume required 226
   whirling disease 120–121, 236–237
   white spot disease 235
   world production 223
   Yersinia ruckeri 150

Rainbow trout fingerling syndrome   106–107
    treatment   135
Ram ventilation   8
Ramirez dwarf virus, ornamental fish   364
Rancid dietary lipids   96, 157, 239–240, 390
Recirculation systems   49–50, 193
    for eels   49, 312
    environmental advantages   58
    gas bubble disease   203
    hygiene   314
    for prawn hatcheries   278
    water quality   312
Record keeping
    in broodstock selection   252, 268
    in channel catfish production   254
    in diagnosis and treatment   69, 131, 133, 135, 188,
        206, 241
    of dose calculations   135
    of feeding patterns   154
    importance of   36, 154, 198, 245
    in ornamental fish culture   362
    in prawn culture   283, 295
Recreational ponds
    algal blooms   399
    management   395–399
    water quality   399
Rectum   17
Red diseases, of eels   315–316
Red sore disease, of game fish   404
Red spot (red fillet) syndrome, of channel catfish   262
Red-ear sunfish   397–398
Renibacterium salmoninarum, and bacterial kidney
        disease (BKD)   107, 199
Renin–angiotensin system   25
Reproduction, crustacean   30
Reproductive system   26–27
Respiration
    eased by benzalkonium chloride   135
    normal   6–9
Respiration abnormal   71
Respiratory distress syndrome   8
Respiratory system, crustacean   29
Restaurant trade   54
Reticuloendothelial system   11, 21
Rice paddies, and prawn farming   284
Rickettsia infections   107–108, 288
Roach, as forage fish   398
Rodlet cells   7, 16, 17
Romet   147, 150, 266, 407
Root effect   10, 19
Rotenone treatment, cod   347
Rotifers, as live feed   51, 155, 276, 329–330, 348,
        380
Rotifers *see also* feed, live

Running water ongrowing systems   45–47
Rust disease   366

Saccharase   16
Saddleback lesions   106, 108, 200, 258–259
Safety
    of consumer   176
    and health equipment   54
    of operators   33, 138, 176, 193, 211, 212, 244, 293,
        376
Safety considerations, and treatment compounds   176,
        362
Safety margins, in anaesthesia   162, 164
Salinity   170, 182–183
    in control of infection   393, 407
Salmo trutta see Brown trout
Salmon
    Chlamydia infections   107
    hatchery   43–44
    jaw deformities   128
    lymph heart   15
    migration   24
    parr   44–45
    summer lesion syndrome (SLS)   95
    Vibrio anguillarum   104
Salmon *see also* Atlantic salmon
Salmon louse *see* Sea louse
Salmon pox   97–98
Salmonicola spp.   117
Salmonids
    aeration equipment   50
    aquaculture   31
    bacterial kidney disease, erythromycin treatment
        148
    benzocaine dosage   164
    blood fluke   125–126
    broodstock   36, 156
    Chilodonella infection   112
    drug doses   147
    feed, artificial   51, 155
    feeding patterns   170
    flagellate parasite   126
    flesh pigmentation   158–159
    flukes   126
    furazolidone treatment   148
    general management   31–36
    goitre   96
    hatchery   36–37, 43–44
    Ichthyobodo infection   111–112
    infectious haematopoietic necrosis (IHN)   99
    infectious pancreatic necrosis (IPN)   99
    jaw teeth   16
    larval development   44, 51

Salmonids—*continued*
  low tolerance of contamination   57, 64
  metomidate anaesthesia   166
  nematode parasites   125
  ongrowing systems   45–47
  oxytetracycline treatment   149
  pyloric caeca   18
  Romet treatment   150
  Salmonicola infection   117
  tagging   167
  transference of fry   37–38
  Triaenophorus infection   124
  vaccines available   143
  viruses   99–100
  whirling disease   120–121
Saltwater eel disease   316
Sampling
  bacteriological   80–81, 207
  of live fish   75, 219, 372, 373
  regular   334
  selection for   72
  of small fish   79–80
Sand particles, danger to fish   89, 94
Sanguinicola   125–126
Sanguinicola spp. infection
  of carp   305
  of ornamental fish   368
Saprolegnia   108
Saprolegnia infection
  of Atlantic salmon   199, 200–201
  of carp   303
  of channel catfish   263
  clinical signs   234
  cotton wool appearance   200, 365
  of eels   318, 319
    treatment   325
  of eggs   234
  of game fish   404
  of ornamental fish   365
  of rainbow trout   234
  treatment and control   108, 212
Sarafloxacin hydrochloride   150
Scaleless fish, compounds toxic to   141
Scales   2, 6
Schreckstoff cells, of carp   4, 5
Scophthalmus maximus see Turbot
Scotland, salmon farming   193–221
Scyphidia infection   114
  control   114
  in eels   321
  in ornamental fish   367
Sea cages   47–49
  for cod   348–349
  Coho syndrome   108

  design and construction   48, 194, 219, 225
  excess food and waste products   57–58
  exposure to parasitic fauna   110
  feeding methods   52
  fibrosarcoma outbreaks   100
  furunculosis outbreaks   103
  for halibut   340
  location   182, 194
  mortality removal   197–198
  net fouling   32
  in Norwegian fjords   179–180
  observation difficult   206
  for rainbow trout   225–226, 228
  in Scotland   194
  for sea-bass and sea-bream   381
  storm damage   48
  treatment methods   67, 134, 137
  for turbot   41
  vibriosis outbreaks   234
Sea louse (*Caligulus* and *Lepeophtheirus*)   117–119
  in Atlantic salmon   197, 199, 202, 203
  cod   353
  control   66, 67, 118, 217
  counting   210
  epizootics   118
  in game fish   405
  as intermediate hosts   307
  in Norway   188
  in sea-bass   388
  secondary infection   127, 200, 203
  treatment   67, 118–119, 137, 186, 188, 212
    stressful to fish   205
Sea water
  in land-based tanks   194
  in prawn hatcheries   277
  sterilisation   181
Sea-bass
  Acanthostomum inbutiforme infection   387
  Aeromonas spp. infection   383
  Amyloodinium spp. infection   385
  antibiotic treatment   392
  antiparasitic treatment   392
  aquaculture systems   380
  bacterial infections   383–384
  birnavirus   382
  broken neck syndrome   390–391
  cage farming   47
  Caligulus spp. infection   388
  cannibalism   389
  Chlamydia infections   107
  clinical diagnosis   391
  Colobomatus spp. infection   388
  Colponema spp. infection   385
  crustacean parasites   388

Sea-bass—*continued*
  Cryptobia spp. infection   385
  Dactylogyrus spp. infection   387
  deformities   389
  Diplectanum aequans infection   387
  disease prevention   393
  Edwardsiella spp. infection   384
  Eimeria spp. infection   385–386
  Epibdella spp. infection   387
  fatty liver   390
  feeding hierarchy   389
  fungal diseases   384
  gill flukes   387
  grading   389
  Gyrodactylus spp. infection   387
  Henneguya spp. infection   386
  husbandry   380–381
  Ichthyophthirius multifiliis infection   384
  infectious pancreatic necrosis (IPN)   382
  jaw teeth   16
  larval rearing   44
  leeches   388
  legislation   381
  Lernatropus spp. infection   388
  lordosis   389
  lymphocystis   381–382
  myxobacteria infection   384
  Myxobolus spp. infection   386
  natural history   379–380
  Nerocilia spp. infection   388
  Oodinium infection   112
  parasitic diseases   384
  Pasteurella spp. infection   106, 384
  quinaldine sulphate anaesthesia   165
  sunburn   389–390
  swim-bladder problems   388
  Tracheolobdella lubrica infection   388
  trichodiniasis   386
  vaccination, vibriosis   393
  veterinary approach   379–394
  vibriosis   383
  viral diseases   381–383
  vitamin deficiencies   391
Sea-bream
  Aeromonas spp. infection   383
  Amyloodinium spp. infection   385
  antibiotic treatment   392
  antiparasitic treatment   392
  aquaculture systems   380
  bacterial infections   383–384
  cage farming   47, 101, 381
  Chlamydia infections   107
  Chlorormyxum spp. infection   386
  Chondrococcus infection   106

  clinical diagnosis   391
  Colponema spp. infection   385
  crustacean parasites   388
  Cryptobia spp. infection   385
  Cryptocariasis spp. infection   386
  Dactylogyrus spp. infection   387
  deformities   389
  disease prevention   393
  distended gut syndrome   382–383
  Edwardsiella tardiella   105
  Eimeria spp. infection   385–386
  epitheliocystis   386–387
  Ergasilus spp. infection   388
  fatty liver   390
  fungal diseases   384
  Furnestia echeineis spp. infection   387
  gill flukes   387
  gill rot   384, 387
  Gyrodactylus spp. infection   387
  Haemogregarina spp. infection   386
  helminth parasites   388
  husbandry   380–381
  Ichthyophthirius multifiliis infection   384
  infectious pancreatic necrosis (IPN)   382
  jaw teeth   16
  Kudoa spp. infection   386
  Labratrema minumus infection   387
  larval rearing   44
  leeches   388
  legislation   381
  lipoid liver degeneration   390
  lordosis   389
  lymphocystis   381–382
  lymphocystis disease virus (LDV)   101
  microspora infection   386
  Microtyle infection   387
  mineral requirements   158
  myxobacteria infection   384
  myxosporea infectiom   386
  natural history   379
  neoplastic conditions   389
  nutrional diseases   390
  Oodinium infection   112
  papilloma   383
  parasitic diseases   384–388
  Pasturella piscicida   106
  Pleistophora senegalensis   386
  Polylabris tubicirrus infection   387
  Pycnadenoides senegalensis infection   388
  sunburn   389–390
  systemic granuloma   390
  trichodiniasis   386
  veterinary approach   379–394
  vibriosis   383

Sea-bream—*continued*
   viral diseases 381–383
   vitamin deficiencies 391
   white stripe disease 389
Seals *see* Predation
Seasonal variation, oxygen levels 196, 265
Sedation, before transport 219
Seine netting 53
Sekoke disease, of carp 308
Selective breeding 110, 128
Self-inflicted trauma 71
Sensory organs 22–24
Separation of age classes 31, 194, 200, 216
   for parasite control 118, 121, 126
   in prawns 294
Septicaemic vibriosis, eels 316
Seriola quinqueradiata see Yellowtail
Serological tests 84
Seven freedoms 217–219
Sex distinction 26
Sex hormones 26
Sharks, metomidate anaesthesia 166
Sheatfish
   branchiomycosis 302
   as food fish 297
Shell disease, prawns 288
Shellfish, international trade 54
Shoaling behaviour, normal and abnormal 71,
   171
Shock sydrome, rainbow trout 157
Shrimp, aquaculture *see* prawns
Shrimp meal, in salmonid diet 158–159
Shrimps
   essential fatty acids for 157
   feed for 156
   formalin treatment for ciliate parasites 138
Siamese fighting fish 366
Side-swimming 71
Silage, fish waste 156
Silurus glanis see sheatfish
Silver carp, *Hypophthalmichthys molitrix* 297
Silver eels *see* eels
Site selection 198, 293
Size disparity 169, 196
   as cause of starvation 95–96, 156
   in eels 39
Skin
   anatomy 4–6
   damage 94, 95, 170
   relatively impervious 11
Skin flukes 115–116
   formalin treatment 138
   of ornamental fish 367
Skin lesions 73, 91

Slaughter, disposal of by-products 216
Slaughter methods 53, 171, 219
   anaesthetic overdose 219
   for examination of marine invertebrates 85
   and fish welfare 36
   humane 219
   for pet fish 171
   for sampling 72, 206–207
   in Scotland 198
   stunning and pithing 220
Slime disease, of ornamental fish 366
Smallmouth bass 399
Smoked fish industry 53, 198, 223
Smoltification 32, 38, 179, 194
Smolts 44–45
   aquaculture 179, 180
   failure to thrive 128
   grading and counting 52–53
   salt-water challenge 220
   transfer to sea 38, 196
   transportation 54
Snails, as intermediate hosts 124, 238, 353, 405
Snakehead rhabdovirus 101
Sodium chloride (salt) 141–142
   administration 142
   dosage 142, 212
   in ectoparasite treatment 141–142, 187
   ornamental fish 376
   in transportation of live fish 255
   in treatment of koi 142
Sodium thiosulphate, in transportation of live fish
   255
Soft shell syndrome, prawns 290
Soft-rayed fish 1, 3, 6, 9
Soles, *Entobdella* infection 116
Sound and pressure 10–11, 170–171
Spaerospora renicola infection, in carp 303–304
Sparus aurata see Sea-bream
Spawning
   of channel catfish 252–253
   of halibut 342
   hormone-induced 396, 400, 401
   inhibited by dimetridazole 142
   of striped bass 401, 402
Spawning containers 44, 253, 399
Spawning tanks, for prawns 278
Sphaerospora spp. 122
Sphaerospora spp. infection
   in Atlantic salmon 199, 200–201
   in channel catfish 261–262
Spinal cord 21–22
Spiny-rayed fish 1, 3, 6, 9
Spleen 18, 20, 79
Sporozoan parasites, of eels 319

Spring viraemia of carp   300–301
    clinical diagnosis   308
    clinical signs   100
    control   100
    notifiable disease   174, 300
    in ornamental fish   362–363
    prophylaxis   301
Staining of bateriological preparations   85
Starling's law   15
Starter feeds   155
Starvation
    before handling   196, 218
    before slaughter   53
    before transport   219, 255
    before treatment   131, 137
    causes   95
    signs   95
Static pondfish ongrowing systems   45
Statutory control, of effluents   58
Statutory controls
    in dichlorvos treatment   138
    for treatment   131
Statutory controls *see also* withdrawal period
Steelhead   223
Sterile plastic loops   81–82
Sterilisation
    in recirculation systems   49–50
    of sea water   181
Stock origin   198
Stock records *see* Record keeping
Stocking density
    in aquarium systems   360
    for Atlantic salmon   189–190, 197
    and disease prevention   33, 66, 70, 110, 214, 215
    economic considerations   32–33
    for eels   313
    and fin damage   203–204
    and *Ichthyophthirius multifiliis* infection   305
    in Norwegian aquaculture   182, 189–190
    for prawns   294
    for striped bass   402
    for turbot   330
    and water quality   57, 183, 197, 218
    welfare considerations   169
Stomach   15, 16
Stomatopapillomatosis, in eels   315
Storm damage, to sea cages   47–48
Streptococcus spp.   107
    MIC data   147
Streptococcus spp. infection
    in game fish   406
    in rainbow trout   232
Stress
    in eels   314
    in game fish   408
    minimisation   218, 244–245
    reduced by anaesthesia   161
Stress factors, physical   66
Stress reactions, of fish   161
Stress testing
    Aeromonas salmonicida   38
    for furunculosis   103, 198, 211, 220
    for infectious pancreatic necrosis (IPN)   333
Stress-induced disease   57, 70, 91, 98, 99, 101, 110,
        127, 232, 234, 256, 262–263, 315
Stressful procedures
    grading   196
    handling   215
    transportation   254–255
    treatment   131
    underfeeding   156
    vaccination   143
Striped bass
    ammonia tolerance   403
    columnaris disease   406
    commercial production   401–404
    crappie   407
    Diplostomum spp. infection   405
    eye fluke   405
    feed   403
    as food fish   393
    as game fish   395–396
    in vitro fertilisation   402
    infectious pancreatic necrosis (IPN)   407
    legislation   404
    lymphocystis   407
    pasterellosis   406
    pond systems   402
    spawning   401, 402
    stocking densities   402
    taxonomic classification of hybrids   401
    transportation   404
    vibriosis   406
        vaccine   408
    water quality   403
Sturgeon   91
Sudden death syndrome   127
Sulphadrugs   147–148
Sulphonamides   185, 243, 374
Summer lesion syndrome (SLS), salmon   95
Sunburn   95, 170, 363, 389–390
Sunfish   393, 397
Supersaturation *see* Gas bubble disease
Surplus fish, slaughter   219
Suspended solids
    acceptable levels   218, 227
    and gill damage   62, 64, 66, 94, 170, 182
    and gill disease   89

Suspended solids—*continued*
  increased by storms   71
  neutralise potassium permanganate   141
  in Scottish waters   196–197
  settlement control   228
Swabs   81
Sweden, fish health legislation   229
Swim-bladder
  fibrosarcoma   98
  infection, in eels   322–323
  inflammation
      in carp   100, 303–304
      in ornamental fish   363, 364
  normal anatomy   9–10
  problems, in sea-bass   388
Swimming, normal and abnormal   4, 71, 91, 171, 304,
      320
Symphysodon discus (discus), *Capillaria* infection   143
Systemic granuloma, sea-bream   390

Table scraps, unsuitable food   362
Tail rot
  and *Chondrococcus psychrophila* infection   106
  and *Saprolegnia* infection   108
Tank systems
  for anaesthesia   162
  design   133, 219
  for halibut   340
  hygiene   32, 216, 331
  for prawns   276–279
  for rainbow trout   225
  for salmon hatcheries   193
  for striped bass   402
  for treatment   131–132
  for turbot   331
Tapetum   23
Tapeworms
  in Atlantic salmon   199, 203
  in carp   305–306
  Caryophyllaeus spp.   126
  Diphyllobothrium spp.   124
  Eubothrium spp.   126, 188, 203, 213
  in game fish   405–406
  Ligula spp.   124
  in ornamental fish   368
  Proteocephalus spp.   405–406
  treatment   186
Taste buds   24
Tea-seed cake   283, 292
Teeth   16
Teleosts, definition   1
Tench
  antibiotic treatment   142

aquaculture   297
branchiomycosis   302
as forage fish   398
parasitic infections   303
pond systems   358
sensitivity to treatment compounds   138
Terramycin   266, 407
Testis   27
Tetracyclines   243
Tetrahymena spp. infection   113, 366
Tetramicra spp. infection, in turbot   333–336
Thelohanellus spp. infection, in carp   304
Therapeutic agents *see* Treatment
Therapy *see* Treatment
Thermal injury   166
Thirst   170, 217
Threadfin shad, as forage fish   398
Thrombocytes   19
Thymus   21
Thyroid   24–25
Tilapia
  Edwardsiella tardiella infection   105
  effects of aflatoxin   98
  as forage fish   256, 398
  Oodinium infection   112
Tinca tinca see Tench
Tissue analysis   88, 209
Tissue culture techniques   87–88
Tissue fixation   78
  for invertebrates   86
Toltrazuril   336
Top dressing, with pharmaceuticals   147
Toxic gases   32, 60, 369
Toxicity
  of dietary components   96–97
  of treatment materials   67, 135, 164, 370
Toxins
  endogenous   94–95
  exogenous   96–97
  and ornamental fish   363, 369
  safe levels in food   175
Tracheolobdella lubrica infection, sea-bass   388
Tranquillisation *see* Anaesthesia
Transmission
  of bacterial kidney disease (BKD)   199
  of infectious haematopoietic necrosis (IHN)   99
  of infectious pancreatic necrosis (IPN)   199
  of prawn pathogens   294
  of *Renibacterium salmoninarum*   107
  of viral haemorrhagic septocaemia (VHS)   99
Transportation
  of channel catfish   254–255
  of eels   313
  of game fish   408

Transportation—*continued*
    of halibut   340–341
    of live fish   54, 89, 219, 255
    of ornamental fish   363
    sedation for   163
    of smolts   38, 54
    stressful procedure   171, 254–255
    of striped bass   404
    of tissue samples   79–80, 88
    of turbot   40
    water quality   171, 254, 254–255
Trash fish
    as carrier of infection   107, 108, 200, 234, 333
    as feed   155
    pasteurisation   337
Treatment
    in aquaculture   131–152
    of Atlantic salmon, in Norway   186–187
    availability of therapeutic agents   91, 242
    of carp   308
    of channel catfish   266
    of cod   355
    collective   131
    EC legislation   173, 176–177
    of eels   324–325
    environmental considerations   131, 176
    of halibut   343–344
    individual   131, 373–374, 376
    licensed
        best choice   144
        in Norway   189
        of ornamental fish   362
        of turbot   331
        in UK   144
    licensing   144, 147, 176, 242, 246
        of dichlorvos   138
        of trichlorophon   137, 138
        in the UK   211
        in the USA   266, 407–408
        of vaccines   246
    management aspects   153–154
    need reduced by good husbandry   58, 66
    for *Oodinium* infection   112
    procedures   131
    of rainbow trout   242–244
    safety aspects   362, 376
    statutory record of drug use   36
    stressful to fish   57, 211, 218
    toxicity   66–67, 95, 96, 370
    of turbot   331, 336
    unlicensed
        of ornamental fish   373–374
        for prawn diseases   292
        welfare considerations   218

    use of tanks   131–132
    veterinary   131, 211, 218
Trematode parasites
    of carp   305
    of halibut   344
Triaenophorus spp. tapeworms   124, 368
Tribrissen   188
Tricaine methanesulphonate   72, 164–165, 171, 186, 220, 373
Trichlorophon   137, 186
    toxic to characins   138
Trichlorophon/mebendazole treatment, goldfish   137
Trichodina complex   113–114
Trichodina complex infection
    in Atlantic salmon   199, 201
    in channel catfish   260
    chloramine-T treatment   135
    clinical signs   114
    in cod   352–353
    control and treatment   114, 135, 138, 260, 393
    in eels   320–321
    formalin treatment   138
    in ornamental fish   367
    in rainbow trout   235–236
    in sea-bass and sea-bream   386
    in turbot   332
Trichogaster trichopterus see Gourami
Trichophyra infection   114–115
    in channel catfish   261
    control   115
    in eels   321
    in ornamental fish   367
Trimethoprim   147–148
Tropical fish, metomidate anaesthesia   166
Trout
    fingerlings   44–45
    hatchery   43–44
    infectious pancreatic necrosis (IPN)   230
    pyloric caeca   16
    veterinary approach   223–247
    viral diseases   230
    whirling disease   44
Trout *see also* brook trout; brown trout; rainbow trout
Trypanoplasma   125
Trypanoplasma infections
    in carp   303
    clinical signs   303
    in tench   303
Trypanosma   125
Trypanosoma infection
    of eels   319
    of ornamental fish   366
Trypsin digest test   88
Tuna, anaesthetic administration   162

Turbot
Aeromonas spp. infection 333
algal blooms 334
Alteromonas spp. infection 333
antibiotic treatment 336
aquaculture
commercial secrecy 327
environmental control 328
flow rates 328
and *Lactobacillus* spp 329
light intensity 328
systems 327–328
water sources 328
bacterial diseases 333
treatment 335–336
bacterial septicaemia of larvae 331–332
blood sampling 335
Bothriocephalus infection 334
treatment 336
broodstock 40, 328
cage systems 47, 328
Chondrococcus spp. infection 333
chlorine poisoning 328, 334
clinical diagnosis 334–335
deformities 333
depigmentation 332
disease 331–334
disease prevention 336–337
disease-free stock 337
ectoparasitism 332
eggs 328
feed 331
artificial 329
live 40, 327, 328–330, 336
fin rot 332
Flavobacterium spp. infection 333
formalin treatment 336
fungal infections 333
furunculosis 333
gill necrosis 93
grading 41, 337
granulomatous hypertyrosinaemia 334, 336
growth rate 330
haemogregarine infection 334
hatchery 327, 328–330, 336–337
hepatorenal syndrome 334
herpesvirus 101
herpesvirus scophalmi virus 333
high-value species 327
husbandry 40–41, 328–331
Ichthyoboda spp. infection 332
Ichthyophonus infection 333
in-feed medication 336
infectious pancreatic necrosis (IPN) 333

kidney 335
larval rearing 44
legislation 331
marketable size 330
microsporidial infection 333–334
mortality removal 337
neoplastic conditions 334
nursery 327–328, 330
nutritional diseases 334
opportunist pathogens 331–332
oxytetracycline 336
parasitic diseases 332, 334
treatment 336
pseudo-albinism 332
Pseudomonas spp. infection 333
sea cages 41
stocking density 330
tank systems 328
Tetramicra infection 333–334, 335
treatment 336
transportation 40
treatment, licensed 331
Trichodina spp. infection 332
veterinary approach 327–338
vibriosis 104, 331–332, 333, 383
vaccination 337
viral diseases 333, 335
water temperature 327
yellow 334

UK
availability of vaccines 143
fish health legislation 198, 229
treatment licensing 144, 211
Ulcer disease
brook trout 103–104
goldfish 364
Ulceration 73
in ornamental fish, treatment 376
and vibriosis 199–200
Ulcus syndrome, cod 350, 354
Ultimobranchial gland 25
Ultrasound diagnosis, halibut 343–344
Ultraviolet radiation 95, 170, 200, 218
Ultraviolet sterilisation, in eel recirculation systems 314
Underfeeding
of Atlantic salmon 189–190
causes stress 156
and starvation 95
Urine, crustacean 30
Urolithiasis 158

Uronema 113
Uronema spp. infection, of ornamental fish 367
Urophysis 21, 25–26
USA
    channel catfish culture 249
    fish health legislation 229
    treatment licensing 266, 407–408
Uvilifer spp. infection, largemouth bass 405

Vaccination 143–144
    of carp 143, 309
    of channel catfish 269
    duration of effect 143–144
    of eels 325–326
    for enteric redmouth (ERM) 105, 143, 217, 246
    equipment 54
    for furunculosis 103, 143, 185, 217, 246
    for gaffkaemia 143
    for Hitra disease 143
    immersion method 190
    minimun size of fish 143
    in Norway 190
    of ornamental fish 377
    of prawns 293
    of rainbow trout 245–246
    safety considerations 177
    for sea lice 66
    side effects 191
    stressful 143, 190
    for vibriosis 105, 143, 185, 217, 246, 337, 393,
        408
    for yersiniosis 191
Vaccines
    administration 143, 144
    currently available in UK 143
    development 58, 246
Vandalism, ornamental fish 66
Veins 15
Velvet disease 366, 405
Vent, imflammation 74
Veterinary approach
    to carp 297–309
    to channel catfish 249–270
    to cod 345–356
    to eels 311–326
    to game fish 393–408
    to halibut 339–344
    to ornamental fish 357–377
    to prawn culture 271–295
    to salmon farming
        in Norway 179
        in Scotland 193–221

    to sea-bass and sea-bream 379–394
    to turbot farming 327–338
Veterinary examination, work space 72–73
Vibrio spp. 104, 105, 234
    drug resistance 152–153
    and haemorrhagic septicaemia 104–105
    identification 83–84
    MIC data 147, 149, 150
    virulence 294
Vibriosis
    acute and chronic 104–105
    of Atlantic salmon
        in Norway 185
        in Scotland 199–200
    clinical signs 200, 234
    of cod 351–352, 354–356
    control 105
    diagnosis 104–105
    of eels 316
    luminous, of prawns 286
    of prawns 286–288
    and predator damage 200
    of rainbow trout 234
    Romet treatment 150
    sarafloxacin hydrochloride treatment 150
    in sea cages 234
    in sea-bass and sea-bream 383, 393
    stress-induced 190
    in striped bass 406
    of striped bass 408
    transmission 144, 181
    treatment 105
    of turbot 331–333, 337, 383
    and ulceration 199–200
    vaccination 143, 185, 217, 246, 337, 393,
        408
Vibrostat 0/129 test 83–84
Viral aetiology
    for infectious salmon anaemia (ISA) 128
    for pancreatic disease 127
Viral diseases 98–101
    of Atlantic salmon 185, 199
    of carp 300–301
    of channel catfish 256–257
    of cod 350, 354
    economic importance 98
    of eels 314–315
    of game fish 407
    of ornamental fish 363–364
    of rainbow trout 242
    of sea-bass and sea-bream 381–383
    source of infection 98, 119
    of trout 230
    of turbot 333, 335

Viral erthyrocytic infection, of sea-bass and sea-bream 382
Viral erythrocytic necrosis (VEN), of cod 350
Viral haemorrhagic septicaemia (VHN)
   clinical signs 230
   of Coho salmon 230
   transmission 230
   of trout 230
Viral haemorrhagic septicaemia (VHS)
   clinical signs 99
   control 99
   notifiable disease 174
   of rainbow trout 99
   of sea-bass and sea-bream 382
   of turbot 333
Viral kidney disease, of eels 315
Virology 87–88, 209, 324
Viruses
   of carp 100
   of catfish 100
   implicated in papilloma 98
   of salmonids 99–100
   transmission 98
Viscera, necroscopy features 77, 207–209
Vitamin deficiencies 96–97, 155
   of carp 307–308
   of prawns 290
   of sea-bass 391
   of sea-bream 391
Vitamin requirements 157–158
   of rainbow trout 239, 240
Vitamins, added to feed 155
Volume
   calculation 133–135
   of Norwegian salmon farms 180
Vorticella spp. infection
   in eels 321
   in game fish 404
   in ornamental fish 367

Waste products
   and biological oxygen demand (BOD) 62, 196
   as cause of disease 70, 107
   of crustaceans 30
   from aquaculture 228–229
   from prawn hatcheries 285
   nitrogenous 6, 94
   phosphorus content 228
   removal 31–32, 57
   toxic 363
   and water quality 57, 63

Water
   buffering capacity 180–181, 220, 314
   contamination 57, 65
      by drugs 176
   oxygen levels 182–183, 218
   pH 180–181, 218
Water analysis 89
Water flow
   in gills 8
   rate 218
   requirement 31–32
   in treatment 132
Water hardness
   effect on anaesthesia 164
   effect on toxicity 63, 64, 67
   effect on treatment 138, 142, 165
Water levels, lowered for treatment 131, 132
Water management, in prawn culture 280–281, 283–284
Water quality
   in aquarium systems 357–358, 360–361
   in Atlantic salmon farming 180–181, 196–197
   and bacterial gill disease 199
   basic requirements 58–66, 218
   in carp ponds 307
   in channel catfish culture 250–251, 264–265
   crucial to fish health 31, 57, 66, 70, 91
   and disease control 122, 214–215
   in eel culture 313
   and gill disease 89
   in marine farming 197
   and parasitic disease 110
   in prawn culture 281, 291, 294–295
   in rainbow trout culture 226–229
   in recirculation units 312
   in recreational ponds 399
   in smolt farms 180
   and stocking density 183, 197
   sudden changes 89
   in turbot hatchery 336–337
   welfare considerations 169, 170
Water sources
   for channel catfish culture 251
   and heavy metals 64
   in Norway 180–181
   and parasitic disease 110
   for prawn culture 279–280
   in rainbow trout farming 226
   for transportation hauling tanks 254
   for turbot farming 328
Water temperature
   and anaesthesia 164
   in aquarium systems 359
   and bacterial kidney disease (BKD) 232

Water temperature—*continued*
  and disease   70
  and eel infections   313, 317
  and fish feeding   169–170, 256
  and heart rate   15
  high
    and *Aeromonas* infection   234
    and *Branchiomyces* infection   108
  and infectious haematopoietic necrosis (IHN)   99
  and *Lernaea* infection   117
  low, and disease   40, 104, 106
  and quinaldine sulphate treatment   165
  and rainbow trout   227
  stratification   64
  sudden changes   64, 91–93, 170, 218, 219
  for transportation   255
  and turbot   327
  and vaccination   190
Water treatment systems   49–50
Waterfowl, and carp production   297
Weather conditions
  and disease   70
  effect on fish   66, 205
  and treatment   138
  and water quality   196
Welfare considerations   217–219
  in aquatic veterinary medicine   169–171
  legislation   173
  for ornamental fish   362, 363
Wels (*Siluris glanis*), antibiotic treatment   142
Whirling disease
  in earth pond systems   121
  in Norway   184, 185
  notifiable disease   174
  of salmonids   44, 120–121, 236–237
White catfish, *Ictalurus catus*   252
White grub, of game fish   405
White head disease   383
White perch, *Pasteurella* spp. infection   406
White spot disease *see Ichthyophthirius multifiliis* infection
White stripe disease, of sea-bream   389
White-lip disease   263–264
Whitefish, branchiomycosis   302
Wild fish
  as carriers of disease   121, 193, 216, 230, 233, 267, 295, 314, 386, 388
  overexploitation   284–285
Winter kill (winter fungus, winter mortality), channel catfish   263

Winter sore   104
Withdrawal period
  for anaesthetics   162
  for antibiotic treatment   145
  for benzocaine   164
  for co-trimazine   148
  for licensed products   211
  in Norway   189
  for oxolinic acid   149
  for oxytetracycline   150
  for sarafloxacin hydrochloride   150
  for tricaine methanesulphonate   165
Wound repair
  crustacean   29
  temperature dependence   5
Wrasse, as cleaner fish   66, 119, 215, 352

Xanthophyll   159

Yeast
  as immunostimulant   153
  as source of pigments   158
Yellow eels *see* Eels
Yellow grub   124, 405
Yellow turbot   334
Yellowtail (*Seriola quinqueradiata*)
  amoxycillin treatment   147
  Benedenia infection   116
  Pasteurella piscicida infection   106
  Streptococcus infection   107
Yersinia ruckeri   105
  and enteric redmouth (ERM)   231
  MIC data   149, 150, 153
Yersinia ruckeri infection
  co-trimazine treatment   148
  in Norway   185
  Romet treatment   150
  sarafloxacin hydrochloride treatment   150
  vaccination   191
Yolk-sac fry, problems   128

Zinc-deficiency cataract   96, 241
Zooplankton, as halibut feed   341